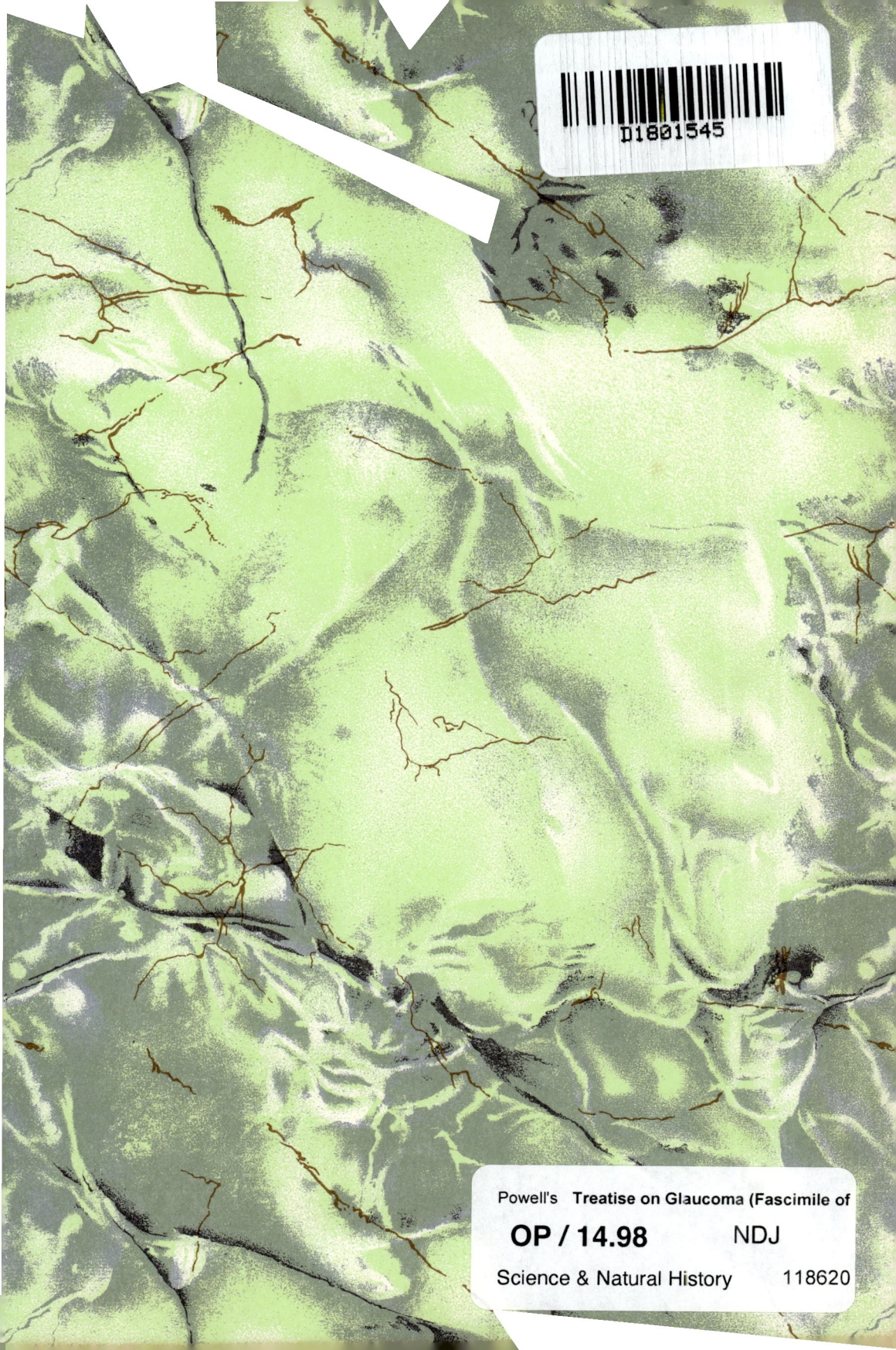

Powell's Treatise on Glaucoma (Fascimile of
OP / 14.98   NDJ
Science & Natural History   118620

A TREATISE ON GLAUCOMA

COLLECTOR'S EDITION
LIMITED TO
THREE-HUNDRED NUMBERED COPIES

THIS VOLUME IS NUMBER *51*   OF THREE-HUNDRED

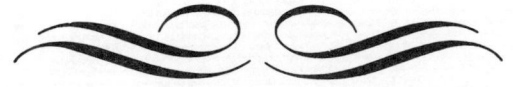

A TREATISE ON
GLAUCOMA

by

ROBERT HENRY ELLIOT

(Fascimile of 1918 Edition)

ROBERT E. KRIEGER PUBLISHING COMPANY
1979

ORIGINAL EDITION 1918
REPRINT WITH NEW INTRODUCTION
1979

PRINTED AND PUBLISHED BY
ROBERT E. KRIEGER PUBLISHING COMPANY INC.
645 NEW YORK AVENUE, HUNTINGTON, NEW YORK 11743

©COPYRIGHT 1979 – INTRODUCTION BY
ROBERT E. KRIEGER PUBLISHING COMPANY INC.
LIBRARY OF CONGRESS NUMBER 78-20807
ISBN NUMBER 0-88275-842-X

Library of Congress Cataloging in Publication Data

Elliot, Robert Henry, 1864-
   A treatise on glaucoma.

   (Classics in opthalmology)
   Reprint of the 1922 ed. published by H. Frowde, London in series: Oxford medical publications.
   1. Glaucoma.   I. Title   II. Series
[DNLM: WW290 E46t 1922a]
RE871.E44   1979   617.7'41   78-20807
ISBN 0-88275-842-X

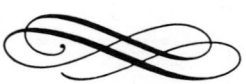

ALL RIGHTS RESERVED

INTRODUCTION

by

PAUL HENKIND, M.D., Ph.D.

The history of glaucoma in modern times, from 1850 on, is one of the most astonishing in all of ophthalmology. Many texts in use today suggest that we can knowingly diagnose and manage patients with that complex of conditions known as glaucoma. It is true that we have tools which help to quantitate ocular pressure, the extent of the visual field, and the exact amount of cupping of the optic nerve head; we can distinguish by gonioscopy between open and narrow angles and the clinician today is certainly better informed about the glaucomas than were his predecessors. However, he knows little more about the pathogenesis of the most common form of the condition, open angle glaucoma, than his teacher or his teachers' teachers.

Dr. Robert Henry Elliot (1864-1936), one of that band of Englishmen whose lot it was to serve the Empire in India, was the outstanding glaucoma expert in the English-speaking world in the early 20th century. He was not content only with operating upon countless thousands, an opportunity easily afforded a surgeon working with the seemingly endless population, but wanted to know more about the disease that blinded so many of his patients. He was a meticulous observer and studied the subject of glaucoma with intelligence and diligence. He developed the trephine operation for glaucoma and fully understood the need for filtration if it was to succeed. By no means a bench scientist, he digested all the basic information that laboratories could provide and rendered a useful summary.

It is regrettable that few ophthalmologists of recent times have taken the opportunity to read this wonderful book. There are sections which have not stood the test of time but much of what it contains is as apt today as when Elliot first penned it and, had they read it, they would be less likely to come up with "new" discoveries. This book will be a revelation to those who encounter it for the first time and they will not soon forget it.

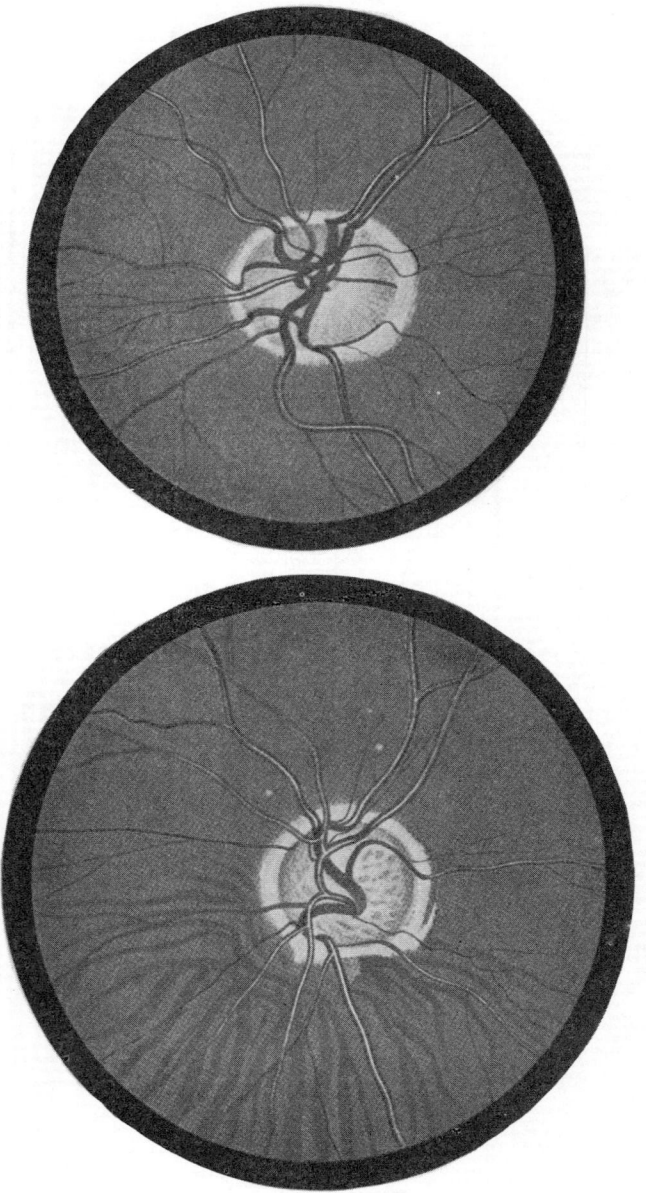

GLAUCOMATOUS CUPPING OF THE OPTIC DISC.

Both Illustrations show well (1) the bending of the vessels over the edges of the discs, (2) the haloes of surrounding choroidal atrophy, and (3) the stippling of the floors of the cups.

(Reproduced by kind permission of Mr. Adams Frost from his Ophthalmoscopic Atlas, Oxford Medical Publications, London.)

OXFORD MEDICAL PUBLICATIONS

A TREATISE ON
GLAUCOMA

BY

ROBERT HENRY ELLIOT
M.D., B.S.(Lond.), Sc.D.(Edin.), F.R.C.S.(Eng.)
LIEUT.-COLONEL I.M.S. (RETIRED)

LATE SUPERINTENDENT OF THE GOVERNMENT OPHTHALMIC HOSPITAL, MADRAS
LATE PROFESSOR OF OPHTHALMOLOGY, MEDICAL COLLEGE, MADRAS; AND
LATE FELLOW OF THE UNIVERSITY OF MADRAS
LECTURER IN OPHTHALMOLOGY, LONDON SCHOOL OF TROPICAL MEDICINE
OPHTHALMIC SURGEON TO THE SEAMEN'S HOSPITAL SOCIETY, AND TO THE
HOSPITAL FOR TROPICAL DISEASES, ENDSLEIGH GARDENS, LONDON

WITH 213 ILLUSTRATIONS AND FRONTISPIECE

LONDON
HENRY FROWDE AND HODDER & STOUGHTON
THE *LANCET* BUILDING
1 BEDFORD STREET, STRAND, W.C. 2

First Edition . . . *1918*
Second Edition . . *1922*

PRINTED IN GREAT BRITAIN BY MORRISON AND GIBB LTD., EDINBURGH

To
E. C. I. E.

PREFACE TO THE SECOND EDITION

I MUST commence with an apology for the long delay in bringing out a second edition. It has been due to the fact that I am obliged to do my literary work in my spare time, and that the amount of labour involved in following up the many additions to the literature of Glaucoma during the past four years has been very great.

I have altered the title, for I have given my book a more ambitious scope than before. I have felt it was more than a textbook that was wanted. There are so many questions in connection with glaucoma which are still unanswered, and there is still so very much work to be done, that I have felt that the aim to be kept before me was the writing of a book which would enable a reader to recognise the stage to which any part of the subject has been brought by the work of those who have preceded him. It is my hope that, in this way, I shall be able to be of assistance to those who desire to advance our knowledge by a further study of the many problems still awaiting solution, and thus shall, even in some small measure, succeed in stimulating research. I am convinced that the man or the profession, that rests content with the knowledge bequeathed by the past, is bound to move backwards instead of forwards. The opportunities for research in connection with glaucoma are immense, and I would commend this subject to all who have the privilege to be teachers in medical schools. It is for them to inspire their students and to direct their energies along such lines.

Then again I have had a second object before me :

Often and often in the treatment of patients suffering from glaucoma, questions have arisen in my mind to which I could find no answer. It has accordingly been my endeavour to marshal the knowledge at our disposal in orderly array, so that any point of doubt or difficulty can be decided, if possible, for the inquirer by a reference to the work that has been done in the past, much of which has lain hidden in works which are very inaccessible to most of us.

A third object has been kept before me, and one which many would have expected me to have placed first : I have sought to give a full, clear, and consecutive account of my subject, so that those who desire to master it as a whole may be able to do so by a perusal of my pages. In this sense the work is a textbook, but, as I have explained under my two previous headings, in a wider sense it is much more.

I have striven consistently to give credit where credit is due, and to put forward the views of others as freely and as fully as my own, even when I differ from them. There must always arise in such a work as this, questions of precedence and differences of opinion as between different surgeons: My rule has been to state the facts, quoting verbatim as far as possible from the authors themselves, and to leave the inferences to the reader.

A feature of this edition has been that the references are placed at the end of each Part of each Chapter, and that they have been made so full that anyone who works from them, as a starting-point, can easily obtain access to the whole literature of the subject.

An effort has been made to bring each section of the book thoroughly up to ·date. Fresh papers have been included even while the proofs have been in the Press right up to January 1922. Considerable additions have been made, and parts of the book have been practically

PREFACE TO THE SECOND EDITION

rewritten. It is possible that, despite every effort to the contrary, important papers have been overlooked; if this has been the case, I shall sincerely regret it. The literature has been so enormous that no one can feel confident that omissions have not occurred. The number of illustrations has been raised from 158 to 213 and Frontispiece, though even this does not indicate the true increase, since a number of the old figures have on several occasions been included under one number instead of under two or three.

It remains for me to make acknowledgment of the great help I have received from my many correspondents all over the world. I appreciate their suggestions and the many kind things they have written more than I can tell them. I have also to express my indebtedness to those who have helped me by the specific acts of kindness enumerated below :

The *American Journal of Ophthalmology* permitted me to reproduce the illustration found in Fig. 53.

Professor Bailliart supplied the block of his ophthalmodynamometer (Fig. 111), and sent me kind personal communications.

The *British Journal of Ophthalmology* gave me permission to copy the illustrations appearing as Figs. 6, 159, and 160.

Dr. Gradle furnished the block of Fig. 106.

Dr. McLean furnished the block of Fig. 107.

Messrs. Zeiss furnished the blocks of Figs. 29, 45, 113, and 114.

Professor Morax furnished the blocks of Figs. 24–27, 40–43, 104, 108, and 109.

Dr. Luther C. Peter and the Editor of the *Archives of Ophthalmology* gave me permission to copy the illustration which appears as Fig. 50.

Professor Schiötz furnished me with the photograph for Fig. 105B.

Mr. Edgar Stevenson furnished me with the photograph reproduced as Fig. 117.

Mr. A. Hugh Thomson permitted me to make use of the illustration reproduced as Fig. 44.

The Council of the Ophthalmological Society of the United Kingdom supplied the blocks of Figs. 44, 86–93, and 203–210.

Messrs. Weiss supplied the blocks of Figs. 72, 73, 110, 157B, and 184.

I have kept two acknowledgments to the end. I should be remiss indeed if I were not grateful to my Publishers for their invaluable help in all matters connected with the production of the book, which has always been freely and generously placed at my service. Lastly, Mrs. Elliot has helped me from start to finish, not only with photographs and drawings, but in every possible way. Without her assistance I could not have brought out this second edition, and should not have attempted to do so.

ROBERT HENRY ELLIOT.

54 WELBECK STREET, LONDON, W. 1,
23rd January 1922.

PREFACE TO THE FIRST EDITION

It has been my ambition for many years, to write a book on Glaucoma, which might be helpful to other students of the subject. It was only when I began to study carefully and systematically the vast literature available, that I realised how great the task really was, and how chaotic were many of the prevailing views. I found that much had been taken for granted without sufficient evidence; that incorrect data had been confidently built upon; that the same terms had been used in different senses by different writers, and that many other sources of confusion had been introduced.

For three years I have patiently and steadily striven to unravel the tangle, to separate the true from the false, to learn the views of those who are best qualified to speak, to weigh their opinions against each other, and to strive to winnow out the wheat from the chaff. In doing so, I have been amazed at our ignorance of many important points; I have striven to give everyone a fair hearing, to eliminate all prejudice from my judgments, to give full credit where it is due, but unhesitatingly to reject anything and everything which appears to me unworthy of credence, be the authority for it what it may. In doing so, it has been my earnest endeavour to avoid giving offence. I repeat that it is my desire to help the honest student, and in striving to do so, I have certainly helped myself to a clearer comprehension of this great subject. It has been my aim and object to state each case as clearly and as simply as possible, while at the same time, putting my facts forward in as readable a manner as I could.

The experience of years has left me as fully convinced of the value of sclero-corneal trephining as when I penned the first edition of my monograph on that subject ("Sclero-corneal Trephining in the Operative Treatment of Glaucoma," George Pulman & Sons Ltd. First Edition, 1913; Second Edition, 1914). In the present volume, however, I have endeavoured to take a much wider view and to present not only my own individual ideas, but those also of all surgeons, who have left any mark behind them. I have studiously refrained from burdening the reader with statistics. Those who are interested in such figures will find them given at length in the second edition of "Sclero-corneal Trephining" and in my summaries of the year's work on Glaucoma in the Ophthalmic Year Books of 1913 to 1916. A perusal of these articles will show how vast the subject is.

I have endeavoured to acknowledge the sources of the valuable help I have received in the pages of the book, but there are certain special matters that I desire to mention.

The editors of *The Ophthalmoscope, The Ophthalmic Review*, and *The Ophthalmic Record* have courteously permitted me to reproduce as chapters of this volume the articles which have appeared in their pages. Those articles have been extensively rewritten to bring them up to date, and for that purpose the current literature has been carefully surveyed, inclusive of that for the year 1917.

The Council of the Ophthalmological Society and the Editorial Committee of the *British Journal of Ophthalmology* have kindly permitted me to reproduce certain illustrations from their Transactions and Journal.

My book has been enriched by the kindness of Mr. Priestley Smith, who with his usual generosity, has allowed me to make use of a number of his classic illustrations.

To Mr. Treacher Collins I am indebted, not only for the

PREFACE TO THE FIRST EDITION

loan of many beautiful specimens, but also for the opportunity to discuss with him some of the difficulties with which I have been confronted in the course of my study of the subject.

To Professor Bjerrum, Professor Roenne, and Dr. Sinclair my thanks are due for the generous way in which they placed their perimetric material at my disposal.

I am much indebted to Mr. Adams Frost and to Messrs. Henry Frowde and Hodder & Stoughton for very generously allowing me to reproduce as my frontispiece the well-known coloured illustrations of the glaucoma cup, which appear in the "Adams Frost Atlas of Ophthalmology." I deeply appreciate their liberality in doing so.

Professor Arthur Thomson has likewise most generously allowed me to make use of the very beautiful illustrations which appeared in his articles in *The Ophthalmoscope*.

Messrs. Weiss and Messrs. George Spiller have very kindly furnished me with blocks which they were good enough to prepare for the purpose.

A number of the illustrations are from original photographs by Mrs. Elliot, to whom I am also indebted for much help in the proof-reading and in other ways.

The difficulties of bringing out the book in war time have been very great, and I therefore feel that I must express my indebtedness to Mr. H. L. Jackson of Messrs. H. K. Lewis & Co. Ltd. for the valuable assistance he has given me.

ROBERT HENRY ELLIOT.

54 WELBECK STREET,
  CAVENDISH SQUARE,
    LONDON W.,
      1918.

CONTENTS

CHAPTER		PAGE
I. PRELIMINARY		1
PART I.	Introductory	1
PART II.	The Anatomy of the Parts concerned in Glaucoma	3
PART III.	Historical	18
II. THE INTRA-OCULAR PRESSURE AND THE TENSION OF THE EYE		23
PART I.	The Terms used	24
	The Physical Conditions regulating the Intra-Ocular Pressure	27
PART II.	The Bearing on Intra-Ocular Pressure of the Continuous Flow of Fluid through the Chambers of the Eye	40
	The Changes in the Chamber Pressure which attend Some Forms of Glaucoma	45
	The Source and Method of Production of the Intra-Ocular Fluid	49
	Magitot's Views	55
PART III.	The Relationship of Systemic Blood-Pressure to Intra-Ocular Pressure	59
	The Relationship between the Intra-Ocular Blood-Pressure and the Intra-Ocular Fluid Pressure Outside the Vessels	64
III. THE ÆTIOLOGY OF GLAUCOMA		83
PART I.	Introduction	84
PART II.	The Pathological Anatomy of Glaucoma	87
PART III.	The Pathological Anatomy of Glaucoma (*continued*)	102
PART IV.	The Causes of Glaucoma	121
IV. THE DIAGNOSIS OF GLAUCOMA		149
PART I.	Introductory	149
	The Stages of Glaucoma	152
	The Clinical Course of a Simple Attack	155
	The Clinical Course of a Congestive Attack	159
PART II.	The Signs and Symptoms of Glaucoma, considered from an Anatomical Point of View	166
PART III.	Subjective Phenomena	224

CHAPTER			PAGE
Part IV.	The Visual Field		228
Part V.	The Visual Field (continued)		294
Part VI.	Tonometry		317
	The Examination of the Light Sense		338
V. Secondary Glaucoma			346
Part I.	Introductory		347
Part II.	Ætiology		347
Part III.	Treatment		385
VI. Congenital Glaucoma and Some Allied Conditions			400
VII. The Medical Treatment of Glaucoma			442
VIII. Iridectomy in Glaucoma			458
Part I.	The Opinions of the Old Masters		458
Part II.	The Views of Modern Surgeons		473
Part III.	The Technique of the Operation of Iridectomy for Glaucoma		483
IX. The Newer Operations for Glaucoma			487
Part I.	The History of the Newer Operations for Glaucoma		488
Part II.	Preparations for Operation		504
Part III.	Sclerotomy for Glaucoma		510
Part IV.	Lagrange's Operation		511
Part V.	Holth's Operation		515
Part VI.	Herbert's Operations		522
Part VII.	Scleral Trephining (Fergus's Operation)		526
Part VIII.	Sclero-Corneal Trephining (Elliot's Operation)		531
Part IX.	Modifications of Sclero-Corneal Trephining suggested by Various Surgeons		559
Part X.	Complications which may be met with during a Glaucoma Operation		571
Part XI.	After-Management of Patients operated on for Glaucoma		578
X. The Pathology of Filtration			603
Part I.	The Filtering Scar in the Treatment of Glaucoma		603
Part II.	The Histology of the Trephined Disc in Glaucoma Operations		618
Appendix. A New Instrument for measuring the Diameter of the Cornea			639
Index of Names			641
Index of Subjects			646

LIST OF ILLUSTRATIONS

Glaucomatous Cupping of Optic Disc	*Frontispiece*

FIG.		PAGE
1.	Meridional Section through the Anterior Portion of the Eye	4
2.	Showing the Blood Supply of the Ciliary Body and of the Adjoining Parts . . . . . *facing*	5
3.	Canal of Schlemm reconstructed	6
4.	Ditto	7
5.	Optic Nerve Entrance	12
6.	Canal of Entrance of Optic Nerve	13
7.	Lamina Cribrosa	15
8.	Ditto	15
9.	Ditto	16
10.	Manometer for Estimation of Intra-Ocular Pressure	25
11.	The Filtration Angle	74
12.	Diagram showing Pump Action on Canal of Schlemm	75
13.	Section through Pectinate Ligament	78
14.	Diagram showing Valvular Action of Channels in Pectinate Ligament	79
15.	Mechanical Closure of Filtration Angle in Acute Glaucoma	103
16.	The Angle of Chamber opened and closed	104
17.	Filtration Angle closed by Adhesion : Acute Glaucoma	105
18.	Compression of Iris Stroma	107
19.	Iris atrophied, and Ciliary Processes retracted	107
20.	Section of Normal Eye	109
21.	Section of Glaucomatous Eye	109
22.	Blocking of Pectinate Ligament by Cells	114
23.	Shallowing of Angle of Chamber preceding Glaucoma	114
24.	Œdema of Cornea in Acute Glaucoma	169
25.	Ditto	170
26.	Corona of Light round a Flame	176
27.	Druault's Experiment	179
28.	Ditto	180
29.	Ulbrich's Drum	188

LIST OF ILLUSTRATIONS

FIG.		PAGE
30.	Ectropion Uveæ	190
31.	Section of Glaucomatous Cup	197
32.	Paper Device to illustrate Points in Connection with Glaucomatous Cupping	*facing* 203
33.	Ditto . . . . *do.*	203
34.	Ditto . . . . *do.*	203
35.	Ditto . . . . *do.*	203
36.	Diagram of Glaucoma Cup . . . . *do.*	208
37.	Diagram of Physiological Cup . . . *do.*	208
38.	Diagram of Atrophic Cup . . . . *do.*	208
39.	Coloboma of the Optic Nerve . . . *do.*	208
40.	Glaucomatous Cup	209
41.	Ditto	210
42.	Coloboma of the Optic Nerve	211
43.	Coloboma of Sheath of Optic Nerve	212
44.	Large Intra-marginal Cup	215
45.	Corneal Microscope and Slit-lamp	220
46.	Normal Visual Fields (Sinclair)	230
47.	Normal Visual Fields (Bjerrum)	230
48.	Papillo-Macular Bundle in Cross Section of Optic Nerve	233
49.	Distribution of Nerve Fibres on Retina (Baas)	234
50.	Distribution of Nerve Fibres on Retina (Peter)	236
51.	Ditto	237
52.	Ditto, enlarged	238
53.	The Fundus by Red-free Light	239
54A.	Early Shrinkage of Nasal Field	241
54B.	Later Stage of above	241
55.	Field in Late Chronic Glaucoma	243
56.	Ditto	243
57.	Visual Field, Left Eye : Late Chronic Glaucoma	244
58.	Ditto, Right Eye	244
59.	A Sectored Field : Chronic Glaucoma	245
60.	Remnant of Visual Field : Late Chronic Glaucoma	245
61.	Defects in Nerve Bundles corresponding to Field Defects of Next Figure	246
62.	Bjerrum's Sign and Roenne's Step	247
63.	Colour Fields in Chronic Glaucoma	248
64.	Fields showing Bjerrum's Scotomata (Sinclair)	250
65.	Ditto	251
66.	Ditto	252

LIST OF ILLUSTRATIONS

FIG.		PAGE
67.	Fields showing Signs of Optic Atrophy (Sinclair)	252
68.	Bjerrum's Screen on Stand	253
69.	Bjerrum's Screen on Spring Roller	254
70.	Marks' Recording Scotometer	255
71.	Author's Scotometer	258
72.	Author's Head-rest	259
73.	Author's Pointer	259
74.	Form for recording Scotometer Readings	260
75.	Scotometer Chart, Blank	261
76.	Normal Blind Spots charted	262
77.	Scotometer for Use with Bjerrum's Screen	263
78.	Author's Large Perimeter	264
79.	Bjerrum's Scotoma (absolute)	265
80.	Bjerrum's Double Arcuate Scotoma	265
81.	Roenne's Glaucoma Fields	266
82.	Ditto	269
83.	Seidel's Sign	271
84.	An Early Scotoma charted by Means of the Author's Scotometer	273
85.	The Same Field Ten Days after Operation	273
86.	Author's Scotometer Chart	275
87.	Ditto	276
88.	Ditto	277
89.	Ditto	278
90.	Ditto	279
91.	Ditto	280
92.	Ditto	281
93.	Ditto	282
94.	Paracentral Scotomata separated from Blind Spot	288
95.	Charts showing Progress of Central Scotomata (Van der Hoeve)	289
96.	Ring Scotoma (Van der Hoeve)	291
97.	Hemianopic Field : Chronic Glaucoma (Bjerrum)	291
98.	Central Relative Scotoma (Bjerrum)	292
99.	Bow-shaped Remnant of Field (Bjerrum)	292
100.	Quadrantic Defect of Field (Bjerrum)	293
101.	Anatomical Distribution of the Nerve Fibres in the Retina	302
102.	Field of Vision	308
103.	Schematic Section of Eye	309
104.	The Principle of the Schiötz Tonometer	319

LIST OF ILLUSTRATIONS

FIG.		PAGE
105A.	Schiötz Tonometer (Original Model)	320
105B.	Ditto (New Model)	321
106.	Gradle's Tonometer	322
107.	The McLean Tonometer	322
108.	Application of the Schiötz Tonometer	330
109.	Ditto	331
110.	Tonometric Chart	336
111.	Bailliart's Ophthalmo-dynamometer	337
112.	Author's Light Sense Apparatus	341
113.	Zeiss' Photometer	343
114.	Ditto (in Section)	344
115.	Wound of Cornea : Secondary Glaucoma	349
116.	Perforating Ulcer of Cornea : Secondary Glaucoma	350
117.	Staphyloma of Cornea	351
118.	Ditto	352
119.	Fistula of Cornea	353
120.	Ditto, Higher Magnification	353
121.	Annular Posterior Synechia	354
122.	L'iris bombé	355
123.	L'iris bombé	355
124.	Anterior Dislocation of Lens	356
125.	Nucleus of Cataract, freely movable between Chambers	356
126.	Anterior Dislocation of Lens	357
127.	Lens Nucleus impacted in Angle of Anterior Chamber	358
128.	Lateral Dislocation of Lens	359
129.	Ditto, Higher Magnification	360
130.	Posterior Dislocation of Lens	361
131.	Reclined Cataract	361
132.	Blocking of Angle of Chamber by New Formation	362
133.	Epithelial Cyst of Anterior Chamber	369
134.	Ditto, Higher Magnification	369
135.	Downgrowth of Epithelium along Track of Wound	371
136.	Capsulo-Corneal Synechia	371
137.	Tumour of Iris and Ciliary Body	376
138.	Tumour of Iris	377
139.	Sarcoma of Choroid	378
140.	Vitreous Streamers	392
141.	Buphthalmic Child	404
142.	Section of Buphthalmic Eye	405
143.	Ruptures of Descemet's Membrane	406

LIST OF ILLUSTRATIONS

FIG.		PAGE
144.	Ruptures of Descemet's Membrane, in Section	417
145.	Fœtal Condition of Angle of Chamber	419
146.	Iridectomy for Glaucoma	485
147.	Madras Eye Bandage	509
148.	De Wecker's Sclerotomy	510
149.	Lagrange's Operation	512
150.	Ditto	512
151.	Ditto	513
152.	Ditto	513
153.	Holth's Forceps	516
154.	Holth's Keratome	516
155.	Holth's Double Hook	516
156.	Holth's Iris Forceps	516
157A.	Holth's Punch-Forceps	517
157B.	Ditto (New Model)	517
158A.	Diagram of Holth's Operation	517
158B.	Ditto	517
158C.	Ditto	517
159.	Diagram of Holth's New Operation	520
160.	Section of Eye to show Holth's New Operation	521
161.	Herbert's Wedge-Isolation Operation	523
162.	Ditto	523
163.	Herbert's Small Flap Operation	524
164.	Ditto	524
165.	Ditto	524
166.	Herbert's Triple Small Flap Operation	525
167.	Ditto	525
168.	Ditto	525
169.	Early Incision in Sclero-Corneal Trephining	533
170.	Present Incision in Sclero-Corneal Trephining	533
171.	The Flap in Sclero-Corneal Trephining	535
172.	Disc Forceps for Trephining	546
173.	Diagram of Parts concerned in Trephining	553
174.	Ditto	554
175.	Ditto	555
176.	Ditto	556
177.	Bowman's Trephine	560
178.	Stephenson's Trephine	560
179.	Author's Trephine	560
180.	Gray Clegg's Slotted Trephine Blade	561

LIST OF ILLUSTRATIONS

FIG.		PAGE
181.	Lang's Trephine	561
182.	Pusey's Trephine	561
183.	Butler's Trephine	561
184.	Young's Trephine	562
185.	Von Hippel's Trephine	562
186.	Vogt's Motor Trephine	563
187.	Taylor's Motor Trephine	563
188.	Desmarres' Knife used in Splitting the Cornea	564
189.	Lang's Knife for Splitting the Cornea	564
190.	Stephenson's Knife for Splitting the Cornea	564
191.	McReynold's Corneal Wedge	564
192.	Von Mende's Flap	565
193.	Dupuy-Dutemps' Flap	565
194.	Hill Griffith's Flap	566
195.	Photo of Filtering Scar during Life	568
196.	Ditto	569
197.	Method of Fixation of Eye by Traction of Thread	572
198.	Filtering Scar after Removal of Eyeball	606
199.	Filtering Scar in Section	607
200.	Ditto	608
201.	Ditto	609
202.	Ditto	610
203.	Ditto	620
204.	Trephined Disc in Section	623
205.	Ditto	624
206.	Ditto	625
207.	Ditto	626
208.	Ditto	628
209.	The Splitting up of Descemet's Membrane	630
210.	Excrescences on Descemet's Membrane	631
211.	Ditto, under Higher Magnification	632
212.	The Splitting up of Descemet's Membrane	635
213.	The Author's Microscope for the Measurement of the Cornea	639

A TREATISE ON GLAUCOMA

CHAPTER I
PRELIMINARY

SUMMARY
PART I
INTRODUCTORY.
PART II
THE ANATOMY OF THE PARTS CONCERNED.
PART III
HISTORICAL.

PART I

Introductory

THE term " glaucoma " is not the title of any one single disease. It is rather a convenient clinical label for a large group of *pathologic* conditions, the distinctive feature common to all of which is a rise in the intra-ocular pressure.

The causes of these conditions are many and varied, the pathological findings are most diverse, and the difference in the symptoms presented is so extraordinary, that very careful study is required to detect the bond which serves to unite these very dissimilar manifestations of disease in a common category.

When we speak of the hardness of a glaucomatous eye, or of its rise in tension, we are referring to the outward manifestations of an increase of the fluid pressure within the globe. To this increase all the causes of glaucoma lead up ; on it every sign and symptom of the condition depend.

If the rise in pressure can be traced to the action of some antecedent local disease, we speak of the glaucomatous condition as *secondary*; failing this we term it *primary*.

The presence of an increase in intra-ocular pressure necessarily brings about some measure of interference with the free escape of blood from the interior of the eye to the surface. So long, however, as such interference does not give rise to obvious congestion of the eye or of its conjunctiva, we speak of the condition as " *simple* or noncongestive glaucoma." When evidence of interference with the venous return makes its appearance, the disease is said to be " *congestive.*" The term " inflammatory," though often used in this connection, is erroneous and should be dropped.

The classification of all cases of glaucoma into three groups—viz., the *acute*, the *subacute*, and the *chronic*—has been productive of much confusion, owing to the difference in the way in which these terms have been used by writers on the subject.

Those cases which present the signs and symptoms of severe congestion, as a result of a steep rise in intra-ocular pressure, may reasonably be spoken of as acute, the term subacute being reserved for those in which the evidence of congestion is less pronounced. To define a chronic case is more difficult. All that the term really implies is that the condition has lasted for some time ; but, in accepted usage, it is also understood that the case is not in an acute or subacute stage. Any glaucomatous eyeball, whether of the simple or of the congestive type, may fall into this category. The point to be emphasised is that there is no such thing as acute, subacute, and chronic glaucoma. Any glaucomatous eye may be in an acute, a subacute, or a chronic stage, and may readily pass from one to another of these stages, and back again into that from which it sprang ; but to speak of acute, subacute, and chronic glaucoma, as if we were dealing with so many clinical entities, is wrong and misleading.

Part II

The Anatomy of the Parts concerned in Glaucoma

Before we can study the processes of disease in an organ, or the methods of combating them, it is essential that we should make ourselves acquainted with certain anatomical details of the structures concerned.

The ciliary body and the parts adjoining it are " the cockpit " of glaucoma. A study of Figs. 1 and 11 (*v.* pp. 4 and 74) will make a number of important points clear ; a few of the more essential anatomical features demand some attention.

The Conjunctiva.—It will be noted in the illustration (Fig. 1) that the subconjunctival tissue is continued well in advance of the sclero-corneal junction. It is along this layer that we work in " splitting the cornea " in the operation of trephining, and the looseness of the tissue just referred to explains the ease with which that manœuvre is conducted.

Schlemm's Canal (Figs. 1 to 4 and 11) lies at the junction of the cornea and sclera, close to the inner surface of the corneo-scleral envelope. It is separated from the aqueous chamber only by the loose open network of the pectinate ligament (Figs. 1 and 11). Fluid can pass readily from the chamber to the canal through the open spaces of this meshwork, but there is no direct connection between the canal and the chamber. The anatomy of these parts has recently been very carefully worked out by Maggiore, and some points of special interest deserve a reference here. He has reconstructed a schematic section of the area (Fig. 2) from a large number of serial sections, in order to show the connections of the various vascular plexuses of this important neighbourhood. This figure is worthy of the careful study of all who are interested in the anatomy of glaucoma.

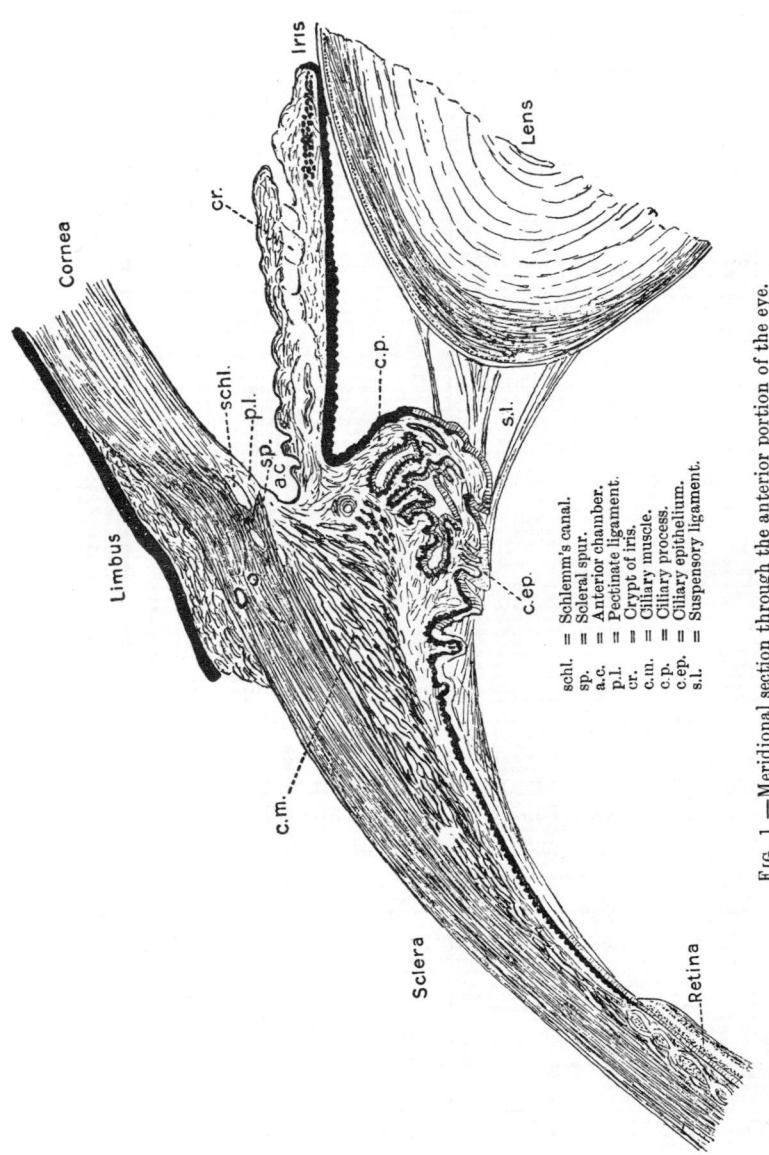

Fig. 1.—Meridional section through the anterior portion of the eye.
(Modified from Fuchs.)

schl. = Schlemm's canal.
sp. = Scleral spur.
a.c. = Anterior chamber.
p.l. = Pectinate ligament.
cr. = Crypt of iris.
c.m. = Ciliary muscle.
c.p. = Ciliary process.
c.ep. = Ciliary epithelium.
s.l. = Suspensory ligament.

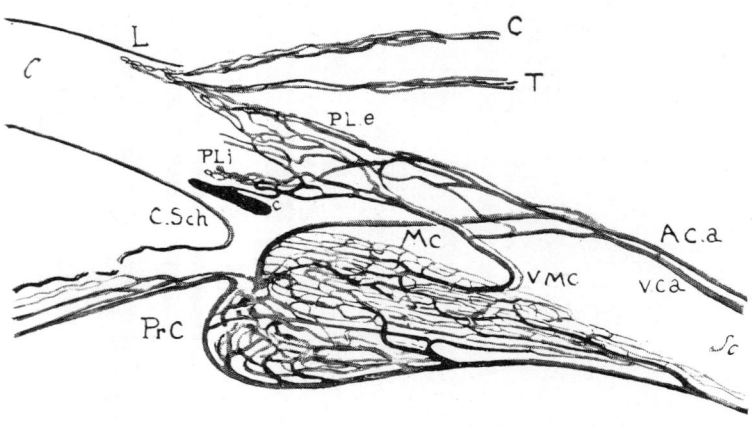

Fig. 2.—Reconstruction of a schematic section, showing the blood supply of the ciliary body and the parts adjoining it. The connection of the various vascular plexuses is shown. L, limbus; C, conjunctival plexus of vessels; T, plexus of vessels in Tenon's capsule; PL.e, episcleral plexus; PLi, intrascleral plexus; C.Sch, canal of Schlemm, with small collector vein, c; Ac.a, anterior ciliary artery; VCa, anterior ciliary vein; Mc, plexus in ciliary muscle; VMc, vessels of the ciliary muscle; PrC, ciliary processes; Sc, sclera.

In addition, he has made a plaster reconstruction of the canal of Schlemm, and photographs of parts of this are shown in Figs. 3 and 4, which are as interesting as they are instructive.

He finds that the canal has a complete endothelial lining. Under normal conditions, it contains clear lymph only, and no blood corpuscles ; but it is evidently a vascular structure, and it is joined to the deep pericorneal vascular plexus by 20 to 30 connecting trunks, which have a very small lumen, and only appear as slits. This deep plexus (Fig. 2, PLi) is formed of numerous veins with a few slender and scanty arterial twigs. As is well known, it plays a leading part in glaucoma.

Maggiore's pathological studies of this area are also interesting, as tending to show that blood corpuscles and inflammatory cells have a strong tendency to work their way from the angle of the anterior chamber, through the spaces of the pectinate ligament, into Schlemm's canal. Similar observations have been made by earlier investigators, especially in connection with free cells detached from malignant growths of those parts of the uveal tract, which abut on the aqueous chamber. The inference from this evidence favours the hypothesis of the outflow of fluid at the angle of the anterior chamber. The point is of interest as the very existence of a drainage flow by way of the angle of the anterior chamber, has recently been challenged. It is difficult to take such a challenge very seriously.

The Scleral Spur (Figs. 1 and 11) lies between the pectinate ligament anteriorly and some fibres of the ciliary muscle posteriorly. A contraction of these fibres will pull back the spur and tend to open wide the canal of Schlemm. As soon as muscular contraction ceases, the pectinate ligament, being elastic, will draw the scleral spur back into place, and so close the canal of Schlemm (Arthur Thomson). It will be shown later (Chapter II. Part III.) how this pump action, by its constant repetition during the waking hours, draws the fluid from the anterior chamber into the canal of Schlemm, and then sweeps it on again from the canal into the neighbouring veins.

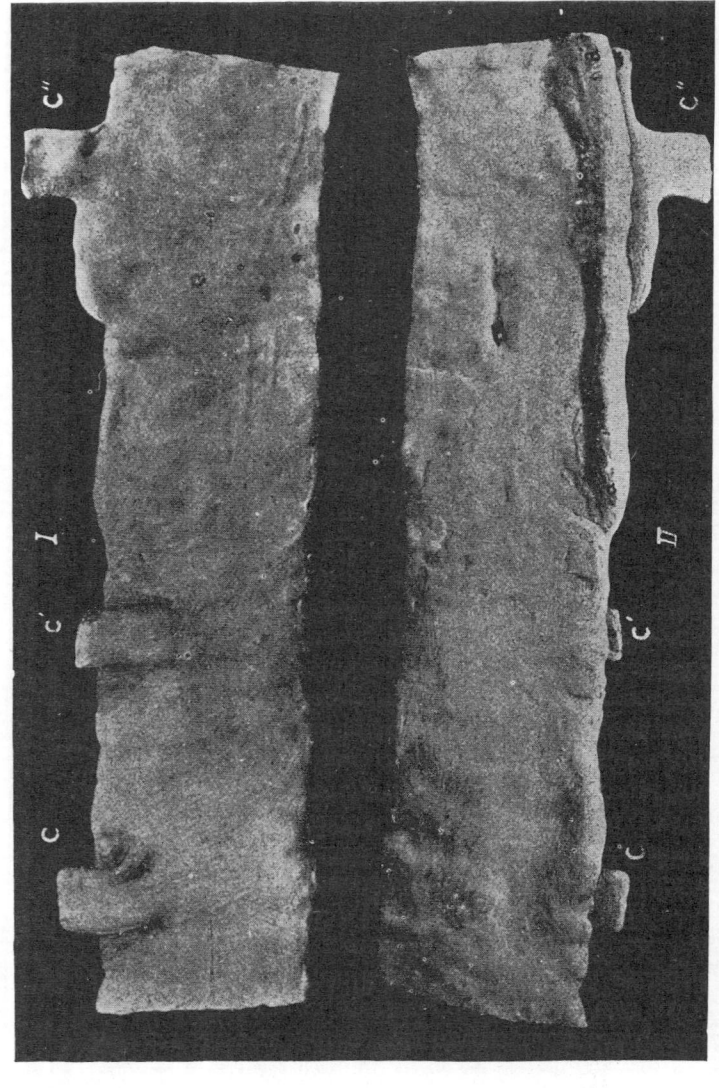

FIG. 3.—Photographs of a Plaster Reconstruction of the Canal of Schlemm. I shows the superficial (corneal aspect), and II the deep aspect. c c' c" are collector vessels entering the canal at various angles. Save for a small tubular projection a a', the canal of Schlemm is here composed of a single tube.

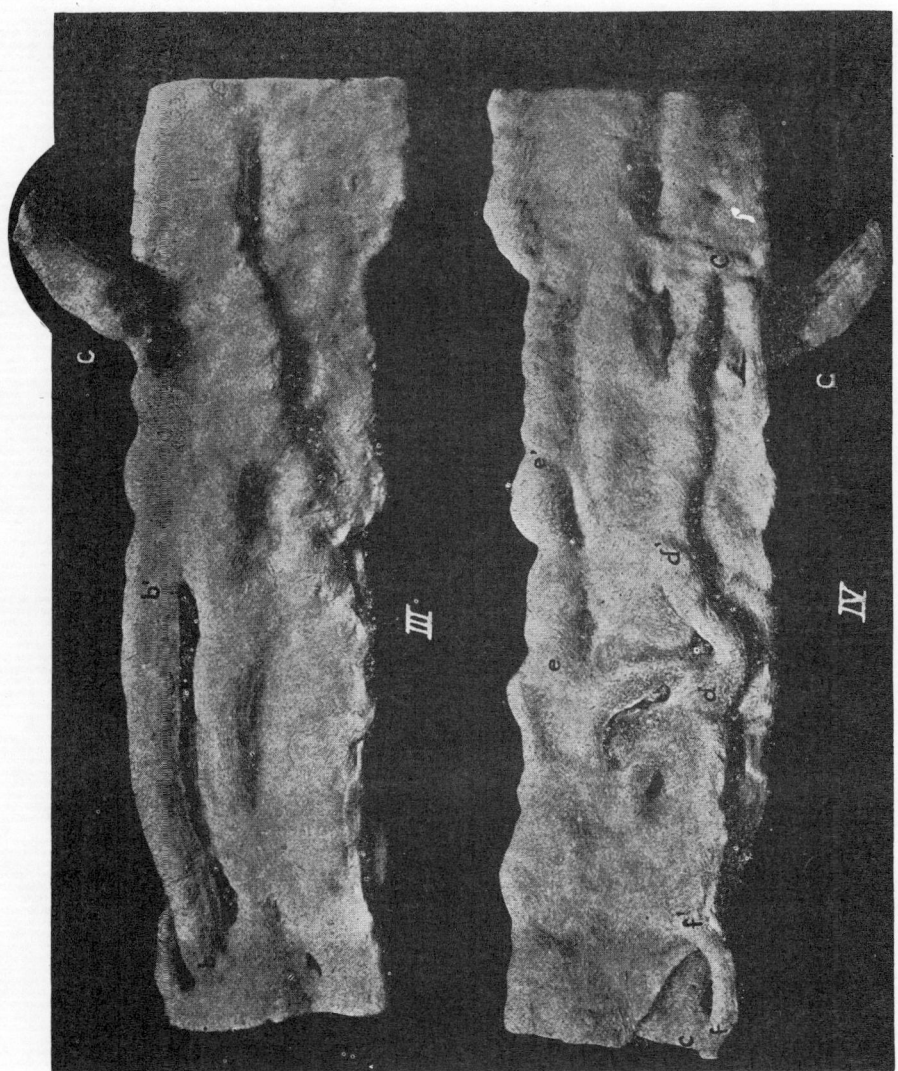

Fig. 4.—Photographs similar to those of Fig. 3, but differing in that the canal is no longer single but is broken up to a certain extent, the result being the formation of tubules b b', d d', e e', f f'; c c show collectors as before.

The Anterior Chamber has an almost exactly circular contour, while the cornea is oval in shape with its long axis transverse ; the consequence is that the extent of the angle of the chamber concealed by the scleral border varies considerably in different directions. Rochon-Duvigneaud worked this matter out with great care and gave the following measurements of the interval between the transparent edge of the cornea on the one hand, and the angle of the anterior chamber on the other : (1) above the cornea in the vertical axis, 2·25 mm. ; (2) below the cornea in the same axis, 2 mm. ; (3) to the nasal or temporal side of the cornea in the horizontal axis, 1·25 mm. These measurements naturally vary in individual eyes, and the author's researches showed that in the smaller and lighter Indian patient they are slightly less than those obtained on European subjects by the French worker. The importance of a knowledge of these facts to the surgeon, who has to consider the various operations for glaucoma, is too obvious to need emphasis.

The Angle of the Chamber (Figs. 1 and 11) is at the best of times a narrow space. Inasmuch as the outflow of the aqueous fluid takes place in this neighbourhood, it is most important that the angle should remain widely open. Its patency may be infringed in several ways :—

1. *Extreme dilatation of the pupil*, by crowding the membrane out to its periphery, tends to fill up the angle, and so to impede the passage of fluid through it.

2. The *ciliary body* may become swollen by congestion with blood. If it does so, its apices move forward. A glance at the illustration (Fig. 1) will show that, if this happens, these apices will press upon the base of the iris, and push the latter forward against the cornea, thus closing the angle. A second point may be learnt from this drawing : If the apices of the ciliary body move forward, the attachments of the suspensory ligament of the lens do the same ; this, obviously, will allow the lens to advance, and so to press on the base of the iris. In this connection Figs. 21 and 23 may be profitably consulted now.

3. As life advances, the *lens* enlarges, whilst the tunic

of the eye remains stationary in size. The swollen lens tends to press the iris forward, and so to occlude the angle, just as in the previous case.

4. When the iris and cornea are brought into close apposition, in one of the ways above described, their adjacent surfaces are apt to be glued together by the *exudate* they throw out. In this way a permanent obliteration of the angle may be brought about.

The Iris.—On the anterior surface of this membrane are found pit-like depressions, the crypts of the iris (Fig. 1), which lead to the depth of the iris stroma, and which place its tissue spaces in free communication with the cavity of the aqueous chamber. In this stroma the fluid comes into intimate contact with the thin-walled iris veins, and passes into the latter, probably by osmotic action. The crypts are of importance when the angle of the chamber is in an early stage of closure, for the fluid from the chamber can enter through them and find its way along the iris stroma to the neighbourhood of the pectinate ligament, across which it then passes to enter Schlemm's canal.

The Ciliary Body.—Whilst few authorities now accept the suggestion that there are definite tubular secretory glands in this body, it is believed that its lining cells have the power of taking up fluid transuded into their neighbourhood from the capillary vessels, and passing it across on to the free surface by a definite act of secretion.

The view usually accepted is that the fluid thus poured out passes by two streams, one backward into the vitreous, and the other inward and forward into the posterior division of the aqueous chamber; thence it finds its way through the pupil into the anterior division of that chamber, and flows outward all round to reach the angle.

The ciliary body presents a large surface of attachment to the sclera. This is of interest in connection with the operation of *cyclodialysis*, the purpose of which is to tear the former structure away from the latter over the area marked out by a limited incision; the pectinate ligament is obviously divided during this step. The object aimed at is to open up a communication between the anterior chamber in front and the suprachoroidal space behind, by means of the detachment of the ciliary body.

The *vessels and nerves* which supply the ciliary body and iris pass forward between the choroid and the sclera. In this course they are exposed to the full force of the intra-ocular pressure, since they lie against the hard unyielding scleral coat.

There is a free communication between the vascular system in the interior of the eye and that on its surface through the *perforating vessels*, which pierce the sclera close behind the cornea. Morax has discussed the nature of these anterior ciliary vessels which are so constantly found dilated in subacute glaucoma. He appears to lean to Heerfordt's view that these are arterial and not venous, but he has had some difficulty in making up his mind on the subject. The author has devoted some attention to these vessels, and is strongly inclined to believe that they are venous and not arterial for the following reasons : (1) If a length of the vessel is rendered bloodless and pressed on with spatulæ at two distant points, it fills quite as readily, if not more readily, from the direction of the eyeball than from the opposite one. (2) When one of these vessels is cut during an operation, the bleeding from it is never pulsatile. (3) When quite a large trunk of this kind is examined under very high magnifications, with a corneal microscope, not the faintest trace of pulsation can be detected.

The whole of the choroidal and retinal circulation lies between the fluid contents of the eye and the unyielding sclera, and must suffer whenever the pressure within the eye is increased. The arterial and venous circulations react differently. The pressure diminishes the amount of blood entering the eye through the arteries, and also that leaving it through the veins. The effect is to diminish the arterial supply and to establish a condition of venous congestion. If the pressure rises slowly, the circulation can adapt itself to the change of conditions, and the glaucoma remains simple. If, on the other hand, the increase in pressure is a rapid one, no such adaptation is possible, and an attack of congestive glaucoma is the result. This, however, is possibly far from being the whole truth. It seems probable that the anatomical conditions, governing the escape of the venous blood from the eye, and those of the reservoirs into which this blood is passed immediately after its exit, exercise a profound influence on the incidence of the vascular factor when high tension supervenes. To this point we shall return on a later occasion.

It is important to bear in mind that there are two quite separate and independent vascular systems within the eye. Of these, one cares for the retina and the retrobulbar segment of the optic nerve, whilst the other is responsible for the uveal tract, the sclera, and some part of the episcleral tissue. The most important channels for the uveal tract are the posterior ciliary arteries, which are about 20 in number. The long posterior and the anterior ciliary arteries contribute more modestly to the arterial supply. The veins are two or three times more numerous than the arteries, and are of much larger calibre. They arise suddenly from the fusion of about fifteen capillaries which meet in a small vortex, and in turn form larger vortices, called "venæ vorticosæ." The anterior segment of the eye is also rich in veins; this is especially true of the ciliary region, the ciliary processes being almost entirely made up of bunches of veins. In spite of the seemingly large number of anastomoses between the anterior and posterior venous systems, the suppression of either leads to a marked venous stasis of the eye (Magitot).

The fluids of the eye are of three kinds: (1) The blood, (2) the lymph, and (3) the aqueous humour. The aqueous humour differs from the other two in containing very little albumin and a high percentage of sodium chloride, whilst they contain much albumin and less salt. This matter will be dealt with at more length when we are discussing Magitot's views on the origin of the aqueous humour.

The Entrance Canal of the Optic Nerve.—The scleral coat is perforated for the passage of the second cranial nerve into the globe. The hole is, however, not clean punched out, but is partially blocked by a fibrous membrane, the *lamina cribrosa*, which, as we shall presently see, is a thinned out portion of the scleral tissue. It has neither the thickness, measured antero-posteriorly, nor the density of the scleral coat; in addition to this, it is perforated by a number of apertures for the transmission of the bundles of fibres of the optic nerve. It is not strange therefore that this should prove the weakest part of the wall of the eye, and consequently that which is the first to yield under a rise of intra-ocular pressure. If the neighbourhood of the ciliary body may be described as the " cockpit " of glaucoma, this area equally merits the title of the " graveyard " of that disease, for it is here that there lie hid the dead and wasted nerve-heads, killed by the fatal intra-ocular pressure.

The canal is divided for anatomical purposes into a choroidal and a scleral portion. The inner or choroidal opening of the canal is about 1·5 mm. in width; it may be taken to be bounded by the margin of the opening in the choroid, and by the contiguous part of the sclera. The outer opening, or scleral foramen, as is well known, is usually much wider than the inner; its boundary is formed by the outermost layers of the sclera. An antero-posterior section through this part of the eye shows the optic nerve and its canal presenting roughly the appearance of a truncated cone with its base external, and its truncated end internal (Fig. 5). The explanation of this lies in the fact that the fibres of the optic nerve lose their medullary sheaths as they pass through the scleral coat of the eye; at the same time, the coarse intraneural septa disappear; the bulk of the nerve consequently diminishes considerably from without inward. From such considerations it is easy to understand the shape of the advanced glaucoma cup with its overhanging edges and with the apparent interruption in the continuity of the blood vessels which emerge from it, as seen by the ophthalmoscope. A reference to Fig. 31 and to the Frontispiece will make these points additionally clear.

The wall of the canal is formed by a whitish fibrous

tissue, which, in the choroidal part of the tube, is clearly distinguishable from the uveal layers, but which, in the

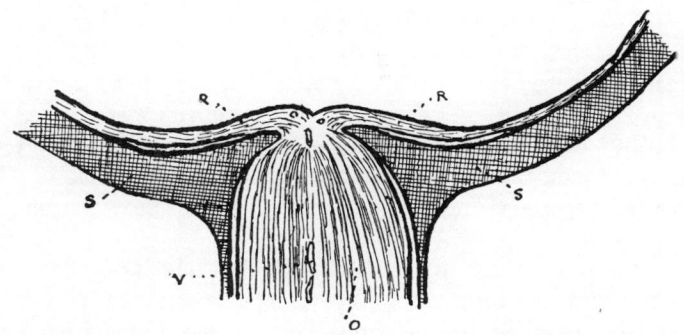

Fig. 5.—Optic nerve entrance. (Drawn by E. E. from a lantern projection of a slide.)
R. Retina; S. Sclera; O. Optic nerve; V. Central vessel.

sclerotic portion, blends with the adjacent sclera, with which it appears to be continuous. It is as though the

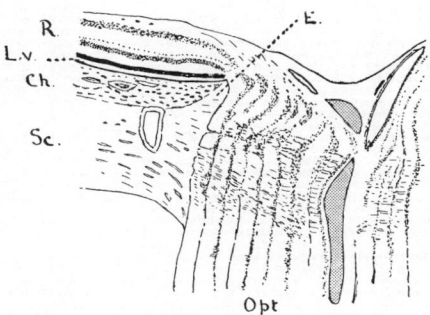

Fig. 6.—Semi-diagrammatic representation of lining of the canal of entrance of the optic nerve. R. Retina; Ch. Choroid; L.v. Lamina vitrea of choroid. The inturned selvedge edge E of the scleral tissue, which lines the choroidal part of the canal, ceases at the lamina vitrea. Sc. Sclera; Opt. Optic nerve. (Modified from Salzmann.)

sclera around the inner foramen ended in a selvedge edge, which is carried up clear to the membrane of Bruch; scleral tissue thus lines the whole of the optic canal (Fig. 6).

There has been much dispute as to the exact nature of this lining, and for this reason Salzmann has preferred to describe it by the indefinite and non-committal name of " the border tissue." It is generally accepted that fibrous tissue elements from this border tissue extend into the framework of the optic nerve, and so help to form the cribriform plate. Differences of opinion exist (1) as to whether elements derived from the choroid take any part in the formation of the fibrous tissue framework of this part of the nerve, and (2) as to the exact part played by other tissues.

It is important to understand that the framework or scaffolding of this part of the nerve is derived from two sources—(1) the mesodermal, which we have just been discussing, and (2) the ectodermal. The latter tissue is usually spoken of as " neuroglia " or " glia." Considerable differences of opinion exist as to the exact relationship of these two sets of tissue within the intra-ocular portion of the optic nerve. Such discussions are to a large extent academic. It is, however, of much greater and of more practical interest to note that the supporting tissue found in this portion of the nerve varies very greatly both in its distribution and in its amount. Thus, according to Fuchs, we find in some cases a tendency for a large amount of this tissue to lie in bundles along the direction of the length of the nerve, and so to run from before backwards, whilst in others it consists of sheets or laminæ, which cross the nerve trunk at right angles to its course and which may, and often do, run clean across all round from the marginal ring of the canal of the optic nerve to the central vessels. Moreover, these laminæ may vary in number, in strength, and in completeness. These points are well illustrated by a comparison of Figs. 7, 8, and 9. In Fig. 7 it will be observed that the large number of strong lamellæ, superposed upon each other, give the lamina cribrosa a considerable depth as measured from before backward, whilst in Figs. 8 and 9 the paucity of lamellæ has diminished the depth of that membrane. Nor is this all that can be learnt from these illustrations. The strength of the individual lamellæ, apart altogether from their number, is obviously greater in the nerve depicted in Fig. 7 than in Figs. 8 and 9. Still

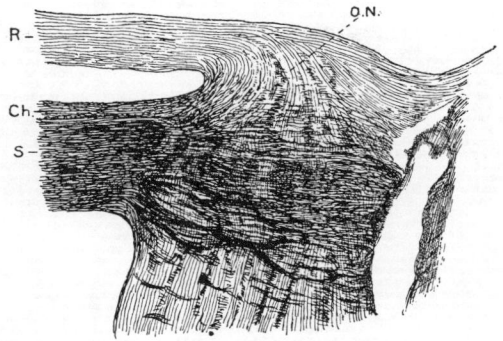

FIG. 7.—The transverse lamellæ are here very strong and are also very numerous. The result is that they build up a thick strong lamina cribrosa. The longitudinally placed glial elements are relatively poorly marked in this drawing.

one more point, the lamellæ are not always of even strength right across the section of the nerve; indeed they appear

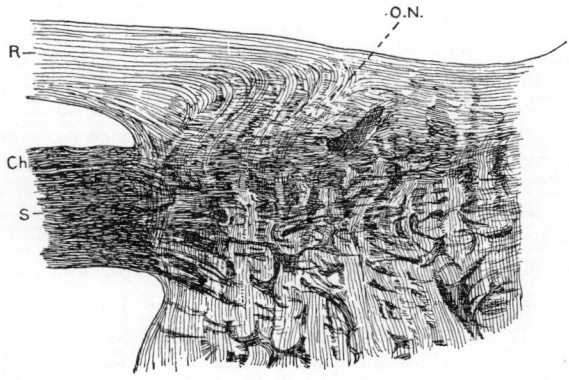

FIG. 8.—The transverse lamellæ lie mainly in the anterior part of the optic canal, and are not very strong, as compared with the glial tissue which lies in bundles along the length of the nerve.

to vary widely in this respect. If one may illustrate the point: In one case the membrane may be attached to the canal all round its circumference and may stretch across the whole section of the nerve; in another, only a part of the membrane may be present, the remainder being wanting or weak. Granted then such differences in the number, thickness, and completeness of the individual lamellæ, it must be at once obvious that not only will there be great differences in the resistance to pressure of the laminæ cribrosæ thus built up in different eyes, but also that similar differences will surely be found in different parts of this membrane, even in the same eye. Fuchs

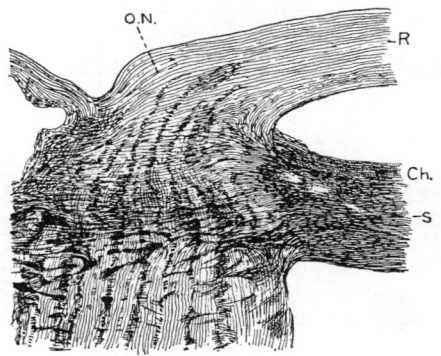

FIG. 9.—This resembles Fig. 8, except that the transverse lamellæ lie mainly in the posterior part of the canal (the usual arrangement) and the longitudinally placed glial bundles are not quite so strongly in evidence.

FIGS. 7, 8 and 9 are diagrammatic representations, constructed from Fuchs' microphotographs, and modified in accordance with the text of his article to make the points he emphasises clearer. The lettering is the same in all.

R. Retina; Ch. Choroid; S. Sclera; O.N. Optic nerve.

believes that those laminæ cribrosæ, whose elements are mainly made up of transversely running lamellæ (Fig. 7), must be much more resistant to pressure applied, as intraocular pressure always must be, along the axis of the nerve, than are those in which the bulk of the tissue is built up of bundle-like elements, which run in the direction of the long axis of the nerve (Fig. 8). This proposition is self-evident, for the transverse lamellæ, tethered as they are to the sides of the canal of the optic nerve, will check even the slightest tendency to a push of the nerve directly backwards, whilst the bundles, which run in the axis of the nerve, will readily be displaced, along with the structures between which they lie.

There is another point, of which we were not ignorant, but which has been emphasised for us by Fuchs in his paper under reference, viz., that the situation of the lamina cribrosa varies greatly in different eyes. This of course depends (1) on the position at which the various connective tissue lamellæ, which between them form the lamina, find their attachment to the walls of the optic canal, and (2) on the number of these lamellæ. Figs. 7, 8, and 9 illustrate these points clearly. For convenience' sake, we shall take them in reverse order. In Fig. 9, the lamina cribrosa lies in what is usually described as its normal position, *i.e.*, in the posterior segment of the canal. In Fig. 8 it lies almost wholly in the anterior portion of the canal. Fig. 7 forms a contrast with both of the preceding ones, since in it the lamina appears to occupy practically the whole length of the canal.

It is obvious, as Fuchs has pointed out, that these variations in anatomical structure must greatly influence the ophthalmoscopic appearances presented by different cases of optic atrophy, unaccompanied by increase of pressure; in the first case taken above (Fig. 9), the cup would be much deeper than in either of the others (Figs. 7 and 8), that is, if we assume that the underpressed anterior surface of the lamina cribrosa forms the floor of the cup.

We shall have to return to this subject when discussing the diagnosis and pathology of the glaucoma cup. Many of the other points which have been dealt with in this section, will be taken up at greater length in their appropriate places.

REFERENCES

ELLIOT, R. H.—" The Yielding of the Optic Nerve-head in Glaucoma," *Brit. Journ. Ophth.*, July 1921, vol. v. p. 307.

FUCHS, E.—" On the Lamina Cribrosa," *Arch. f. O.*, 1916, vol. xci. Part III.

MAGGIORE, L.—" The Canal of Schlemm in Man," *Annal. di Ottal. e Clin. Ocul.*, May–June 1917.

MAGITOT, A.—*Ann. d'ocul.*, vol. cliv. pp. 272, 334, 385; and *Amer. Journ. Ophth.*, 1918, vol. i. p. 587.

MORAX, V.—*Glaucome et Glaucomateux*, Gaston Doin, Editeur, 8 Place de L'Odeon, Paris, 1921, pp. 88 and 89.

ROCHON-DUVIGNEAUD.—*The Topography of the Angle of the Anterior Chamber*, Paris, 1892.

SALZMANN, M.—*Anatomy and History of the Human Eyeball*, trans. by Dr. E. V. L. Brown, Univ. of Chicago Press, Chicago, 1912, pp. 90 and 91.

THOMSON, A.—*The Ophthalmoscope*, 1910, vol. viii. p. 608; and 1911, vol. ix. p. 470.

Part III

Historical

To review the history of glaucoma would be a task which would far transcend the limits of the present work. Interesting as such an undertaking might prove, it would yield the reader little of practical value in return. Hence the decision to take up but a few of the outstanding landmarks of the subject, and to deal with them only in the rough. They loom so large in the dim back pages of the history of ophthalmology, that it would be a poor compliment either to the great names linked for ever with them, or to the reader's intelligence, to accord them any different treatment.

Over four centuries before the dawn of the Christian era, Hippocrates, in the course of his aphorisms, enumerated the diseases of advancing years, and mentioned the " glaucoses " as amongst the known affections of the eyes (ὀφθαλμῶν καὶ ῥινῶν ὑγρότητες, ἀμβλυῶπιαι, γλαύκωσες, καὶ βαρυήκοιαι). Such knowledge as he possessed of the subject was very hazy, and he did not even distinguish from cataracts the conditions, which we now class under the heading of a pathological increase in intra-ocular pressure. The Greek and Latin writers who followed him had learnt one important fact at least, that a great practical difference existed between the various groups of morbid conditions which they recognised as being situate behind the pupil, and there giving rise to blindness; for they had found that some of these were very favourable from the operative standpoint, whilst others were most unfavourable. The former they spoke of as " suffusions " (ὑπόχυσις), and the latter as glaucomata. Such were the doctrines accepted by Galen, Rufus, Paulus Ægineta, and many of the old writers of the early Christian centuries, and they constitute the first really big addition to the heritage of the knowledge bequeathed us by the past. We have to pass over many centuries before we come to anything fresh of real value in the writings on glaucoma, which in the interval are taken up with barren discussions as to whether the lens or the vitreous is the real seat of the disease, or with other speculations equally wide of the mark.

The invention of the ophthalmoscope by Helmholtz in the year 1851, was destined to open up an entirely new path for the diagnosis of glaucoma, and was soon followed by Adolph Weber's clinical discovery of cupping of the disc. Hard on the heels of this work came Heinrich Müller's confirmation of the discovery as a result of his studies of the pathological anatomy of the eyeball. Too much credit cannot be given to Mackenzie for blazing the trail which led to these important findings, for, more than a quarter of a century earlier (1830), he had drawn attention to the hardness of glaucomatous eyes, had maintained that this hardness was due to overfilling of the globe with fluid, and had suggested paracentesis of the aqueous, or preferably of the vitreous chamber, with a view to the therapeutic withdrawal of fluid from the eye. About the same time, Albrecht von Graefe discovered the venous and the arterial pulse in the retinal vessels, and observed their dependence on the increase of the intra-ocular pressure, whilst Donders showed that the same phenomena can be produced in healthy eyes by means of digital pressure on the globe. Coccius added the observation that the harder the eye, the more easily is the arterial pulse produced in it by the pressure of the finger. Bowman, recognising the value of these discoveries, made a number of examinations of hard, of normal, and of soft eyes, and introduced his finger-tip method of taking the ocular tension, together with the use of the three now familiar degrees, above and below the normal respectively. Amongst the many who contributed to the literature of glaucoma at this time, von Graefe stands out pre-eminent for his great discovery of the value of iridectomy in congestive cases, but apart altogether from this, his keen powers of clinical observation enriched the science of ophthalmology for all time. In close relationship with his work must be mentioned the name of his ardent disciple de Wecker, who strenuously fought the rising tide of opposition, which threatened at one time prematurely to engulf his master's valuable method. De Wecker has a higher claim still on our admiration, for it was he who practically introduced Stellwag's sclerotomy, and it was he—let us remember this above all else—who first realised what von Graefe only dimly apprehended—viz., the value of the filtering scar, and who set himself to find a method whereby a permanent filtration of the intra-ocular fluid could be established through the coats of the eye. This dream of his was an inspiration of genius to which we probably owe all the progress that has lately been made. That he failed to attain his end is true, but his was the powerful prophetic vision, that from his Pisgah height turned men's eyes to the Land of Promise and of Hope, which was to be reached by the future conquest of glaucoma.

For the moment we must leave this attractive subject to study the physiological researches, which have laid truly and well the foundations for the pathological study of glaucoma.

Leber's classic work established the secretion of the intra-ocular fluid by the ciliary body and the method of excretion of that fluid. This paved the way for the work of Max Knies and Adolph Weber, who working independently and following the clue given by Leber, simultaneously discovered the very important fact of the closure of the angle of the anterior chamber by the adhesion of the iris base to the cornea, in cases of glaucoma. Then followed the work of Priestley Smith, who not only adopted and gave publicity to these valuable discoveries, but made the subject his own and enriched it by a lifetime of careful and painstaking research.

Once again we must hark back to the fruitful year of 1876 to do honour to the name of Laqueur of Strasburg, for the introduction of the use of meiotics in the treatment of glaucoma, and for the courage with which he maintained his stand in the teeth of the opposition which it aroused. He was fortunate to have the veteran Snellen amongst his powerful supporters.

It would be impossible here even to outline the extraordinarily valuable work which has been done on the changes in the visual fields in glaucoma; but our résumé would be incomplete without the mention of three honoured names—those of Haffmans of Utrecht, who worked under the guidance of Donders in 1860, of Bjerrum of Copenhagen, and of his pupil Roenne.

In conclusion we must speak of the wonderful interest which has been taken in all subjects connected with glaucoma during the past twenty years. The description of Heine's cyclodialysis in 1905 had been preceded by Herbert's efforts two years earlier to obtain a filtering scar, but it was left to Lagrange in 1906 to introduce the operation of sclerectomy which has made his name a household word throughout the ophthalmological world. He it was who materialised the dreams of von Graefe and de Wecker, and who converted their longing foresight into the practical triumphs of the surgery of to-day. All the modern filtration operations, from which we hope so much, are the indirect offspring of his genius. It is therefore fit and right that a summary of the history of glaucoma, which opened with the name of " The Father of Medicine " should close on that of the great Frenchman, Lagrange.

REFERENCES

BJERRUM, J.—*International Congress of Medicine*, Berlin, 1890.
BOWMAN, SIR W.—*Brit. Med. Journ.*, Oct. 11, 1862.
COCCIUS.—*Ophthalmometrie und Spannungsmessung*, Leipzig, 1872.
DE WECKER, L.—*Soc. franç. d'ophtal. Congrès de* 1901. See also article by R. H. Elliot, *The Ophthalmoscope*, 1916, vol. xiv. pp. 509 and 573.

DONDERS, F. C.—*Archiv f. O.*, vol. i. pt. 2, p. 75.
HAFFMANS.—*Bijdrage tot de Kennis van het Glaucoma*, Utrecht, 1900.
HEINE, L.—*Deut. medizin. Woch.*, vol. xxi., 1905.
HERBERT, H.—*Trans. O.S. of U.K.*, 1903, vol. xxiii.
HIPPOCRATES.—*Aphorisms*, sec. iii. 31.
KNIES, M.—*Archiv f. O.*, vol. xxii. pt. 3, p. 163.
LAGRANGE, F.—*Rev. général d'ophtal.*, 1906.
LAQUEUR, L.—*Archiv f. O.*, 1876, vol. xxiii. pt. 3, p. 149.
LEBER.—*Ibid.*, 1873, vol. xix. pt. 2, p. 87; and Graefe-Saemisch, *Handbuch der Ges. Augenheilk.*, vol. ii. pt. 2, p. 302.
MACKENZIE, W.—*Practical Treatise on the Diseases of the Eye*, Longman, Brown, Green and Longman, Lond.
MÜLLER, H.—*Archiv f. O.*, 1856, vol. iv. pt. 1, p. 377.
ROENNE, H.—*Ibid.*, vol. lxxi. pt. 1, p. 52.
SMITH, P.—*The Pathology and Treatment of Glaucoma*, J. & A. Churchill, Lond., 1891.
VON GRAEFE, A.—*Archiv f. O.*, vol. i. pt. 1, p. 373; and vol. ii. pt. 2, p. 202; and *New Sydenham Soc.'s Monographs*, 1859.
WEBER, A.—*Archiv f. O.*, vol. ii. pt. 1, p. 141; and vol. xxiii. pt. 1, p. 1.

CHAPTER II

THE INTRA-OCULAR PRESSURE AND THE TENSION OF THE EYE

SUMMARY

PART I

THE TERMS USED.
THE PHYSICAL CONDITIONS REGULATING THE INTRA-OCULAR PRESSURE.

PART II

THE BEARING ON INTRA-OCULAR PRESSURE OF THE CONTINUOUS FLOW OF FLUID THROUGH THE CHAMBERS OF THE EYE.
THE CHANGES IN THE CHAMBER PRESSURE WHICH ATTEND SOME FORMS OF GLAUCOMA.
THE SOURCE AND METHOD OF PRODUCTION OF THE INTRA-OCULAR FLUID.
MAGITOT'S VIEWS.

PART III

THE RELATIONSHIP OF SYSTEMIC BLOOD-PRESSURE TO INTRA-OCULAR PRESSURE.
THE RELATIONSHIP BETWEEN THE INTRA-OCULAR BLOOD-PRESSURE AND THE INTRA-OCULAR FLUID-PRESSURE OUTSIDE THE VESSELS.
    The Osmotic Theory of the Removal of Intra-ocular Fluid.
    Professor Thomson's Pump-action Theory.

PART I

IT is not possible to take up the study of the source of the intra-ocular pressure without being profoundly struck by the wide divergence between the views of those who have written or spoken on the subject. Part of the confusion which has arisen would appear to be due to an avoidable vagueness in the use of terms, part to an effort to argue the question on the basis of *schemata* which are not wholly apposite, and part to attempts to draw deductions before sufficient data are available. We are not yet in a position to pass final judgment. All we can do is to endeavour to straighten out the facts from the fictions which have gathered round them, whilst avoiding the temptation of being led to found dogmatic theories, where the present state of our knowledge does not appear ripe for such decisive treatment.

Terms

It will clear the ground if we begin by defining some of the terms which are in constant use in this discussion.

Pressure[1] is defined as the force exerted by one body on another by its weight, or by the continued application of power, viewed as a measurable quantity, the amount being expressed by the weight upon a unit of area.

Tension[1] is defined as a constrained condition of the particles of the body when subjected to forces acting in opposite directions away from each other, thus tending to draw them apart, balanced by forces of cohesion holding them together; the force or combination of forces acting in this way, especially as a measurable quantity (the opposite of compression or pressure).

In the light of the above definitions, we can discuss two terms which have often been confused with each other, and have consequently been used in the wrong sense, viz., intra-ocular pressure and ocular tension.

The *intra-ocular* pressure is the pressure (usually measured in mm. of Hg.) at which the intra-ocular fluid stands within the eye. It can only be measured by means of a manometer (Fig. 10), and the readings obtained are easily vitiated by errors in experimental technique.

The *tension of an eye* is a measure of the state of tension of its tunic, and can be estimated either digitally or by means of a tonometer. Of the latter instruments the Schiötz (Fig. 105) is the prototype of all the best models now in use. The tension of an eye is frequently confused with the

[1] The definition is from the New English Dictionary (Oxford).

INTRA-OCULAR PRESSURE AND TENSION

intra-ocular pressure, and this confusion has been deepened by the fact that every effort has been made to ensure that the modern tonometer shall give a reading which as nearly as possible indicates the pressure of the fluid within the chambers of the eye. This pressure is, however, only one of several factors which go to make up the tension of the ocular tunic. The thickness and the distensibility of that tunic, the surface area of the organ, and possibly other factors as well, enter into the question.

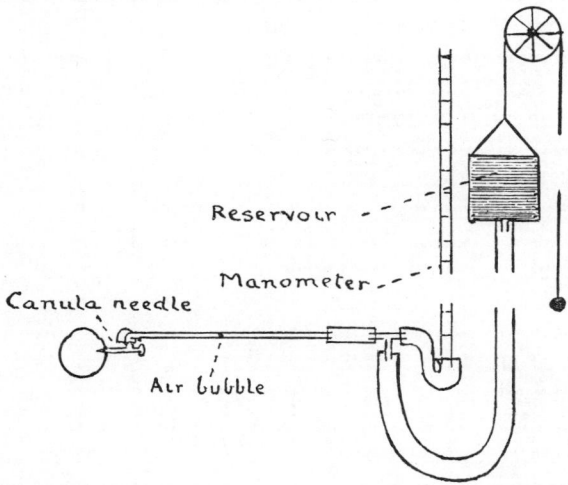

FIG. 10.—A diagrammatic representation of the principal parts concerned in an estimation of intra-ocular pressure, by means of a manometer. The needle is seen within the eyeball. (Modified from McLean.)

Elastic,[1] that spontaneously resumes (after a longer or a shorter interval) its normal bulk or shape, after having been contracted, dilated, or distorted by external force.

Rigid (in physics), theoretically such as to resist change of form, when acted on by any force.[2]

Closed, shut up,—inclosed.[2] The meaning conveyed is that nothing can pass into or out of a box, sphere, or other structure, which is said to be *closed*.

[1] The definition is from the New English Dictionary (Oxford).
[2] The definition is from Annandale's Concise English Dictionary.

Filtering scar.—This term has been used as though it were synonymous with the term fistulous scar. It might possibly be desirable to separate the two in view of the opinion held by some ophthalmologists, that filtration may take place through a spongy cicatrix, in which no actual fistula can be found to exist. Without admitting that such a condition actually exists, yet in deference to the opinion of those who think differently (Herbert and others), and to save confusion in debate, it might be well to speak of a scar in which an actual fistula can be seen to be present, or is believed to be present, as a *fistulous scar*, whilst reserving the term *filtering scar* for the condition (of the existence of which actual proof is wanting) in which the fluid is supposed to traverse a mass of spongy cicatricial tissue in order to reach the subconjunctival space. If this terminology were accepted, the escaping fluid should likewise be called *fistulous* or *filtering* fluid, as the case might be. It is, however, unlikely that it will be adopted, as there is little to be said in its favour.

Schemata.—In reading the various discussions on the subject of the intra-ocular pressure, one is struck with the ingenuity which has been displayed in the efforts of writers to reduce the physical conditions they believe to be present to *schemata*, in the hope that they will thereby simplify the comprehension of the problems involved. Not less striking, if more diverting, is the uniformity with which each such *schema* is unhesitatingly rejected by another thinker. It is obvious that there are lessons to be learnt from a consideration of these phenomena. *Schemata* may obviously be of use, but it would appear that such use is very restricted. They may possibly help to clear up some doubtful points, but it would seem certain that little reliance can be placed on them for large deductions. Nor is this surprising, when we remember that there are physical and anatomical facts in connection with the eye which are still under dispute. Moreover, the exact reproduction of the complex conditions which enter into the make-up of even the dead eye, demands an expenditure of money, thought, labour, time, and skill, which is beyond the means of most, if not of any, experimenters. When on to this is grafted all that the phenomena of life imply, and we may mention amongst other things the behaviour of nerves and of muscular tissue under varying conditions, we find ourselves confronted with a situation which is enough to give pause even to the most enthusiastic.

The Physical Conditions Regulating the Intra-ocular Pressure

The eye has, in recent years, been not infrequently spoken of as " a closed sphere, with rigid walls, and of fixed contents "; and arguments as to its behaviour, under various conditions, have been built on the assumptions contained in the above description. It is, therefore, necessary to insist most strongly (1) that the eye is *not* a closed sphere, (2) that its walls are *not* rigid, and (3) that *its contents vary* in volume under conditions both of health and disease.

The eye is *not* a closed sphere. Fluid is freely entering it from without and is as freely leaving it from within. This fluid, be it observed, is not contained merely in the vessels of the organ, but passes out from those vessels into the cavities of the eye. From these cavities it passes back again into the vessels and so leaves the globe. This procession of fluid through the eye goes on throughout life, and if it stops or is interfered with, the health of the eye is at once endangered. It is therefore difficult to understand how anyone can entertain the view that the eye is a " closed sphere "; and it is obvious that any *schema* founded on such an assumption must be open to grave criticism.

The eye is *not* a rigid sphere. Its walls are distinctly distensible and elastic. This is a very material point in all our considerations. We have no wish to use terms in any strained sense, and we take the definition already given of the word rigid, believing that it represents the sense in which it is usually employed in our language, viz., theoretically such as to resist change of form, when acted on by any force.

The contents of the eye are *not* fixed. On the contrary, we believe that they are constantly varying in volume, and that these variations in volume determine the degree of tension of the ocular tunic, as tested either by the fingers or by the tonometer.

At first sight, it would appear tempting to take up and discuss each of these headings separately, reviewing the evidence bearing on each in turn. Further consideration, however, shows that to do so would involve repetition and confusion, and it has therefore been resolved to group them all together. In doing so, we approach the subject from various and widely different points of view, for the topic has proved of interest to the physicist, to the physiologist, to the pathologist, and to the clinician.

(*a*) The difference in feel between various eyes is marked, even under the conditions of health; and when we come to deal with abnormal conditions, this difference is still more accentuated. In the healthy eye we feel a sense of elasticity or resiliency of the ball, such as we are accustomed to find in a moderately distended rubber ball, *e.g.*, in a rather slack football or tennis ball. Under digital examination we can dimple its walls, and feel them spring back into place as soon as the force we exert is removed. If we now turn our attention to a globe which is shrinking under the influence of an attack of cyclitis, we find that it feels like a soft bag of fluid. Its coat is obviously not rigid, and its contents are not of the same volume as those of a normal eye. It may be answered that in such a case the alterations that have taken place in the tunic of the eye affect the proposition so far as the rigidity of that structure is concerned; but this argument will obviously have no bearing on the change in volume observed; nor, so far as the tunic is concerned, will it meet the case of an eye from which a large vitreous escape has taken place during the course of a cataract extraction; and yet the way in which such a globe collapses shows conclusively that its walls are not rigid. We shall find even more instructive the case of a hypotonic eye (with a Schiötz reading corresponding to a tension of 8 to 15 mm. of Hg.) such as may sometimes be met with after one or other of the modern sclerectomy operations. Such a globe is closed to the outer surface, but fluid is passing freely from its interior through the breach in the scleral coat, into the subconjunctival space. It feels soft to the fingers and the tonometer reading is low. Should the hole in the sclera fill up, the evidence of the passage of fluid from the inside of the eye into the subconjunctival space disappears, the eye hardens and the tonometer reading goes up. We shall return to this subject again shortly. For the moment we pass on to consider the feel of a high tension eye, such as that just described. The rise in tension may be so slight as to be inappreciable to finger estimation, or so great that the surgeon describes the eye as being " as hard as stone." As we review these variations in the feel of a globe, ranging from flaccidity to stony hardness, what is the most natural explanation which presents itself to our minds ? The obvious answer will be that the feel of the globe is an expression of the tension of its coat, and that the degree of that tension is largely determined in the instances before us by the volume of the fluid contents of the eye. In other words, the evidence of our senses, trained in the everyday actions of life, indicates clearly to us that when handling an eye, we are not dealing with a sphere which possesses a rigid wall, or with one with fixed contents.

(*b*) It is possible to carry the argument still farther by means of a simple experiment. If an eye is connected with a manometer (Fig. 10), by means of a needle passed into the interior of the globe, the pressure within the globe can, by a simple arrangement, be made to vary at will, say from 5 mm. of Hg. up to 80 mm. or more. From time to time during this process of raising the pressure, the tension of the globe can be taken with the fingers. If this is done, the eye is found to pass, as the pressure rises, from a soft bag of fluid to a hard tense sphere, varying just as we have shown it does under clinical conditions. We can, in fact, duplicate the changes in the feel of the globe with which our clinical experience has made us familiar. The globe obviously becomes tenser both to sight and feel, and it is evident that the increasing pressure is in part at least an expression of an increase in its fluid contents, of its passage, in fact, from a soft bag of fluid to a tensely filled sphere. In any case we can eliminate the pressure of the column of fluid as a causative factor, by shutting off the tap which connects the interior of the eye with the source of pressure, before making each observation; if we do so, we shall not find any change in the feel of the eye. A point to be emphasised is that during the earlier stages, the increase in volume of the contents of the eye is appreciable to the senses, whilst, as will be shown later, the volume is still increasing, up, at least, to a point at which the pressure stands at 80 mm. of Hg.

(c) It has been suggested that the dimpling of a normal eye under digital manipulation, is effected by the expulsion of a certain quantity of blood from within the globe, under the pressure of the fingers. It may be open to question whether a sufficient quantity of blood could be expelled in this way to give rise to the amount of dimpling one is familiar with. But even if it were possible to accept this explanation for the normal eye, how can we explain the fact that a high tension eye will not dimple at all under the fingers? Is it to be believed that the rise in the pressure within the vessels feeding the eye—from, we will say, 25 mm. to 80 mm. of Hg.—suffices to make the globe so hard that we cannot dimple it, or that we can do so only by exercising considerable and (clinically) unjustifiable pressure? It is necessary to put this question so clearly that there can be no possibility of a mistake about our answer to it. We can readily understand that if the rise in tension of the globe is due to overdistension of its tunic with fluid, dimpling is impossible, for the fluid is incompressible, and the coats have reached their maximum (or very near it) of distension. But can we say that if the hardness is due to an increase of the intra-ocular blood-pressure, the effort to expel the blood from the ocular vessels against an increased blood-pressure of 55 mm. of Hg., would call for the exercise of so much force as we know has to be exerted ? It scarcely seems credible that this can be so.

(*d*) We return now to consider more at length an important point to which allusion has already been made above. It is practically universally admitted that if a means is provided whereby the contained fluid can effect a free escape from the interior of a glaucomatous eye into the subconjunctival space on the outside of the globe, the tension of the eye is lowered, and that so long as fistulisation is maintained, the tension will not again rise to pathological limits or, at least, will only do so under rare and very exceptional conditions. To put it in other words, if we provide a means whereby the contained fluid can freely escape from the interior of a glaucomatous eye into the subconjunctival space on the outside of the globe, we *ipso facto* reduce the tension to normal or subnormal limits. So long as fistulisation of the eye is maintained, the tension can not and will not rise again to pathologic limits. This is the underlying principle of all the modern operative methods for the relief of glaucoma. De Wecker was one of the first to grasp this idea, and the outcome was that he devised the operation of sclerotomy, a procedure which is admitted to have been an advance on older methods, but which fell into disrepute, because it was found that as soon as the wound healed soundly, which it generally did sooner or later, the escape of fluid through the scar ceased, and the tension of the eye rose again to pathological limits. The same criticism has been widely offered on Herbert's ingenious operations, subject, however, to the important modification that the technique of these methods has proved superior to that of de Wecker's procedure in establishing, or in endeavouring to establish, a permanent flow through the wound. And so too with Holth's operation, with Lagrange's operation, and with trephining. Be the method what it may, it is a fact established by clinical experience, that the effect of any operative procedure, in maintaining a reduction in ocular tension, can only be counted on so long as the artificial outlet for the escape of the aqueous fluid is kept inviolate. Once let the channel become closed up, by cell proliferation, or by structure prolapse, and a return of the rise in tension may be confidently expected. On the other hand, if too large and too free a channel is cut in the ocular tunic, the escape of fluid is so rapid that a condition of hypotonus is established. Indeed, so real is the latter trouble—it need hardly be spoken of as a danger, for there is no definite evidence that it is dangerous—that surgeons have been driven to modify their technique in such a way as to adapt it to the various conditions of the eyes under treatment. Their endeavour has been to graduate the size of the channel established for the drainage of the imprisoned fluid, in accordance with the needs of the individual case.

In considering the above facts, it must be borne in mind that the one factor, which the modern operation alters, is the rate of escape of fluid from within the eye to the subconjunctival space. Except indirectly, the pressure of blood within the eye is not interfered with. When the intra-ocular pressure tends to rise, be the cause of that tendency what it may (whether increased secretion, diminished outflow, or raised blood-pressure), the result must obviously be an increased outflow through the artificial channel in the tunic. If the outflow be sufficiently rapid, then a rise in intra-ocular pressure cannot take place. If this argument be accepted, it becomes clear that the essential factor in the success of all of the modern operations for glaucoma lies in a control of the volume of the intra-ocular contents.

(e) The criticism may be offered that in the preceding paragraphs we have been discussing conditions which are found to exist in eyes, which not only were pathologic to start with, but which have in addition been altered in the mechanism of the circulation of their nutrient fluid, by grossly artificial means. It is therefore of great interest to recall some observations made by Starling before the Royal Society of Medicine in 1913. He said: "We have studied the conditions which alter the rate at which fluid escapes from the eyeball. Why does one not always find a permanent rise of intra-ocular pressure with a rise of arterial pressure ? The association is certainly seen, but it is by no means constant. The explanation is probably found in some experiments by Henderson (Erskine) and myself. If we try the effect of raising the intra-ocular pressure artificially, we find that a little time after raising the pressure to 50 or 60 mm. Hg., filtration becomes more easy, as if additional channels had been opened up, or pre-existing channels enlarged. A similar change might occur in the normal eye, and in this way the intra-ocular pressure might be kept at a normal height, although the arterial pressure was permanently raised." If we accept these observations, there is strong reason for thinking that the *modus agendi* of the modern operation is an imitation, a crude one perhaps, of the age-long and beautifully compensated methods, whereby nature has provided against harm being done to the delicate structures of the eye by the inevitable fluctuations of intra-ocular blood-pressure. In both cases the underlying principle of the measure is an alteration in the volume of intra-ocular contents. Nature then has shown her agreement with the modern surgeon's estimate that the contents of the eye are neither fixed nor incapable of alteration.

(*f*) The subjects discussed in the previous section have led the way to a consideration of the influence of massage on the eye. It has long been known that massage of the eyeball is a very valuable adjunct to the treatment of a case of glaucoma, both before and after operation on the globe. More recently the subject has been systematically studied by various surgeons, and amongst others by Carpenter and by Schoenberg. These observers, working independently of each other, both lay stress on the fact that the fall in tension observed in different eyes after the use of massage, varies greatly both in the rate and in the ease of its production ; they believe that a delay or a diminution in the reduction of tension may point to a threatening of glaucoma. Carpenter goes so far as to suggest that a normal index of filtration should be worked out by experiments, and thinks that if this is done we shall be in a better position to diagnose doubtful cases. The question naturally arises as to how massage effects a reduction in the tension of an unoperated eye. Three possible explanations present themselves : (1) That the rate of excretion of the intra-ocular fluid is accelerated by the movements conducted ; (2) that the intra-ocular blood-pressure is lowered, and the amount of blood in the eye decreased by the removal of venous blood from the globe ; and (3) that the intra-ocular mechanism, which is presumed by Magitot and others to control vaso-constriction in the choroidal, vascular tunic, is brought into play and so determines a fall in intra-ocular pressure by diminishing the bulk of that coat. It will be observed that any one of these explanations involves an alteration in the volume of the fluid contents of the eye. It would seem to be practically certain that massage (properly conducted) must lead to an increase in the freedom of escape of venous blood from the eye, and to a change in the tone of the intra-ocular vessels, for we know that it has a similar action in other parts of the body. If so, the actual volume of blood in the organ, and the intra-ocular blood-pressure would both be reduced. A consideration of what happens when massage is applied to an eye which has been previously subjected to a successful trephining operation, throws some light on the subject. Some years back the author called attention to the following experiment which has been often repeated and confirmed by others since then. The tension of a recently trephined eye is taken with a Schiötz tonometer ; then the amount of pitting of the conjunctiva in the neighbourhood of the trephine hole is carefully noted after pressure with a probe. Free massage is employed, and the tension and pitting are again noted. It is now found that the tension has distinctly fallen, and the conjunctival pitting is markedly increased. The obvious explanation of these results is that the massage has pressed fluid out from the interior of the eye (*i.e.*, from the aqueous chamber) through the trephine hole into the subconjunctival space. The fall in tension has in fact been brought about by a reduction of the fluid contents of the eye. This reduction may be partly due to expression of blood from the veins, but it is certainly also in part due to the escape of the aqueous fluid itself. There would appear to be at least a strong presumption, that what happens through the artificial channel of a trephine wound, may likewise happen through the normal channels for excretion, since the phenomenon of reduction of ocular tension is observed in both cases.

(g) It is the experience of competent pathologists that there is a difference between the feel of an eye excised for glaucoma, and of one removed for conditions in which the tension is not raised. They state that if the globe reaches them quickly and without any delay, they can tell the difference between the two, because the former feels harder than does the latter. It is quite obvious that, if this statement is a correct one, we can eliminate blood-pressure as a factor in producing the feeling of hardness. It is evidently a question of the volumetric contents of the globe, or of the rigidity of its coats. There is a further observation which sheds light on the problem, viz., that if a glaucomatous eyeball is thrown down on the floor after removal, it " bounces," whilst a normal tension globe will not do so, or at least that the former will bounce much more markedly than the latter will. The writer cannot claim to have made the experiment, but he has met with those who have either seen it done, or else have actually done it, and the facts are vouched for by observers of absolutely the first rank. That the experiment is unfavourable to the preservation of pathological specimens is immaterial to our present argument. The obvious inference from it would appear to be that the eye behaves like other elastic globes (e.g., a tennis ball or a football), and that its elasticity is increased, within certain limits, by an increase in the distension of its coats ; in other words by an increase in the volume of its contents. In drawing this inference, sight is not lost of the fact that the contents in the case of the ball are gaseous, whilst those of the eye are liquid.

(*h*) In studying more particularly the question of the *rigidity* of the eye, there are certain observations and experiments which demand our careful attention. It is at the same time of the utmost importance that we should bear in mind the definition [1] already given of the word "rigid." Adamük, von Hippel, Grünhagen, and other competent observers long ago showed that stimulation of the cervical sympathetic caused a rise in intra-ocular pressure. Parsons considered that the cause of this rise of pressure was the contraction of the unstriped muscle contained in the orbit, and his finding was supported by Henderson and Starling. More recently, Lederer, of Würzberg, has shown by manometric readings that the contractions of the recti and of the oblique muscles raise the intra-ocular pressure. He explains this action by the suggestion that when any muscle and its antagonist act, they draw back the globe against the orbital contents. Again, it is a matter of common and undisputed knowledge that digital pressure temporarily raises the intra-ocular pressure, as can be seen by the behaviour of the retinal vessels. It is equally well known that prolonged manipulation or bandage pressure will very appreciably lower the tension of an eye. In the face of such facts, and especially of those which concern the rise in tension under the influence of extrinsic muscular, or of digital pressure, it does not seem logical to speak of the tunic of the eye as "a rigid case."

(*i*) Closely allied to the above observations, are those in which the intra-ocular pressure is altered, whilst the extra-ocular pressure remains constant. For instance, when the operation of paracentesis is performed on an eye, the anterior chamber empties, the cornea falls back on the support of the lens and vitreous body, and the change in curvature of the front of the eye is obvious to any observer; after a short delay the chamber re-forms, and the curvature of the cornea is evidently restored. Take another

[1] Rigid, such as to resist change of form when acted on by any force.

INTRA-OCULAR PRESSURE AND TENSION

instance: Every surgeon is familiar with the cases of the "inelastic eye," met with from time to time after extractions. The same phenomenon may sometimes, though rarely, be noticed to occur after any operation (*e.g.*, iridectomy) which lets out the aqueous fluid. The sucking of an air-bubble into the eye, or the filling up of the chamber with aqueous fluid from an irrigator, will at once restore to the cornea its normal convexity; let out the fluid once more and the cornea again becomes concave forwards. To apply the term "rigid" to the cornea under such circumstances would be clearly incorrect, since it very readily changes its form under the influence of a force acting on it either from its anterior or from its posterior surface. It has been said that "the eye is sufficiently rigid for physiological purposes," and that it "might more or less be regarded as a rigid box." These vague statements are difficult to answer since it is hard to understand their precise meaning. It is, however, quite possible to push the argument still farther, and to disarm even such vague suggestions as these by a consideration of what we know of the circulation of the fluid within the eye. We shall do so.

(*j*) Koster showed that when the pressure within an eye was raised from 20 to 70 mm. of Hg., the intra-ocular contents increase by $\frac{7}{1000}$ of their normal volume. He also showed that this expansion was a gradual one, corresponding with the gradual rise in the internal pressure. The inference that an increase of $\frac{7}{1000}$ of the volume of an eye would be accompanied by a rise in intra-ocular pressure corresponding to 50 mm. of Hg., seems fairly obvious, *i.e.*, if other conditions remained the same. The actual increase in the volume of the globe in the above experiment is one of 45 c.mm. There has been a tendency to speak of this quantity as if it were negligible. A little consideration will show that this attitude is far from being beyond criticism. The cubic contents of the aqueous chambers of the eye have been estimated at from 0·23 to 0·40 of a c.c. The amount of the fluid which leaves the eye per minute has been variously computed at from 5 to 7 c.mm. per minute. It may therefore be calculated that the time which it takes for the whole contents of the anterior chamber to escape, cannot be less than 33 minutes, and may be as much as 80 minutes. In any case the rate of flow is very slow indeed. The knowledge of this fact is obviously of great importance if we would comprehend aright the significance of Koster's figures. A quantity of 45 c.mm. sounds very little, but it is equal to something between $\frac{1}{5}$ and $\frac{1}{9}$ of the total contents of the aqueous chamber. Moreover it represents a quantity of fluid which is said to take from $6\frac{1}{2}$ to 9 minutes to escape from the chambers of the eye. Looked at in this light it can no longer be brushed aside as *une quantité négligeable*. In the same connection must be mentioned Affleck Greeves' observations on pigs' eyes. The principal interest of his communication lies in the fact that the increases in volume observed corresponded closely with the increases in the intra-ocular pressure, thus agreeing with Koster's observations on the human eye.

(*k*) It is of interest to turn from these physiological measurements of very limited stretching of the eyeball to those instances of very extensive stretching of the globe which we meet with constantly in our practice. Many ophthalmologists (including Ischreyt, Levinsohn, and Sattler) think that there is in some cases, at least, a connection between high intra-ocular pressure and the stretching met with in myopic globes. The author is strongly inclined to believe that there is much more in this view than has hitherto been generally recognised. In buphthalmos the overstretching of the globe is still more marked, and here the assumption that it is preceded by a pathological change in the tunic of the eye itself is still more doubtfully accepted. It may be contended that the large globes met with in myopia, megalo-cornea, and buphthalmos, are all developed in the young eye. Their very existence, none the less, remains as a protest against the statement that the tunic of the eye is rigid.

Before proceeding any farther, it is convenient to pause here to sum up our conclusions :

(1) The teachings of physics, physiology, pathology, clinical experience, and surgery seem all to be in agreement on the subjects we have been discussing.

(2) The eye is *not* a closed sphere, since there is a constant flow of fluid through its chambers. This fluid passes into it from without, and again leaves it in due course. Arguments founded on the assumption that the eye is a closed sphere, must be received with the gravest doubt; for, since the premises are incorrect, the deductions therefrom are not likely to be reliable.

(3) The tunic of the eye is *not* rigid. On the contrary it is very susceptible to the influence of forces acting either from within or from without, and readily changes its form thereunder. Moreover, it is both elastic and distensible. The degree of elasticity and that of distensibility may be small, but these properties are distinctly present, and their existence cannot be disregarded without the introduction of serious fallacies into the argument.

(4) The contents of the eye, so far from being fixed, are continually varying in volume, both in health and disease. These variations determine (*a*) the measure of distension of the ocular tunic, (*b*) the tension of the eyeball (as measured digitally or by means of tonometers), and (*c*) the intra-ocular pressure. The factors which determine the rise and fall in the volume of the intra-ocular contents will be discussed later in this chapter. They are somewhat complicated, and include not only those which help to strike the balance between the secretion (the term is used without prejudice) and the excretion of the intra-ocular fluid, but those also which decide the volume of blood present in the different sections (arterial, capillary, and venous) of the intra-ocular vascular system.

REFERENCES

ADAMÜK, *C. f. d. Med. Wiss.*, 1866; *Ann. d'ocul.*, 1867, vol. lviii.
CARPENTER, J. T.—*Penn. Med. Journ.*, vol. xvii. p. 264, and *Ophth. Year Book*, vol. xi. p. 201.
GREEVES, A.—*Proc. Roy. Soc. Med.*, Feb. 5, 1913.
GRÜNHAGEN.—*Berl. Klin. Woch.*, 1866.

HENDERSON, E. E. AND STARLING, E. H.—*Journ. of Physiology*, vol. xxxi.
KOSTER, G.—*Archiv f. O.*, vol. xli. p. 2, and Parsons' *Pathology of the Eye*, vol. iii. p. 1042.
LEDERER, R.—*Arch. f. Augenheilk.*, vol. lxxii. p. 1, and *Ophth. Year Book*, 1912, vol. ix. p. 193.
MAGITOT, A.—*Ann. d'ocul.*, vol. cliv. pp. 211, 272, 334, 385; *Amer. Journ. Ophth.*, vol. i. p. 587; *Brit. Journ. Ophth.*, vol. ii. p. 93.
PARSONS, J. H.—*The Pathology of the Eye*, vol. iii. p. 1056.
SCHOENBERG, M. J.—*Journ. Amer. Med. Assoc.*, vol. lxi. p. 1098; *Arch. Ophth.*, vol. xlii. p. 117; *Ophth. Year Book*, vol. x. p. 170.
STARLING, E. H.—*Proc. Roy. Soc. Med.*, 1913, vol. vi. No. 3.
VON HIPPEL, E.—Parsons' *Pathology of the Eye*, vol. iii. p. 1056.

PART II

On the Bearing on Intra-ocular Pressure of the Continuous Flow of Fluid through the Chambers of the Eye

There is a statement which has been so often repeated unchallenged, that it is in danger of being accepted without due examination, viz., that the pressure in the aqueous and vitreous chambers is the same throughout. Let us first examine certain beliefs, which, in spite of the fact that they have recently been vigorously attacked (Magitot, Roemer) are still widely, if not almost universally, accepted by ophthalmologists. The fluid which fills both chambers of the eye is secreted or transfused from the ciliary body; we need not now enter into the question whether this is a true secretion or a transfusion, as it does not affect the point at issue. This fluid again passes out of the chambers of the eye and back into the blood vessels in the neighbourhood of the angle of the anterior chamber, and (probably in a lesser degree) through the crypts of the iris. Whether the escape of the fluid is due to the pull of osmosis, to the push of pressure, or to a pump-action, is immaterial to our present argument. So far we are on ground which most ophthalmologists will hold to be indisputable. The very fact that there is a flow argues that there is a difference in pressure, which is at its maximum in a comparison of the area of secretion (using the term without prejudice) with that of excretion. In other words, the highest pressure must obviously be at the area of secretion, and the lowest at that of excretion, whilst between the two there is a gradual fall. The difference is so slight that no instrument yet devised has been able to detect or to measure it. Nevertheless, the first principles of hydrodynamics assure us of its existence. If a simile might be permitted, it would be that of a man standing at the edge of one of our large reservoirs, into which water enters at the sides, and from which it leaves by one or more funnel-opening surface pipes near the centre. To the careless spectator there is a sheet of what appears to be still water; but a closer observation will satisfy him that the fluid is entering the tank at the sides, and leaving it at the centre. A slight movement of the water at the centre and sides assures him of this, and he therefore knows that there must be a difference of level between the two; the centre must be a little lower than the sides, and yet apart from the movement of floating objects, he might find it impossible either to demonstrate or to prove this in such a way, as to satisfy one who did not share his knowledge of the laws of moving water. How much more difficult would it be to take points between the two extremes and to demonstrate the difference of level between them, and yet it exists along every inch of the whole stretch of water! To apply the simile, the difficulty—nay, the impossibility—of demonstrating a difference of level between the different parts of the interior of the eye does not for a moment weaken our absolute confidence that such a difference exists. We have to remember that the teaching of the most reliable investigations would appear to be that only about 5 c.mm. of aqueous leave the eye in a minute, and that it probably takes about 48 minutes to excrete the small amount of fluid found at any one moment in the anterior chamber; indeed, it is quite likely that even these low estimates may be well in excess of the actual facts. We can thus easily realise how extremely slow the flow of the nutrient fluid of the eye must be, and how little chance we have of being able to measure it by so crude a method as a manometric estimation of the pressure in the chambers of the eye. None the less we believe that fluid is poured out from the ciliary body into the anterior portion of the vitreous chamber, and into the periphery of the posterior division of the aqueous chamber, and that it then makes its way, owing to a slight difference of level, through the pupil to the angle of the anterior chamber, from whence it effects its escape. That the current may be immeasurably slow does not affect the argument one jot; there *is* a difference of pressure and there *is* a current, and the direction of the latter is as already indicated.

Nor is this all the evidence at our disposal. We can first learn a valuable lesson from the cases of ring synechia with *iris bombé*. The bellying forward of the iris is very clear evidence that the pressure behind it is greater than that in front. Probably the difference in pressure between the area of secretion and that of excretion, which we referred to above, is here slightly exaggerated by the damming back of the fluid at the pupil, though it must be very doubtful if a manometer experiment could show it even in this case. If now we perform an iridectomy, or even an iridotomy, however small, we find that the bulging of the iris ceases, and the membrane lies flat. We have here an experiment, planned for us on a scale far more delicate than any we could devise, to show conclusively that the intra-ocular pressure is not uniform throughout the chambers of the eye. So far from it being safe to assume that the pressure in the aqueous and vitreous chambers is the same, we see clearly from this clinical observation that the pressure is not the same throughout the extent of even one chamber alone. We can learn yet another lesson of the same nature from this little surgical experiment, for no sooner do we establish a free communication between the reservoirs of fluid which lie in front of and behind the iris, than the tension of the globe shows a marked and permanent fall. It is obvious that the aqueous, dammed back behind the iris, has now been allowed to find its normal outlet, presumably at the angle of the anterior chamber—yet another argument in favour of the view of an onward flow of the fluid contents of the eye.

The suggestion may be put forward that we are dealing here with a pathological condition, inasmuch as the closure of the pupil shuts the fluid in the posterior chamber off from access to the anterior chamber. It might conceivably be urged that from the moment we open up a channel between these two chambers by iridectomy or by iridotomy, all evidence of a difference in pressure at once ceases. Such an argument cannot, however, be advanced, even for a moment, in explanation of Ulbrich's valuable observations on a case, in which nature had provided a living manometer, which showed any differences in pressure between the two divisions of the aqueous chamber. In the inner lower quadrant of the iris there was a partial coloboma, closed by a delicate membrane, which could be seen to bulge forward into the anterior chamber, and backward into the posterior chamber at irregular intervals. A close study of these movements revealed that they represented the passage of fluid forward from the posterior to the anterior chamber through the pupil. So slight were the differences of pressure involved, that this flow was not continuous. After each escape forward of a gush of fluid a variable time was seen to elapse, before the pressure rose high enough to force even so slender a barrier as was imposed by the contact of the iris margin with the lens capsule. Nevertheless the lesson is plain for all to read, that even in conditions of health there are differences in pressure between the two divisions of the aqueous chamber, and that these differences in pressure have a most important bearing, both on the rate and on the direction of the flow of fluid in the eye. Inasmuch as the fluid from the vitreous chamber must presumably pass through the posterior chamber to reach the anterior, it is obvious that the pressure stands at the highest level in the vitreous chamber, and at the lowest in the anterior chamber, the posterior being intermediate between the two. This is self-evident, for otherwise no flow could take place.

The possibility that the fluid in the vitreous chamber may have its source in osmotic action, does not appear to affect the proposition. If an excessive amount passes into that chamber, be the method of its passage what it may, the pressure within the cavity will rise relatively to that in the posterior chamber, and *vice versa*. The important fact is, that so long as there is a flow from the vitreous cavity through the posterior into the anterior chamber, we have no alternative but to assume that it is following in its course *a line of descending pressure*.

Many years ago, the author saw in Madras a case similar to Ulbrich's. In this the living manometer was furnished by an atrophic patch in the iris, the result of an old inflammation. The bulging of this patch under pressure of fluid from behind and its subsidence at intervals could be easily watched.

Before leaving this subject, we may recall the evidence afforded by the varying depths of the anterior chamber in certain pathological conditions. Treacher Collins has pointed out that such variations are indications of differences in pressure between the aqueous and vitreous cavities, and has illustrated his point by reference on the one hand to the shallow anterior chamber of glaucoma, as representing an increased pressure within the vitreous cavity, and on the other hand to the deep anterior chambers found in hypotonic eyes, as affording an evidence of an increase in the pressure in the aqueous chamber relatively to that in the vitreous chamber. Later, Collins has carried these observations a stage farther, and has shown that, under experimental conditions, differences in pressure may occur in different parts of the same eye during life. He had a number of rabbits trephined by Colonel Kirkpatrick, some in front of the ciliary body and some behind it ; later, at varying periods, the animals were killed and the globes prepared and sectioned. In every case hypotony was produced, and as a consequence there was an effusion of serum into the chambers of the eye. The important point was that the extent of this effusion varied in different parts of the eyes according to whether the anterior or posterior chamber had been opened. It therefore appeared to be a fair deduction that not merely had the general intra-ocular pressure been reduced throughout the eye, but further that the amount of lowering had varied locally within the globe, and this too during life.

These considerations lead us by natural steps to a short study of some further work on the subject, which, though frankly pathological, has, nevertheless, a strong bearing on the elucidation of the physiological problems before us.

The Changes in Chamber Pressure which attend Some Forms of Glaucoma

Priestley Smith has established experimentally the fact that the same sequence of events (viz., pushing forward of the diaphragm of the eye, shallowing of the chamber, and obstruction of the angle of excretion), with which we are familiar in acute glaucomatous attacks, will follow if we raise the pressure in the vitreous chamber above that which is present in the aqueous chamber. It may be said that the differences in pressures with which he worked were probably in excess of those which exist in the eye, though in the necessary absence of manometric observations of glaucomatous eyes, we cannot certainly affirm that this is so. The important point is that we know from these experiments what will happen, if the pressure in the vitreous chamber rises above that in the aqueous chamber, and we also know that such a difference in the two pressures can be established, by artificial means at least.

If the above premises are conceded, and it is difficult to understand how they can be disputed, we may pass on to a practical application of the knowledge so gained. In glaucoma, especially if acute, we meet with a shallowing of the anterior chamber, which is evidently due to a pushing forward of the diaphragm of the eye. The obvious explanation would appear to be that there has been an accumulation of fluid in the vitreous, as compared with that in the aqueous chamber. There is strong clinical evidence in support of this interpretation of the phenomenon, for the performance of an iridectomy in a case of acute glaucoma can be made both safer and more easy by the performance of a preliminary sclerotomy. In this operation, a knife is passed through the sclera into the posterior chamber of the eye, and is then rotated in such a way as to allow of the escape under the conjunctiva of some of the imprisoned fluid. If we are content to wait for ten to fifteen minutes, we find that the tension of the globe falls, and the anterior chamber deepens ; at the same time we observe that fluid passes out from the eye through the puncture and accumulates under the conjunctiva. The explanation which naturally suggests itself, and which is of course by no means new, is that the release of fluid from the vitreous chamber has in some way reopened the usual channels of communication between the vitreous and aqueous chambers, and possibly has at the same time opened up the channels of excretion of fluid from the eye. It would appear that the normal condition, in which the difference in pressure between the anterior and posterior divisions of the eye is present but immeasurably small, has been again restored in the place of the abnormal state which was represented by an overfilling of the vitreous as compared with the aqueous chamber.

Whilst on this subject, we may with profit consider the bearings of another and an allied clinical observation : Those who do many trephine operations are familiar with the fact that at the close of the procedure, the eye, which has softened with the escape of the aqueous fluid, sometimes shows a sudden and rapid hardening, due to the effusion of fluid, presumably from the choroidal vessels, into its interior ; at the same time, the anterior chamber becomes so shallow as to be practically non-existent, clearly showing that the effusion lies behind the diaphragm of the eye. If the patient be kept quiet in bed, the time will come, in the majority of cases, when the tension will fall, and this fall will be both rapid and marked as soon as the anterior chamber becomes converted from a potential into an actual cavity, in other words, as soon as the angle of the chamber opens sufficiently to permit the trephine hole to take on the function for which it is intended, viz., that of draining away the excess fluid accumulated within the eye.

We start then with the clinical observations (1) that the first incident in the development of an acute glaucoma is most frequently a distension of the vitreous chamber at the expense of the aqueous chamber, and (2) that the *status quo* can often be restored by letting out a few drops of fluid from the overloaded vitreous reservoir. It is much more difficult to carry the matter a stage farther on, in the attempt to find a solution to the questions : How is this distension brought about ? and how does the tapping of the posterior chamber of the eye produce the effect we have under consideration ? It is necessary to seek a solution of these problems. Before doing so, however, it is desirable to remind ourselves of certain elementary physiological facts. The secretion (using the term without prejudice) poured out by the ciliary body is believed to find its way by two main routes, viz., (1) more or less forward into the posterior division of the aqueous chamber, and (2) backward into the vitreous body. Collins' recent work on hypotony, already referred to, has shed an interesting confirmatory light on this hypothesis. It is presumed that the fluid from the latter of these two streams eventually finds its way forward through the suspensory ligament to join the anterior stream in the posterior division of the aqueous chamber, from whence the united volume of fluid is directed forward through the pupil, on its way to the angle of the anterior chamber, and to the crypts of the iris. As has already been intimated, another possibility is that the fluid in the vitreous body is changed by diffusion between it and that in the posterior chamber. It is also conceivable that alterations in the osmotic properties of the vitreous body may strongly influence the rate and direction of this diffusion, and consequently the relative pressures in the vitreous and aqueous chambers. In any case the fluid, in its passage forwards from the vitreous body, must traverse what we may call "the straits " of the perilental space. Priestley Smith has shown how these straits may be closed to its passage by the growth in bulk of the lens on the one shore, and by the swelling of the ciliary body on the other. When this closure is effected, the fluid continuity of the vitreous and aqueous chambers is interrupted, and a relatively impervious diaphragm is then stretched across between the two reservoirs of fluid. Assuming that his data are correct, it requires little imagination to see what will follow. He has elaborated the argument (in his book on *Glaucoma*, p. 130), and has there cited other possible factors in the production of the obstruction to the flow of fluid. If we can accept his views, we find a ready and simple solution of our problem. Even if we do not accept them, other ways in which the circumlental straits can be blocked readily suggest themselves. The obstruction may possibly be brought about by a change in the degree of permeability to fluid of the superficial layers of the vitreous body, of the hyaloid membrane, or of the suspensory ligament. Also, there are, as we have suggested above, those who think that an altered constitution of the fluid which finds its way into the vitreous body under glaucoma conditions, may lead to a change in the osmotic power of the vitreous, and so to a swelling of this jelly-like structure. The objection has been raised that on the first principles of hydrostatics, it is not possible to have a difference in pressure in different parts of the fluid mass in a closed cavity. Once again, the answer is both obvious and simple, viz., that it is not a question of hydrostatics in a closed chamber, since we are dealing with a mass of moving fluid. It is a question of hydrodynamics. This is the key to the mystery, or to what has very unnecessarily been made a mystery. The difference in pressure between the fluid at its areas of secretion, and of excretion, premises a movement of the fluid mass. Anything which stands in the way of that movement, as the closure of the perilental straits would do, will exaggerate the difference of pressure between the fluid in the vitreous body and that in the chamber. Any step which will lower the pressure in the vitreous chamber, and thereby lessen ciliary congestion, will pave the way for a reopening of the normal channels of communication between the two chambers. We repeat once again that sight has too often been lost of the fact that our problem is one of hydrodynamics and not one of hydrostatics. We are not dealing with a closed chamber, but with one through which fluid is passing continuously, even if very slowly. This cardinal fact modifies all our conceptions on the subject. To lose sight of it is to miss the crux of the whole question.

In closing this subject, it is of interest to refer to a recent paper by Parker, who has developed the same thesis in an endeavour to establish the existence of two types of glaucoma upon the assumption that either the anterior or the posterior lymph system is the more seriously involved. He holds that, when the lens and iris are in their normal position, the indications are that the obstruction is to the outflow along the anterior system, the fluid moving towards the posterior outlet only. On the other hand, when the lens and iris are displaced forward, and a shallow chamber results, he thinks that the probability is that the posterior system is blocked, and that the flow is forward towards the anterior chamber.

The Source and Method of Production of the Intra-ocular Fluid

The intra-ocular fluid is derived from the blood. Apart from its nutrient and dioptric functions, it plays an important rôle in maintaining the normal pressure of the eye, and thereby keeping the tunic of the globe in a suitable condition of distension. It is the generally accepted belief that this fluid is poured out from the ciliary body, but there is considerable difference of opinion as to whether it is a filtration or a true secretion. Closely connected with this question is that of the exact part of the ciliary body which produces the fluid.

Experimental research has shown a close relationship between the amount of intra-ocular fluid secreted, and the difference recorded at the same time, between the systemic blood-pressure and the intra-ocular pressure ; and this has been taken to indicate that the process is to be regarded as one of filtration, and not one of secretion. It has further been contended that, inasmuch as the intra-ocular fluid is practically free of proteins, the pressure required for the purpose must be one of at least 30 mm. of Hg., *i.e.*, the difference between the intra-ocular capillary pressure and that of the intra-ocular fluid must be one of at least 30 mm. of Hg. The advocates of the filtration theory were wont to maintain that there was no difficulty in the way of supposing that such a difference of pressure can and does exist within the eye. To this supposition the secretionists demurred, believing that the pressure in the intra-ocular capillaries is lower than has been assumed (*Proc. Roy. Soc. Med.*, Sec. on Ophth., February, 1914). Unfortunately there is no known method of accurately estimating this capillary pressure. This subject has recently come in for a good deal of study. Priestley Smith's estimate was based on admittedly approximate calculations, which were to some extent vitiated by uncertainties in the data employed. He took the pressure in the retinal artery, at its point of entrance, to lie between 90 and 100 mm. Hg., and the exit pressure in the central vein to be on an average not less than 25 mm. Hg. He reckoned that the fall in pressure in the two halves of the circuit could be determined from the relative cross-sectional areas of the arteries and veins. Working from this point of view, and with certain reservations, he concluded "that in a healthy eye, with a chamber pressure of 24 mm. Hg., the pressure in the retinal capillaries is probably not far removed from 40 mm. Hg."

Bailliart, working with his ophthalmo-dynamometer (Fig. 111), has, in his latest communications, placed the systolic and diastolic arterial pressures in the retinal artery at 70 and 30 mm. Hg. respectively. He argues that *the capillary pressure must be lower than the diastolic arterial pressure, as otherwise the retinal circulation could only be carried on during a part of the cardiac cycle.* It must therefore be lower than 30 mm. Hg., and higher, or at least not lower than 20 mm. Hg., the latter being the figure he has fixed on as approximately representing the normal intra-ocular pressure. From these data, he would argue the probable capillary pressure as about 25 mm. Hg.

Magitot, who has worked with Bailliart, offered two years earlier a different set of figures. He placed the retinal arterial pressure at 70 mm. Hg., the venous at 40 mm. Hg., and the ocular pressure at 25 mm. Hg.

The difficulties of the subject will be still better appreciated from the fact that Duverger and Barré, who worked with Bailliart's instrument, put the systolic retinal arterial pressure at 100 mm. Hg., and the diastolic at from 50 to 60 mm. Hg. We cannot review all these figures without feeling that we have still much to learn, and that we shall do well to take to heart Rochon-Duvigneaud's advice to let our theory-building wait on the further advance of our knowledge. How sound this is must be obvious to anyone who has read the very recent controversy on the height of the intra-ocular pressure. Into the details of that controversy it would be superfluous to enter, but the outstanding facts are that Schiötz gives the limits of normal intra-ocular pressure at between 15 and 25 mm. Hg., whilst McLean puts the lower limit at 22 and the upper at 40 mm. Hg. When two of the ablest and most experienced workers on the subject differ so markedly on so fundamental a point, it would be obviously unwise to attempt to dogmatise on the further issues that hang upon it.

Not the least important of the recent contributions to the subject is Bailliart's suggestion that our estimate of the capillary pressure in the retina must be based on that of the diastolic, and not on that of the systolic arterial pressure.

It is pertinent to mention here a further objection which has been raised to the filtration theory, viz., that the anatomical conditions demanded for the presumed filtration of the fluid do not exist, and that, presupposing that the fluid were expressed as suggested through the capillaries of the ciliary processes, it would find itself, not in the chambers of the eye, but in the connective tissue spaces of the ciliary body, the easiest method of escape from which would be *not* through the lining epithelium of the ciliary body, but towards the angle of the anterior chamber. The reply to this has been that it is not possible to argue a physiological problem on the basis of anatomical observations alone, and that such data require the support of experimental work before they can be accepted.

The important fact to bear in mind would seem to be that, other things being equal, the production of the intra-ocular fluid varies directly with the height of the blood-pressure in the vessels of the eye. From this it would appear that we must either look on it as a filtration under pressure, or else assume that the secretory cells are sensitive either to the variations in local blood-pressure, or to the volume of tissue fluid transuded into the spaces of the ciliary processes.

Those in favour of the filtration theory would locate the seat of production of the intra-ocular fluid at the ciliary processes ; whilst those who think there is a true secretion, believe that the *pars plana* of the ciliary body takes no small share in the work. They point to the existence of the glands described by Treacher Collins, and to the morbid exudation which can be traced from the neighbourhood of the *pars plana* into the vitreous under certain conditions, as showing that this part of the body is capable of active secretion. Moreover, the ciliary processes are covered by a well-marked columnar or cubical epithelium, the cells of which are as well formed as are those of the salivary glands or of other secreting structures. They urge that there is therefore no *a priori* reason to dispute the possibility of the intra-ocular fluid being looked on as a true secretion. It has been further suggested that part of this secretion takes place forwards from the anterior portion of the ciliary body into the aqueous chamber, and part backwards from the posterior portion of the body into the vitreous.

Others, however, take the view that the ciliary body does not resemble a true gland in its general anatomical features, and that the tubular depressions of the *pars plana* bear only a superficial resemblance to true tubular glands as these are met with elsewhere.

If the fluid transuded from the ciliary body contains albuminous matter, as it does in certain pathological conditions, the lining layer of epithelium strips off in large bullæ. Treacher Collins has pointed this out as clear evidence that the cells which compose it cannot be looked on as constituting an inert membrane, since in thus stopping the passage of albuminous matter they show that they have some selective power.

One of the most recent, and at the same time one of the most ardent, advocates of the secretion theory is Seidel, who has studied the influence of muscarin, eserin, and pilocarpine—both locally applied and injected into the blood-stream—on secretion and absorption in the body generally and in the eye in particular. The action of these drugs can be inhibited by atropin. His experiments lead Seidel to believe that there is in the eye a specific organ of secretion, and that the pouring out of the intra-ocular fluid is not the result of a passive physical process, but of the active co-operation of living cells. He mentions a number of histological peculiarities, which are found in the epithelial cells of the ciliary region, and which differentiate them from other cells; he considers that these peculiarities are the anatomic expression of the physiological differentiation to which they owe their special secretory power.

There would seem to be a tendency to arrive at a happy compromise, and whilst insisting that filtration under pressure plays an important rôle, to admit that the fluid thus poured out in the neighbourhood of the lining membrane of the ciliary body, may be actively passed through by the epithelial cells to the surface of the membrane. If this theory ultimately finds favour, the production of the intra-ocular fluid will have to be regarded as a combination of pressure-filtration and of secretion. In the present state of our knowledge, it would be most unwise to dogmatise, since the data available are insufficient. We must therefore be content to await the progress of further research, and we can do so with the greater equanimity, since the interest of the question is largely an academic one, as will be understood from the following considerations. If we look on the process as one of filtration, requiring a high capillary blood-pressure, we must remember that work is done in this filtration ; to get the fluid through requires that work should be done, and by the time the fluid has passed through it has lost some of the energy with which it started its journey ; it has fallen in fact to, or nearly to, the level of the intra-ocular pressure. On the other hand, if the fluid is a true secretion, that secretion is an active vital process ; the cells actually do work, and there is therefore no loss of energy involved ; for that matter the pressure of the fluid secreted might easily rise above that of the intra-ocular pressure. The assumption, on the part of the secretionists, that the initial pressure in the capillary vessels is low, is of course not inconsistent with their view that the normal tension of the eye may be maintained by the process of secretion. It is even possible that a tension far above the normal might be produced by the same agency.

To summarise our conclusions :

(1) It is essential to bear in mind, that in dealing with the physical conditions governing the behaviour of the intra-ocular fluid, as it passes into and out of the eye, we have to do with a body of *moving water*, and that the laws to which we must appeal are those of hydrodynamics, and not those of hydrostatics.

(2) There are distinct, though slight, differences of pressure at various points in the mass of fluid within the eye, the highest pressure probably lying at the area of production of the fluid, and the lowest, certainly, at that where it is excreted.

(3) The above conclusions are borne out by the teachings both of physiology and of pathology.

(4) The question whether the intra-ocular fluid is poured out by an act of secretion, or by a process of pressure filtration, is still *sub judice*. Possibly the action is a

INTRA-OCULAR PRESSURE AND TENSION 55

combined one, pressure and secretory activity each taking a part therein. Fortunately, the interest involved is academic, rather than practical.

Magitot's Views

The paragraphs, that have so far constituted this Part II., stand much as they appeared in the first edition of this work, despite the fact that a new element has been introduced into the case by the very interesting work of Hamburger, Magitot, and others. A résumé of that work will now be given. Magitot is an iconoclast, whose object is to upset all our preconceived ideas on the subject now under discussion, and to induce us to reconsider the very foundations of our belief. It may be asked why the whole chapter has not been rewritten, with the interpolation of this new work and with an endeavour to consider it side by side with the older theories. The answer, the apology if you will, is that, after very careful consideration, the task has seemed to the author to be one of too great difficulty in the present stage of our knowledge. He is bound to confess that while Magitot's work has interested him most deeply, and has opened up important avenues of thought and speculation, he is very far from being able to accept it in its entirety. At the same time, he has found the greatest difficulty in forming an opinion as to how much of it should be accepted and how much rejected. Every radical departure from beliefs which we have long cherished is apt to provoke our opposition, and the history of all the great advances in medical science has been punctuated with incidents which we should be glad now to forget, and which might always have been avoided had the leaders of scientific thought been ever heedful of the advice Gamaliel tendered to the Council at Jerusalem, advice which he coupled with the warning, which for our present purpose may be more pointedly rendered by the alteration of a single word, "Lest haply ye be found even to fight against truth." With this in his mind, the author will endeavour to summarise Magitot's conclusions, striving to do so as fairly and impartially as possible. He would, however, advise any who are personally interested in the subject to study the French originals, or failing that, the excellent résumés to which references are given at the end of this Part.

Magitot's researches have led him to look upon the eyeball as a closed space, which has an internal pressure of 25 mm. Hg., and which is traversed by arteries with a pressure of 70 mm. Hg. and by veins with a pressure of 40 mm. Hg. He believes that the aqueous humour is of the same nature as the cerebro-spinal fluid and the perilymph of the ear, and therefore quite different from the lymph of the eye with which it neither mixes nor comes into direct contact. He points out that the eye possesses independent lymphatic channels for its anterior and posterior segments, and that these are represented, like those of the encephalic centres, by the perivascular sheaths. He maintains that the aqueous humour is secreted at the beginning of life by special neuroglial cells, and that the quantity necessary to replace that which is absorbed, is obtained by a process of dialysis from other glial cells. He denies *in toto* its origin from the ciliary body. He points out that it contains very little albumin and a high percentage of sodium chloride, while serum and lymph contain much albumin and less salt. He regards the high percentage of salt as a proof of the dialysis of the fluid. The aqueous, he says, has a triple rôle, (i.) optic and static, (ii.) nerve-protecting, and (iii.) lens-conserving.

He lays great stress on the rôle of the choroidal tunic in influencing intra-ocular pressure, and pertinently points out that this tunic is really about four times as thick as post-mortem sections show it to be; the erroneous appearance presented is due to the collapse of the choroidal vessels after death. He maintains that the real purpose of this vascular reservoir, with its free arterial supply, is the maintenance of the normal tonus of the eye. He considers that the blood supplied through it is controlled by centres of three kinds—(1) bulbar, (2) thoracic or cervico-cephalic, and (3) peripheral. The last-named are situated in the choroid itself, and consist of a rich plexus of nerve cells. It is these which control the local variations of the blood supply to the interior of the eye. He does not believe in the perpetual secretion of the aqueous humour or in its escape at the angle of filtration, and he attacks with a truly catholic zeal all the accepted beliefs dear to ophthalmologists. We may, for the moment, anticipate what we have to say later on this subject, so far as to state, that those who have worked with Bailliart's instrument have failed to find evidence to justify this hypothesis of the existence of local centres for the regulation of intra-ocular pressure.

It would be impossible to follow Magitot here through the many phases of his argument. He insists on the whole subject being dealt with as a question of normal physiology, and takes exception to the important rôle which pathology and therapeutics have played in our conceptions of the subject. The author would, however, point out that the course which Magitot thus criticises, and which our predecessors have consistently followed, is justified by the rarity with which experiments can be performed on the living eyes of man. In the previous pages some of the very important pathologic evidence has been reviewed, and it would seem rash indeed to forsake teachings so pregnant with guidance as these have proved to be.

That the great choroidal reservoir, with or without the system of nervous control which Magitot believes it to possess, may exercise a powerful influence on intra-ocular pressure, and especially on its variations from time to time, almost goes without saying. It would, however, seem probable that the object of all this mechanism is rather to prevent variations in intra-ocular pressure than to produce them. It seems easier to conceive of it as a regulating mechanism of the pressure conditions within the eye, than as the cause of those conditions. It is obvious that this mechanism will be at its best when the eye is young and healthy. If the author rightly understands Magitot, the glaucomatous rise in pressure should, according to him, be ascribed to vascular changes in the choroidal reservoir. It is easy to see how grief, fear, exhaustion, and other nervous influences might modify the pressure within the eye through this reservoir, but is there not another factor at work ? For answer, let us take the hardest globes we know—those with long-standing glaucoma, and showing a pressure of 80 mm. Hg. and more—and consider for a moment the physical conditions present. The uveal tract is thinned in all its parts, until it often has become a skeleton of its former self. Can it then be the source of the pressure ? Certainly not ! On the other hand, the absolute obstruction to the escape of fluid, whether at the closed angle, or through the atrophied iris, furnishes a ready explanation of the high pressure produced, even in the presence of a greatly diminished secretion of intra-ocular fluid.

Once again be it said that Magitot's writings are of sufficient interest to command the respectful study of all who are attracted by this subject, but that, in many respects, they fail to carry conviction to the author's mind. He would, however, be far from wishing to prejudice others in the matter, and would again commend these very interesting papers to every student of the causes of variations in intra-ocular pressure.

REFERENCES

BAILLIART, P.—*Ann. d'ocul.*, Nov. 1919, vol. clvi. pp. 694–695.
COLLINS, E. T.—*Proc. O.S. of U.K.*, 1917 ; *ibid.* 1918.
DUVERGER AND BARRÉ.—*Ann. d'ocul.*, 1919, vol. clvi. p. 704.
GALLAVARDIN.—Quoted by Bailliart.
HAMBURGER, C.—*Ann. d'ocul.*, 1919, vol. clvi. p. 695 ; *The Nutrition of the Eye*, 1914 ; and *Klin. Monatsbl. f. Augenheilk.*, 1920, vol. lxv.
MAGITOT, A.—*Ann. d'ocul.*, 1917, vol. cliv. pp. 211, 272, 334, and 385 ; *Amer. Journ. Ophth.*, vol. i. p. 587 ; *Brit. Journ. Ophth.*, vol. ii. pp. 53 and 93.
PARKER, W. R.—*Amer. Journ. Ophth.*, vol. i. p. 628 ; *New York Med. Journ.*, vol. cviii. p. 91 ; *Ophth. Year Book*, vol. xv.
ROCHON-DUVIGNEAUD.—*Ann. d'ocul.*, 1919, vol. clvi. p. 705.
ROEMER, P.—*Textbook of Ophth.* Urban & Schwarzenberg, Berlin und Wien, 1919.

SMITH, P.—*The Pathology and Treatment of Glaucoma.* J. & A. Churchill, London, 1891.
SEIDEL.—*Klin. Monatsbl. f. Augenheilk.*, vol. lxi. p. 330; *Brit. Journ. Ophth.*, 1918, vol. ii. pp. 257–272.
ULBEICH.—*Bericht der Ophth. Gesell. zu Heidelberg*, 1907.

PART III

The Relationship of Systemic Blood-Pressure to Intra-ocular Pressure

The consensus of opinion would appear to be that experimental investigation has established the existence of a distinct relationship, under ordinary conditions, between the systemic blood-pressure and the intra-ocular pressure. Speaking in general terms, the two may be said to rise and fall together. It would, however, be a very great mistake to suppose that the intra-ocular pressure servilely follows the vagaries of the general blood-pressure; nor would anyone, who understands the elements of the physiology of the subject, expect such a sequence of events. It is the more necessary to draw attention to this point, since it at times appears to have been lost sight of. From some of the communications which have appeared, one would almost gather that a rise in general systemic pressure must logically be followed by a corresponding rise in intra-ocular pressure. This we know is not the case. It seems necessary, under the circumstances, to remind ourselves of certain elementary facts which will be admitted by most ophthalmologists.

(1) In studying the arterial pressure in any organ, we must take account, not merely of the state of the arterioles in that organ, but also of that of the arterioles in other and distant areas, *e.g.*, a dilatation of the arterioles of the eye might, if associated with a heavy fall of pressure in the splanchnic area, be accompanied not by a rise, but actually by a fall in intra-ocular pressure.

(2) The capillary pressure, which after all is the pressure which most concerns our argument, is much more influ-

enced by changes in the venous than in the arterial pressure, be the organ what it may ; for the ever-varying peripheral resistance of the arterioles has to be reckoned with in the latter case ; whereas no corresponding barrier exists between the capillaries and the veins. How true this is may, perhaps, be best judged by a consideration of the work done by Duverger and Barré, and by Velter. This will be dealt with at greater length in the next section. All that we need say at present is that these observers found a remarkable want of correspondence between the variations in the arterial blood-pressure within the eye, and those of the intra-ocular fluid-pressure.

(3) The number of influences at work in affecting the blood-pressure is not only very large, but those influences may be very complicated, especially in the sense that they may act selectively on certain organs, altering the *status quo* in them out of all proportion to their action on other parts.

In the light of these principles, it is comparatively easy to understand what otherwise might appear to be contradictions. Take for instance the statements made by Casolino with regard to his work on the behaviour of the ocular pressure under the influence of various drugs which modify the arterial systemic pressure : The inhalation of nitrite of amyl caused only slight lowering of the arterial pressure, and very marked lowering of the intra-ocular pressure. The first effect of adrenalin was to raise both the arterial and intra-ocular pressures, whilst later the latter fell again. Strophanthus caused a rise in arterial and a fall in intra-ocular pressure ; and so on. Again Rollet and Curtil found that the instillation of adrenalin, especially in inflamed eyes, produced a marked fall of intra-ocular pressure ; this is hardly surprising, for the local vaso-constriction produced, must sensibly diminish the volume of blood present in the eye, and therefore *ipso facto* the total fluid contents of the organ. First Wessely and later Roemer and Kochmann found an actual rise in intra-ocular pressure, coincident with the sinking of the systemic blood-pressure, under the influence of nitrite of amyl. The leading lesson, which such experiments with drugs seems to teach, is that the relationship of intra-ocular pressure to blood-pressure is a very complicated one, and only to be understood by a most careful study of all the factors which enter into the problem.

Next we may take up the influence of advancing age on intra-ocular pressure, and contrary to what might have been expected, we learn that it is apparently negligible. In spite of the fact that the systemic pressure rises in most individuals as life advances, the tension of the eye would appear to show no corresponding alteration. This was first found by Langenhan and Engelmann, and was later confirmed both by Craggs and Taylor, and by Toczyski. Magitot went a step farther, when he recorded his observation that, on the average, the intra-ocular pressure is lower in the elderly than it is in the very young. Still more recently, McLean has written as follows: "The normal young adults I tested—those not above twenty-five years of age—frequently presented intra-ocular pressures of between 35 and 40 mm. Hg.; whilst those of more advanced years—those above sixty—frequently gave readings below 30 mm. Hg. of intra-ocular pressure." Vaughan's evidence is equally practical: He followed 20 cases of glaucoma for a period of two years, and was unable to find evidence that variations in the degree of hypertension depended on alterations in the blood-pressure. These observations show most strikingly, that in seeking to understand how the pressure is maintained within the eye, we must look far wider than to the blood-pressure alone.

From conditions of health we pass to those of disease. Craggs and Taylor found a number of subjects whose systemic blood-pressure (taken at the arm) was between 180 and 208 mm. of Hg., who yet presented a normal ocular tension, and who had no sign or symptom of glaucoma. On the other hand, they observed a number of cases of glaucoma with very high ocular tension (70 to 80 mm. of Hg.), who nevertheless had normal blood-pressures for their ages. They "conclude that high arterial tension is not a necessary and apparently not even a leading factor in the ætiology of glaucoma." In the same year Lobo, discussing the "inflammatory glaucoma" of hot countries, emphasised the fact that arterio-sclerosis does not play an important part in its ætiology. More recently, Fourrière's observations endorsed and supported those made by Craggs and Taylor. H. Sattler, too, is included amongst those who have not found a higher average blood-pressure among the glaucomatous than amongst the non-glaucomatous of the same age ; and he points out that those who are suffering from diseases associated with a high blood-pressure are not specially prone to glaucoma ; their eye troubles are of another kind, being usually due to local diseases of the vessel walls ; nor has he seen glaucomatous attacks which could be directly attributed to an increase of blood-pressure during violent muscular exercise. On the contrary, as he points out, the exhaustion and heart failure which follow over-exertion, mental depression, and weakening diseases, *e.g.*, influenza, are frequently associated with glaucoma. In a similar connection, Priestley Smith has shown that chronic excess of blood-pressure in the larger vessels is no evidence of a like excess of pressure in the capillaries which secrete the intra-ocular fluid ; on the contrary it is associated with increased resistance in the arterioles, and hence with an insufficient capillary circulation.

Foster Moore, attacking the question from the clinical standpoint, believes that " in some cases of arterio-sclerosis with a high general blood-pressure, this high pressure is so damped down by thickening and rigidity of the vessel walls, or by subendothelial proliferation, that the pressure in the retinal vessels is not raised, and may be instead below the normal." His general findings are very like those of Craggs and Taylor, but he goes farther than they did, and says that " general arterio-sclerosis is not a causative factor in simple primary glaucoma, and an attempt to reduce the general blood-pressure in such cases is not likely to improve the condition of the eye, in which the local blood-pressure may already be below the normal."

Bailliart has recently carried this argument of Moore's

a stage farther still. He points out that to treat a patient, who shows evidence of high tension in his retinal arteries, with drugs which lower the general blood-pressure, is to invite disaster ; for any fall which occurs in the general pressure is here brought about simply as a result of vaso-dilatation. In consequence, the pressure will rise in the veins and capillaries, and the patient will therefore be more than ever exposed to the danger of local hæmorrhages. Again, when the glaucoma symptoms are due, as Bailliart believes they may be, to a spasm of the retinal arterioles, which limits the blood supply to the capillary circulation, strychnine, being a vaso-constrictor, simply increases the trouble. What is needed in these cases is such treatment, by drugs or otherwise, as is calculated to open up the capillary and venous circulation in the affected eye.

Not the least interesting of the many papers which have appeared on this subject, is from the pen of A. MacRae. His most salient points can alone be quoted : (1) His statistics " are not uniformly either in favour of or against the theory that the average blood-pressure in glaucoma is high," but they " tend to oppose it." (2) He points out that " what we measure with the Riva Rocci type of apparatus is the blood-pressure, plus the resistance of the artery to the obliteration of its lumen ; and this latter may form no inconsiderable part of the reading." He argues that inasmuch as we cannot with certainty measure the real blood-pressure, it is premature to attempt to decide the existence of a relationship between it and the intra-ocular pressure. (3) He shows, as the result of experiments which he made, that whilst exercise considerably heightens the general blood-pressure, it leaves the intra-ocular pressure untouched. (4) He believes that " an altogether exaggerated importance has been given to the blood-pressure as a factor in maintaining or increasing eye tension."

Magitot's views on this subject have already been dealt with at the close of Part II. of this chapter and need not be again detailed. Up to a certain point, they appear to be shared by Bailliart, who holds, that within physiological limits, the intra-ocular and the retinal arterial pressures move up and down together, and that the front-rank cause of retinal arterial hypertension is a rise in the general blood-pressure. Duverger and Barré (together) and Velter, who have worked with Bailliart's instruments and along his lines of research, whilst agreeing with him in the latter opinion, differ strongly from him in the former, for they have not found any relationship on either side between the retinal arterial tension and the intra-ocular pressure. Thus, their evidence, so far as it goes, is opposed to the view that the fluid pressure within the eye is directly dependent upon the vagaries of the general blood-pressure, and this quite apart from any consideration of the complications introduced by arterial sclerosis. Amid such a welter of discordant opinions, it is obvious that the only course open to us is to await the accumulation of evidence, which will doubtless in time be forthcoming.

To conclude our consideration of this very interesting subject, we know that a rise in venous blood-pressure is favoured by a weak or slow heart, and by any factor which obstructs the free return of venous blood, and so favours venous congestion, and the observations and opinions above recorded must be read in the light of this knowledge. It would seem likely that in estimating the importance of the rôle played by increased intra-ocular blood-pressure in affecting the pressure of the intra-ocular fluid, we must look to the venous rather than to the arterial side of the system.

The Relationship between the Intra-ocular Blood-Pressure and the Intra-ocular Fluid-Pressure Outside the Vessels

The whole subject of the pulse in the vessels of the eye has, during the last few years, been very carefully studied and discussed by a number of writers (Bailliart, Henderson, Magitot, Duverger and Barré, Velter, Priestley Smith, the author, and others). Much of this literature has a

INTRA-OCULAR PRESSURE AND TENSION 65

very close bearing on the problems of glaucoma, and will well repay study by any who are really interested in the subject. There are, however, a few points which deserve a more detailed reference inasmuch as they bear closely on our present topic.

(1) The ophthalmoscopic examination of a number of normal eyes reveals the fact that a spontaneous pulse is present in over 50 per cent., and that in nearly 25 per cent. of the remainder, it can be readily produced by exerting light digital pressure on the globe. It has long been realised that such a pulse can only appear when the intra-ocular pressure and the pressure in the central vein in the eye are very nearly in equilibrium. During arterial systole there is a slight rise in intra-ocular pressure, and during diastole a slight fall in the same. These changes are due to the influx of an additional volume of arterial blood into the eye with systole, and to its escape during diastole. The small alternate increase and decrease thus brought about in the fluid contents of the eye causes the venous pulse: During diastole the venous pressure is above the intra-ocular pressure, and the blood flows outward in an uninterrupted current; whereas during systole the small increase of pressure is sufficient to make the escape of the venous blood more difficult; the flow is thus momentarily checked, and then goes on again. The repetition of this constitutes the venous pulse, and is clear evidence that the intra-ocular and venous pressures are normally very evenly balanced. If this were not so, this phenomenon would not be observed.

(2) If we exert firm digital pressure on an eyeball through the lids, and then remove the finger, we find that in most cases a spontaneous pulse, previously present, disappears. If we once again press gently on the eyeball the pulse reappears; or again, if we wait for a while, it reappears spontaneously. In the former case, our gentle added pressure has once more brought up the intra-ocular pressure close to the venous pressure; in the latter case, the original condition of close balance between the two has been resumed under natural conditions. We have

here one more lesson on the close relationship between the two, and at the same time we have an indication of the existence of a compensating mechanism, which keeps the two pressures together when for any reason they tend to separate.

(3) If, instead of exerting firm pressure on an eye with the finger, we press on it quite gently, watching the vessels in the optic disc the while, we notice that a segment of the vein, nearest its point of exit, becomes blanched. This does not require more than light pressure, but the amount of force used is quite an appreciable quantity; one can keep the finger on the lid, raise it gently so as to lessen the pressure exerted, and observe the vessel refill; or again, one can increase the pressure and see the vessel become colourless over a gradually increasing length of its course—from the exit point peripherally—as one weighs heavier and heavier on the eye with the finger. The many other interesting phenomena, which can thus be observed, are dealt with at some length in the author's communication, the reference to which will be found at the end of this Part.

From such observations it has been deduced that the pressure of the blood in the trunk of the retinal vein is slightly above the pressure of the intra-ocular fluid in which it lies. So far we would appear to be on firm ground, for if the venous pressure were not above that of the ocular fluid, the exit flow from the vein would be impeded exactly as it is in the above procedure.

The clinical experiment we have described was duplicated in the laboratory by Prof. Leonard Hill, when " he opened one of the vortex veins in the eye of a cat, allowed the blood to escape from there, and forced Ringer's solution to run into the aqueous, by raising the pressure bottle; the outflow from the vein stopped when the aqueous pressure was raised to the arterial pressure." He was carrying out under laboratory conditions the same experiment which we surgeons use in our practice, except that he pushed it farther than we do, viz., to the stoppage of all circulation, whereas we think it better to stop with the production of the arterial pulse, *i.e.*, at the level of diastolic arterial pressure.

The above experiment of Hill's was, after all, but a variation of the much earlier observations of von Schultén. The latter watched the retinal circulation of albino rabbits through a magnifying ophthalmoscope, whilst the intra-ocular pressure was gradually raised, and at the same time measured, by means of an injection-manometer. The blood-pressure was simultaneously observed in the opposite carotid artery. He was thus enabled to note (1) the point at which the venous circulation was interfered with, viz., at a pressure of 50 to 60 mm. Hg.; (2) that at which the flow through the retinal and choroidal arteries became intermittent, viz., at a pressure of from 90 to 120 mm. Hg., and (3) that at which the systolic arterial pressure was overcome (10 to 20 mm. Hg. higher than the last measurement), as evidenced by the cessation of the arterial flow. The estimate for the retinal and choroidal arterial pressure was a small but variable degree lower than that found simultaneously in the opposite carotid. Priestley Smith has criticised these experiments, and pointed out that the very fact of compressing an artery raises the pressure of the blood in the vessel, before it arrests the onward flow; consequently the chamber pressures recorded above are probably higher than those normally prevailing. He thinks that the mean pressure in the retinal arteries of the rabbit may safely be taken to be from 90 to 100 mm. Hg., and that, in all probability, the same estimate may be accepted for man. This is, however, still an open question.

It has sometimes been assumed that the pressure in all the veins leaving the eye must be the same at their points of exit. If this were certainly correct, it would be of interest, since we can, as above shown, form some estimate of the relationship between the intra-ocular pressure and the blood-pressure in the proximal part of the retinal vein. The matter is probably not of very great moment, but it is as well to bear in mind that the assumption may not be *absolutely* correct. Speaking in general terms we know that as the blood passes from the smaller to the larger veins in its flow towards the heart, the pressure steadily falls, and that " the larger the vessel, the lower the blood-pressure " is a good general rule. The large size of the canal of Schlemm, as compared with that of the retinal vein, would suggest that possibly the pressure within the former vessel may be lower than that in the latter. The same remark applies to the vasa vorticosa. At first sight this suggestion seems to open up very attractive possibilities, for if we assume that the pressure in the canal of Schlemm is lower than that in the central retinal vein, we can explain to ourselves the method of escape of the intra-ocular fluid into that canal. Thus, we might argue : The pressure in the retinal vein being a little higher than that of the intra-ocular fluid, the vein is kept patent, and its flow can continue ; again, the pressure in the intra-ocular fluid being a little higher than that in the comparatively large canal of Schlemm, the drainage of fluid into that canal from the interior of the eye is quite simply explained. We are here confronted with a difficulty, for if the pressure in the canal of Schlemm is less than that in the anterior chamber, it would appear likely that the canal would promptly be closed by pressure from without. The reply to this has been that inasmuch as this canal lies in the substance of the resistant wall of the sclera, and is lined merely by a thin layer of endothelium, it is kept permanently patent by the rigidity of the tissue in which it is situated, despite the fact that the pressure within it is slightly lower than that outside it. In further support of this contention, we may cite the well-known fact that in microscopic sections, Schlemm's canal is always found patent. Moreover, we know from Bailliart's work, that even the central retinal vein can remain patent, presumably by the resistance offered by its coats, when the pressure within it is less than that of the intra-ocular fluid outside. There is, however, one weak point in the above argument. If the pressure in this canal is less than the intra-ocular pressure, whilst that in the veins into which it empties is greater than that pressure, we are obviously presupposing a flow from a lower pressure to a higher one, which is an impossibility. On the other hand, if the thin-walled veins at their points of exit have not a higher pressure than the intra-ocular fluid, we can only suppose that they would be closed at such points by the excess of pressure, unless we assume that the efferent vessels from Schlemm's canal are, like the canal itself, prevented from collapsing by the rigidity of the walls which surround them.

Nor is this the only difficulty we meet with. It is generally accepted that a considerable quantity of intra-ocular fluid escapes through the iris veins. This assumption is firmly based on the results of anatomical investigations supported by the data furnished by experiments. Now these veins are thin-walled, and it seems very likely that they will collapse if the pressure outside them is greater than that within their lumina; so that the arguments, which might conceivably carry some weight when applied to Schlemm's canal, will hardly carry so much weight here.

We may put the question thus: If we are to assume that the intra-ocular fluid escapes from the eye under pressure by a process of filtration, the necessary corollary of this assumption must be, that the pressure of that fluid is slightly higher than the pressure for the time being in the canal of Schlemm, and in its efferent veins, and that the mechanical arrangement of the parts saves their walls from collapse. To assume that the pressure in the canal is equal to that of the intra-ocular fluid is impossible, for under such circumstances, no flow of fluid would take place. It is an elementary law that an equality of pressure can lead only to stagnation. The condition is one which is illustrated for us in everyday life, when an over-filled basin empties down to the level of its waste pipe, and then stands steadily at that line until more fluid is added, or until a fresh method of exit is provided for the water present. It would be equally impossible to suppose that fluid flows from the canal into its outflow veins against the force of a higher pressure in the latter.

If then we reject the idea that there is a constant, negative pressure within the canal of Schlemm, and the vessels which lead out from it, we must fall back, either on the view that osmotic influence explains away our difficulty, or on Arthur Thomson's theory that the ciliary muscle, by its action on the scleral spur, sucks the fluid from the anterior chamber into the canal of Schlemm, and then drives it on into the neighbouring veins by means of a pump-action. We shall consider each of these possibilities in detail.

The Osmotic Theory

According to this, the intra-ocular fluid is sucked into the canal of Schlemm and into the iris veins, as a result of osmotic action. For the acceptance of such an explanation, an equality of pressure inside and outside the vessels would be unimportant; indeed the fluid might easily be drawn into them against the push of a higher pressure within their walls. Dealing with other parts of the body, Starling has shown that, provided a vein is sufficiently thin-walled, fluid will readily pass into it from the tissues, even though the pressure within it may be in excess of that outside. The determining factor is the relative richness in diffusible contents of the two volumes of fluid.

There is a point to which we must allude at this stage. The supposition, that fluid passes from the anterior chamber into the canal of Schlemm by osmosis, obviously demands that there shall be a difference in the osmotic properties of the fluids in those two areas. If it be true, as some have suggested, that the contents of the canal are identical with those of the anterior chamber, then osmosis is obviously impossible. There is, however, no proof that this is the case. Some have even maintained that this canal is a venous sinus, whilst all are agreed that it is in very free communication with the neighbouring veins, and that at times it is found to contain blood. Salzmann says of it " a slight circulatory disturbance during life is probably quite sufficient to fill it partially or entirely with blood owing to its open communication with the veins." It

INTRA-OCULAR PRESSURE AND TENSION 71

therefore requires no great stretch of imagination to assume that osmosis is possible between the fluids circulating in the anterior chamber and in the canal of Schlemm, especially when we remember how slow the movement of fluid is in both of them, and therefore how little difference in osmotic properties is required.

We have to some extent been prepared to accept the idea that the escape of the intra-ocular fluid is due to osmosis, by the researches which have been carried out during recent years by a number of observers. A very short review of this work will therefore be germane to the discussion. According to Roemer, the subconjunctival injection of fluid in the eyes of dogs led to a rise in tension. He explained this on the supposition that the fluid found its way into the anterior chamber, and there produced alterations in the osmotic and chemical state of the vessels within the eye. Craggs found, that in man the influence of subconjunctival injections of normal saline solution was very uncertain, and that in some cases the injections were followed by a rise in tension, as measured by a Schiötz tonometer. Verderame supported Roemer's findings, but went farther and showed that the more concentrated the fluid injected and the greater its bulk, the more distinct was the rise of tension observed in the eye. Others have recorded similar observations. Roemer's suggestion that the saline injection fluid finds its way into the anterior chamber is sanctioned by what we know of the behaviour of drugs, such as cocaine, when solutions of them are subconjunctivally injected.

Hertel's work, though closely allied to the above, attacked the problem from a different standpoint, since he injected certain soluble substances, *e.g.*, glucose and sodium salts, into the blood-current of men and animals, or else administered them in large doses by the mouth. The effect in either case was a very marked fall in intra-ocular pressure, which he satisfied himself was not due to a fall in the general blood-pressure. He attributed it to the osmotic abstraction of water from the interior of the eye, brought about by the high concentration of the active substance in the blood. He found that the normal tension returned to the eye with the readjustment of the concentration of the blood, and that this return could be hastened by the injection of isotonic or hypotonic saline solutions. Moreover, he found that a distinct though transitory fall in intra-ocular pressure could be brought about in the glaucomatous eyes of men and animals by the injection into the blood-stream of concentrated saline solutions. Hertel has further suggested that the hypotony of diabetic coma is to be attributed to the abnormally high sugar and acetone contents in the blood, and not, as had been suggested, to any special tension-reducing substance in the serum; and he has proposed that the condition should be met by the free intravenous injection of normal saline solution. From an experimental point of view in normal animals, he did not find it easy to reduce the tension of the eye by dilution of the blood, for hæmolysis follows any attempt to inject water or low saline solutions intravenously, and the drinking of water, even in large amounts, produces very little effect on the concentration of the blood, and on the tension of the eye. Sattler spread the *ægis* of his clinical opinion over these experiments, whilst uttering a warning that such treatment, as Hertel had suggested, might not be free of risk. Closely allied to Hertel's work was that of Tristaino, who, moved thereto by the clinical experience of Weekers, experimented on rabbits in order to ascertain the power of intravenous injections of a solution of chloride of calcium in reducing ocular tension. His experiments are the more interesting in that they go far to confirm Verderame's findings, for he discovered that the rapidity, the intensity, and the duration of the effect produced were all proportional to the amount of the drug administered, and to the frequency of its administration.

It might be unwise to strain the lessons to be learnt from this mass of interesting work, but it seems probable that we can make the following tentative deductions:—
(1) That the therapeutic overloading of the blood with

certain soluble substances, is capable of producing such a change in the osmotic relationship between it and the intra-ocular fluid, that a fall in the intra-ocular pressure is thereby brought about ; and (2) that a converse therapeutic change, which either enhances the saline contents of the intra-ocular fluid as compared with those of the blood, or diminishes the latter as compared with the former, may be a factor in bringing about a rise in the intra-ocular pressure.

It must be admitted that the grounds for the second deduction are clinically not quite so satisfactory as those for the first.

We thus open up fields of inquiry both as to the possible influence of pathological alterations in the osmotic behaviour towards each other of the blood and intra-ocular fluid, and also as to the conditions under which the normal escape of fluid takes place from the cavities of the eye into the blood vessels.

Professor Arthur Thomson's Pump-action Theory

Professor Arthur Thomson's theory was set forth at length in *The Ophthalmoscope*. The reader is referred to his original article in that journal for details. We shall first take the anatomical foundations of his argument.

The meridional fibres of the ciliary muscle are inserted into the posterior surface of a projecting rim of scleral tissue. This rim in section appears as a small triangular area of condensed scleral tissue, the so-called scleral spur. The base of this process is confluent with the inner surface of the sclera, just outside the filtration angle. Its apex points forward and inward towards the outer wall of the iridial angle ; to its anterior sloping margin are attached the bundles of the trabecular tissue of the pectinate ligament, formed by the splitting up of Descemet's membrane, whilst from its posterior edge arise the meridional fibres of the ciliary muscle (see Fig. 11).

When the muscle contracts the spur will be drawn back by a lever action, just as one would pull open a door.

74 GLAUCOMA

A diagrammatic representation of the arrangement is shown in Fig. 12.

The pectinate ligament formed by the breaking up of

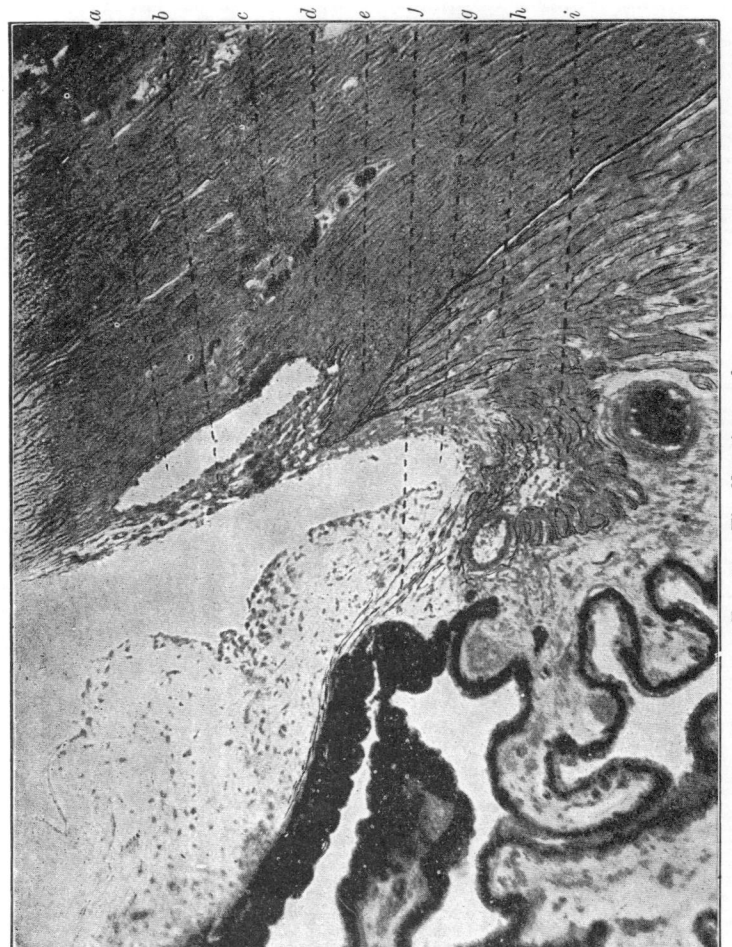

Fig. 11.—The filtration angle.

a, Canal of Schlemm; *b*, trabecular tissue of pectinate ligament; *c*, scleral vein; *d*, dense scleral tissue; *e*, scleral process or spur projecting inwards and forwards from the sclera close behind the canal of Schlemm; *f*, radial muscular fibres of the iris extending outwards below the iridial angle; *g*, iridial angle; *h*, meridional fibres of the ciliary muscle; *i*, circular fibres of the ciliary muscle.

(*By kind permission of Professor Arthur Thomson, M.A., M.B., F.R.C.S., and the Oxford Press.*)

the membrane of Descemet has its spaces lined everywhere by an extension of the endothelial layer which covers the posterior surface of Descemet's membrane. These spaces intervene between the angle, or sinus of

INTRA-OCULAR PRESSURE AND TENSION

the anterior chamber, and the canal of Schlemm. The latter consists merely of an endothelial lining resting immediately on the surrounding tissue, and not provided with any other definite wall.

" It will thus be seen that the scleral spur is intermediate

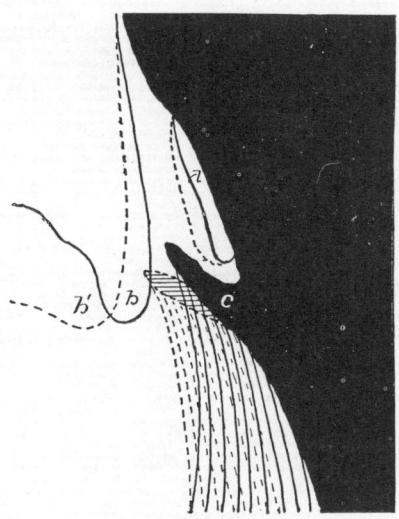

FIG. 12.—A diagram to show how, by the backward displacement of the scleral process, induced by the action of the ciliary muscle, the lumen of Schlemm's canal is enlarged. (Arthur Thomson.)

a, Schlemm's canal.

b, The iridial angle when the ciliary muscle is relaxed and the scleral process is drawn forward by the elasticity of the pectinate ligament.

c, The scleral process or spur, with the pectinate ligament attached in front and the ciliary muscle behind.

The solid outline represents the parts when the muscle is inactive. Under these conditions, for the sake of clearness, the canal of Schlemm is represented as open, though much narrower than when the ciliary muscle is contracted, as indicated by the dotted lines.

in position between a contractile tissue posteriorly, and an elastic tissue anteriorly ; or, expressed in another way, that whilst the meridional fibres of the ciliary muscle by their contraction can pull the spur backwards and inwards, the elastic tissue attached to its anterior surface will by its resiliency tend to counteract this and pull it forwards and outwards again. We are thus provided with an admirable arrangement whereby the lumen of Schlemm's canal can be modified under different conditions.

"There are three muscles which may exercise an influence on the position of the scleral spur, pulling it backwards and inwards ; these are the meridional and circular fibres of the ciliary muscle, and the sphincter muscle of the pupil. The former act in accommodation, and in their action are usually associated with the contraction of the pupil. The resultant of the combined action of these muscles is such as to draw the scleral spur backwards, and owing to its lever-like connection with the inner surface of the sclera, also inwards, with the consequent result that the fibres of the pectinate ligament which are attached, as has been described, to the anterior surface of the scleral spur are put on the stretch. Further, in consequence of the intimate connection of the fibres of the pectinate ligament with the inner wall of Schlemm's canal, of which, in fact, they form the inner wall, it follows that that wall is forcibly pulled inwards, and the lumen of Schlemm's canal is thereby increased. In this way a negative pressure is established within the canal into which fluids will pass along the line of least resistance. When the muscles afore-mentioned cease to contract, the pectinate ligament by its inherent elasticity pulls the scleral spur forwards and outwards again, thus mechanically effecting the collapse of the inner wall of the canal of Schlemm against its outer wall, and so restoring it to the ordinary influences of the intra-ocular pressure."

Thomson claims that the action he has described can be imitated, and demonstrated by gentle traction in a suitable direction made under a dissecting microscope. He holds that, apart altogether from the elastic recoil of the pectinate ligament, the shape of the scleral rim is such as to cause it to return to its position of rest by elastic rebound as soon as the muscular pull on it is relaxed. The induction of a negative pressure within the canal of Schlemm will naturally lead to the accumulation of fluid within it along the channels of least resistance. As the result of the observations of earlier writers, " it seems clear that whilst fluid may pass freely from the anterior chamber into the canal of Schlemm and so onwards into the surrounding veins, it is, under ordinary conditions, highly improbable that that fluid, once having entered the canal of Schlemm, can return from that canal into the aqueous chamber."

We have therefore to discover " the manner in which a valve-like action may be brought to bear on the channels connecting the canal of Schlemm and the interspaces of the pectinate ligament. These latter appear as a series of channels parallel to the inner wall of Schlemm's canal : posteriorly, as displayed in Figs. 13 and 14, they bend round to enter the posterior edge of the canal, but be it noted that since this arrangement of vessels lies within the receding angle, formed by the anterior edge of the scleral spur and the inner surface of the sclera itself, it follows therefore that when the scleral spur is pulled inwards by the action of the ciliary muscle, these channels will be uncurved and somewhat straightened, so as to render more easy the flow of fluid through them ; when, however, on the relaxation of the muscular contraction, the scleral spur is pulled forwards again by the elasticity of the pectinate ligament, the angle between it and the sclera proper will become narrower, the small channels will become acutely bent and so blocked, and thus a valve-like action will be induced, which will, under these conditions, prevent any return flow from Schlemm's canal." When by the retraction of its inner wall a negative pressure is established within the canal of Schlemm, fluid will, under normal conditions, more readily enter it from the aqueous chamber than from the surrounding venous circulation, because the channels of communication between the canal and the aqueous chamber are freer and more open than those between the canal of Schlemm and the surrounding veins. The result is, that following each contraction of the ciliary muscle, there is a rush of fluid into the canal of Schlemm from the anterior chamber. When the elastic rebound of the pectinate ligament and of the scleral spur

78 GLAUCOMA

come into play, "the pressure so exercised will assist in the expulsion of the fluid contained in Schlemm's canal onwards through the channels which connect it with the

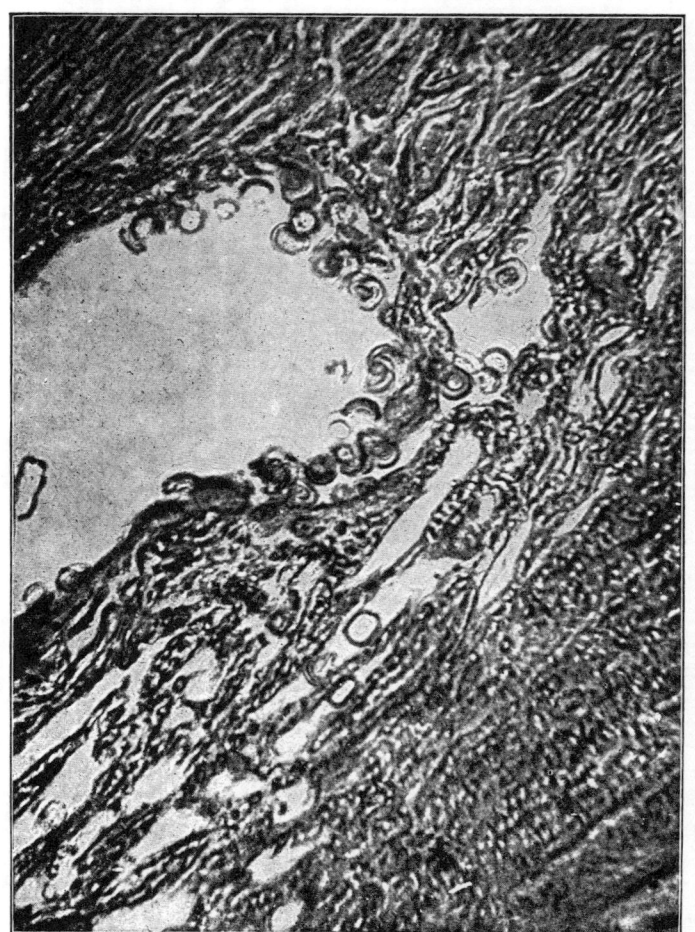

Fig. 13.—A section passing through the trabecular tissue of the pectinate ligament and the posterior circumference of Schlemm's canal. (Arthur Thomson.)

Within the canal a number of red blood-corpuscles are seen clinging to its walls; to the left of the canal our blood-corpuscles may be seen lying in channels within the trabecular ligament. The path by which these corpuscles have left the canal of Schlemm is shown in the section near the lower left-hand side of the canal, where some of the corpuscles have been arrested in their passage through a channel which is there displayed.

venous circulation, since, as has been proved experimentally, although it is possible to inject Schlemm's canal from the scleral veins, it is not possible to force the injection back from the canal into the anterior chamber. This

INTRA-OCULAR PRESSURE AND TENSION 79

return flow is checked, as has been explained, by the more abrupt bending, or kinking of the connecting channels passing from the interspaces in the pectinate ligament into the hinder part of Schlemm's canal, as they lie in the receding angle between the scleral process and the sclera itself, which angle being narrowed by the return of the

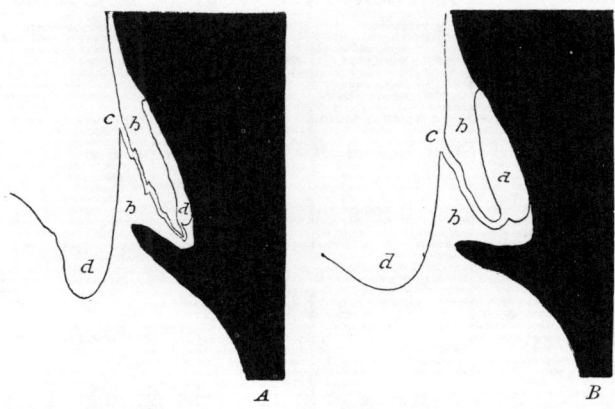

FIG. 14.—Diagrams to illustrate how the channels in the pectinate ligament are kinked and compressed when the scleral process is drawn forward, and how they are opened and straightened when the scleral process is pulled back, thus imparting to them a valvular action. (Arthur Thomson.)

A illustrates the conditions when the scleral process is pulled forward by the elasticity of the pectinate ligament.
B when the scleral process is pulled back by the action of the ciliary muscles.

a, The canal of Schlemm.
bb, The trabecular tissue of the pectinate ligament with—
c, A lymph channel running irregularly through it.
d in A, Represents the iridial angle when the scleral process is pulled forwards and the pupil dilated.
d in B, When the scleral process is pulled back and the pupil contracted.

scleral process to the position of rest, will naturally lead to a compression of the channels which lie within it." (Fig. 14.)

Thomson suggests that if this theory is rejected, "it is easy to imagine how the lymph spaces around the angle may be provided with a system of valve-like openings, which, whilst affording no opposition to a flow in one direction, may by the forcible opposition of their lips, offer an efficient block to any return in an opposite direction, particularly if the flow in the opposite direction be at an increased pressure. Just such an increase in the pressure might be induced by the elasticity of the pectinate ligament itself."

The above description has been given largely in Professor Thomson's own words. The proposition requires no advocacy, since it will recommend itself to every thoughtful mind, as a sane, well-reasoned, and obvious interpretation of anatomical data, the presentation of which carries conviction in every line. There is, however, one point which must be made quite clear. This muscular arrangement, which Thomson describes, can presumably only be supplementary to other factors for the removal of lymph from the eye, for it can only be in vigorous action during the waking hours. In this we find an analogy with the arrangement which prevails for the removal of lymph from other parts of the body by means of active muscular movements when the subject is awake. Whether, however, he wakes or sleeps, the movement of lymph goes on continuously in all his organs, under the influence of the driving power of the heart, and of the action of osmosis. It is of interest that our views with regard to the eye should have fallen into line with what is known of the rest of the body, since it lends an air of probability to our arguments.

An added interest is derived from the fact that, in the chronic type of glaucoma, the symptoms of increased pressure come on during sleep, and are manifested when the patient first awakes. As soon as he begins to call his iris and ciliary muscles into active operation, the mists, rainbows, etc. pass away. The deduction is obvious. We shall revert to this subject again in later chapters (pp. 97 and 171).

It must be admitted that the subject bristles with difficulties on every side, and that the time is not yet ripe for dogmatic decision. Indeed it may well be doubted whether it ever will be ; for the processes we are studying do not lend themselves, either to direct observation, or to experimental control. Under the circumstances, the only course open to us is to face the difficulties, to acknowledge our limitations, and to await the hoped-for advent of a wider knowledge. Meantime we may endeavour to summarise our conclusions, fully mindful of the fact that they will not meet with universal acceptation. The knowledge of this is far from acting as a deterrent, for on so recondite a subject, honest criticism and free discussion can only make for good.

(1) Whilst the systemic blood-pressure tends, as it rises and falls, to exert a corresponding influence upon the intra-ocular pressure, this influence may be masked, or even wholly neutralised, by a number of other factors.

(2) The high blood-pressure of general arterio-sclerosis is not necessarily, or even usually, associated with a high intra-ocular pressure, and is emphatically not a factor in the causation of glaucoma.

(3) The venous exit-pressure throughout the eye must always be a little in excess of the intra-ocular pressure, if the circulation of blood is to be satisfactorily maintained. It is therefore very difficult to assume that the pressure in Schlemm's canal can be below that of the intra-ocular pressure, and that the channel is held open against a negative pressure by the rigidity of the structures which surround it, unless the same assumption is extended also to the veins which lead out from it.

(4) It seems probable that osmotic action plays a large part in the transference of fluid from the anterior chamber into the canal of Schlemm and the iris veins, and that this action is strongly reinforced during the waking hours by the pump action described by Thomson.

REFERENCES

BAILLIART, P.—*Ann. d'ocul.*, 1919, vol. clvi. p. 690.
CASOLINO, L.—*Arch. di Ottal.*, 21st year, p. 588.
CRAGGS, H. C., AND TAYLOR, C. G.—*The Ophthalmoscope*, 1913, vol. xi. p. 350.
DUVERGER, C., AND BARRÉ, J. A.—*Arch. d'opht.*, Feb. 1920, p. 71.

ELLIOT, R. H.—*Brit. Journ. Ophth.*, 1921, vol. v. p. 481.
HENDERSON, T.—*Trans. O.S. of U.K.*, 1914, vol. xxxiv. p. 309.
HERTEL, E.—*Archiv f. O.*, 1915, vol. xc.; *Brit. Journ. Ophth.*, 1918, vol. ii. p. 634.
HILL, LEONARD.—Discussion, *Proc. Roy. Soc. Med.*, vol. vi. No. 3, p. 53.
MCLEAN, W.—*Arch. Ophth.*, 1920, vol. xlix. p. 304.
MACRAE, A.—*The Ophthalmoscope*, 1915, vol. xiii.
MAGITOT, A.—*Ann. d'ocul.*, 1917, vol. cliv. pp. 334, 385; *Brit. Journ. Ophth.*, 1918, vol. ii. p. 93.
MOORE, F.—*R.L.O.H. Reports*, May 1915, vol. xx. part 1.
ROEMER, P.—*Centralb. f. p. Augenh.*, vol. xxxviii. p. 200.
ROEMER, P., AND KOCHMANN.—*Berl. Ophth. Gesell.*, Nov. 1913; *Centralb. f. p. Augenh.*, vol. xxxviii. p. 9.
SALZMANN, M.—*The Anatomy and Histology of the Human Eye Ball*, translated by E. V. L. Brown, University of Chicago Press, Chicago, 1912.
SATTLER, H.—*Berl. Klin. Woch.*, 1913, Nos. 49 and 50; *Ophth. Rev.*, 1914, vol. xxxiii. p. 89.
SMITH, PRIESTLEY.—*Brit. Journ. Ophth.*, May 1918, p. 257.
STARLING, E. H.—*Principles of Human Physiology*, 3rd edition. J. & A. Churchill, London, 1920.
THOMSON, A.—*The Ophthalmoscope*, 1911, vol. ix. p. 470.
TOCZYSKI, F.—*Klin. Monatsbl. f. Augenh.*, June 1912, p. 727.
TRISTAINO, B.—*Arch. di Ottal.*, vol. xx. p. 589; *Ophth. Year Book*, 1913, vol. x. p. 172.
VAUGHAN, H.—*Journ. Med. Soc.*, New Jersey, vol. xiv. p. 386.
VELTER, E.—*Arch. d'opht.*, Feb. 1920, p. 88.
VON SCHULTÉN.—*Archiv f. O.*, vol. xxx. part 3, p. 1.
WEEKERS, L.—*La Clinique Ophtal.*, June 10, 1912.
WESSELEY, K.—*Thirty-eighth Ophth. Congress*, Heidelberg, p. 116.

CHAPTER III

THE ÆTIOLOGY OF GLAUCOMA

SUMMARY

PART I
INTRODUCTION.

PART II
THE PATHOLOGICAL ANATOMY OF GLAUCOMA.
1. CHANGES IN THE VORTEX VEINS.
2. DISEASE OF THE VESSELS.
3. SCHNABEL'S CAVERNOUS ATROPHY.
4. FIBROSIS OF THE PECTINATE LIGAMENT.
5. HYDROPHILISM.

PART III
THE PATHOLOGICAL ANATOMY OF GLAUCOMA (*continued*).
6. CLOSURE OF THE FILTRATION ANGLE.
7. SHALLOWING OF THE ANTERIOR CHAMBER.
8. THE DIMENSIONS OF GLAUCOMATOUS EYES.
9. THE CONTINUOUS GROWTH OF THE LENS THROUGHOUT LIFE.

PART IV
THE CAUSES OF GLAUCOMA.
1. AGE.
   Anatomical changes,
   Degenerative changes,
   Hydrophilism,
   Autogenetic intoxication,
   The influence of the secretions of the ductless glands,
   Changes in the vascular system.
2. SEX.
3. HEREDITY.
4. ERRORS IN REFRACTION.
5. MYDRIASIS.
6. NERVE SHOCK AND STRAIN.
7. FEBRILE DISEASES.
8. INJURIES.

Part I

Introduction

A PERUSAL of the modern literature of the ætiology of glaucoma is suggestive of a mental kaleidoscope, in which outstanding and not infrequently discordant data are viewed from innumerable angles. At first sight the picture seems attractive, and one which satisfies the casual observer. When, however, he endeavours to get at close quarters with the subject, he finds that it bristles with difficulties. The more he studies it, the more dissatisfied he is likely to become with the present state of our knowledge. The reasons for this would appear to be manifold :

(1) Some of our principal data do not rest on a basis of universal acceptation, but still remain the arenas of vigorous dispute. (2) Few, if any, eyes are submitted to a microscopic examination at a very early stage of the disease; most, if not all, of our material is from globes far advanced in glaucoma, an exceedingly large percentage being taken from blind painful eyeballs. In such material the tissue-changes which are causative of glaucoma, are obscured and overlaid by those, which are consequent upon the morbid processes that have been at work. Under these circumstances, it is impossible to distinguish with certainty between cause and effect, and yet, we not infrequently see articles in which these considerations are overlooked, with the result that dire confusion exists in the mind of the writer and is spread to some at least of his readers. (3) There is a widely existent confusion between the ætiology, the pathogeny, and the pathological anatomy of the disease. It is true that this confusion is not peculiar to the study of glaucoma, but it is markedly accentuated in this disease, owing to the reasons mentioned in our two previous headings. An endeavour to seek more precise definition in our terminology appears likely to be of benefit and will therefore be attempted. *Pathology* has been

defined [1] as "that part of medicine, which explains the nature of diseases, their causes and symptoms." A more restricted meaning is given to the term by those who would understand by it merely the study of pathological anatomy. To avoid ambiguity, however, it will be better always to speak of this branch as *pathological anatomy*. *Pathogeny* is defined [1] as "the science of the generation and development of disease," whilst *ætiology* [1] is "an account of the causes of disease." It is fatal to clear thinking to confuse these three.

We cannot start, as we would like to do, from the teachings of the pathological anatomy of glaucoma, to reason out either its ætiology or its pathogeny. If we do so in the present state of our knowledge, we shall be in danger of building on sand. Our study of the pathogeny of the disease must necessarily be a clinical one, whilst our views on its ætiology have been based on clinical observation, tempered by a study of the changes produced both in the eye and in the organism by those conditions of life, which our observations lead us to believe are causative of the disease. (4) There is a subsidiary element of confusion, which it will be convenient to discuss here. Some writers in speaking of the causes of glaucoma, include under this heading anatomical changes, such as the continued growth of the lens throughout life, or the fibrosis of the pectinate ligament. The question may fairly be raised as to whether these are *causes* of glaucoma. Do not the causes of glaucoma lie farther back in the advance of age, and in those degenerative processes which are inseparable from the wear and tear of a living organism? It is a nice point and one which is of comparatively little importance, provided that we clearly recognise the true position of affairs; but to draw up a list of the causes of glaucoma, and to include in that list the anatomical changes produced by antecedent degeneration or disease, side by side with the names of those causative conditions, is illogical in theory and confusing in practice. (5) The term "Glaucoma" is not the title of a single disease.

[1] Annandale's *Dictionary*. Blackie and Son Ltd., 1901.

It is rather a convenient, clinical label for a large group of conditions, the distinctive class feature of which is that of a rise in intra-ocular pressure. The ætiology differs widely in different cases; the pathological anatomy of the globes, when they come to dissection, shows no less variation; whilst the difference in the symptoms which are presented is so great, that it would be difficult without careful study, to recognise the strong bond that has served to unite all these cases in a common category. That bond, we repeat, is the rise in intra-ocular pressure. To this rise all causes lead up. In this rise of pressure, be its source what it may, every sign and symptom we meet with in glaucoma, finds a ready explanation; whilst the variations met with in the different types of the disease are explained with equal facility by the interplay of those anatomical and pathological conditions which vary so widely in different eyes, and which thereby profoundly influence the rate in the rise of the intra-ocular pressure in any individual case. Once such a rise is established, it dominates the whole of the picture from a clinical point of view. Indeed, it not seldom does so to the exclusion of a just consideration of the ætiological factors of the situation. It is necessary then to keep clearly in mind, that in dealing with cases of glaucoma, all causes of the condition, however diverse they may be, lead up to the one central feature of a rise in the pressure within the eye. On the other hand, every characteristic sign and symptom of the disease can be traced back to this same central feature. A rise in the tension of the eye is the hub of the glaucoma wheel. To alter the metaphor, it is the junction through which all lines must pass, whether of ætiology or of clinical course. We must not allow this to blind us to the fact, already stated, that glaucoma is not a disease, but a collection of widely different pathological conditions.

All the different factors, which from time to time have been cited as causes of glaucoma, may ultimately be classified under one or other of two headings:—(1) Those which influence the balance of secretion and excretion of the intra-ocular fluid, and (2) those which directly or indirectly determine a change in the vascular conditions prevailing within the eye.

To this statement we shall on more than one occasion have to return. There is no single assertion in connection with the pathology of glaucoma, which equals it in importance. Before, however, we address ourselves to the serious study of the ætiology of the disease, we must first learn all that pathological anatomy has to teach us, and this despite the fact already stated that anatomical data alone would furnish a very insecure foundation for the superstructure we desire to raise.

Part II

The Pathological Anatomy of Glaucoma

Much that has been written in the past on the pathological anatomy of glaucoma has now merely an historic interest. For this, faulty observation and premature deductions have been largely responsible. Cause and effect have been confused, an undue influence has been ascribed to conditions which have been found to be present, and imagination has not infrequently been allowed far too much licence.

We shall take up in turn the more interesting observations which have been made, and discuss their present status in the light of recent knowledge. In doing so, it will be convenient to start with those which can be most easily dismissed, and to pass gradually up to those which now seem to be most worthy of attention.

1. Changes in the Vortex Veins

Birnbacher and Czermak found extensive changes both in and around the vortex veins in glaucomatous eyes. The vessels, the lymph spaces surrounding them, and the sclera in the neighbourhood showed considerable cellular infiltration, whilst the endothelium of the veins had undergone great proliferation. It was argued that such changes would obstruct the flow through these veins, lead to congestion of the areas drained by them, and thus bring about a rise in the intra-ocular pressure. An air of probability was lent to the suggestion by the fact that various observers had found that ligature of the venæ vorticosæ in animals led to a very marked increase of the intra-ocular pressure. Probably the most interesting work on the subject is that of Koster, who, after summarising the results of those who had preceded him, gave his own findings.—When all four veins were ligatured, very high tension immediately came on ; the pupil dilated, the anterior chamber became shallow, especially at its periphery ; the iris vessels filled with blood ; and a marked swelling of the ciliary body could (in albino rabbits) be readily seen with the ophthalmoscope. Three weeks later the eyes appeared normal, except that the periphery of the iris remained adherent to the margin of the cornea. When two or three, instead of all four, of the vorticose vessels were ligatured, the iris thickened and came forward *only in the region corresponding with the ligatured vessels*; and it could be observed that *the ciliary body was swollen in the same region and not elsewhere*. The degree of glaucoma was much milder than in the earlier quoted experiments.

It cannot be denied that these observations are full of suggestive interest, but they have been robbed of much of their force by A. W. Stirling, who has shown that so far from the anatomical changes described by the Austrian observers being constantly met with in glaucoma, they are in reality very rare indeed in connection with that disease.

The statement has also been made that appearances, precisely similar to those recorded by Birnbacher and Czermak, are to be seen in eyes which are free from all suspicion of high tension. It is, however, hard to trace the authority for this assertion.

Heerfordt went a step farther than anyone had done before and suggested, on very insufficient evidence, that acute glaucoma was due to an obstruction to the intra-ocular circulation, located in the sinuses into which the vortex veins empty. The idea seems an extravagant one.

It would be rash to assert that obstruction to these large veins might not, in some cases at least, be a determining factor in the onset of a glaucoma, for which other changes had possibly prepared the way ; but it would be safe to say that modern ophthalmological opinion does not lay any very serious stress on the rôle of the changes we have been discussing.

2. Disease of the Vessels as a Cause of Glaucoma

From the earliest days, a number of observations have been placed on record as to œdematous and vascular conditions seen in the posterior pole of the eye, and it has been suggested that these might stand in a causal relation to rise in tension. Such suggestions still crop up sporadically, in which the writers, on the strength of the various evidences of venous congestion which are so familiar in glaucoma, maintain that it is " a vascular disease." They, however, fail to bring forward any fresh evidence on the subject. There are few conditions in which cause and effect are more easily confused than in glaucoma, but surgical opinion has long decided, that all the evidences of vascular disturbance, on which these writers lay so much stress, find a ready explanation in the *results* of an increase of intra-ocular pressure. Fifty years ago von Graefe wrote : " The great distension of the retinal capillaries is also, in my opinion, caused by the escape of the venous blood being impeded through the increased pressure." It is extremely unlikely that this verdict will ever be seriously questioned, unless some new and cogent facts are brought forward for the purpose. Mere speculation will certainly carry little, if any, weight. Nothing that has been here said is to be taken as affecting the rôle of venous congestion in determining a rise in intra-ocular pressure, or that of the interplay between the vascular factors and those which control the relationship between secretion and excretion of the aqueous fluid.

3. Schnabel's Cavernous Atrophy of the Optic Nerve

In the year 1892, Schnabel advanced the view that the cupping of the glaucomatous disc was due, not to an increase of the intra-ocular pressure, but to an "active atrophy" of the nerve itself. He considered that the lamina cribrosa was not pushed back by pressure from within, but that it was pulled back from without by the shrinking of the wasting nerve. In that part of the nerve, which lay within the scleral canal, he observed the presence of microscopic holes, which by enlargement and coalescence, led to the formation of what he described as a "cavernous degeneration." As the morbid process progressed, the spaces became larger, until at last a single huge cavity—the cupped disc—was left. In association with these changes, there was a proliferation of vascularised connective tissue, which subsequently shrunk and became more condensed. Other writers have confirmed Schnabel's observations, so far as they concern the existence of a cavernous degeneration in a limited number of cases of glaucomatous cupping, and have described septum-like projections into the floor of the cup in some of these. The latter appearances evidently represent the partitions between neighbouring "caverns," at a very late stage of their coalescence.

It was not very long, however, before two facts appeared to emerge in an unmistakable manner from the increasing mass of observations which had been laid before ophthalmologists, viz., (1) that cavernous degeneration of the optic nerve is met with in eyes which have never been subject to an increase in internal pressure, and (2) that no signs of it are to be found in many, if not in most, glaucomatous globes. This matter was practically thrashed out in a discussion on a paper read by Schnabel in Vienna in 1908. His most interesting points were :—

(1) That where an increase of tension was absent, the lamina cribrosa was not displaced, and (2) that a progressive cavernous atrophy might occur after the completely successful reduction of a rise in ocular tension by means of an iridectomy. These propositions were admitted by the meeting, and ratified later by ophthalmological opinion, but his consequent contention that glaucomatous cupping was not due to an increase of intraocular pressure, was rejected then, and has never since come into favour. The most important item of evidence against such a view is to be found in the behaviour of the glaucoma cup, in certain cases, after a successful reduction of ocular tension by means of a filtering operation (successful iridectomy being included in this category). Holth has dealt in a very interesting manner with this subject. He has shown that von Graefe was the first to observe a transitory levelling of a glaucoma cup, after the performance of a successful iridectomy. Since then, others also have noticed the same phenomenon, whilst to Axenfeld belongs the credit of having drawn prominent attention to the subject in recent times. Holth has repeatedly seen complete and *permanent* disappearance of the glaucomatous excavation after successful filtration operations. Axenfeld has had a similar experience, and many other surgeons have since confirmed the observation in their own practice. The author has now seen it in quite a number of instances; indeed he is disposed to look on it as a by no means uncommon event. Nor is the evidence merely ophthalmoscopic, for both Holth and Butler have established their clinical findings on the subject by the anatomical examination of eyes which had been successfully sclerectomised.

Von Graefe's work on the subject not merely claims priority over all other, but is of peculiar interest, since his acute power of clinical observation led him to notice that the phenomenon was far the most clearly in evidence in one particular group of cases, viz., in those where acute symptoms supervened on a previous chronic glaucoma. He thought that in such cases the previous chronic disease brought about a condition of the optic nerve, which led to its yielding readily and rapidly under an access of pressure. The cupping thus produced showed, in his experience, a greater tendency to recede, once the element of markedly increased pressure was withdrawn, than did that which was the outcome of a slow prolonged increase of intra-ocular pressure. He adds : " In this way I saw deep cavities change within a week into flat basin-like depressions."

Lange, too, has made some very interesting observations in this connection. He has seen a diminution in the depth of glaucoma cups, not only after operation, but also after the use of meiotics. In one case the depth of the cupping varied from time to time with the changes in the tension of the eye. The writer has seen a similar case.

It is the rule to find, that after the performance of a successful filtration operation, undertaken for the relief of tension, the visual acuity ceases to fall ; indeed, in a certain percentage of cases, a more or less decided rise in vision is met with. At the same time the fields may be expected to enlarge ; sometimes, indeed, to a very considerable extent. These changes for the better are independent of any diminution in the depth of the cupping of the disc. It is, however, equally beyond dispute that in a definite, but fortunately small, proportion of cases, the optic atrophy and the resultant affection of vision continue to progress, despite the most ample relief of tension. Indeed, this may occur even in cases in which the depth of cupping shows decided diminution, as a result of the lowering of the intra-ocular pressure. Such instances have been made much of, and seen in an altogether false perspective by some surgeons, whilst they have been ignored by others. It is true that they are but seldom met with, but they do occur, and this fact demands an explanation. To assume on that basis, as has been done, that operations which lower the pressure within the eye are useless, or that an increase of intra-ocular pressure is not the paramount feature of glaucoma cases, is futile.

Schnabel was led astray when he advanced the view that the cupping of the disc was the result of essential changes in the nerve, apart altogether from pressure. The cupping of the disc met with in glaucoma is the direct result of an increase of intra-ocular pressure. His theory was an extravagant one, but the work he did was of great value for this reason, if for no other, that it drew attention to these cases of the continuance of atrophy of the nerve, after the prime cause of that atrophy had been removed. To explain the phenomenon in question, we may tentatively put forward several possible suggestions :—(1) That in these cases, the trouble from the first is an atrophy of the nerve, quite independent of pressure (what has been called an " essential atrophy "), and that the anatomical change is of the cavernous type ; (2) that the two conditions, viz., atrophy from pressure, associated with cupping, and some form of primary (or essential) atrophy occur together, as the result of accidental circumstances ; it is conceivable that in the weakened condition of the nerve the excess of pressure required might be very slight ; and (3) that the tendency to atrophy of the nerve is for some reason present in a latent form, and that it is enabled to assert itself, as a result of the injury the nerve has sustained in consequence of the pressure to which it has been subjected. It is possible that in different cases any one of these three may be the correct explanation, but the writer thinks that probably the last-named is most frequently the correct solution. This view will be best explained by a reference to a recent case in his own practice.—A patient was sent to him for consultation, in whom, in spite of a perfectly performed and successful trephining, the visual fields were steadily diminishing, and vision was failing ; the tension of the eyes was distinctly below normal, and free filtration was taking place. A search for a source of auto-intoxication suggested more drastic dental attention than the patient had yet received. His teeth were all removed, with the result that the fields showed a very early increase in both eyes, and central vision at the same time improved. The explanation would appear to have been that the nerve had been so damaged by the glaucoma, that it was rendered unable to resist the attacks of the poison produced autogenetically in the pyorrhœic area. It is likely that other intoxications may act in a similar manner. The lesson to be drawn is, that when we find an atrophy of the optic nerve progressing in spite of the relief of tension by a suitable operation, we should search diligently for a source of autogenetic intoxication, and treat the same vigorously whenever it is found. If this be done, then Schnabel's work will have been of considerable value, even although we may reject as fantastic his explanation of the phenomena he observed.

It remains to be added that Fleischer believes (*a*) that Schnabel's cavernous excavation is an atrophy arising from infiltration of the nerve with lymph, and (*b*) that the presence of this fluid is caused by circulatory stasis, associated with a marked rise in the tension of the eye. Fuchs apparently holds somewhat similar views (see Chapter IV. Part II.), and so does Gilbert.

Ischikawa has examined ten glaucomatous eyes and found Schnabel's " caverns " in the five cases which were of recent origin, but not in the other five which were of longer standing; he believes that the caverns are characteristic of glaucoma, as Schnabel claimed they were, and that they form a specific class of disease of the optic nerve; this begins as an œdema of the nerve fibres, which later become dissolved and thus form the caverns; the glaucomatous excavation is due to the coalescence and subsequent disappearance of these caverns; the latter are not found in any other diseases, with the exception of high myopia, in which he attributes them to mechanical factors. It is one thing to postulate that changes which may accompany glaucoma are specific or semi-specific in character; it would be quite another to assume, as Schnabel erroneously did, that an increase of intra-ocular pressure was not concerned in their origin.

It seems not impossible that we have still much to learn on the subject, in spite of the fact that it has been

THE ÆTIOLOGY OF GLAUCOMA

freely canvassed by ophthalmologists for nearly a quarter of a century. Indeed, the lesson, when learnt, may prove to be both valuable and important.

4. Fibrosis of the Pectinate Ligament

T. Henderson has advanced the view that a structural change in the pectinate (or cribriform) ligament is responsible for an obstruction to the ready access of the aqueous fluid to Schlemm's canal. His main points are as follows :—

(1) The cribriform ligament is a continuation of the inner lamellæ of the cornea ; it is composed of regular and evenly disposed interlacing fibres ; and it ends as the ligament of origin of the ciliary muscle.

(2) The angle of the anterior chamber has for its boundaries, the cribriform ligament in front, and the iris root behind, the ciliary body being thus excluded from reaching the anterior chamber at all.

(3) The cribriform ligament is purely cellular at birth and undergoes increasing sclerosis as life advances, until, in old age, its fibres come to resemble those of the adjacent sclera.

(4) It "is nothing more than a regular and open network, formed of interlacing fibres, which are a direct continuation of the longitudinal and circular bundles of the sclera about the venous sinus of Schlemm's canal."

(5) The spaces in the cribriform ligament are directly continuous with those between the corneal lamellæ, and the ligament is to be looked on simply as a very open part of the corneo-scleral envelope.

(6) The results of sclerosis of the ligament are : (a) To reduce the contrast between the cribriform ligament and the surrounding corneo-sclera to one of magnitudes of fibres only, and (b) to reduce the interspaces and alveoli of the retiform tissue. The thickness of the ligament itself, as it lies between the anterior chamber and Schlemm's canal, is unaffected.

(7) On anatomical grounds alone, a free communication

is postulated between the anterior chamber and the suprachoroidal space, along the posterior portion of the cribriform ligaments.

(8) The sclerosis of the ligament creates an increasing mechanical obstruction, which predisposes to glaucoma by impeding the access of aqueous both to Schlemm's canal and to the venous channels traversing the suprachoroidal space.

(9) Again, on anatomical grounds, it is assumed that the action of the ciliary muscle in accommodation is to facilitate the escape of the aqueous into the suprachoroidal space, and thus to produce a physiological deepening of the anterior chamber.

It is one thing to admit that this sclerosis of the pectinate ligament may offer an obstacle to the free escape of aqueous from the eye, always provided that other conditions remain constant, and so may predispose the organ to a rise in tension. It is quite another thing to agree with Henderson that we have here the chief of the predisposing anatomical causes of glaucoma. According to his own showing, the fibrosis is universal; on the other hand, we know that glaucoma is a not very common disease, although the tendency to it increases with age. We do not even find that the intra-ocular pressure rises with the advance of age, as we should expect it to do, if these fibrotic changes really oppose a constantly increasing resistance to the passage of aqueous from the eye; indeed all the evidence before us is to the effect that it is decidedly lower in the elderly than it is in young adults. Moreover, as Priestley Smith has pointed out, Henderson's theory does not account for the shallowing of the anterior chamber met with in so many of our glaucoma cases, nor for the equally characteristic closure of the filtration angle. The danger of arguing a physiological problem on purely anatomical grounds is well recognised, and all that we can safely admit is that the sclerosis of the pectinate ligament, the existence of which has not, we believe, been disputed, may well be one of the predisposing causes of glaucoma, inasmuch as it may tend to upset the balance normally held between

THE ÆTIOLOGY OF GLAUCOMA

the secretion and excretion of fluid from the eye. To go farther would be to outrun our facts.

The treatment of this subject would be incomplete without a reference to the valuable writings of Professor Arthur Thomson. These have already been quoted in the previous chapter, but some repetition may be pardoned in view of the fact that their true value has not yet been fully appreciated. It is impossible to give more than a brief abstract of the principal parts of that section of his work, which immediately affects the question at issue :—

(1) He evidently prefers to retain the time-honoured name of "the pectinate ligament"; there are obvious advantages in following his lead in this matter. (2) He describes this ligament as consisting of an open meshwork of fibro-elastic tissue, which can be traced forward into direct continuity with the homogeneous elastic layer of Descemet. If the latter membrane be traced backwards, it is found to break up into a number of fibrillæ, arranged in a brush-like fashion. Under meridional section, the appearance presented is that of the triangular area of trabecular tissue, long familiar to us as the pectinate ligament. Thomson is satisfied that the spaces within this tissue are lined by extensions from the layer of endothelial cells, which covers the posterior surface of Descemet's membrane. The majority of fibres of this ligament are attached to the front of the scleral process, whilst the meridional division of the ciliary muscle is inserted into the posterior surface of that spur. (3) By the aid of anatomical observation, assisted by admittedly rough experiments on dead eyes, he has evolved the theory, that the escape of fluid from the anterior chamber into the canal of Schlemm, and again from that vessel into the neighbouring veins, is the result of a pumping action, in which the muscles of the ciliary body and of the iris draw back the scleral process and so open both the canal of Schlemm and the trabecular spaces of the pectinate ligament. Again the elasticity of this ligament and of the scleral spur itself tends to close both the spaces and the canal, and so to drive the aqueous fluid onward into

the surrounding veins. This is admittedly a deduction, and must be taken as such, but the excellence of Thomson's preparations, and of his photographs of them, as well as his reputation as an anatomist, carry a measure of conviction, which is materially strengthened by the fact that his arguments are as simple as his method of presenting them is lucid. Some of the work on this subject put forward in recent years has been so involved, and so difficult to understand, that it has tempted one to doubt whether the writers had really mastered the arguments they presented. It is refreshing to turn from such studies to the products of Professor Thomson's pen. In the light of what he has written, whilst it is still conceivable that an encroachment on the trabecular spaces of the pectinate ligament may be an important factor, it seems still more likely that a want of elasticity in these thickened fibres may greatly mar the usefulness of the parts for the function which Thomson ascribes to them. In other words, the regular pump action, whose motive force is supplied by the muscles of the ciliary body and of the iris, may be hampered both in contraction and in the subsequent rebound by any change which damages the extensibility and the elasticity of the pectinate ligament. In this way a predisposition to glaucoma may presumably be established.

The author had an opportunity of studying the anatomy of the pectinate ligament on a number of corneo-scleral discs which he had removed during trephining operations. The specimens again and again showed most clearly the breaking up of the membrane of Descemet into the brush-like fibrillæ described by Thomson. This point will be clear to anyone who will study the micro-photographs reproduced in Figs. 206, 207, 209, and 212.

5. Hydrophilism

The studies of Fischer on the production of œdema by the action of acids or alkalies on the colloidal tissues of the body, led him to apply his conclusions to the explanation of the causation of glaucoma. According to him,

THE ÆTIOLOGY OF GLAUCOMA

this condition is an œdema of the eyeball, in which the amount of water held by the hydrophilic colloids of the eye is increased. He did not distinguish between the individual structures, but thought the whole globe participated in the change. He believed that the most important causative factor of such an hydrophilism was an increase in the amount of acid present in the organ, and that the recognised exciting causes of an attack of high tension were those which might be expected to lead to an abnormal production or accumulation of acid in the eye. Ruben, who repeated the experiments, agreed with Fischer's main contentions, but found that the swelling under acidosis involved the sclera and cornea, but not the vitreous. He thought that in this way a shrinking of the intra-ocular capacity was brought about, and that hence an increased pressure of the contents of the eye resulted. It would naturally suggest itself, that if such a swelling of the coats of the eye actually did occur, the efferent vascular channels would probably suffer more than the afferent, owing to their thinner walls, and that thus an obstruction to the escape of fluid and of venous blood from the eye might take place, which would be much more important than the mere reduction of intra-ocular contents, for the latter might be easily compensated so long as the channels of fluid-escape remained open. It is of interest, in this connection, to recall the fact that Maynard, in Calcutta, saw over twenty cases of glaucoma, associated with a wave of epidemic dropsy. The observation may possibly have a bearing on our present subject. The obvious criticism of the view of the case presented by Fischer and by Ruben is (1) that in glaucoma we do not find evidence of that swelling of the ocular tunic which their theory demands; this subject has been considered by Ischreyt, who carefully measured the thickness of the sclera in glaucomatous eyes; (2) that the strength of acid concentration with which they worked would not be found *in vivo* in the tissues; and (3) that it does not necessarily follow that a very much diluted acid will produce the same results, or even the same class of results, as a comparatively concentrated one. What is more, even had they confined themselves to claiming that the swelling produced led to an obstruction of the efferent channels, it would still have been incumbent on them to bring forward anatomical evidence of such a change. Nor have they been more fortunate in the results of the treatment which has been based on their theory. Thomas claimed that the tension of a glaucomatous eye could be reduced by the subconjunctival injection of a solution of sodium citrate. This therapy was founded on Fischer's finding that certain salts (amongst others, sodium citrate) have the power of preventing the absorption of water from acid solutions. He was supported by Sedwick, Grandclément, and McCaw; other surgeons have, however, been less fortunate in their results from this form of treatment. The majority of ophthalmologists have found that the remedy does *not* reduce the tension in glaucoma, and that it may even seriously aggravate it.

More recently, Scalinci has championed Fischer's theory so far as " irritative glaucoma " is concerned. He adopts the view that the first stage in this affection is an œdema of the vitreous, arising from the tissue colloids possessing an abnormal affinity for water, due to an increase in their acid contents, there being either an excessive production, or a defective elimination of acid. It is quite true that a distension of the vitreous is apparently not infrequently the first incident in an attack of glaucoma; but, as has been pointed out above, there appears to be reason to think that the vitreous body is not itself hydrophilic. In any case, it is quite clear that the profession has not hitherto shown any general inclination to adopt the hydrophilic theory; the evidence in its favour has seemed too scanty and too weak. This is, however, quite a different thing from the assumption that there is no germ of truth lying hidden in the views we have been discussing. The causes of glaucoma are doubtless very diverse in different cases, and it would be as rash as it would be uncalled for to deny all value to views, which do not appeal strongly to us either as individuals or as a profession.

REFERENCES

BIRNBACHER AND CZERMAK.—*Archiv f. O.*, 1886, vol. xxxii. part 2 ; and *Ein Beitrag zur Anat. d. Glaucoma Acutum.* Graz, 1890.
BUTLER, T. HARRISON.—*The Ophthalmoscope*, vol. xii. p. 468.
ELLIOT, R. H.—" Histology of the Trephined Disc in Glaucoma Opera tions," *Trans. O.S. of U.K.*, 1918, vol. xxxviii. p. 227.
FISCHER, MARTIN H.— Pflüger's *Archiv f. Physiol.*, 1909, vol. cxxvii., abstracted in *Ophth. Rev.*, 1910, vol. xxix. p. 72.
FLEISCHER, B.—*Thirty-eighth Ophth. Congress*, Heidelberg, p. 110.
FUCHS, E.—*Klin. Monatsbl. f. Augenh.*, Jan. 1911.
FUCHS, E.—" On the Lamina Cribrosa," *Archiv f. O.*, 1916, vol. xci. part 3.
GILBEET, W.—*Archiv f. O.*, vol. xc. p. 76.
GRANDCLÉMENT, E.—*Clinical Ophthalmology*, vol. xviii. p. 275.
HEERFORDT, C. F.—*Ophth. Rev.*, vol. xxx. p. 196.
HENDERSON, T.—*Glaucoma.* Arnold, London, 1910.
HOLTH, S.—*The Ophthalmoscope*, 1911, vol. ix. p. 494; *ibid.*, 1912, vol. xii. pp. 347–354.
ISCHIKAWA.—*Arch. Ophth.*, vol. xliv. part 3, p. 339 ; *ibid.*, vol. lxxxvii. part 3, p. 429.
ISCHREYT, G.—*Ibid.*, July 1908, p. 441.
KOSTER, W.—Von Graefe's *Archiv f. O.*, 1895, vol. xli. part 2, p. 30.
LANGE.—*Klin. Monatsbl. f. Augenh.*, vol. l.
MCCAW, J. A.—*Ophth. Rec.*, June 1915 ; and abstract, *Brit. Journ. Ophth.*, 1918, vol. ii. p. 281.
MAYNARD, F. P.—*Indian Med. Gaz.*, 1909.
RUBEN, L.—*Thirty-eighth Ophth. Congress*, Heidelberg, p. 133.
SCALINCI, N.—*Actes du XII Congrès International d'Ophtalmologie*, Petrograd, 1914.
SCHNABEL, W. J.—*Arch. f. Augenh.*, 1892, vol. xxiv. ; and *Wien. Med. Woch.*, 1900.
SCHNABEL, W. J.—*Zeitschr. f. Augenh.*, April and June 1908.
SEDWICK, W. A.—*Ophth. Rec.*, vol. xxi. p. 187.
STIRLING, A. W.—*R.L.O.H. Reports*, 1893, vol. xiii. p. 419.
THOMAS, H. G.—*Journ. of Ophth. and Oto-Laryngol.*, vol. v. p. 205.
THOMSON, ARTHUR.—*The Ophthalmoscope*, 1910, vol. viii. pp. 608 et seq.; *ibid.* 1911, vol. ix. pp. 470 et seq.; *The Anatomy of the Human Eye*, Clarendon Press, Oxford, 1912.
VON GRAEFE, A.—*Archiv f. O.*, Berlin, 1858, B. IV. Abth. 2, S. 127.
VON GRAEFE, A.—*New Sydenham Soc. Proc.*, 1859, p. 368.

Part III

The Pathological Anatomy of Glaucoma (*continued*)

6. Closure of the Filtration Angle

No discussion of the part which the filtration angle plays in the causation of glaucoma would be complete without the mention of four classic names :—Leber, who, in 1873, first demonstrated the function of this angle as the filtration area of the eye ; Knies and Weber, who, working independently on the clue thus afforded them, discovered simultaneously the frequency with which the angle of the anterior chamber was obstructed in glaucomatous eyes (A.D. 1876) ; and Priestley Smith, whose careful, painstaking, and accurate life-work has made to science a contribution of nearly everything worthy of credence that is to-day comprised in our knowledge of the pathology of glaucoma. So true is this statement that the writer feels the impossibility of fully acknowledging his indebtedness to Mr. Priestley Smith in what appears in the following pages. There is no branch of the subject that has not been illumined by his researches. The work that he did in his early years has never yet been seriously challenged, and commands to-day, as it rightly should, the practically unqualified acceptance of all those who are best fitted to give an opinion on the subject. His views may be summarised as follows :—

(1) Closure of the filtration angle is, in all early cases, caused by the *base of the iris* being *pressed against the periphery of the cornea*. At first, the closure thus brought about is simply mechanical (Fig. 15). The surfaces are in apposition, and the free escape of aqueous is thus impeded, but no more ; for the fluid from the aqueous chamber can readily make its way along the meshes of the loose iris stroma, and can thus find a free passage through the open mouths of the crypts of the iris into the loose structure of the cribriform ligament, and thence

into Schlemm's canal. Such is the condition with which we have to deal in the very early stages of a case of congestive glaucoma, and up to quite a late stage in simple glaucoma.

(2) The apposed surfaces of *iris base and corneal periphery become adherent to each other* as the result of a plastic exudation thrown out between the two membranes (Fig. 16, *B*). This occurs very early in acute cases (Fig. 17), more slowly in the subacute, and only after a considerable lapse of time in the simple glaucomas. In

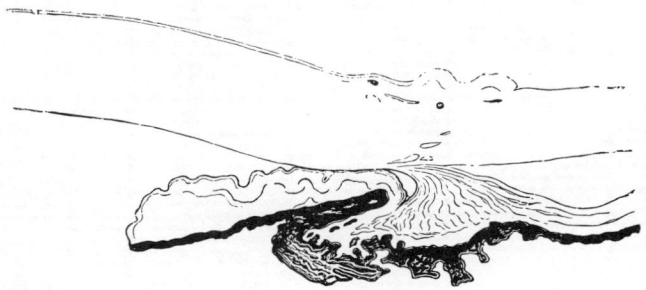

FIG. 15.—Primary glaucoma: acute; recent. (Priestley Smith.)
Ciliary processes swollen and advanced; iris base pressed against cornea, but not adherent to it. The eye was excised ten days after the beginning of the attack. It had been affected previously with senile cataract, nearly mature. At the time of excision: T+3; great pain and injection; V=0; anterior chamber very shallow; pupil dilated and irresponsive to eserin.

all alike, however, it is merely a question of time, for closure of the filtration angle occurs sooner or later in nearly all, if not in all, unrelieved primary glaucomas. As might have been expected, the firmness of the adhesions formed varies greatly in different cases. In the simple attacks, not merely do these adhesions appear late, but they are so easily broken down that the manipulation of the eye, necessary for microscopic examination, is often sufficient to detach the iris base from the cornea, and thus to give a false impression of openness of the angle, which belies the true condition that existed *in vivo*. In any case, the adhesions first formed may be very peripheral and may

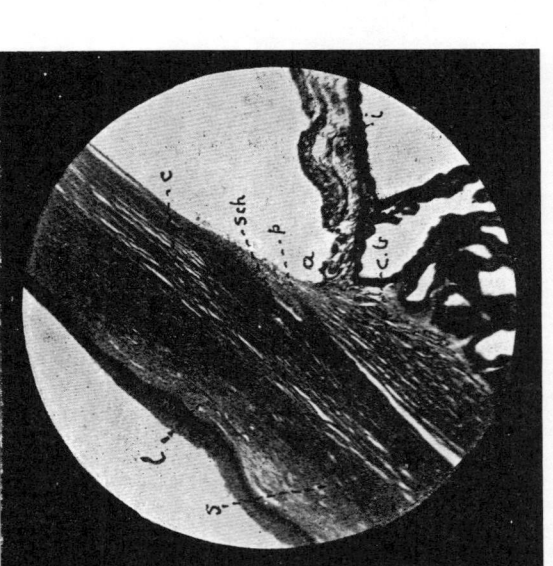

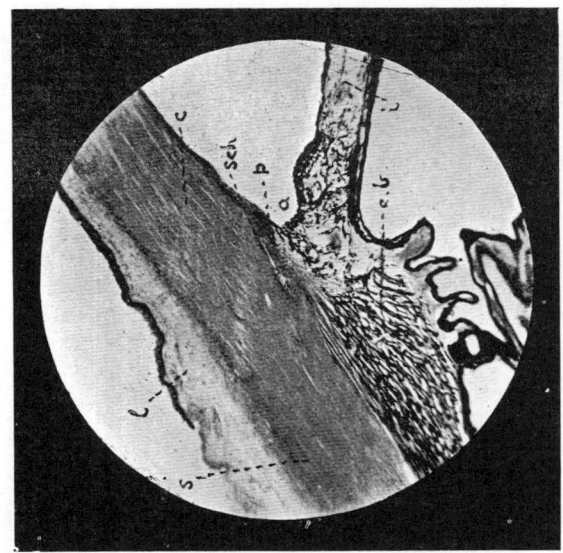

Fig. 16.—Angle of chamber: *A*, Open; *B*, Closed.

s, Sclera; *l*, limbus; *c*, cornea; *sch*, canal of **Schlemm**; *p*, pectinate ligament; *a*, angle of chamber; *c.b*, ciliary body; *i*, iris. Note that in *A* the angle is widely open, and the pectinate ligament is freely bathed by the fluid of the chamber; whilst in *B* the base of the iris is adherent to the pectinate ligament, thus shutting the canal of Schlemm off from the aqueous fluid.

(*From original photos by E. E.*)

not extend round the entire circumference of the eye.
As time goes on the belt of adhesion widens and becomes
firmer and firmer, whilst the whole periphery of the
anterior chamber eventually becomes involved.

(3) A further stage is believed to have been reached
when the *iris tissue* is not merely in contact with and
sealed to the periphery of the cornea, but is also *firmly
compressed* against it in such a way as to occlude the
spaces which normally allow the free passage of fluid
through the iris stroma (Fig. 18). How important
this compression may be will be better understood by

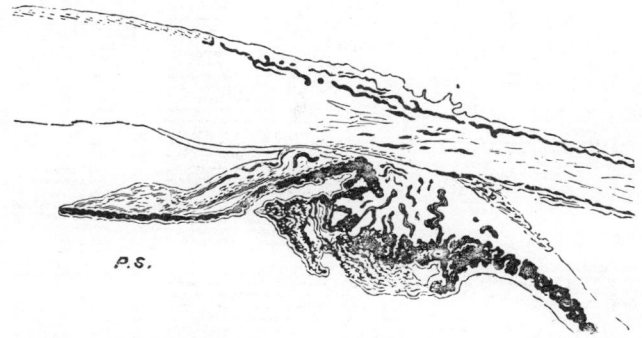

FIG. 17.—Primary glaucoma: acute; duration about 12 months.
(Priestley Smith.)

Filtration angle closed by adhesion; ciliary processes moulded into a wedge-like form by compression between lens and iris.

a reference to the writings of Hamburger, who compares a healthy iris to a "suction sponge" with its pores directly immersed in the aqueous. Anyone who is accustomed to examine the iris through a high powered corneal microscope, with the aid of an efficient illumination, such as that provided by the Gullstrand slit lamp, will be perfectly prepared to accept the simile used by Hamburger as being probably an accurate presentation of the condition present. For our fuller knowledge of the results of compression of the iris, we are indebted to Fuchs, who first described it in connection with glaucoma, secondary to leucoma adherens. He pointed out, that so long as the iris tissue remains normal in structure, which it may do even after it has become adherent to the cornea, the fluid from the anterior chamber can find its way freely along the loose meshwork of its stroma, and thus pass from it into and through the ligamentum pectinatum. This is the more easily possible, since "in many places, corresponding to the peripheral crypts, the anterior layer of the iris is absent, and the aqueous humour contained within the iris is therefore in immediate contact with the ligament." In the cases Fuchs studied, the determining factor of the onset of glaucoma was the state of the iris, which "looked normal or even a little distended in cases with normal tension, whilst it was compressed and atrophied in cases with excess of pressure." He considered "the atrophic change to be the effect—not the cause—of the hypertonia." Priestley Smith has applied Fuchs' observations to cases of ordinary glaucoma; he would appear to be perfectly correct in doing so. The third stage then, would be that of compression of the adherent iris. Such compression would have a double effect :—(i.) It would impede the normal excretion of fluid, by opposing a barrier to its passage through the iris stroma, on its way to the pectinate ligament and so to the canal of Schlemm, and (ii.) it would interfere with the vascular circulation throughout the tissue of the iris, and thus pave the way for the next stage of the process, viz., atrophy of the iris.

(4) *Atrophy of the iris tissue.*—This late stage, like every other of the processes we have been describing, is reached much earlier in the acute and subacute forms of glaucoma than in the simple chronic form. It is merely an expression, as has already been suggested, of interference with the normal circulation through the part (Fig. 19).

(5) The final stage is a *drawing back of the iris when the ciliary processes retract*; this process may be so extreme as to lead to the iris being greatly stretched or even torn through, as may be seen in Fig. 19.

The question, which next presents itself to our notice, is the very important one :

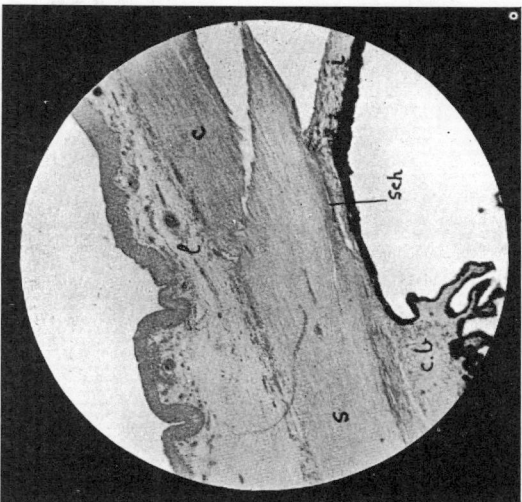

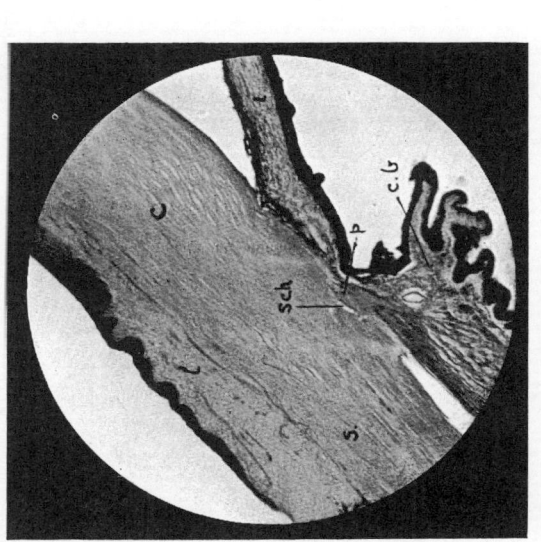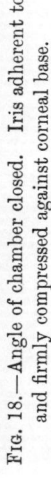

Fig. 18.—Angle of chamber closed. Iris adherent to and firmly compressed against corneal base.

Note the indentation opposite the pectinate ligament; this is due to the greater yielding at this spot under pressure, the spaces in the pectinate ligament being thereby closed.

Fig. 19.—Angle firmly closed. Iris and ciliary body atrophic; the latter much retracted. The scar of an unsuccessful operation wound is seen.

s, Sclera; l, limbus; c, cornea; sch, canal of Schlemm; p, pectinate ligament; a, angle of chamber; c.b, ciliary body; i, iris.

(The above two figures are from original photos by E. E. of specimens kindly lent by Mr. Treacher Collins.)

How is the Closure of the Filtration Angle brought about?

The answer varies with the form of glaucoma we are discussing. We will therefore take each in turn.

(1) In congestive glaucoma, the ciliary processes are enlarged, owing to the increased supply of blood to the parts, and their apices extend farther forward than usual. They thus come into contact with the iris anteriorly, and sometimes with the lens margin internally, and so may acquire a wedge-like shape from compression between these two structures (Figs. 15 and 17). Moreover, the processes become thickened transversely, with the result that the spaces between them are narrowed or obliterated. This explains the pushing forward of the iris base which occurs so early in congestive cases, and which is accompanied by a corresponding shallowing of the anterior chamber. But this is not all. The position will be more easily appreciated if we put it thus :—(*a*) The congestion of the ciliary processes leads to their turgescence ; (*b*) the result is a displacement forwards and inwards of their apices ; (*c*) this carries the iris directly forwards and so tends to jam its base against the periphery of the cornea ; and (*d*) it, at the same time, causes an advancement of the lens in its zonule, which helps to shallow the anterior chamber. A vicious circle is thus established. At the same time, the changes which will be discussed in the next paragraph, are operative also in the cases we have been discussing, but are thrown into the shade by the manifestations of the congestive process.

(2) In simple glaucoma, the displacement forwards of the iris is a result of the enlargement and advance of the lens, which take place as life progresses (Fig. 21). In the early stages, these changes involve no serious compression of the iris ; fluid can still gain access to the pectinate ligament through the open iris crypts, even when the iris and cornea are in actual contact peripherally. Later on, as the tension increases, the area of iris contact grows wider, the channels in the iris stroma gradually become

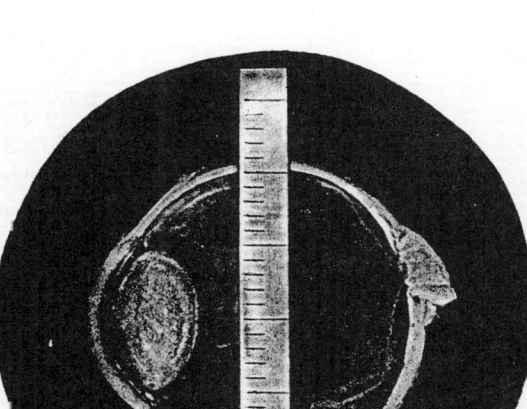

FIG. 21.—Primary glaucoma: horizontal section. Age 60. Refraction, Hm. = 4 D., about. (The healthy fellow eye has Hm. = 4 D., and the patient is confident that the two eyes were alike before the attack.) Glaucoma of subacute type began about eight months ago, and the eye became quite blind with severe pain and congestion about one month before excision.

In order to realise fully the exceptional relations of the lens in this eye, one ought to imagine the atrophied ciliary body replaced by one of ordinary size. (Priestley Smith.)

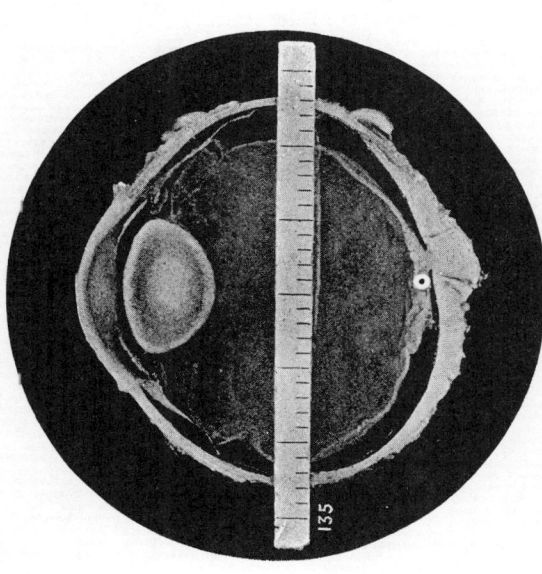

FIG. 20.—Healthy eye: horizontal section. Age 25. Refraction emmetropic. (Priestley Smith.)

compressed and closed, and the applied surfaces become adherent to each other. These adhesions may, however, be so slight that they readily separate during the preparation of the eye for examination. In the final stages of simple chronic glaucoma, congestive attacks, sometimes very mild in character, may supervene, due to the increased compression to which the iris is subjected.

In all cases of glaucoma alike, the relative size of the eye is an important factor ; this will be dealt with later under its appropriate section. Nor must vascular, secretory, and degenerative conditions be left out of count, but these too will find a mention each in its proper place. For the present, we are concerned with the pathological condition of the angle of the chamber, and the questions which arise therefrom.

To summarise in the briefest possible manner what has gone before, we may say :—(1) That all forms of glaucoma (with certain rare exceptions which will be discussed later) are eventually brought about by a closure of the filtration angle ; (2) that such a closure is due (*a*) in congestive cases to a swelling of the ciliary processes, and (*b*) in simple cases to an alteration in the size and position of the lens.

In order to make the position quite clear, we shall now, even at the cost of some repetition, set down categorically the evidence for and against the above propositions, commencing with that in their favour, and then passing on to that which is adverse to them :

(1) Closure of the filtration angle occurs at some stage in nearly all, if not in all, cases of primary glaucoma, provided the condition remains unrelieved.

(2) It appears (clinically) to be an early feature of the acute and subacute forms of congestive glaucoma ; in these it becomes permanent if left alone ; but if relieved, the angle reopens, and the glaucoma passes away.

(3) The common antecedents of an acute attack of glaucoma, *i.e.*, nervous and vascular disturbances, as well as the consequences of the ill-advised use of mydriatics,

THE ÆTIOLOGY OF GLAUCOMA

find a ready explanation on the theory of closure of the angle, but not otherwise.

(4) Closure of the angle is "the one common feature in the morbid anatomy of secondary glaucoma" (Parsons).

(5) In simple glaucoma, a peripheral adhesion is almost always present in the final stage of the complaint, and appears to arise, as in acute glaucoma, from a pushing forward of the iris base by the ciliary processes.

(6) A closure of the angle, as the result of very slightly raising the vitreous pressure above that in the anterior chamber, can be demonstrated in the dead eye; it at once stops all passage of fluid through the eye, and is associated with a shallowing of the anterior chamber.

(7) A marked shallowing of the anterior chamber is a feature common, sooner or later, to both the simple and the congestive types of glaucoma.

(8) In all forms of glaucoma, a small size of the eye is found to be a prevalent feature. The influence of this on closure of the angle will be discussed shortly in the appropriate section.

(9) Slight contact between the iris base and the cornea will account for doubtful, slight, and varying rises of tension at an early stage in chronic cases; whilst later, a slowly increasing compression of the iris base will explain (*a*) the gradual rise in tension often met with, (*b*) the slow formation of a peripheral and widening band of iris adhesion, and (*c*) the ultimate access of pain and congestion.

(10) The fundamental process at work seems to be the same in almost all cases of glaucoma, although the rate of progress of the rise in pressure and the part borne by vascular disturbances vary very greatly in different eyes.

Criticism of the Foregoing Evidence

The evidence we have just adduced, in favour of the supposition that a closure of the filtration angle is the cause of glaucoma, is not beyond criticism.

(1) It may be suggested that the *actual anatomical evidence is scanty*, and that we have relied largely on

clinical data in order to form a conception of the pathological conditions, which our train of reasoning would lead us to believe is present. This is partly true, and the explanation is fairly obvious, for (i.) we seldom if ever get material for investigation at an early stage of glaucoma ; (ii.) it is very difficult to obtain a view of the iris base and of the ciliary processes in the living eye ; and (iii.) when the globe is removed for examination, the relationship of the parts is greatly altered, (*a*) by reason of the loss of blood, which necessarily takes place, (*b*) by changes in the pressure within the globe on its removal, (*c*) by changes occurring under hardening reagents, or under freezing and thawing, and (*d*) by further changes which take place when the hemisphere is divided into yet smaller parts before cutting.

(2) In addition to all this, *one worker may criticise another's methods* of preparation of specimens, and by showing that his technique is faulty, may maintain that his deductions are unreliable. This line has been taken with reference to Priestley Smith's work, and it has been suggested that there have been two sources of fallacy therein, viz. :—(i.) A possible want of strict meridionality in the sections made, and (ii.) an absence of sufficient serial sectioning to justify a correct reconstruction of the parts. Priestley Smith has answered these objections, detailing his method of preparing specimens in doing so. The most important point is that some of the eyes have been examined after an equatorial section, which permits the ciliary region to be studied by the naked eye from behind, and so avoids the source of fallacy to which objection has been taken.

(3) It has from time to time been *suggested that the closure of the filtration angle is a consequence and not a cause of glaucoma.* A review of the arguments in favour of the closure of the angle being causative of the rise in intra-ocular pressure has been put forward above, and each surgeon must draw his own conclusions. To the writer's mind, the evidence, although circumstantial, is overwhelming.

(4) It has been pointed out that *a closed angle is sometimes found in eyes which have never been hard,* and the inference has been drawn that under the circumstances it would be wrong to conclude, that closure of the angle leads to a rise in ocular tension. The suggestion is that it is merely an accidental coincidence. The reply to this is, (i.) that in some of these eyes an artificial exit for the escape of fluid exists ; *e.g.*, the presence (*a*) of a minute fistula, or (*b*) of what has been termed a " pseudo-cornea," in which the new tissue, stripped of endothelium, is no longer impervious to fluid ; (ii.) that in others the secretion of the ciliary body has been arrested by disease ; and (iii.) that in still others, the iris, though in contact with the pectinate ligament, and adherent to it, has never been compressed, and consequently has not really interfered with the access of the aqueous to Schlemm's canal.

(5) On the other hand *an open angle has been demonstrated anatomically in eyes blinded by glaucoma.* Such instances present no real difficulty. Each case must be dealt with and explained on its own merits. (i.) In some of the eyes, it is suggested that an albuminous fluid, unfit for filtration, has replaced the normal aqueous. (ii.) In others a closure of the angle, which existed during life, has been broken down in the course of the preparation of the specimen. Priestley Smith examined 54 eyes, which had been lost by primary glaucoma, and found that only 5 of them had an open angle ; of these, 3 showed a displacement of pigment, which strongly suggested that the separated surfaces of iris and cornea, found in the laboratory, were really in contact in the living eye ; the remaining 2 were probably cases of secondary glaucoma. (iii.) In serous iridocyclitis, the cells which are derived from the inflamed parts, may pass forward into the anterior chamber, and be found in large numbers in the meshes of the pectinate ligament (Fig. 22). It requires very little effort of the imagination to believe that such a process may greatly interfere with the normal course of the escape of fluid from the sinus of the chamber. The closely allied topic of blocking of the angle of the chamber by particles

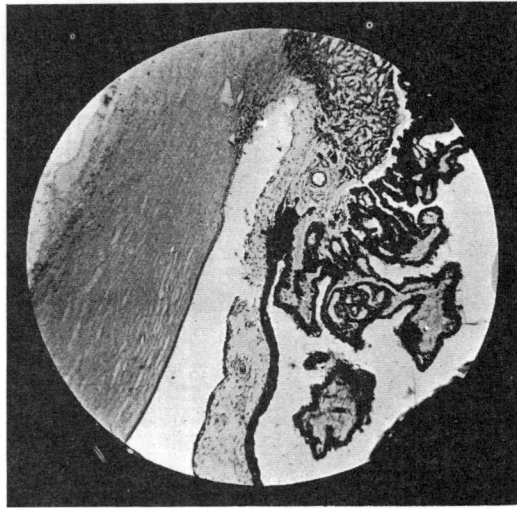

FIG. 23.—Narrowing of angle of chamber preceding glaucoma.

The fellow eye was glaucomatous; this eye had not yet shown signs of glaucoma, but the pressure of the congested ciliary body on the base of the iris is evidently in danger of cutting off the sinus from the rest of the chamber, and so of obstructing the ocular filtration.

(*Photo by E. E. from specimen kindly supplied by Mr. Treacher Collins.*)

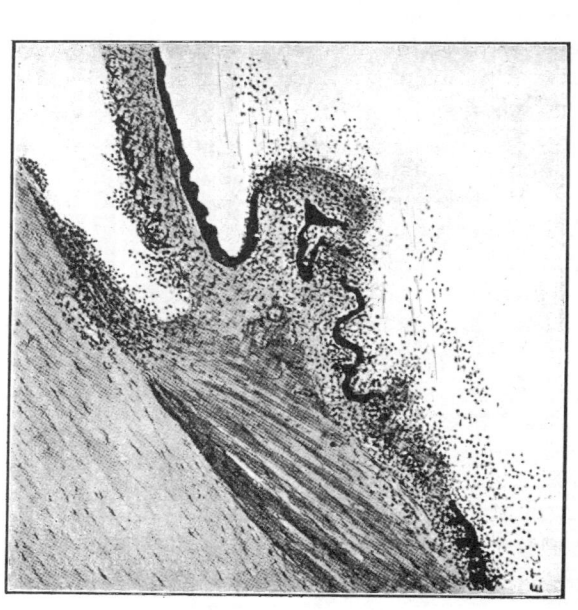

FIG. 22.—Section showing the ciliary body and angle of the anterior chamber in a case of serous cyclitis.

The vascular tissue on the inner surface of the ciliary muscle is much infiltrated with inflammatory cells. The pigment epithelium lining the ciliary body shows areas of degeneration. Cellular inflammatory exudate is shown on the inner surface of the ciliary body and about the angle of the anterior chamber. The mesh of the ligamentum pectinatum is filled with cells, and accumulations of them have formed on the back of Descemet's membrane and on the anterior surface of the iris. (*Kindly supplied by Mr. Treacher Collins.*)

of iris pigment has been dwelt on at length by Koeppe, Schieck and Levinsohn, and the claim has been put forward that an observation of this process during life may enable a very early diagnosis of glaucoma to be made. The subject will be again taken up in the chapter on Diagnosis (p. 219). (iv.) When the integrity of the vitreous body is interfered with, strands of hyaloid material may pass forward into the angle of the chamber (*e.g*, after laceration of an after-cataract), or modified vitreous cells may be found in the meshes of the pectinate ligament (*e.g.*, after traumatic dislocation of the lens into the vitreous) (Hudson). Either of these conditions might easily be conceived as opposing a mechanical barrier to the normal escape of fluid from the eye. (See Chapter V. Part II.)

7. SHALLOWING OF THE ANTERIOR CHAMBER OF THE EYE

A shallowing of the anterior chamber of the eye is an anatomical feature which is met with, sooner or later, in the vast majority of cases of glaucoma. The subject has frequently been referred to in the preceding pages, and it has been pointed out that the phenomenon we are now discussing occurs very early in acute and in subacute congestive glaucoma, and at a much later period, but still with great constancy, in the simple form of the affection. It is very closely associated with the closure of the angle of the chamber. The pressure on the iris base, which leads to the latter, must obviously have the effect of diminishing the depth of the chamber. The shallowness so produced favours a wider adhesion between the iris base and the periphery of the cornea. We here meet with yet another instance of the establishment of a vicious circle in the evolution of this disease. It is sometimes pointed out that cases are seen in every clinic, in which the anterior chamber is not perceptibly shallowed in eyes which are the seat of unquestionable glaucoma. This subject has been dealt with in the previous section. In addition to what has there been said it must be remembered that it is not always easy to decide whether the angle of the chamber is interfered with or not. It does not necessarily follow that a chamber, which is shallow centrally, has its angle obliterated, or that a chamber which has a fair depth centrally, has a free angle. The use of modern diagnostic methods will, however, sometimes help us to decide these points. This matter will be dealt with in a later chapter, and need not detain us now.

Mr. Priestley Smith, in a personal communication, kindly placed at the writer's disposal the following summary of his views on the shallowing of the anterior chamber. It is felt that it would be a work of supererogation either to comment on the statement, or to attempt to add to it, and it is therefore published exactly as it has been received, with merely a cordial acknowledgment of the kindness which prompted the sending of it:

" In primary glaucoma the anterior chamber is usually shallow. In the main this is a pre-existing and predisposing condition—a cause rather than a consequence—as proved by the fact that persons suffering as yet in one eye only, usually have a shallow chamber in both. It is a physiological condition proper to the life-period in which primary glaucoma commonly arises. The explanation lies, in part at least, in the continuous growth of the lens. That the chamber is shallower in some eyes than in others at the same time of life may be explained by the fact that lenses belonging to the same life-period, differ considerably not only in total bulk but in the ratio of their axial and transverse diameters ; some are relatively thick but small transversely, others thin and wide.

" Another possible cause for the senile shallowing of the chamber, and for individual differences, is this :— The lens is held in position chiefly by the innumerable cords which pass at various angles from its peripheral zone to the ciliary processes, and—as experiments have shown—when the processes advance the lens advances with them. Now the processes alter in size and shape with the advance of life ; they are more prominent and bulky in the old than in the young; moreover individual eyes belonging to the same life-period present great differences in this respect.

" It is likely that these changes in the processes involve change in the position of the lens.

" But the physiological shallowing of the chamber is only half the question. In acute congestive glaucoma the chamber becomes shallower *during the attack*. The iris no doubt is partly responsible; it becomes thicker as the pupil dilates; it may thicken still more through venous hyperæmia; its periphery is carried forward by the swollen processes. But this is not all. The chamber becomes shallower in the area of the pupil; the lens moves forward. Why is this? High pressure in the chamber does not explain it unless we assume an excess of vitreous over aqueous pressure.

" We know that a slight excess of this kind suffices to displace the lens and processes, to close the filtration angle, and therewith to arrest escape of fluid from the eye. A likely cause for such excess in acute glaucoma is found in the condition of the circumlental space. In elderly people the space between lens and processes is narrowed by the increased volume of the lens; it is further narrowed, sometimes in marked degree, by the increased bulk of the processes. The grooves between the processes become narrower for the same reason (Hess); during an acute glaucoma the processes are turgid with blood and have been found jammed against each other laterally and against the lens. Under these conditions it is likely that vitreous fluid is unable to enter the aqueous chamber —that it is imprisoned behind the lens and drives it forward.

" This explanation, suggested by the writer many years ago, is, however, not the only possible explanation. When the ciliary processes (in the rabbit) are rendered turgid by ligaturing the vortex veins, their apices advance and the lens advances with them (Koster). The same result has been obtained by cauterising the limbus of the eye externally, and when only one-half of the circle was cauterised the swelling of the processes was limited to this half, and the lens was tilted forward *at this side only* (Grönholm). These observations, the latter especially, suggest that when the processes become turgid and advance, the lens is carried forward by reason of its attachment to them.

"In any case they show that extreme swelling of the processes even in a healthy eye (of a rabbit) shallows the chamber, 'closes the filtration-angle, compresses the base of the iris, and arrests the escape of fluid from the chambers, so as to produce an exaggerated picture of acute glaucoma."

It remains to add that Morax holds a different view about the shallowing of the anterior chamber in glaucoma. He believes that, whilst it is an important sign in the acute and subacute attacks of the disease, it has no significance outside these limitations, save in the cases of secondary glaucoma, in which the iris is involved.

8. The Dimensions of Eyes in Glaucomatous Patients

According to Priestley Smith—

(1) The eyes of women are, on the average, a little smaller than those of men ; this is in correspondence with the relative size of the bodies in the two sexes.

(2) The eyes of glaucomatous persons are, on the average, a little smaller than those of the non-glaucomatous. He found the average horizontal diameter of the cornea to be 11·17 mm. in the glaucomatous, and 11·6 mm. in the non-glaucomatous.

(3) The last statement is equally true of the acute and of the chronic forms of the disease.

(4) Smallness of the eye is not an ever-present factor in primary glaucoma, but it is a determining factor in a considerable number of cases, and must be taken into account in any complete explanation of the disease.

(5) It is due to defective growth, and not to senile shrinkage of the eye.

THE ÆTIOLOGY OF GLAUCOMA

(6) There is no hard and fast line between eyes which are a little below the normal in size, and those which can be unhesitatingly classed as microphthalmic. All intermediate forms can be traced without difficulty. The percentage of very small corneas is much greater in the glaucomatous than in those with healthy eyes.

(7) The decisive factor in determining the onset of glaucoma is not the absolute size of the eye, but its size relative to that of the lens it contains. The subject must therefore be again considered when dealing with the next section.

9. THE CONTINUOUS GROWTH OF THE LENS THROUGHOUT LIFE

Thomson has found that " in the full time fœtus, the cornea amounts to about one-fifth of the circumference of the globe on section ; its transverse diameter measures about 10·6 mm. in the specimens examined, so that there is comparatively little increase in its growth requisite to reach the adult proportions. It follows then that the increase in the size of the globe after birth is mainly due to an expansion of the scleral part of the eyeball and of its contents." Again, according to Priestley Smith, the cornea increases little, if at all, in its diameters after the age of five, and possibly diminishes slightly after forty. The sclera is probably fully grown somewhat before the rest of the body. It is obvious that, since these two structures determine the size of the eye, the growth of the globe ceases even before that of the body generally. The lens, on the contrary, continues to increase in size up to an advanced period of life ; nor need this difference between it and the rest of the globe cause us any surprise, since it is ectodermal in origin, whilst they arise from the mesoderm.

" The salient fact is that while the lens grows larger as life advances, the globe does *not*, so that the older the eye becomes, the more likely it is to suffer from the disproportion in question ; and the smaller it is, the earlier in life is the disproportion likely to arise " (Priestley Smith). Now an enlargement or an advance of the lens tends to push the iris base into contact with the periphery of the cornea, a tendency which will obviously be exaggerated in eyes with a restricted corneal periphery (Fig. 21). The consequences would be easy to foretell, viz., (1) at an early stage, a mechanical closure of the angle of the chamber, leading to an obstruction to the free flow of fluid towards the canal of Schlemm, and (2) at a later period, a compression of the iris tissue, resulting in a still more serious interference with the excretory currents of the eye.

It is probable that the changes we have just been discussing are operative in the causation of all attacks of glaucoma, but it is in the chronic non-congestive forms that the rôle of changes in the size or position of the lens bulks the largest. In the congestive attacks they are overshadowed by the evidences of the vascular storm, whilst in the simple cases they are not thus obscured.

REFERENCES

FUCHS, E.—*The Ophthalmoscope*, 1908, vol. vi. pp. 742–746.
GRÖNHOLM, V.—Abstract in Nagel's *Jahresbericht* for 1901, p. 552.
HENDERSON, T.—*Glaucoma*. Edward Arnold, London, 1910.
HESS, C.—*Arch. f. Augenh.*, 1910, vol. lxvii. p. 341; and abstract in *Ophth. Rev.*, Jan. 1913.
HUDSON, A. C.—*R.L.O.H. Reports*, vol. xviii. part 2.
KOEPPE, L.—*Heidelberg Ophth. Congress*, 1916; and *Arch. of Ophth.*, vol. xlvii. p. 106.
KOSTER, W.—Von Graefe's *Archiv f. O.*, 1895, vol. xli. part 2, p. 30.
LEVINSOHN, G.—" Pathogenesis of Glaucoma," *Klin. Monatsbl. f. Augenh.*, 1918, vol. lxi. pp. 174–180.
MORAX, V.—*Glaucome et Glaucomateux*, Librairie, Octave Doin, Paris, 1921.
SCHIECK.—*Klin. Monatsbl. f. Augenh.*, 1918, vol. lxi. p. 332.
SMITH, PRIESTLEY.—*Glaucoma*, 1891 (J. & A. Churchill); " Glaucoma Problems," *Ophth. Rev.*, 1910, 1911, and 1912.
THOMSON, ARTHUR.—*The Anatomy of the Human Eye*, p. 9. Clarendon Press.

Part IV

In the two preceding parts of this chapter, we have discussed certain factors in connection with the pathological anatomy of glaucoma, and we are now in a position to investigate the ætiology of the disease. Other pathological points remain for consideration, but these are being reserved for the sections to which they appear most appropriately to belong.

We shall now take, one by one, the factors, which are usually accepted as causative of glaucoma, and study each in turn, bearing in mind throughout that a pathological access of ocular tension may be determined either by (a) an interference with the balance normally held between secretion and excretion in the eye, or (b) by an obstruction to the escape of blood from the eye, or (c) by a combination of these influences.

The Causes of Glaucoma

(1) **Age.**—Age takes precedence over all known causes of this disease. Of this there can be no shadow of doubt. Priestley Smith's researches settled the question nearly a quarter of a century ago : To quote his words—the frequency of glaucoma increases "slowly at first, more rapidly later in each decade, until about the sixtieth year. Between sixty and seventy, it is about as frequent as between fifty and sixty. After seventy its frequency diminishes." It must be obvious, that the figures for the later decades of life cannot be rightly compared with those for the earlier, in estimating the frequency of the disease, because for each succeeding decade, the number of persons living is rapidly contracting until, after seventy, it is very small indeed. Moreover, the old are, for a variety of reasons, unable or unwilling to seek help to the same extent that younger people do.

More recently Haag has analysed a series of 1032 cases of primary glaucoma. He found that 4 occurred in the first decade of life, 16 in the second, 26 in the third, 74 in the fourth, 176 in the fifth, 288 in the sixth, 329 in the seventh, 116 in the eighth, and 3 later. He thus supplies a very interesting confirmation of Priestley Smith's work, which in its turn was founded on no less than 1000 cases, scattered through the practice of a large number of surgeons. The fact that Haag's figures are from a single clinic and are serial, lends them an additional value.

Kagoshima's recent statistics, taken from 21,455 private patients, though less detailed than the foregoing, are in close agreement with them.

It is one thing to decide, that beyond any shadow of doubt, the advance of life stands in a strong causal relationship to glaucoma, but quite another to form in one's mind, a clear and orderly conception of the inner meaning of this connection. In order to do so, we must pass in review all the possible factors of the case, and endeavour to attribute to each its share in the whole. It should, at the same time, be carefully remembered that our arguments must, in the absence of better data, be founded very largely on inferences drawn from clinical observation. This has been said before in the course of this book; it is repeated here, not with a view of casting doubt on the deductions arrived at, which the writer believes to be sane and well founded, but in order that we should at no time lose a sense of the true position we occupy. If the conclusions arrived at are to carry conviction, it is obvious that they must be reached by simple, logical and obvious processes of thought.

How does the Advance of Life cause Glaucoma?

That is the question we must now put, and the possible answers are so many, that it will be necessary to consider them under a number of headings and sub-headings :—

(A) Advancing age may act by bringing about *alterations in the anatomical conditions* of the parts. Amongst such we may class the following :—(*a*) Enlargement of the lens; (*b*) slackening of the zonule of the lens, allowing an advance of its anterior surface, or of its whole bulk;

and (c) thickening of the fibres which constitute the pectinate ligament.

It is not only conceivable, but it is also probable, that each one of these factors is operative, to a greater or less extent, in most cases of glaucoma. They have already been discussed, and it is therefore unnecessary to deal with them any further now.

(B) Next to be considered is the *influence of degenerative changes*. Under this heading we include (a) an increase in the volume of fluid secreted by the eye, as a result of:—
(i.) Nervous irritation of secretory fibres, (ii.) degeneration of glandular elements, or (iii.) alterations in the vaso-motor conditions present ; and (b) an alteration in the nature of the secretion poured out by the ciliary body.

We shall take these in turn.

(a) An increase of secretion may be conceived to be the result of one or another of the factors enumerated, or of a combination of several factors. The view that an increase in the amount of fluid poured into the eye might bring about a pathological rise in tension, first saw the light in the days of von Graefe and Donders. The former attributed the excess of fluid so produced to a serous choroiditis, whilst the latter was in favour of the theory, that an irritation of the secretory nerves of the eye was to blame. During the years which followed, many workers and writers took the same line. The bibliography has been excellently surveyed by Parsons. After a time these views fell into disrepute, and long remained so, under the influence of the overshadowing rôle accorded to the obstruction offered to excretion by the closure of the angle. Quite recently, however, there has appeared an inclination on the part of prominent ophthalmologists to reconsider this question. Priestley Smith has spread the ægis of his advocacy over the long discredited views of Donders in the following words :—" Over-production of the intra-ocular fluid is at least a possible cause of chronic glaucoma—as suggested long ago by Donders." About the same time, Bjerrum (1912) advanced the view that glaucoma arises from an inflammatory process, which especially affects the ciliary body, and so leads to hyper-secretion from that structure. Two years later Kuemmell gave utterance to almost identical views on this subject. Still more recently, Verhoeff, writing in connection with the question of the efficiency of the drainage of the eye after sclerostomy operations, raised the question of " the rate of total secretion against a given pressure," and said " it by no means necessarily follows, that because two glaucomatous eyes have equal intra-ocular pressures, their rates of secretion will be equal, especially against equal lower pressures." The above remarks of Verhoeff's are primarily directed to the question of the prognosis after operations for glaucoma, but they have a much wider interest, inasmuch as they show the recurrence of a tendency amongst leading pathologists to lay stress on variations in secretory activity as a possible factor in the causation of glaucoma. The fact that ophthalmologists, so widely scattered as those whose names have been mentioned above, and each with so high a reputation in pathology, should have given utterance to the views that have been mentioned, is in itself sufficient to make us seriously review the position; and indeed, there would seem to be much in favour of the idea that excess of secretion may be not infrequently a factor, and sometimes a very powerful factor, in the causation of glaucoma.

The writer has been not a little impressed by a recent case in his own practice, in which a perfectly smooth trephining operation was complicated by an injury to the patient's eye from the hat of a lady visitor. The chamber filled with blood, which soon cleared away, but, in spite of quite good filtration, the tension remained high. There were probably other features in the case, but it was difficult to exclude the possibility that an increased secretion had resulted from the injury.

Prima facie, there would appear to be no reason why any one of the three factors we have mentioned should not be productive of an increase in secretion. Indeed, the analogy with other organs is all in favour of our hypothesis.

THE ÆTIOLOGY OF GLAUCOMA 125

It may be argued that the secretory function of the ciliary body is still under dispute. This matter has already been discussed in an earlier chapter. The conclusion there arrived at, after a careful consideration of the arguments on both sides, has been that the production of the intra-ocular fluid is probably to be regarded as a combination of pressure filtration and active secretion. If this view be the correct one, and there is good reason to think it is, then it requires but a little stretch of the imagination to believe that nervous impulses, such as we know by direct experiment powerfully influence the salivary and other glands, must also be taken into account in dealing with the ciliary body. This is admittedly a deduction, but inasmuch as the conditions present render any direct observation of the intra-ocular secretion impossible during life, at least with the means at present at our disposal, we are necessarily thrown back on deduction, and indeed it seems unlikely that we shall ever have a better foundation to build on.

In support of the suggestion that degenerative changes in the ciliary body may lead to excessive exudation in the chambers of the eye, Priestley Smith, in the article above quoted, has evoked the analogy of the kidney in chronic nephritis, and has maintained that even although fresh channels of excretion may be opened as a result of the increased force of secretion, the result will inevitably be a rise in intra-ocular pressure, due to the fact that the fluid is secreted under pressure higher than the normal.

As to the influence of alterations in vaso-motor control within the eye, it has been shown experimentally, that irritation of the fifth nerve or of the sympathetic may be productive of a marked increase of intra-ocular pressure. This has, quite reasonably, been attributed to the influence of local vaso-motor dilatation. In this connection, we have to take account of the powerful influence of nervous conditions on the progress of an attack of glaucoma. It is well known that sleeplessness, anxiety, fatigue, hunger, and other similar factors may determine the first onset of an attack of glaucoma, or may convert a simple into a congestive form of the disease. Again, we are all too familiar with the fact that very slight injuries to the head may eventuate in a wholly unexpected attack of glaucoma. Bearing in mind that a tendency to a loss of vaso-motor control is a constant accompaniment of the advance of life, it is not difficult to explain these phenomena. Once again, it is true that we are depending on deduction, but the physiological basis of our hypothesis would appear to be well founded and reliable.

To assign to any individual case the rôle played by cell degeneration, by nervous excitation of secretion, or by vaso-motor disturbances would be obviously impossible; but we can at least conclude that the two latter will, as a rule, lead to more transitory and erratic rises in tension, whilst degeneration of the glandular elements will tend to favour a slowly progressive and permanent condition of hypertonus.

(b) An alteration in the nature of the secretion poured into the eye has been adduced as one of the possible causes of primary glaucoma. It is generally assumed that such a change in the chemical constitution of the aqueous is a powerful factor in the production of hypertonus, secondary to chronic and subacute forms of iridocyclitis. From time to time, the suggestion has been made that a similar factor may be at work in some of the cases which are usually accepted as being primary in origin. Such a supposition has two strong points in its favour :—(1) That the border-line between certain cases of acknowledged secondary glaucoma, and certain other cases which are usually classed as primary glaucoma, is sometimes a very narrow one indeed; and (2) that in cases of congestive glaucoma, phenomena closely allied to those which characterise inflammation appear with great frequency. The readiness with which the formation of synechiæ occurs after operations for glaucoma is one of the many evidences of this.

It might be suggested that the question could be settled by experiments. A perusal of the work of Uribe Y. Troncosco, Scalinci, and others, negatives this suggestion.

THE ÆTIOLOGY OF GLAUCOMA

The difficulties of such a form of research are very great, and most surgeons will probably agree that, unless and until new methods are found of investigating this very difficult subject, comparatively little positive evidence of any value is likely to be forthcoming.

Priestley Smith has put forward the following hypothesis, which is best reproduced in his own words:—
" Chemically the aqueous and vitreous fluids are nearly, but not quite, identical, and they both proceed from the ciliary body; but, as already pointed out, they are probably produced by different zones, the aqueous by the processes, the more sluggish vitreous by the non-plicate zone. It is likely that senile degeneration may attack these zones separately or unequally, and that vitiation or overproduction of the vitreous fluid may occur with normal production of the aqueous. In the final stage of chronic glaucoma there is certainly sometimes undue retention of fluid in the vitreous chamber, for the aqueous chamber becomes inordinately shallow, and the vitreous, if we examine it in the bisected eye, shows signs of serous infiltration—but here again we must beware of mistaking consequences of high pressure for initial causes." In support of his position he cites some experiments made by Wessely, who, by injections into the vitreous, obtained an atrophy of the retina, choroid, and *pars plana*, with but little involvement of the ciliary processes. The vitreous body was totally abolished, while the production of the aqueous fluid was apparently unaffected.

These ideas are interesting and attractive, but manifestly and admittedly speculative. Once again, then, the only scientific position to take up is that of open-minded agnosticism. The time is not yet ripe for dogmatic assertion.

(c) It has been suggested that glaucoma is caused by a *pathological tendency to hydrophilism on the part of the tissues of the eye*. This tendency is supposed to be brought about by an overloading of the tissues with acid products of metabolism. It has been assumed that the tissues swell in consequence of the increased absorption of water.

If, for the sake of argument, we suppose that these premises are correct, we should not find it difficult to imagine, that the swelling of the tissues might impede the exit of the intra-ocular fluid by narrowing the channels of excretion, and that it might, at the same time, obstruct the circulation by constricting the blood vessels as they pass into or out of the eye ; in that case, the veins would evidently suffer sooner and more than the arteries, and a condition of venous congestion would thus be set up. It is well known that, as life progresses, the elimination of waste products from the tissues becomes increasingly difficult ; and so, if we were once to grant what Fischer and his followers have claimed, we should find the advance of years dominating this factor, as it does so many others. The influence of hydrophilism can, however, only be accepted with hesitation and reserve. As the subject has already been discussed in Part II. of this chapter, it need not be pursued further.

(D) Closely allied with the subject of the preceding section, is that of the various morbid conditions, which lead to *autogenetic intoxication*, and which are associated with low forms of inflammation. These may be conceived of as acting :—(*a*) By obstructing the paths of exit of the ocular fluids, or (*b*) by hampering the ciliary muscle and so lessening the action, which, on Arthur Thomson's authority, we presume that structure possesses of removing lymph from the eye. (See previous chapter.)

This matter has been admirably put by S. D. Risley in the following words :—" Glaucoma is a disease, coming on at an age when wear and tear, harassing vicissitudes, misfortunes, exposure, overwork, and vicious living have sapped the physiologic foundations of life ; when infections have found entrance to the structure of the organism through the doorway of the epithelium ; and when a variety of toxic, auto-intoxic, and other influences have set up vascular and cardiovascular disease, associated nephritis, uveitis, high blood-pressure, etc. Glaucoma, in fact, rarely occurs in individuals in good general health."

Again, Lagrange, always interesting and far-sighted in

his views on glaucoma, has said that an eye attacked by hypertension is a sick eye in a sick body. It is not merely a hypertonic, but also a sclerosed, dystrophic organ, which shares its troubles with the rest of the body—a body in which renal and cardiac disease, the calculous and arthritic diatheses and neuropathy play leading parts. The secretions of the organ are toxic and anisotonic, whilst the channels of excretion are blocked. Indeed, the cases which find a place in the group we are now discussing, are those which are most likely to be confused with, and which indeed are separated only by a fine boundary-line from one class of the secondary glaucomas. Once again, overshadowing the accepted or the suggested causes of the disease, we find the malign, relentless spectre of the advance of years.

Hertel's work on the influence on ocular tension of altered conditions of the blood has been dealt with in the previous chapter. There we spoke of the changes produced in the course of physiological experiments. We now turn to study the possibility that similar conditions may be set up as the result of pathological processes. Hertel thought that a morbid diminution of the concentration of the blood might play an ætiologic part in glaucoma. He studied young patients suffering from this disease, selecting those, who in other respects appeared healthy, and who presented a normal blood-pressure, and found in a number of such that the osmotic concentration and the albumin contents of the blood were below normal, whilst patients who suffered from nephritis, and whose blood concentration was high, had low ocular tensions, despite their high blood-pressure. His inference was that "thinning of the blood," whether sudden or chronic, might bring about a pathological rise in intra-ocular pressure. He believed that the escape of water from the vessels depends not only on the osmotic concentration of the blood, but also on the permeability of the blood vessels. He pointed out that psychic stimuli and cold increase the escape of water from the vessels, and so tend to cause glaucoma, whilst warm baths and blood-letting increase the reception of water from the tissues, and so act favourably on the course of the disease. The bearing of this work on the subject of auto-intoxication is obvious. It has this further charm, that it gives an element of precision to the somewhat vague and nebulous ideas which most of us hold on the relationship between the congeries of conditions which we label auto-intoxication and the onslaught of glaucoma.

The same may be said of E. von Hippel's work, in the course of which he supplemented a general clinical examination of the patient by the use of the Abderhalden reaction. The anatomical and serological conditions found present in glaucoma cases, suggested to him that a disturbance of the organs of internal secretion might be a causative factor of the disease.

(E) During the last few years, much attention has been concentrated on *the influence of the secretions of the ductless glands* on the problems of health and disease, and there have not been wanting suggestions that glaucoma, like many other affections, is caused or influenced by aberrations in the quantity or quality of these secretions. It is quite certain that no observant physician or surgeon of experience would be prepared to deny the possibility thus suggested. Hertel believes that the osmotic ebb and flow of the body fluids—inclusive of those of the aqueous and vitreous chambers—is influenced by the thyroid gland; he thinks that certain phases of the secretion of this gland may predispose to the occurrence of hypertension in the eye. Such suggestions may be termed speculative, but they are undoubtedly attractive, and may well yield a harvest in the future. The author would only add his conviction that it will in all probability be a mistake to confine attention or investigation to any one alone of the ductless glands.

(F) As life advances, widespread, deep-seated, and extensive *changes* take place *in the vascular system*. There can be no question that these have a very considerable bearing on the causation of glaucoma. Looked at from the standpoint of physiological possibilities, it suggests itself, that a pathological rise in the intra-ocular pressure may be due to one or more of the following factors :—(i.) An increase of the vascular pressure in the body generally ; (ii.) a similar increase localised in the eye ; (iii.) a lowering of the vaso-motor control in the body generally ; and (iv.) a similar change in the eye specially. In discussing this subject, the best course would appear to be to advance to our conclusions by a process of elimination, a plan which we shall accordingly adopt.

(i.) *Is arterio-sclerosis a factor in the causation of glaucoma ?*—A very few years ago the answer to this question would have been emphatically in the affirmative. The line of reasoning appeared perfectly clear. Arterio-sclerosis, like glaucoma, is a disease whose occurrence becomes much more frequent as life advances. With it is associated a rise in the systemic blood-pressure. The intra-ocular pressure is fundamentally dependent on the systemic blood-pressure and, in conditions of health at least, it follows that pressure. What could be more natural than to conclude that arterio-sclerosis should bring about a rise in the ocular tension ! Nor was the matter left to supposition alone, for various observers brought forward evidence to show that the systemic blood-pressure was higher in glaucomatous subjects than in healthy people of the same age. The inference appeared to be that the raised blood-pressure *was* a factor in the causation of glaucoma. Within the last few years, however, a number of investigators have shown that these views had been too readily accepted. Kraemer and Alexandre were amongst the earliest to voice independently the view that the relationship between arterio-sclerosis and glaucoma had been too lightly assumed. This subject has been discussed at length in the previous chapter, and we need not repeat what has there been said. It suffices to say that well-founded medical opinion to-day answers the question that heads this section in the emphatic negative, and holds that there is no obvious causal relationship between arterio-sclerosis with its attendant rise of systemic pressure and the onset of glaucoma.

Before leaving the subject we may mention that

Kleczkowski stated, some years back, that the blood of glaucomatous patients could be shown to contain adrenalin; his work was founded both on biological and on chemical tests. The subsequent investigations of Löhlein, of Vogt and Jaffé, and of Kusama and Nakano, have altogether failed to confirm any such finding, which was apparently due to faulty technique.

(ii.) As to the influence of an *increase of vascular pressure localised in the vessels of the eye*, all that can be said is that whilst it is a factor which we cannot exclude, and which indeed may on occasion be of very great importance, our present methods do not permit us to investigate the subject, and it would therefore be most unwise to dogmatise on what we so little understand.

(iii. and iv.) Finally we may take together the question of *loss of vaso-motor control* in the body generally and in the eye specially. It is universally accepted that interference with the normal circulation through the globe is a leading feature of congestive glaucoma. It has also been contended in the previous pages that vascular disturbances play a not unimportant rôle in the simple cases as well. All that we know of the exciting causes of glaucoma is in conformity with the view that the great majority of them act by interfering in one way or another with the vaso-motor control, either in the body generally, or in the eye individually, or in both. Pass in review a list of these causes :—Cold, hunger, starvation, sleeplessness, nervous or bodily exhaustion, anxiety, sorrow, constipation, bronchitis, cardiac or hepatic obstruction, and so on ! Are they not one and all of them calculated to interfere with the quiet, even interplay of physiological function, and to lead to disturbances of the vascular balance, and especially to congestion in one part or another of the nervous system ? Does not the passage of years, with all that it connotes, play into the hands of the enemy, by rendering the body less able to resist all those constantly recurring shocks, at which youth laughs, but to which age must sooner or later succumb ? Lastly, does not every influence which tends to restore a quiet, even control of the vascular system, find its place in our repertoire for the non-operative treatment of glaucoma ?

(2) **Sex.**—With regard to the influence of sex on the incidence of glaucoma, it may be questioned whether we have anything of value to add to what Priestley Smith taught us nearly a quarter of a century ago. Females suffer in rather larger numbers than males ; the ratio given by that writer was 56·9 per cent. against 43·1 per cent. It is of interest to compare these figures with those recently given by Kagoshima from Japan, where the precentages work out at 61·9 for women and 39·09 for men. The chronic, non-congestive cases are found perhaps a little in excess in males as compared with females, whilst the congestive forms are nearly twice as common in the latter as in the former. The unstable condition of the female nervous system at the time of the climacteric is probably sufficient to account for this disparity. If, however, we accept this explanation, it is necessary that we should clearly understand whither it logically leads us. It presumably means either that a very large number of potential cases of glaucoma in males never pass the boundary-line to declare themselves by subjective phenomena and other signs and symptoms, or else that they remain simple in nature and are thus overlooked. Probably both events influence our statistics to some extent. In any case, the greater liability of females to congestive glaucoma appears to be due to a wider and more frequent prevalence in them of the exciting as compared with the predisposing factors of the disease. The reflection to which this leads the thoughtful surgeon is obvious : It cries aloud the necessity of keeping the possibility of the occurrence of glaucoma in all its forms in the very forefront of his mind, when examining the eyes of people who are advancing in years. Eye affections of a painful or congestive type in elderly females should always be carefully examined and watched, whilst failing vision, without an obvious cause to account for it, in either sex, and perhaps particularly in elderly men, should invariably be looked on with suspicion, until a definite cause can be assigned for the trouble.

(3) **Heredity.**— The influence of heredity on the incidence of glaucoma is revealed both in the race and in the family. It is probable that the factors at work are not essentially different in the racial and familial manifestations of hypertension. It is usually stated that Jews, Egyptians, and certain races of negroes are specially liable to the disease. Laqueur pointed out that it was no accident, that of three ophthalmologists who had suffered from glaucoma, two of them, himself and Javal, were Jews. It is of interest to consider the various possible modes of action of hereditary influence. Those that most readily suggest themselves are :—(i.) A small size of the eye ; (ii.) a want of normal development, especially of the parts around the angle of the chamber ; (iii.) any conditions which would predispose to nervous or vascular storms ; and (iv.) conditions of environment. We shall take these in turn.

(i.) Priestley Smith has laid great stress on the small size of the eyes affected, especially in relationship to a normal or excessive development of the lens. The writer's experience in South India would lead him to think that glaucoma is a very common disease there. The enormous amount of operative work demanded for the relief of glaucoma is, he thinks, more than can be explained by the very large population catered for, even by such a hospital as that at Madras. He has constantly made the observation there, that the eyes which come on the operating table for hypertension, are decidedly below the average in size. He believes that glaucoma is abnormally prevalent in India, and that the cause of this prevalence has a distinct connection with want of development of the globes. It is not usually stated, but it is the result of Madras experience, that abnormalities of the eye, the result of defective development, are very common in India.

So convinced is Priestley Smith of the ætiologic rôle of the small eye in cases of hereditary glaucoma, that he has suggested that the cornea of any patient coming from a suspected stock should always be measured, with a view to obtaining a clue as to the prognosis. A small measurement would suggest a guarded prognosis, and would indicate that the patient should be carefully kept under observation, whilst the recording of a large corneal diameter would enable the surgeon to set the patient's mind at rest, even though he came from a suspected stock.

The author has been much impressed by the need for an instrument which will measure the corneal diameter with accuracy. The models at present available, inclusive of Wessely's keratometer, seem to him to leave something to be desired. The matter will be dealt with in the chapter on Diagnosis (p. 223).

Lawford has studied the question of familial glaucoma and has established the following points :—(a) It is continuous in descent ; (b) it exhibits the phenomenon of anticipation ; (c) it occurs in all forms ; and (d) it is transmitted by both sexes.

(ii.) A want of normal development of the structures around the angle of the anterior chamber probably plays a part. It seems not unlikely that this factor is more potent in the familial cases than it is in other instances of hereditary glaucoma ; for we know that it is a marked feature in buphthalmos, and that the familial cases provide us with a link between senile and juvenile glaucoma, whilst the latter disease is closely connected with the congenital form of the trouble.

(iii.) From what we know of the great influence exerted on the onset of congestive glaucomatous attacks by those conditions, which favour an instability of the nervous and vascular systems, it would be natural to expect to find such tendencies in races which are peculiarly liable to the disease. It must be confessed that in those mentioned, with the exception of the negroes, such racial peculiarities are not at all obvious. Probably, it is to the predisposing rather than to the exciting factors of glaucoma that we must look for the explanation of racial tendencies of the kind we are discussing.

(iv.) The question of environment opens up a large and interesting field. Has the food of the affected peoples any influence ? The rice-fed and poorly nourished Indians become senile earlier than do Western people. Is it possible that a tendency to tissue degeneration is here indicated ? Again, there is the effect of brilliant sunlight to be reckoned with. And once again, the frequency of glaucoma in peoples, such as the Indians and Egyptians, amongst whom ophthalmias are very prevalent, suggests a possible causal relationship other than that due to perforation and anterior synechia. The possibilities of the suggestion take more definite shape when we remember that Kümmell found that burns of the limbal region were associated with a rise in tension, coupled with a deepening of the anterior chamber. The changes in the same region which are associated with granular ophthalmia may possibly interfere with the normal escape of the intra-ocular fluids. Most of this, however, is but little more than guesswork, and too much stress need not be laid upon it.

(4) **Errors in Refraction.**—It has long been recognised that hyperopia is the commonest refractive error met with in eyes affected with primary glaucoma. The deduction has been drawn that the association is more than accidental, and that a condition of hyperopia stands in a causal relationship to the disease. So strongly has this view been held that Fuchs made the following statement on p. 472 of his fourth edition :—" A disposition toward inflammatory glaucoma appears to belong principally to hypermetropic eyes, whereas strongly myopic eyes are to be regarded as having almost complete immunity against the disease." Priestley Smith has challenged the correctness of this view on the grounds that, (i.) according to Donders, emmetropic eyes become hyperopic after the fiftieth year ; (ii.) small eyes are not necessarily hyperopic ; (iii.) hyperopic eyes are not necessarily small ; and (iv.) hyperopia is more widely prevalent than myopia or even than emmetropia. With regard to the first point, the writer feels doubtful of the correctness of the statement made by Donders. It is true that hyperopia is not at all infrequently found in elderly patients who have all their life been credited with emmetropia ; the same is true of low grades of astigmatism. It is, however, equally true

that a large number of comparatively young patients, who read $\frac{6}{9}$ and over, will be found under a cycloplegic to be hyperopic, or astigmatic, or both. This argument cuts both ways, for it raises the percentage of hyperopes in the population, and so discounts the view that long-sight is a predisposing cause of glaucoma. The writer is extremely diffident about putting forward his own views on such a subject, when they appear to be in opposition to what Priestley Smith has found by statistics, but he holds two cherished beliefs as the result of clinical observation, viz., (i.) that glaucomatous eyes are frequently abnormally small, and (ii.) that the type of eye one commonly meets with in hyperopia is likewise small. He cannot support the latter proposition by statistics, but the observations on which it is founded have been so woven into his clinical experience that he finds it hard to let it go. There can be no question that his views are shared by many good clinicians with large experience and amongst others by Fuchs. He does not quote this as showing they are correct, but merely as putting up a case for further consideration of a difficult and important subject. Several papers which appear to support Priestley Smith's contention, and which have been backed by statistics, have been published in the last few years.

Apart from fairly numerous instances of individual cases of glaucoma occurring in comparatively high myopes, Gilbert, from the statistics of the Munich clinic, found that of 71 cases of simple glaucoma, 62 per cent. were myopic or emmetropic, and 38 per cent. hyperopic; whereas of 115 cases of congestive glaucoma, 77 per cent. were hyperopic, the remainder being equally divided between myopes and emmetropes. He thought the clinical form of the disease to be largely influenced by the state of refraction of the eye. Again, Lange found that 43·3 per cent. of his cases of simple glaucoma occurred in myopes, and Löhlein's researches led him to believe that the myope is just as liable to glaucoma as the emmetrope or hyperope. His statistics showed that in juvenile glaucoma, 50 per cent. of the subjects are myopic. Here, however, we are treading on the question of the relationship of myopia and glaucoma in the young, and of the moot question which of the two is the cause of the other. That must be discussed under another section. Haag's figures from the Tübingen clinic are of interest in this connection : He compared his cases of simple and of congestive glaucoma with each other, and he found that a higher percentage of myopia was present in the former than in the latter. It is obvious that what we really need is a mass of trustworthy statistics of the state of refraction in earlier life of those who subsequently develop glaucoma. Such figures cannot easily be obtained from the out-patient records of hospitals, nor will they come in sufficient volume from the private practice of any one man. It will take time to collect them, but the interest of the subject suggests that it should be done. Even then, the figures will still remain open to some doubt, since it will be extremely difficult to calculate with any degree of accuracy the percentage ratios of emmetropes, myopes, and hyperopes in the class of patients from whom the returns come. We are, however, justified in jettisoning the view that the myope is safe from hypertension. It seems to be quite certain that he is *not*, even though his myopia may be comparatively high. Whether he enjoys a relative immunity is quite another question.

(5) **Mydriasis.**—Anything that causes a dilatation of the pupil tends to block up the angle of the chamber, and so, by causing an obstruction to the outflow of intra-ocular fluid, to raise the tension of the eye. We may divide the causes of dangerous mydriasis into a number of headings : —(i.) The abuse of drugs ; (ii.) the exclusion of light from the eye ; (iii.) the influence of violent emotions ; and (iv.) the effects of depressing diseases or of allied conditions. We shall take up (i.) and (ii.) in turn, leaving (iii.) and (iv.) to be considered incidentally under the appropriate headings.

(i.) *The abuse of mydriatic drugs.*—There is *no* drug which produces mydriasis, which can *safely* be instilled into an eye predisposed to glaucoma, unless the surgeon takes the precaution to neutralise the effect by the subsequent use of a meiotic. Cases are on record in which an access of hypertension has followed the use of each of the following, holocaine, cocaine, euphthalmin, and homatropin. It is true that there are many surgeons of large experience who have been fortunate enough to use mydriatic and cycloplegic drugs in a huge number of instances without ever seeing any evil consequences result. Lagrange recently remarked that in the Bordeaux clinic, they were in the habit of using homatropin in a routine manner, and even to excess, and yet he had never seen a case of glaucoma supervene. Before his time, Badal had freely used atropin in the same clinic and yet in 27 years' experience he had been equally fortunate. In Madras it has long been the custom to use homatropin very freely in the refraction work, and for very many years it has been the routine procedure to instil atropin the night before a cataract extraction. The number of such operations is very large, and yet the author has never seen or heard of glaucoma occurring, either in his own practice, or in that of his predecessors or successors. In spite of this evidence, there can be no question that the danger attending the use of mydriatic drugs is a very real one. That this is so may be gathered from the fact that, in the 3 years since the first edition of this work appeared, no less than 8 cases of glaucoma following medicinal mydriasis have been published in the literature of ophthalmology; a large number of others must have occurred and remained unpublished. A few details of these cases will prove not uninteresting. Two followed the instillation of cocaine (Hamilton, Levinsohn). In one of these only a single drop of 4 per cent. cocaine was used for the removal of a foreign body; an acute congestive glaucoma followed, and would not yield to meiotics. There were 5 cases of glaucoma following the use of homatropin (Desai, Hambresin, Levinsohn, and Levitt). In one of these only a single drop of homatropin solution was used; an acute attack of congestive glaucoma followed. In another there was a similar sequel to the use of homatropin for cycloplegic purposes in spite of the fact that a drop of eserin (1 per cent.) was instilled before the patient was dismissed. One case followed the instillation of 2 drops of a freshly prepared solution of hydrochloride of holocaine (1 per cent) in each eye with an extra drop later in the right eye. A diagnosis of simple glaucoma had previously been made and the drug was used as a preliminary to tonometry. An acute double congestive glaucoma resulted and was not controlled by eserin and other general treatment, and double iridectomy had to be performed.

However rare these cases may be, they are apt to damage very seriously and often very unjustly the reputation of the surgeon concerned. It is therefore all-important that we should not lose sight of the risk that continually hangs over us in the use of mydriatics and cycloplegics, especially in cases in which we have reason to fear that any tendency to glaucoma is present.

There are two important points in connection with this subject which should never be forgotten, viz., (a) that a mydriatic should never be used without first ascertaining the tension of the eye, and the condition of the optic disc ; unfortunately, although all will admit this to be an axiom, the rule is too often broken in practice ; and (b) that no *doubtful* patient should be allowed to leave the surgeon's care until meiosis has been established ; even then he should be provided with a prescription for a mild meiotic to be used at intervals until all danger is past. The necessity for this last injunction will be obvious when it is stated that the meiosis produced (for instance after the use of homatropin) by the instillation of a solution of nitrate of pilocarpine ($\frac{1}{2}$ per cent.) may be markedly in evidence shortly after instillation, but may then gradually pass away, giving place to a mydriasis, which may last for several hours or even for several days. It is necessary to warn the patient to watch his pupils and to instil the meiotic, if need be. This is the more necessary since the mydriasis produced will often long outlast the cycloplegia at which the surgeon aimed. That these instructions are not altogether superfluous may be judged from the fact, that the writer was quite recently consulted by a surgeon, who confessed that he had precipitated an attack of glaucoma by instilling homatropin, in order to examine the refraction of an elderly patient, who had complained of failing eyesight. He had not made an ophthalmoscopic examination before the instillation, as it had not occurred to him that the eye might have been glaucomatous when he first saw it, although subsequent events made it appear probable to him that this was so.

A still graver abuse of drugs is the haphazard instillation of atropin by some practitioners in all doubtful cases of eye disease. Less common, but certainly far more surprising, is the practice in vogue among some ophthalmic surgeons of instilling a weak solution of atropin into the eyes of elderly patients, who are suffering from central cataract, with the object of bringing the periphery of the lens into play and so of improving vision. To the author's mind this custom is indefensible and should be condemned and discontinued. The risk involved is both serious and actual. Any small advantages it may bring are outweighed by the dangers involved. When it is possible to obtain permanent mydriasis by the performance of a small upward iridectomy, which causes the patient no inconvenience, and which lessens, instead of increasing the danger of secondary glaucoma, it seems inconceivable that so dangerous and ill-advised a procedure, as the instillation of atropin under these conditions can be resorted to by ophthalmologists. One of the most unfortunate features of a glaucomatous condition engendered in this fashion, is that it will not yield to meiotics, and operation must be at once undertaken.

Before leaving the drug question, it must be mentioned that dionin has been accused of causing glaucoma, when used in dangerous cases. It is said by Thienpont, that the action is quite independent of any mydriatic effect, and that the rise is temporary and followed later by a fall. He explains this preliminary rise by the congestion of the ciliary body induced by the mechanical obstruction which the action of the drug places in the way of the vascular escape from the anterior portion of the eye. It has been suggested that when using dionin on doubtfully glaucomatous eyes, a meiotic should first be instilled.

(ii.) *The exclusion of light from the eye* is an obvious source of mydriasis. It is well known that an operation for glaucoma on one eye may be followed by the onset of the disease in the opposite, previously unaffected eye, whilst the two are bandaged. This may be in part attributed to the mydriasis induced by the exclusion of light, but it is also at least in part to be set down to the mental shock of the operation, and to the anxiety the patient is necessarily suffering. Nor should the enervating effect of the pain that has been endured before the operation be left out of count. Grönholm, who studied the influence of mydriasis and meiosis on the tension of the eye, concluded that the filtration channels are opened by the act of accommodation, and by contraction of the pupil, and suggested that glaucoma patients should be advised to stay as much as possible in a bright light, and to read, so long as they have any accommodatory power, and as their pupils contract under the influence of light. Arthur Thomson, working independently at the very same time (1911), and approaching the subject from the purely anatomical point of view, came to precisely similar conclusions. As has already been mentioned, he has shown reason to believe that the ciliary muscle and the sphincter iridis, by their contraction, pull on the scleral spur, and in conjunction with the elastic force of the pectinate ligament establish a pump action, whereby the intra-ocular fluid is kept on the move outward. His recommendation was that in glaucomatous cases, the action of the ciliary muscle should be restored by suitable exercises. The main interest for us is, that his communication added an element of scientific precision to the astute clinical advice given by Grönholm, when the latter pointed to exercise of the eyes by daylight as being calculated to remove, or at least to lessen, one of the ætiological factors of high tension. It has long been the author's custom to advise his glaucomatous patients, whilst they are waiting for a decision as to the necessity for operation, or whilst under medical treatment for the disease, to use their eyes freely, short of overtiring them, and to avoid all shades, smoked glasses, etc. He is convinced that this is good practical advice, in spite of the fact that it is in opposition to the recommendations of a large number of eye surgeons.

F. P. Maynard observed that more cases of glaucoma were under treatment during the rainy season in the Calcutta Hospital than at other times, and was inclined to think that the considerable diminution of light which characterises the cold weather in India, was responsible for the development of the seasonal increase in cases of hypertension. The idea seemed so attractive that the writer endeavoured to follow it up in Madras. He was, however, quite unable to find any greater seasonal prevalence of the congestive disease (which obviously is alone in question) after spells of dull weather. The influences which regulate the numbers in which Indians resort to hospitals at different seasons, and the often inevitable delays which take place in the East in bringing what we should recognise as very urgent cases for surgical relief, are amongst the factors which made it quite impossible in Madras, at least, to trace any such influence as Maynard suggested. It is, however, recognised that this evidence is altogether on the negative side, and that the suggestion under discussion may yet prove to be well founded. The observation has been made that glaucoma is more frequent in London during the winter; whilst a similar seasonal prevalence has been noted by Kagoshima in Japan. Before accepting the diminution of light as being the causal factor, it is necessary to take account of cold, wet, privation, and other causes of exhaustion which are always present in the winter season in any large town, either in Northern Europe or in Japan.

(6) **Nerve Shock and Strain.**—We have had frequent need in the preceding pages to refer to the rôle which nerve shock and strain play in exciting an attack of glaucoma in a subject whose eye is anatomically predisposed thereto. Every surgeon knows that any condition which leads to powerful mental excitement, or to exhaustion of the mind or body, is to be numbered amongst the exciting causes of the disease. Many of such patients will give us a history of family bereavement, of haunting fear, of

business anxieties, of long, fatiguing, and anxious night watches, of prolonged mental overwork, of sleeplessness, or of some similar condition or set of conditions, the essence of which is a tendency to nervous exhaustion. Nor must we leave out of our reckoning those cases, in which the second eye becomes glaucomatous whilst the patient is in hospital for operation on the first, for thèse point most instructively to the nature of the agency at work. This is really twofold, viz., (i.) some one or more of the tendencies to ocular congestion, and (ii.) the influence of mydriasis. The former we have discussed at length under a previous section. Of the latter, it is necessary to point out that it may be caused either by strong mental impressions, by nervous exhaustion, or by the shutting off of light from the eyes by means of the bandage.

(7) **Febrile Diseases.**—To those who accept what has been written in the previous section, it can be a matter of no surprise that glaucoma should from time to time be met with after various febrile diseases, and under circumstances which appear to justify our assuming that here cause and effect are in operation. The weakening of the heart's action, and the demoralisation of the vasomotor tone with which we are familiar under such conditions, afford us all the explanation we need. But there is another side to the question. In many infective diseases we are accustomed to find evidence, in certain cases, of the influence of the responsible organisms far from their ordinary and well-recognised areas of activity, and it is therefore in accordance with what we know of pathology, that the eye should sometimes be so attacked by these outlying expeditionary forces of disease. Bacterial or toxic mischief introduced into the system in this way may seriously affect either the vascular arrangements of the eye, or the integrity and efficiency of the excretory passages. Nor is it impossible that the secretory activity of the ciliary body may be pathologically augmented in certain cases, or even that the chemical composition of the excreted fluid may be so altered as to oppose a barrier to its free excretion. Lastly, it is conceivable that the morbid

THE ÆTIOLOGY OF GLAUCOMA

conditions we are describing may favour that presumed state of hydrophilism, on which Fischer and his followers lay so much stress. These considerations bring to mind the association between glaucoma and influenza, as recorded by Fuchs, A. S. and L. D. Green, Menacho, Orcutt, Schipfer, Verderame, and others; between it and epidemic dropsy, as noticed by Maynard; and between it and herpes zoster, as observed by Dubois, Morax, Ten Doesschate, Veasey, Weeks, and others.

Since the first edition of this work appeared in 1918, a good deal of attention has been focussed on this subject, especially in America, with the result that it has come in for profitable and enlightening discussion before various societies.

There is a strong and widespread impression that the so-called " Spanish flue " has been followed in quite an appreciable number of cases by congestive glaucoma, and that this, far from being a coincidence, is a direct result of the special character, which the epidemics of influenza have recently assumed. Some attribute the change for the worse in this disease to the participation of streptococcal and pneumococcal infection with that of Pfeiffer's bacillus. Others surmise that a new and hitherto unidentified organism is to blame. Whatever the explanation may be, the fact remains that a tendency to inflammatory œdema has been strongly marked in all the manifestations of the disease; pneumonia has been common and fatal, and a puffy œdematous condition of the body generally has been a striking feature. It should not therefore be difficult to explain the frequency with which glaucoma—a disease closely connected with unhealthy conditions of the vascular system—has appeared as a complication or early sequela of the disease. The discussion on Orcutt's paper will well repay perusal by anyone who is interested in this subject. Not the least suggestive contribution to that discussion was made by Dr. S. B. Munns, who said, *inter alia*, " Spanish influenza is *per se* a disease of œdema. If the toxins can so alter the vessel wall as to allow too free a passage of serum through it into the surrounding tissues, is it not possible that this may occur in the uvea ? Extensive involvement of the lungs obstructs the pulmonary circulation and thus produces a condition of venous stasis, which may tend to favour the production of glaucoma."

It is of interest here, whilst recording Maynard's observation of the occurrence of a number of cases of glaucoma in the victims of a wave of epidemic dropsy in Calcutta, to quote Manson-Bahr's definition of the latter disease. " An epidemic disease, running its course in from 3 to 6 weeks, and characterised by the sudden appearance of anasarca, preceded in most instances by fever . . . and accompanied by pronounced anæmia. The case mortality varies from 2 to 40 per cent., death being sudden, and depending upon œdema of the lungs, hydrothorax, hydropericardium, or other pulmonary and cardiac complications."

There remains for consideration the method in which herpes zoster ophthalmicus gives rise to glaucoma. This subject was discussed by the American Ophthalmological Society, Atlantic City, 14th to 17th June 1919, the opener being Dr. C. A. Veasey (see References). The speakers included some of the best known names in America—Knapp, de Schweinitz, Verhoeff, Greenwood, Clark, Lamb, Parker, Hiram Woods, Weeks, and Francis—and there was an extraordinary unanimity of opinion that the rise in tension which complicates this disease is due to irido-cyclitis. Two points emerged prominently from the debate : (1) The presence of deposits at the back of the cornea is of valuable diagnostic import, as indicating the cause of the increase in tension; and (2) the correct method of dealing with this class of case is by the employment of mydriatics.

(8) **Injuries.**—It is a well-known fact that an injury, and sometimes a very slight one, either of the eye or of the head, may appear to be the determining cause of an attack of glaucoma. We are not considering now the cases, which would ordinarily be grouped under the heading of secondary glaucoma, and in which some coarse lesion of

one or other of the ocular structures can be demonstrated. The *modus agendi* in these latter cases is simple enough. It is a much more difficult matter to explain why a blow on the head, not necessarily a severe one, should excite an attack of high tension, or why glaucoma should result from a slight abrasion, burn, or other injury of the cornea or of the limbal region. We can only adopt the time-honoured suggestion, that we have here to do with an interference, probably vaso-motor in nature, with the normal circulation of the eye. As has already been said in another section, we know so little of the nervous mechanism of the intra-ocular circulation that the above cannot be claimed to be more than a guess. It is, however, as far as the present state of our knowledge permits us to advance.

REFERENCES

ALEXANDRE.—Paris Thesis, 1912 (see *Ophth. Year Book*, 1913).
BJERRUM, J.—*Klin. Monatsbl. f. Augenh.*, Jan. 1912, p. 42, quoted in *Ophthalmology*, 1912, vol. viii. p. 541.
DESAI, H. M.—*Brit. Journ. Ophth.*, 1919, vol. iii. p. 251.
DONDERS, F. C.—*Accommodation and Refraction of the Eye*, English edition, p. 208.
DUBOIS.—*Klin. Monatsbl. f. Augenh.*, May 1912, p. 601.
FUCHS, E.—*Text-Book of Ophthalmology*, 4th edition, Duane.
GILBERT, W.—*Thirty-eighth Ophthalmic Congress*, Heidelberg, 1912, p. 333.
GREEN, A. S. AND L. D.—*Amer. Journ. of Ophth.*, vol. ii. p. 608.
GRÖNHOLM, V.—*Arch. f. Augenh.*, vol. lxvi. p. 346; *ibid.* vol. lxvii. p. 136. (*Ophth. Year Book*, 1911.)
HAAG, C. — *Klin. Monatsbl. f. Augenh.*, vol. liv. p. 133.
HAMBRESIN.—*Belgian Ophth. Soc.*, Nov. 30, 1919; abstract *Amer. Journ. of Ophth.*, 1920, vol. iii. p. 367.
HAMILTON, R. J.—*Liverpool Med. Chir. Journ.*, vol. xxxvi. p. 156.
HERTEL, E.—*Archiv f. O.*, vol. xc.; and *Arch. Ophth.*, May 1916, vol. xlv. No. 3, p. 301.
HERTEL, E.—"Teaching Concerning Eye-Pressure," *Klin. Monatsbl. f. Augenh.*, vol. lxi. p. 331.
KAGOSHIMA.—*Nippon Gankakai-zashi*, Sept. 1915; and *Ophthalmology*, July 1916, p. 791.
KLECZKOWSKI, T.—*Klin. Monatsbl. f. Augenh.*, Oct. 1911, p. 417.
KRAEMER, R.—Graefe's *Archiv f. O.*, vol. lxxiii. p. 349.
KUEMMELL, R.—*Munch. med. Woch.*, 1914; and *Annals of Ophth.*, April 1915, p. 354.

KUSAMA AND NAKANO.—*Nippon Gankakai-zashi*, Sept. 1915; and *Ophthalmology*, July 1916, p. 790.
LAGRANGE, FELIX.—*Proc. of Seventeenth Inter. Congress of Med.*, London, 1913, Section IX. " Ophthalmology," p. 71.
LAGRANGE, F.—" Discussion on Hambresin's Paper."
LANGE, O.—*Klin. Monatsbl. f. Augenh.*, vol. l.
LAQUEUR, L.—*Ibid.*, June 1910, p. 639. (*Ophth. Year Book*, 1910.)
LAWFORD, J. B.—*R.L.O.H. Reports*, vol. xvii. p. 57.
LEVINSOHN, G.—*Klin. Monatsbl. f. Augenh.*, vol. lxi. p. 174.
LEVITT.—*Amer. Journ. of Ophth.*, Sept. 1917; and *Brit. Journ. Ophth.*, 1918, vol. ii. p. 281.
LOHLEIN, W.—*Thirty-eighth Ophth. Congress*, Heidelberg, 1912, p. 142; *Thirty-ninth Ophth. Congress*, Heidelberg, 1913, p. 97.
MANSON-BAHR, P.—*Manson's Tropical Diseases*, Cassell & Co. Ltd., London, 1921, p. 361.
MAYNARD, F. P.—*The Ophthalmoscope*, 1908, p. 864; *Indian Med. Gaz.*, July 1911.
MENACHO, M.—*Arch. d'opht.*, vol. xiv. p. 569. (*Ophth. Year Book*, 1914, p. 502.)
MORAX, V.—*Ann. d'ocul.*, Feb. 1916.
ORCUTT, D. C.—*Amer. Journ. of Ophth.*, vol. ii. p. 533; *Proc. Chicago Ophth. Soc.*, April 21, 1919.
PARSONS, J. H.—*Pathology of the Eye*, vol. iii. p. 1072. Hodder & Stoughton, London.
RISLEY, S. D.—*The Ophthalmoscope*, 1914, vol. xii. p. 83.
SCHIPFER, L. A.—*Amer. Journ. of Ophth.*, vol. ii. p. 368.
SMITH, PRIESTLEY.—*Glaucoma*, J. & A. Churchill, 1891, pp. 90–94; *Ophth. Rev.*, Jan. 1912.
TEN DOESSCHATE, G.—*Amer. Journ. of Ophth.*, vol. ii. p. 823.
THIENPONT.—*Rev. Int. d'Hyg. et de Therap. Ocul.*, vol. viii. p. 97.
THOMSON, A.—*The Ophthalmoscope*, 1911, vol. ix. p. 470.
VEASEY, C. A.—*Amer. Journ. of Ophth.*, vol. ii. p. 760.
VERDERAME, F.—*Ann. di Ottal.*, vol. xlii. p. 772. (*Ophth. Year Book*, 1914, p. 523.)
VERHOEFF, F. H.—*Arch. Ophth.*, 1915, vol. xliv. No. 2, p. 138.
VOGT, A., AND JAFFÉ, B.—*Klin. Monatsbl. f. Augenh.*, July 1912, p. 23.
VON HIPPEL, E.—*Archiv f. O.*, vol. xc. p. 198; and *Ophthalmology*, April 1916, p. 535.
WEEKS, J. E.—*Trans. Amer. Ophth. Soc.*, 1917, vol. xv. p. 134.

CHAPTER IV

THE DIAGNOSIS OF GLAUCOMA

Part I

SUMMARY :—Introductory.
    The Stages of Glaucoma.
    The Clinical Course of a Simple Attack.
    The Clinical Course of a Congestive Attack.

THERE is a widely prevalent impression that glaucoma is a difficult disease to diagnose. This belief is supported by the fact that, from every land in which modern medicine is practised, the complaint is still heard that patients suffering from an increase of intra-ocular pressure are frequently treated wrongly, or not at all. No country seems exempt from such mistakes. They are reported from Great Britain and the rest of Europe, from Canada, America, Australasia, and Asia. There are few ophthalmologists in large practice who cannot recall quite recent cases in their own experience in which a patient has lost an eye, or even both eyes, in this melancholy and deplorable way. It is said that a generation ago, a distinguished British ophthalmic surgeon stated at a medical meeting, that he felt strongly disposed to take the front page of a leading professional journal and to advertise on it in large letters the leading signs and symptoms of Glaucoma, in the hope of directing the attention of the profession to the danger of overlooking this very serious condition when it occurred in everyday practice. Years have rolled by, and a new generation of medical practitioners fills the places of the men of that era, but it may be questioned whether the mistakes this critic lamented have become any less frequent. When we remember that glaucoma is to be classed among the emergencies of surgical practice, that, as a rule, the diagnosis of an average case is extremely easy, and that the standard of professional knowledge and of professional training has gone up by leaps and bounds during the last 25 years, we are forced to pause and ask ourselves in surprise and wonder for an explanation of a phenomenon so world-wide and so persistent. Is glaucoma, after all, a condition whose manifestations are so subtle and recondite as to require for its correct diagnosis the skill and experience of a highly trained specialist ? There are undoubtedly cases to be met with in which the most careful discrimination is demanded, cases which patient, prolonged observation alone will unravel, and on whose diagnosis able and experienced surgeons may reasonably differ. No one will dispute their existence, but they are few and far between. In the great majority of instances the diagnosis of glaucoma is written large for any medical man to read. So much so that at first sight a mistake would appear to be unpardonable, until we remember the conditions under which the modern medical practitioner works. The wonderful advances of medical science have made a vast difference in his mental equipment ; he has to be a highly educated man, far in advance of his predecessor of a generation ago. But in the increase of his knowledge, and in the enormous breadth of the field he has to keep in view, lie his dangers, so far as glaucoma is concerned. He must be a physician, a surgeon, a gynæcologist, an obstetrician, an ophthalmologist, a toxicologist, a pathologist, a bacteriologist, and an expert in many another field besides. The result is that he has so much to think of, and to remember, that he is in danger of overlooking those things with which he is not in constant touch. He knows the signs of glaucoma well ; and if for any reason he is on the look out for this condition, he will certainly not miss it when he meets it in his practice. But it is a fact, which applies to all alike, that men only see clearly those things which they have been trained to look for, and which they expect to meet with. The sailor discovers a coast-line in the grey haze which the landsman has only interpreted as a cloud on the horizon; the engineer looks down on a distant town, and takes note of the factories it contains, by the observation of phenomena which escape his lay brother; the surgeon recognises the stigmata of hereditary disease in his companion of the railway carriage; and so on with all the other professions. Our point is that the very existence of glaucoma, as a pathologic entity, with which he may have to deal in his very next patient, is crowded out of the thoughts of many a medical man. It is not that he does not know of it, or that he has forgotten its symptoms, but that the bare possibility of its existence has been relegated to the background of his mind, owing to the infrequency of its occurrence in his practice. Nowhere is the saying more true that "fore-warned is fore-armed." A well-known London physician, who has recently passed away, kept pasted above his shaving-glass a short list of the signs and symptoms of glaucoma, in order that he might not fail to diagnose such a case, if he met with it in his practice. His example might be widely followed with profit. Modern surgical methods have revolutionised the treatment of glaucoma, and have made it possible to save a patient's sight, always provided that a diagnosis is arrived at sufficiently early. It is therefore all the more regrettable when a surgeon fails to recognise without delay the evidence of increased intra-ocular pressure, and so lessens the chance of a successful issue to the case. There are very few diseases which are more easily diagnosed than an ordinary attack of congestive glaucoma, and there is certainly no surgical emergency which is more susceptible to early, active, and suitable therapeutic treatment; whilst the modern operations have made the surgical treatment of increased intra-ocular pressure both safe and certain, so far as surgical procedures can ever be said to be either. As for non-congestive glaucoma, if the medical man makes it a rule to think invariably of raised tension as a *possible* explanation of every case of failure of vision, and to keep that possibility in his mind, until a careful examination has ruled it out, he will not have to reproach himself with lamentable mistakes such as we have been discussing.

The Stages of Glaucoma.—It is the usual practice of the text-books to draw a distinction between the so-called prodromata of glaucoma and the attack itself. In spite of the fact that this custom has been hallowed by time, and sanctioned by authority, it is to the writer's mind a wrong one. Once an eye shows signs of glaucoma, even though those signs are nothing more than the rainbows round lights, the transient mists, and the ill-defined headaches and pains in or around the eye, which we have been taught to call prodromal symptoms, *that eye is definitely glaucomatous*, and to hold any other opinion is to bury one's head in the sand. Again, from an etymological point of view, there are objections to the use of the term " absolute " as applied to glaucoma. Indeed, in seeking to classify the stages of glaucoma, without any approach to terminological inexactitude, we are confronted by many difficulties. For the purposes of this book it has been decided to adopt the following scheme :—(1) Early glaucoma, (2) established glaucoma, and (3) late glaucoma. This appears to be both useful and expressive, whilst so far as is possible, it avoids sources of ambiguity and error.

CONGESTIVE AND NON-CONGESTIVE GLAUCOMA.—There is another preliminary point which demands our attention, viz., the necessity of having formed in our minds a clear comprehension, not only of the clinical differences between congestive and non-congestive or simple glaucoma, but also of the widely different conditions, which determine whether or not the vascular factor shall or shall not enter into and dominate any particular case. The radical distinction between the two states lies in the fact, that in the simple cases the changes which bring about the rise in tension have been slowly developed, or else the previously existing anatomical conditions have been such as to oppose the occurrence of any sudden interference with the vascular circulation of the eye, or to compensate for it if it does occur. The ocular blood vessels have therefore had time given them to adapt themselves to their new morbid environment.

THE DIAGNOSIS OF GLAUCOMA

The conditions present in glaucoma have been aptly likened to those which are found in abdominal hernia, with and without strangulation. The comparison seems to present some very interesting analogies. Thus in hernia, a small knuckle of gut, suddenly thrust through a narrow neck, may be strangulated from the first owing to an interference with its blood supply. If, however, the ring is a loose one to start with, or if its walls are readily stretchable, or if the mass thrust through it increases very gradually and so has time to stretch the ring, no strangulation will take place. Acute symptoms may, however, arise at any time, if, owing either to a sudden increase of the hernial contents or to a change in vaso-motor conditions, the return of blood from the hernia is interfered with. Such a vaso-motor change may be local to the hernia or may be general. In the latter case it may affect some or all of the abdominal contents, or even the whole body. Or again, the changes may be both local and general. So likewise, may it be with glaucoma, in which we conceive the position to be as follows :—If the onset of the changes (be they those of fibrosis, of enlargement of the lens, or of any other nature) which oppose the normal escape of fluid from the eye, takes place very gradually, the ocular vessels have time to accommodate themselves to the new conditions. The same holds good, even with a more rapid progress of the pathologic changes, if the anatomical condition of the parts is such beforehand as to favour the free escape of fluid from the eye by the normal channels, or to open up fresh channels for the same purpose. The course of the disease in all these instances will be a simple one. On the other hand, a rapid advance of the process of obstruction of the efferent canals, or an unfavourable anatomical condition of the parts concerned, or even a sudden vaso-motor storm, may pave the way for an interference with the normal escape of blood from the eye, and thereby tend to introduce a congestive element into the case. Thus by augmenting the fluid contents of the eye, it will help to establish a vicious circle whose tendency is to maintain an increase of the intra-ocular pressure. The influence of vaso-motor changes will be here fully as great as we have seen it to be in the case of hernia ; for we have to do with the many conditions which directly affect the blood supply of the head, not forgetting anger, grief, and various other forms of mental excitement, and we have also to take account of all those influences, such as bodily and mental fatigue, which act unfavourably on the whole vascular system, thereby tending to establish conditions which will hamper the normal escape of blood from the tissues. It thus comes about that a case of non-congestive glaucoma may, at any time and with very little warning, pass over into a congestive condition, whilst under favourable circumstances the opposite and happier change may, and not infrequently does occur. The distinction then between the two conditions lies in the presence or absence of obstruction to the free escape of blood from the eye. This, in its turn, depends on the degree of intra-ocular pressure prevailing, and on the anatomical and other conditions present beforehand.

We do not for a moment imply that there is no clinical distinction between congestive and non-congestive (simple) glaucoma. A case which is going to run a congestive course will usually show the so-called prodromata at an early date, and these symptoms will develop in the later stages into the manifestations of the subacute and acute exacerbations of the disease. On the other hand, a case of simple glaucoma may run its course without ever presenting a sign of active congestion, save for the dilatation of the venous circle around the cornea. Our point is that the distinction between the two conditions is not a radical one. It depends on conditions which may at any time alter, and which in doing so will profoundly modify the clinical aspect of the case. An eye which has been the victim of a well-marked attack of congestive glaucoma, may pass into such a state of quietude, that it would be difficult to classify it as other than non-congestive, until the history and the signs of the case have been carefully gone into. On the other hand, as we have already seen, congestive symptoms may supervene in an eye which has long presented the characteristic course of a simple glaucoma. All varieties are met with between that of the fulminating disease, which in a few short hours hurries the eye through a stormy painful course into endless blindness, and that of the simple non-congestive form, whose importance is too often underrated and dallied with, both by the patient and by his medical adviser. The terrible danger of the latter form lies in the fact that the signs and symptoms are so inconspicuous that they are often overlooked or misinterpreted.

The text-book description of an attack of glaucoma frequently presents itself to the student's mind as a hopeless tangle, owing to the fact that the elements of the case are not clearly appreciated. Those elements, at least as the writer sees them, are (1) that the disease is relentless and progressive, (2) that its keystone is a rise of pressure within the eye, (3) that the fundamental causes of this rise are protean, (4) that one and all of them act fundamentally by upsetting the balance between the secretion and excretion of the intra-ocular fluid, and (5) that the entry of the vascular factor into the drama is an accident, though one of the very gravest proportions. If these facts are clearly appreciated, the great variety in the clinical course of the disease will be more easily understood. It appears to the author that the subject may best be dealt with, by first taking a general survey of the principal types of the disease (congestive and non-congestive) from a clinical point of view, and then proceeding to discuss each sign and symptom in turn at greater length. This plan has therefore been adopted.

The Clinical Course of an Attack of Simple or Non-congestive Glaucoma.—It has already been stated that the clinical course of an attack of primary glaucoma varies very widely in different patients. We shall best understand the subject, if we direct our attention in the first instance to the consideration of the class of case in which the glaucoma remains simple (or non-congestive) throughout. The onset is very gradual, the signs of congestion are absent, the patient never suffers a day of pain, and the troublesome headaches, rainbows, and mists, which punctuate the early stages of the congestive form are not even mentioned. The pupil is often found to be dilated, but in not a few instances it is normal or nearly normal in size ; the iris reacts sluggishly, even when the pupil is comparatively small, and may be altogether immobile where marked dilatation is present. Good central vision is often retained to a very late stage, whilst the shrinking of the visual field is well marked. The result is that many of the patients complain that they feel as if they were looking down a tube, and that in consequence they are unable to avoid objects which they meet with when they are on the move. The statement sometimes made that a patient's central visual acuity may be preserved unimpaired, even when his peripheral field has undergone extreme constriction, does not seem to represent correctly the facts of the case. It is probable that central vision is always to some extent affected. It is true that the patient may show $\frac{6}{6}$ vision or even better, but if his record before the disease attacked him could be made available, it would probably be found that the figure mentioned indicates a falling off from what originally was his normal vision. On the other hand a very distinct impairment of central visual acuity is sufficient to justify a doubt, whether the course of the case has throughout been really non-congestive ; it will suggest to the experienced clinician that at some time or another an element of congestion has played a part in the drama of the disease. The effect of this combination of good central and bad peripheral vision has a strong clinical significance. As a patient suffering from simple glaucoma enters the out-patient room, his bearing is characteristic ; he walks hesitatingly, turning his head repeatedly from side to side, in order to safeguard himself from running into or stumbling over objects which may lie in his path. One who suffers from optic atrophy has certain features in common with the chronic glaucoma patient, for in both (1) the disease is bilateral, (2) the pupils are widely dilated, and (3) the eyes are free from congestion. But the atrophic subject's feel-the-way gait with hands outstretched before him, is quite different from the condition we are now discussing. Both patients are sharply distinguished from the man with double immature cataract, who despite his central defect is materially assisted by his broad field as he makes his way to the out-patient's chair. It was the writer's practice in his Indian clinic to impress upon his students the importance of cultivating the power of making rapid diagnoses of the kind indicated, whilst preserving an open mind for the reception of the lessons which a subsequent examination would yield ; and he found that an intelligent student could readily learn to distinguish between the classes of cases above dealt with.

As we have already stated, the disease is a bilateral one. It may affect one eye sooner than the other, and indeed it usually does so, but " the going of the second eye " is as a rule merely a question of time. Men are attacked at least as often as women, and even the young are sometimes to be found included amongst the victims of this disease. The myope is no more immune than the hyperope. When we pass on to the results of an objective examination, we find that there are three signs which for all practical purposes may be said to be invariably present, viz., (1) a cupping of the optic disc, (2) a fall in the normal acuity of central vision, and (3) a characteristic limitation of the visual field. To this " triad of glaucoma signs " we shall frequently have occasion to refer.

An attack of non-congestive glaucoma may pass at any time into a congestive phase. The fact that it has shown no tendency to do so at any time, during a course which is to be measured by years, is not an absolute guarantee for the future. What is more, the disease may lapse back again at the close of a congestive attack, into a close imitation of its old " simple ",form. The thinness of the line, which separates the two varieties of glaucoma, may best be appreciated when we weigh the significance of the fact, that a patient may present in one eye the phenomena of simple glaucoma, and in the other those of the congestive condition.

When we come to discuss the manifestations of congestive glaucoma, we shall find that we are dealing with a much more complex condition, than that which now confronts us in our study of the simple disease. We have begun with the latter, because it presents the phenomena which result from increased intra-ocular pressure in their simplest possible form. Given time for their evolution, all cases of glaucoma, whether simple or congestive, will present " the triad of signs " to which we have referred. The congestive forms will overlay these fundamental manifestations with numerous other signs and symptoms, most of which may be attributed to what we have already spoken of as the " introduction of the vascular factor." Each of these has its own importance, but the members of " the triad " are to be regarded as the essential signs of glaucoma. They should be written large in the memory of everyone who desires to practise medicine without disaster.

It may cause not a little surprise to our readers to find that so far no mention has been made of that most important phenomenon, " an increase in the tension of the globe," which, as we all know, is the outward and palpable sign of an increase of the intra-ocular pressure. The omission has been intentional, as in the early stages of many cases of non-congestive glaucoma a rise in ocular tension is not always to be found on digital or even on tonometric examination. This phenomenon has long puzzled the minds of ophthalmologists, but has, in the light of recent work, ceased to be a mystery. It is probably a mistake to suppose that the clinical course of every attack of simple glaucoma gains strength gradually and evenly as the days pass by. On the contrary, in some cases at least, the simple, like the congestive form, probably, indeed almost certainly, is to some extent intermittent in its advance. Though these intermissions are less marked than those which punctuate the course of the congestive disease, they are none the less to be reckoned with. The writer believes that they are of the same nature ; in other words, that they represent the incursion of the vascular factor in the form of minor vaso-motor disturbances, the intensity of which is such that they give little external evidence of their occurrence. Rightly to understand the matter we must realise that there are two distinct elements to be taken account of :—(1) The slow gradual progress, in the tissues of the eye, of degenerative changes which slowly but surely interfere with the normal excretion of the ocular fluid. (2) The occurrence of vascular storms of slight intensity, which may attract but little attention, and which can only be detected by very careful periodic examination of the patient. If, in these cases, the tonometer is used at frequent intervals, a rise in intra-ocular pressure will sooner or later be found. Apart altogether from these more marked variations, there would seem to be a daily tide of which we must take account. According to Köllner, the intra-ocular pressure in simple glaucoma reaches its maximum between 10 and 11 a.m., and drops rapidly to a minimum between 3 and 5 p.m. ; this holds good whether the eye is under treatment or not. It must, however, be freely admitted that, so far as the patient's feelings are concerned, the course of a simple glaucoma may and often does seem to flow evenly from start to finish. Nor is it uncommon to find amongst uneducated people, that the loss of the first eye passes unobserved, and that the patient only becomes aware that he is losing his sight, when the second eye has already failed to such an extent as to interfere with the ordinary actions of life.

From a clinical point of view we can classify all cases of this disease into the early, the established, and the late. In the middle category come those in which the diagnosis is not in question, since the triad of signs is well marked. Later still, the blind hard eye tells its own tale. It is only in the very early stages that the careful surgeon will be in any doubt. Time, which serves as the enemy of him who fails to be vigilant and watchful, is all on the side of the careful and alert diagnostician. There is no time to be lost, but there is equally no need for rash haste, or for the undertaking of action, except on the basis of a well-founded diagnosis.

The Clinical Course of an Attack of Primary Con-

gestive Glaucoma.—A pronounced attack of congestive glaucoma may begin without previous warning of any kind. More often it is not the opening act of the drama, either being heralded by the appearance, from time to time, of the so-called prodromata, or being engrafted upon and complicating an attack of apparently simple glaucoma. The variation in this respect is extraordinary. One may see an attack of simple glaucoma which has gone on for years before congestive symptoms first make their appearance, and on the other hand there are cases on record, in which surgeons have expressed themselves as convinced that an eye was healthy immediately before its invasion by an acute congestive attack. In the vast majority of cases, however, a careful questioning of the patient will elicit a clear history of what are usually, if erroneously, known as "prodromal symptoms." For months, and even for years previously, the patient has observed that from time to time his vision has become misty, generally for a few hours at a time, but sometimes for much shorter periods. With this has been associated some degree of pain in the eye and headache, together with the appearance of rainbow rings around bright lights viewed in the dark. At the time of these attacks, the Oriental patient not infrequently complains that he has observed in front of his eye flashes of light, which could not be accounted for by physical phenomena. Sometimes these take the form of summer lightning flashes, at others they are compared to dancing fireflies. Not a few speak of a ball of light, which rolls comparatively slowly in front of the eye, whilst yet others complain of the sudden appearance and disappearance of flashing points of light. A few of the more observant will state that in association with these phenomena, they have observed that the pupil of the corresponding eye is dilated, and that the eye is congested. A surgical examination, made during the crisis, will reveal the presence of a steamy cornea and of a shallow anterior chamber. The attacks can usually be traced to periods of bodily exhaustion, to sleeplessness, or to mental worry. Like the asthenopic symptoms which accompany

THE DIAGNOSIS OF GLAUCOMA

errors in refraction, these glaucomatous attacks, for such they undoubtedly are, may be noticed on awaking and wear off as the day advances, or may come on as fatigue deepens in the late afternoon or evening. A symptom not uncommonly present, and one which in not a few cases drives the patient to seek advice, is a sudden increase of presbyopia. This comes in the wake of the attacks, and not infrequently persists in some measure even after their disappearance. If there is one pathological condition more than almost any other, to which the term " relentless " can be applied, it is the one we are discussing. These so-called prodromal attacks are merely the early stage of congestive glaucoma. The progress of degenerative or other changes in the eye is monthly, weekly, daily opposing an increasing barrier to the free escape of fluid from within the globe. The time is rapidly approaching when the disturbance in the balance between secretion and excretion will raise the tension of the globe to the danger point, at which its vascular circulation will be in peril of being seriously interfered with. Any one of the many chance conditions, which are calculated to upset the normal course of the flow of blood through the eye, may now precipitate an access of tension and thus determine the appearance of the signs and symptoms of established glaucoma. In the early stage the recuperative powers of the individual will usually enable him to meet and throw off the attack. The block to his excretory channels is not yet sufficient to make the task a difficult one, and the early onslaughts of the disease are transient and of light severity. As time goes on, however, the attacks become more frequent and more severe ; the intervals lessen and the duration of the crises increases, till each is to be measured by days rather than by hours. But, whether early or late, the process is essentially the same ; the difference is one of quantity, not of quality, and the eye is from the first in the grip of a disease which, though it may vary in the speed of its progress, is nevertheless as resistless as the rising tide. It is true that one meets with cases that have never gone beyond this early stage, which is so falsely spoken of as prodromal. The explanation of this is not difficult. The structural conditions which favour a pathological rise of ocular tension are present in the eye, but their progress is extremely slow, and the patient, guided by wise surgical advice, has learnt to avoid carefully those conditions of life (sleeplessness, fatigue, worry, constipation, etc.), which are calculated to upset the vascular balance of his eye, and thereby to precipitate the occurrence of a congestive glaucomatous attack. There is probably another factor in the case—an anatomical one—which we only dimly apprehend, and which is concerned with the conditions under which the blood escapes from the eye. There can be no doubt that this escape is much more easily hindered in some cases than it is in others, and that on this factor depends, to a large extent, the likelihood or otherwise of the incursion of the vascular factor.

There is a curious psychologic interest in the various ways in which different patients regard the early phenomena associated with commencing glaucoma. In some of them these evoke a casual and interested amusement, whilst in others they inspire an unreasoning and lively terror. Later, when the visual acuity begins to fail and the field of vision shows signs of retracting, a well-founded anxiety drives all alike to seek for medical advice.

Sooner or later the early condition passes into the phase of established glaucoma. The passage from one to the other may be gradual and almost imperceptible, the signs and symptoms of the early stage becoming steadily more pronounced; or, on the other hand, the new phase may be ushered in by a crisis whose severity is such, that the patient and the physician alike, erroneously date the onset of glaucoma from it. Indeed, it is not unusual for such a bout to be one of the most severe the patient has to tell of, for he may have learnt by it to take his illness seriously and to avoid carefully what he now knows to be its exciting causes. The leading symptoms are (1) severe trigeminal neuralgia, usually referred to the eye and forehead, but sometimes to other parts as well; this may be so severe as to give rise to nausea and vomiting; indeed, such cases are not infrequently mistaken for "bilious attacks," with most disastrous results, for the opportunity to apply immediate and suitable treatment is then let slip; (2) a rapid fall of vision; and (3) a marked constriction of the visual field. At the same time it is noted that the eye is distinctly congested; it may even show chemosis; the lids too may share in the hyper-vascularity. The cornea is steamy and insensitive, the pupil is widely dilated and often irregularly oval in outline. The iris appears to be discoloured, though this effect is partly due to its being seen through a steamy cornea and a cloudy anterior chamber; the latter chamber is shallow. The lens has a peculiar green look, from whence the disease has derived the name glaucoma ($\gamma\lambda\alpha\nu\kappa\acute{o}\varsigma$ = sea-green). The eye is very tender, and the patient shrinks from the lightest touch; under gentle examination it is felt to be extremely hard. After a varying period, which may be measured by hours, or even by days (according to the severity of the attack and the treatment accorded to it), the symptoms subside and the acute stage passes off, but the eye is never the same again. It has been permanently, though possibly only slightly, damaged, and every succeeding attack increases the harm done. The subsequent course of events is, however, very varied; in some the organ regains an appearance which a superficial examination might pass as normal, whilst in others a condition of chronic congestive glaucoma is established from this date onward. In any case the downward path of the eye, on its way to blindness, is punctuated by the more or less frequent occurrence of congestive exacerbations of the disease. It will thus be seen that the early attacks may pass gradually into the more severe ones of established glaucoma, or that the latter condition may supervene without any definite history being furnished of the early and slight manifestations of the disease. Or again, the transition from early to established glaucoma may be punctuated by an attack of such severity as to impress itself indelibly on the patient's mind and memory.

In any case the eye is being gradually corralled towards a pronounced condition of chronic congestive glaucoma. This is the logical development of the process; the acute or subacute attacks are mere intercurrent accidents. We have now reached a state of affairs in which every sign of glaucoma is present: The visual acuity is much diminished, the field of vision is contracted, the blind spot is characteristically enlarged, and the tension of the eye is distinctly above normal, though it does not reach the high limits which characterise the congestive exacerbations of the disease. The circumcorneal zone is congested, the perforating vessels are distended, and their points of emergence stand out clearly against the background of the sclerotic; the anterior chamber is shallow; the cornea is clear in the interval between two congestive attacks, but it easily and readily clouds over; it also shows a distinct loss of sensitiveness; indeed, it is usually markedly anæsthetic. The pupil is moderately or even widely dilated, and is frequently of an oval shape, with the long axis of the oval vertical; the iris is sluggish, and if much congestion be present it may take on a greenish hue, doubtless partly due to the state of the cornea and to that of the anterior chamber. In the absence of congestion the colour of the iris is verging towards grey, and atrophic patches tend to make their appearance. In the intervals between the congestive crises, when the cornea and chamber are clear, an ophthalmoscopic examination reveals the cupped disc surrounded by a ring of atrophy, the constricted arteries, the congested veins, the vascular pulsation, and the tessellated fundus, which are met with in glaucoma.

And so at last we come to the third and final scene of this terrible drama. Pushed at first gently, gradually, and imperceptibly on its downward road, hustled later by congestive attacks towards its doom, the eye passes on to blindness, to merit almost the time-honoured classification under the term "absolute glaucoma." Written large over the portals through which it has passed are the words of despair, "Abandon hope all ye who enter here."

THE DIAGNOSIS OF GLAUCOMA

True it is that for many a day the patient will protest that he still has some sight ; his intervals of hopeless gloom are lightened by a curious phenomenon, which may be described as a luminous haze and which may last for hours or even for days at a time. An interesting variant of this phenomenon was met with in one case recorded by de Schweinitz, whose patient, though totally blind from glaucoma, declared that " all things seemed to be a sea of red fire." Even more striking is the fact that patients are to be found, and the writer has met with such, who will protest that there are occasions on which they can sit by a window, look out, and see all the features of a scene with which they were familiar in the days gone by ; and yet on examination the eyes are absolutely blind. To this condition the term " memory sight " may be applied, for the pictures are but the aftermath of visual impressions, which have been stored in the cerebral cortex in a happier past. Such is the power of reflection and of recollection, that the patient's mind is enabled to summon these shadows of earlier impressions and to invest them with all the semblance of a reality. It is indeed a pitiable delusion, born of memory and imagination, of hope and despair. On examination, one finds the porcelain-like bluish-white sclera, against which the dilated anterior ciliary veins show up in vivid contrast, forming an irregular circumcorneal, anastomotic circle ; the cornea may be clear, but it has little or no sensibility ; the anterior chamber is extremely shallow ; the iris has almost receded from sight under the cover of the overhanging limbus, and has assumed the slate-grey tinge of advanced atrophic change. The membrane has only too often been reduced to a mere narrow strip, surrounding and framing a wide pupil, whilst its marginal edge is lined with a black border, the result of an eversion of its posterior pigment layer (ectropion uveæ). The green reflex, the stone-like feel of the eye, and the dead-white, deeply cupped optic nerve-head complete the picture for the time being. Degeneration has yet to play its part. Glassy-looking deposits may cover the cornea, whose surface may become the seat of zonular opacity; or vesicles may develop beneath its epithelium; equatorial staphylomata may make their appearance, and cataract may develop. Even now the unfortunate patient may not be at the end of his sufferings, for severe bouts of pain may attend the congestive attacks, which continue long after all sight has vanished. The condition is that of "the blind painful eyeball of glaucoma." Finally secretion appears to stop, or at least so greatly to diminish that the eyeball shrinks and softens, and the wretched blind sufferer at last finds rest from what seems to him to have been an age-long pain; unless, perchance, he is unfortunate enough to belong to the class of those who have intra-ocular hæmorrhage, ulcus serpens, perforation, irido-cyclitis, and panophthalmitis engrafted on all else they have had to bear. At last then, and a sad long last at that, the curtain falls on phthisis bulbi. A melancholy story indeed! and one to which the failure to adopt a proper treatment has too often largely contributed. The depth of its sadness can only be plumbed by those who remember that glaucoma is a binocular disease, and that it affects in most cases those who, right up to middle or advancing age, have known to the full all the pleasures that flow from sight.

REFERENCES

DE SCHWEINITZ, G. E.—*Diseases of the Eye*, W. B. Saunders Co. Ltd., 8th edition, 1916, p. 375.

KÖLLNER, *Munch. med. Woch.*, 1918, p. 229; and *Ophth. Year Book*, 1918, vol. xv. p. 110.

PART II

The Diagnosis of Glaucoma (*continued*)—The Signs and Symptoms of Glaucoma considered from an Anatomical Point of View

SUMMARY :—The Conjunctiva and Sclera.
             The Cornea.
                Mistiness of Vision.
                Halos round Lights.

THE DIAGNOSIS OF GLAUCOMA

        The various Conditions mistaken for Glaucomatous Halos.
        Anæsthesia of Cornea.
    The Anterior Chamber.
        Its Measurements.
    The Iris.
        Dilatation of the Pupil.
        Changes in its Colour.
    The Ciliary Body.
        Weakness of Accommodation.
    The Lens.
        Alterations in Refraction.
        Cataract.
        The Green Reflex.
    The Optic Nerve.
        Pallor of Disc.
        Cupping of Disc.
        Alteration in apparent Directions of Vessels.
        A dragging over of the Retinal Vessels in a Bundle towards the Nasal side of the Fundus.
        Pulsation in Vessels.
            The Arterial Pulse.
            The Venous Pulse.
        Changes in Calibre of Vessels.
        Various Forms of Cupping.
    The Retina.
    The Choroid.
    Koeppe's Sign.
    The Size of the Globe.

The Conjunctiva and Sclera.—Throughout the whole course of a case of simple glaucoma, the conjunctiva is not perceptibly affected, whilst the sclera only shows one change, viz., a slight enlargement of the anterior ciliary vessels. This enlargement may indeed be only obvious at the points of perforation of these vessels, which stand out as distinct red spots against the white sclerotic background.

In congestive attacks, however, quite a different condition is found, and one which varies greatly according to the severity of the case. If the condition is of slight or moderate intensity, all we see is a zone of circumcorneal congestion, with a little hyperæmia of the neighbouring conjunctiva. But should the case be an acute one, the whole front of the eye may become so overcharged with blood that marked chemosis is produced, and in extreme cases the venous hyperæmia may even spread to the palpebral conjunctiva, whose dusky-red appearance may be such as to suggest an acute attack of conjunctivitis. Under the circumstances, it is not difficult to understand how a mistaken diagnosis of acute conjunctivitis, or of iritis, is sometimes made in these cases.

In the intervals between congestive attacks, the conjunctiva and sclera may resume a normal or nearly normal appearance, inasmuch as the evidence of hyperæmia passes away. But one sure sign remains to testify to the harm wrought by the vascular storm ; this is a permanent enlargement of the anterior veins, most obvious, as in the previous case, at the points where the sclera gives passage to the perforating vessels.

When we reach the stage of late glaucoma, we may find a number of degenerative changes occurring. As a consequence of atrophy, the conjunctiva may become very thin and extremely brittle ; this is of importance, from the point of view of obtaining the flaps used for the various operations undertaken for the relief of tension.

The sclera itself undergoes a curious change of colour, it assumes a delicate bluish-white, porcelain-like appearance, which is highly suggestive of the condition. Further, it may yield over localised areas, evidently due to antecedent inflammation in the deeper parts, thus giving rise to ciliary or equatorial staphylomata. Or again, but rarely, the bulging of the sclerotic coat may affect the whole of the areas which are unsupported by the recti muscles, thus giving the eye a somewhat square shape. We do not, however, meet in adults with the general yielding of the whole coat of the eye, which is so characteristic a feature of juvenile glaucoma.

The Cornea.—In the stage of early glaucoma, we find two symptoms, both of which are referable to an alteration in the condition of the cornea ; these are (1) an *indistinctness of vision*, which the patient describes by saying he feels as if there were a mist before his eyes, and (2) the appearance of *rainbows or halos round bright lights*. Both these phenomena are transient, and are observed only when the eye is in a state of congestion as the result of an interference with its circulation. Two causes have been cited to account for these symptoms, viz., (i.) an overstretching of the cornea, as the result of an increase of intra-ocular pressure, and (ii.) an actual œdema of the membrane. The former is supposed to act by altering the refractive power of the fibrils of the cornea; and the evidence in favour of its existence as a factor is held to lie in the very great rapidity with which the symptoms come on, and again pass away, when the tension rises and falls suddenly; for it has been contended, perhaps on rather flimsy grounds, that such rapid transitions could not be considered to depend upon a change such as œdema, which must necessarily take some time to declare itself, or to disappear once it is present.

The subject of the corneal œdema in these cases has

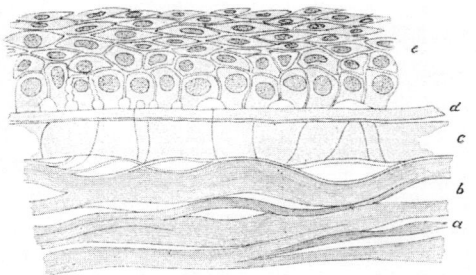

FIG. 24.—Changes in the anterior layers of the cornea, in acute glaucoma, due to œdema (× 441).

e, Corneal epithelium; d, accessory Bowman's membrane, droplets of œdema are seen between this membrane and the epithelium; c, Bowman's membrane; a, lamellæ of cornea, separated by drops (b) of œdema. (Fuchs.)

(*Illustration kindly supplied by Professor V. Morax.*)

been studied anatomically by Fuchs, who finds that the deeper layers of the cornea are unaffected, whilst the lamellæ immediately beneath Bowman's membrane show open spaces due to the accumulation of fluid in that neighbourhood. The layers of the corneal epithelium, and especially the deeper layers, share in the œdematous condition (Fig. 24). Cellular elements, especially leucocytes, can be seen to break through the membrane of Bowman and to form small, sub-epithelial masses. This invasion takes place alongside of the tiny nerve filaments which traverse the membrane on their way to their distribution in the epithelial layer (Fig. 25). The dulness of the cornea in these cases is to be attributed to two factors:—(1) A disturbance of the transparency of the membrane, due to the exuded fluid having an index of refraction different from that of the normal tissues of the part; and (2) an actual irregularity of the epithelial surface as a result (*a*) of certain cells being pushed up more than others by the fluid beneath them, and (*b*) of some of the surface cells being actually destroyed by the œdematous process, minute inequalities being thus left. It is quite probable that the fact that this œdema makes its way, to some extent at least, along the channels in which the nerve filaments lie, has some influence on the anæsthesia of the cornea, which is so prominent a symptom of glaucoma. In the early stage of glaucoma, which we are now discussing, the corneal œdema is essentially transient. It may be so slight as to manifest itself only by the subjective phenomena above recorded; or, on the other hand, it may give rise to a distinct haziness of the corneal surface. The latter is best seen by combining the use of a loupe with that of oblique illumination. In so doing, the beam of light should be focussed *not on* the surface of the cornea, but a little below it. By this manœuvre a ring of light is obtained which shows up a faint corneal opacity much better than the more usual method of focussing the light on the anterior surface of the eye. The haziness of the cornea is usually described as presenting a

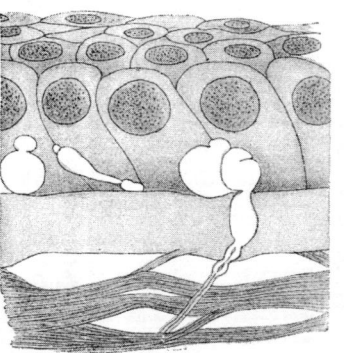

Fig. 25.—Details of the œdematous lesions in the corneal epithelium (× 697). (Fuchs.)

One sees Bowman's membrane (*B*) traversed by the nerve canals, which have been distended by œdema. *E*, corneal epithelium; *cb*, the basal epithelial cells with œdematous spaces; *lc*, superficial layers of the cornea.

(*Illustration kindly supplied by Professor V. Morax.*)

THE DIAGNOSIS OF GLAUCOMA 171

uniform ground-glass-like appearance which is most intense toward the centre of the membrane, and fades peripherally.

It remains to be mentioned that the mists of vision, met with in glaucoma, are not wholly to be ascribed to corneal changes ; on the contrary, as pointed out by Morax, they are due in some, and possibly in a large measure, to the interference with the retinal circulation which is brought about by sudden and transient rises of the intra-ocular pressure.

The subjective aspect of the two symptoms we are considering now claims our attention, and before dealing with each separately, we would pause to make a note of the psychologic interest that attaches to the mental attitude of different people towards these phenomena. Some patients speak of them with amused interest, whilst others are inspired by them with deep alarm.

The *indistinctness of vision* is variously described. Some speak of a cloudiness of the sight, some of seeing as through a haze or smoke, whilst others state that it seems as if there were a fog or mist in the atmosphere ; the more intelligent subjects sometimes volunteer the statement, that when the attacks occur, they are obliged to ask their friends whether the day is misty or not, before they are certain that the phenomenon is subjective. Morax has met with patients in whom the cloudiness of vision takes the very definite form of an impression that the atmosphere is full of soot particles. He also draws attention to the fact that in some cases the sensation of mistiness of vision is quite unassociated with any evidence of the reduction of visual acuity, as shown by test-type examination.

These " mists " are usually most troublesome in the early morning, and pass away as the day goes on, frequently after a few hours or even less. This observation is one of great interest in connection with Professor Thomson's contention that fluid is removed from the eye during the waking hours, as a result of the pump-like action of the iris and ciliary muscles acting on the scleral spur. Such an action must obviously cease, or nearly so, with the advent of sleep. It would therefore suggest itself that sleep would be bad for the glaucomatous patient, whereas we know it is good ; but, clearly, another factor comes into the case, since sleep quiets the circulatory system, and serves to restore its normal condition, which congestive glaucoma so severely disturbs. The balance is therefore in favour of the eye, since the tendency to venous congestion is removed. It may, however, be quite another thing, when we are dealing with a globe, which starts the night not unduly congested, but which is experiencing the difficulties inseparable from a gradual but steady increase in the growing obstruction to the excretion of fluid. The long sleeping hours continuously deprive the organ of its help from the pump-action of the muscles, and so tend to aggravate the want of balance between secretion and excretion. With the advent of morning comes muscular activity, the forced removal of fluid by the pump-action of the ciliary and iris muscles, and the disappearance of the difficulty. As a result the " morning mists " vanish in a short time.

It is well known that the mists of vision and the other signs, which we associate with early glaucoma, are met with in some patients not in the early morning but later on in the day, and especially in the afternoon or evening. If we enquire into the patient's habits, we find that the attacks synchronise with periods of greater or less exhaustion, and that they are often relieved by food, rest, or diversion. A point of considerable interest, and also of diagnostic significance, is suggested by a consideration of the above facts : The occurrence of " morning mists " can best be explained by supposing that there is a primary obstruction to the excretory channels of the eye, and that vascular disturbances are of a secondary nature. On the other hand, the troubles coming on in the afternoon or evening would seem to point to the onset of vaso-motor disturbances, associated with exhaustion of the nervous system, as being the final cause of the attacks. To put it in other words— in the first case we have to do primarily with an obstruction to excretion, and in the second with a condition in which,

THE DIAGNOSIS OF GLAUCOMA 173

from the start, the vaso-motor element is predominant. The distinction between simple and congestive glaucoma and the close interrelation of the two conditions are here most interestingly suggested.

The *halos round lights* are best seen by the patient, when he looks from a distance at a bright light in the dark, and especially at an electric arc light. Two colours at least are usually discernible, an inner blue or violet, and an outer yellow, reddish yellow, or red; a green or greenish yellow band is often seen between them. It is said that the red hues are most in evidence around candle and gas flames, whilst the blue predominate round electric lights. A double halo is said to be sometimes observed, one set of rings lying within the other. Indeed, it seems not improbable that, under laboratory conditions, the observation of this phenomenon would be often elicited. Observers have differed widely as to the size of the glaucomatous halo. Sheard gives it as from 10° to 12°. Others have furnished much lower measurements down to those of from 2° to 2·5°. The author has recently taken considerable trouble to measure such halos, and has found them to vary from 6° 50′ up to 11° 54′. An interesting feature is that they are not even constant in the same eye at different times. We shall return to this subject a little later on.

Another point of interest is that some of the glaucoma patients complain that the halos are dark blue, right out from the centre, with only a fringe of green, yellow, and orange-red. This would appear to be due to the difficulty these patients experience in seeing the central ciliary corona of yellow, which is so obvious to the normal eye as surrounding the source of light. It is suggested that the misty cornea so far diminishes the light admitted that the central area appears dark and therefore indistinguishable from the inner ring of blue. (H. H. Emsley.)

It is well, at this point, to make it clear that all measurements of halos, given in this work, are taken to the outer extremity of the orange-red ring. It is also of interest to record that the rings seen through a steamed glass plate correspond closely in size with those observed in the glaucomatous, and further that the diameter of these rings changes rapidly as the steam dries away, or rather, as the bubbles of condensed water run into each other to form progressively larger aqueous masses. It is generally accepted that the size of the rings, seen by the eye under different conditions, is determined by the diameter of the cells which are optically at fault. If now we accept the view that the glaucomatous halos are a product of œdematous changes in the cells of the corneal epithelium or endothelium, it seems possible that alterations in the size of the droplets formed under the pathological condition present (œdema) may determine a variation in the diameter of the rings seen. We should expect, if this hypothesis is true, that the glaucoma rings would be found to vary according to the condition of the cells which produce them. Thus if these cells were separated from each other by small drops of œdematous fluid, we should expect the resulting halos to be large in diameter ; whereas, if these droplets coalesced and so became individually larger, we should anticipate that the measurements of the halos would diminish. It naturally suggested itself that this might furnish an indication of the stage that the glaucomatous process had reached, and the matter has been carefully studied from this angle, but, perhaps due to the limited number of observations made, it has not so far been possible to come to any definite conclusion.

The persistence of the symptom, and the inconvenience it causes the patients, both vary greatly in different cases. At times the halos are so faint that they have to be carefully looked for, whilst on other occasions the same patient finds that " every tiny flickering flame in the firelight is iridescent with colours." No source of light is then too feeble or too tiny to escape a rainbow crown. It would appear that this condition is especially likely to be established on damp misty days, though it is difficult to say why this should be so.

For the purposes of a clinical test in a darkened room, a candle flame at 5 to 10 feet distance is very serviceable. Ordinary naked electric light flames are most unsuitable, but when placed in a chimney or behind a wide screen, and seen through a 12 mm. ground-glass aperture, they are both efficient and convenient. Most surgeons can command such a source of light, either in their Edridge-Green lamps, or in those they use for retinoscopy. Narrow points of light show the coloured rings excellently, and Sheard strongly advocates the use of the naked bulb of an electric ophthalmoscope for the purpose. It has been stated by a leading authority on glaucoma, that the light-halos may be the only evidence present of the disease. The author cannot concur in such a dictum ; he believes that whenever the rings are seen, careful examination will show other signs of a rise in pressure. The glaucomatous halo is a manifestation, and sometimes a very transitory one, of an œdema of the cornea produced by intra-ocular pressure ; when the pressure is relieved, the œdema disappears and the halos are no more seen. This statement explains the comparative rarity with which we see patients in the halo stage in our consulting rooms ; most frequently we get a history of the rings appearing for short periods, when the patient is tired, and passing away when he gets a meal and rest ; it is only when he comes to us in the course of a congestive attack that we can take him into the dark room, and pin him down to a recognition on the spot of this phenomenon. What is of much greater importance in such instances is that we should be able to demonstrate to him what we mean by "halos," and so prevent him from worrying himself needlessly over phenomena which are of no real importance, but which he may mistake for the pathological manifestation.

This can be done by getting him to look through a glass plate that has been steamed or breathed on, at one of the lights above specified ; he will get a still more vivid idea of the halos through one on which lycopodium has been dusted. Such a plate can be kept for constant use in the dark room, if it is prepared in the following way : A magic-lantern slide cover-glass is dusted over with lycopodium powder, the excess of which is shaken off, the dusted surface is covered with another similar glass, and the two are bound together with lantern-slide binding strips.

Once a patient really understands the nature of the halos, which have a significance in glaucoma, it is much easier to find out whether he really sees them or not. Our next task is a consideration of *the various conditions which from time to time are mistaken by nervous people for halos* ;

(1) On looking at a gas light or other flame at night—especially in a large room, such as a church or hall—one may see it surrounded by a golden haze, made up of radiating luminous beams, some of which are drawn out to considerable length (Fig. 26). This phenomenon may be accentuated by the collection of a small quantity of lachrymal fluid, between the cornea and the lid edge, which forms a tiny meniscus from whose surface the light rays undergo reflection and refraction as they pass into the eye (Morax). If the lid is pulled away from the cornea, the appearance is at once lost ; in any case the phenomenon is innocent of the characteristic spectral coloration.

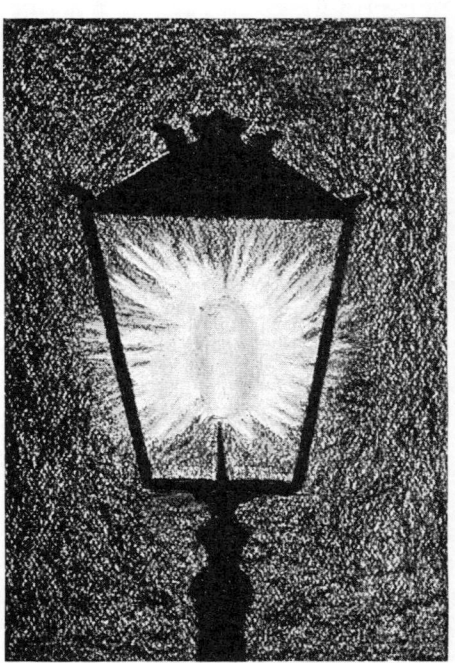

FIG. 26.—The corona of light around a flame ; this is sometimes confused with the coloured halos of glaucoma. It is not a pathologic phenomenon. (Morax.)

(2) Nervous patients who have heard of the glaucoma halos, sometimes persuade themselves that they are seeing them. Such people, as a rule, merely require reassurance in order to make them forget their troubles. In this connection it is interesting to record the frequency with

THE DIAGNOSIS OF GLAUCOMA 177

which we encounter undue nervousness in our glaucomatous patients. This is no doubt partly due to their knowledge of the terrible nature of the disease, and to the mental strain consequently inflicted upon them, but it would almost seem that, as a class, they are unusually nervous. We know this from their behaviour before operation, and even during the procedure, and we see evidence of it long afterwards in the conduct of quite a large group of our successfully operated patients, who come back to us from time to time, with all sorts of fancied ills in connection with their sight, and who, each time, leave our consulting rooms with a renewed lease of the joy of living, the moment we tell them their fears are groundless.

(3) Nervous patients sometimes mistake the scintillating scotoma of migraine for glaucoma halos (Morax). The differential diagnosis is very easily made, even apart from the fact that the former trouble continues even when the eyes are shut, whilst the latter is only in evidence when a patient is looking at a light.

(4) The same point in diagnosis holds for the coloured rings, which many nervous patients see when they close their eyes in the dark, especially after a hard and overtiring day's work. The author has known medical men seriously alarmed by these phenomena.

(5) Patients whose corneæ have become temporarily clouded, as the result of some caustic medical application, often complain of very vivid halos, which pass away when the membranes clear after a night's rest. In Madras, where acute catarrhal conditions are very common, it was formerly the custom to treat these by painting the lids with a 2 per cent. solution of silver nitrate ; after doing so, the corneal epithelium was seen to be cloudy as a result of the action of the drug, and the author was struck with the frequent complaints made by patients, that after each such painting, " the vision was misty and bright lights were seen as if surrounded by halos." He was able to confirm this observation on himself. Treacher Collins has drawn attention to the fact that by dropping a solution of the alkaloid erythrophleine (African arrow-head poison) into the eye, a

similar appearance of rainbows round lights can be produced.

(6) If a bright light is looked at in the dark through a steamy glass, coloured halos are well seen. This may give rise to apprehension in the minds of those who know the importance of this sign. Anyone who wears glasses may see this phenomenon on a foggy night owing to moisture condensing on the surface of his spectacles. Again, the rings may be seen when looking through a steamy plate-glass window from the dark outside, at a bright light far back in a big room. The author specially noticed this when passing the windows of shops lit by a single light at a time when illumination in London was restricted. In either case some alarm may be occasioned, but the matter can be quite simply put to rest, if the spectacles are wiped, or if a part of the window which is not steamy is looked through.

(7) The evidence before us would lead to the inference that the rainbows of glaucoma are due to an interference with the normal condition of the cornea, and not to any change in the lens. This view is supported by the fact that halos are seen by those aphakic eyes which become glaucomatous. At the same time, we must recognise the possibility that changes in the lens may give rise to phenomena indistinguishable from those associated with high tension of the eye. Indeed, Fumiatzew has claimed that rainbow circles round lights can be seen in the early stages of cataract just as readily as in glaucoma. In order to make a differential diagnosis between the two, he advises the surgeon to place before the patient's eye a diaphragm, carrying a hole of the same diameter as that of the patient's pupil under daylight illumination. If the halo is due to nuclear cataract, it will then disappear, but will return again in an intensified form, if the diaphragm is suddenly removed, whilst the patient is still watching the source of light; the latter phenomenon is due to the pupil being caught momentarily dilated. On the other hand, if the halos are due to glaucoma, they are unaffected either by the use of the diaphragm or by alterations in the illumination. If the opacities in the lens are peripheral, the placing of

the diaphragm before the eye dissipates the rainbow, which returns with increased brilliancy when it is again taken away.

(8) The interesting work dealt with in the preceding paragraph was formerly unhesitatingly accepted by ophthalmologists; but a large amount of research has recently been devoted to this subject, and has led us to modify our views, or at least to take up a less decided attitude than our former one. It has been shown that the normal eye can habitually see coloured rings round bright lights in the dark, once its attention has been drawn to them. These halos have been carefully studied by a number of observers (Druault, Morax, Brudenell Carter, Chance, Sheard, Schiötz and others). Carter believes that they are more commonly seen in the aged, and Morax and Druault associate them with dilatation of the pupil. The subject derives an added interest from the indisputable fact, known to many of us, that certain of our patients will see halos when their pupils are artificially dilated, and this in the entire absence of any indication of a rise in ocular pressure. The possibility that this phenomenon may lead to a serious misunderstanding, and may damage a professional reputation, must always be borne in mind. In contrast to the ignorance of the symptoms of glaucoma displayed by some medical men, it is extraordinary that members of the public should often know so much about them as they do. Many of them are well informed about glaucoma halos, and it is essential that the specialist should be on his guard in this matter, both for his own sake and for that of his professional colleagues. If he can show a suspicious patient that his halos are physiological and not glaucomatous, he will often do a very valuable piece of work.

From the practical point of view the differentiation is not difficult : (1) The physiological halos are, in the great majority of cases at least, far less vivid, and far more difficult to recognise than the glaucomatous ones. (2) The former are always present if looked for under suitable conditions, whilst the latter are either only occasionally present, or if constant, are accompanied by other mani-

180   GLAUCOMA

festations of high tension which leave the diagnosis in no possible doubt. (3) The angular diameter of the physiological halos measures 7° to the outer edge of the orange-red. This figure is constant, thus furnishing a striking contrast to that for the glaucoma rings, which, as we have already shown, may vary from under 7° up to nearly 12°.

Druault has suggested a test which Morax claims to be of considerable value: The eye under examination is

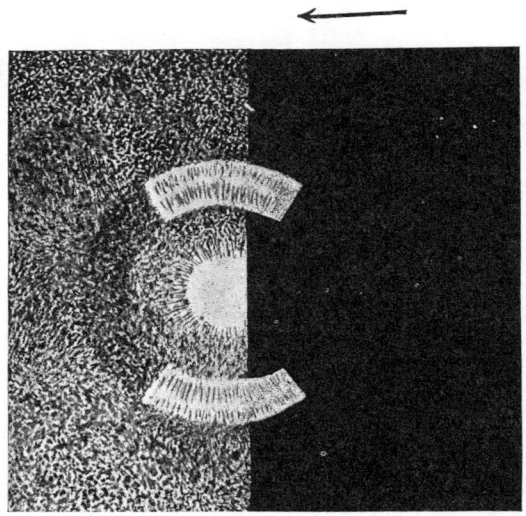

Fig. 27.—Diagram to show Druault's experiment, designed to distinguish between the physiologic and glaucomatous halos. The black screen is moved from right to left; according to Druault two sectors of the ring persisted in the position shown above, the rest of the ring being obliterated, thus indicating that the halo is physiologic. (Morax.)

gradually covered by a straight-edged screen (a piece of darkened cardboard); this is brought in from the side until half the pupil is shut off; when this has been done, part of the coloured ring is still seen, but this is not the part which one might have expected, for the upper and lower quadrants of the luminous circle remain, whilst those to the right and left disappear. He takes this to indicate that the halo is due to diffraction phenomena produced by the

ERRATUM.

I greatly regret to find that I have misinterpreted Professor Morax, and through him Dr. Druault, on page 181. Diagram 28 on that page really represents the change in the halo seen through a lycopodium plate under the advance of a straight-edged screen. The true glaucoma halo on the contrary fades gradually away throughout the whole of its circumference, in proportion as the advance of the screen cuts off an increasing amount of light from the pupil. I would tender a sincere apology for the mistake to Professor Morax and to Dr. Druault. I regret most sincerely that at this date it is impossible to put the matter right in the text.

R. H. ELLIOT.

March 15, 1922.

THE DIAGNOSIS OF GLAUCOMA

lens fibres at the level of the pupil. If, on the other hand, the halo is a true glaucomatous one, and therefore produced by changes in the cornea, the portion which disappears is that which is covered by the screen and that only (Figs. 27 and 28).

So important did this subject appear to the author, that he sought the assistance of Mr. H. H. Emsley, B.Sc., of the Northampton Polytechnic Institute, Clerkenwell,

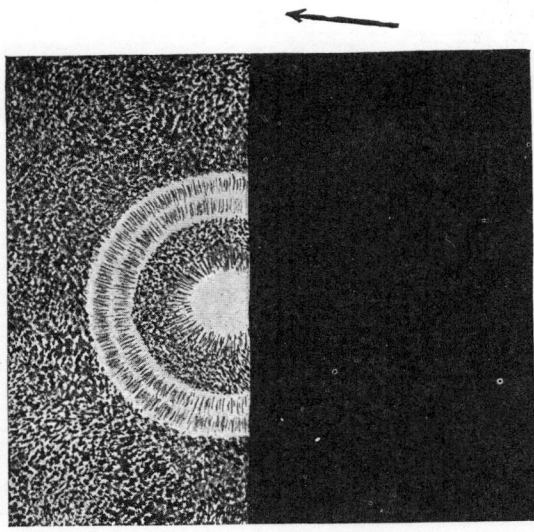

Fig. 28.—Shows the behaviour of the glacomatous halo, when the screen is passed before the eye in the same way as before. Druault claimed that the ring was gradually obliterated, as shown in the figure. (E. E.)

who with his colleague, Mr. Fincham, has kindly made a number of experiments: They found that a stenopaic slit gives better results than the straight-edged screen. When this slit is moved across the area of vision close to a glaucomatous eye, the halo decreases in intensity, and finally disappears simultaneously in its whole circumference, as might have been expected. A physiological halo behaves quite differently. With the slit vertical, and held opposite one border of the pupil, two partial halos are seen at the extremities of a vertical diameter. On a further movement of the slit in a horizontal direction across the pupil, each of these bands divides into two, and these rotate in opposite directions around the circle, finally combining into bands in the original positions, as soon as the slit exposes the opposite border of the pupil. This result is what might have been expected on the assumption that the diffraction halos so seen are due to the radial nature of the structure producing them, which, in this case, is obviously the crystalline lens. These phenomena are much more easily seen by an observer whose pupil is naturally or artificially dilated.

Mr. Emsley would appear to have furnished us with a delicate test whereby we can distinguish between halos due to corneal changes (pathological) and those due to the normal structure of the lens (physiological).

(9) Transient halos round lights are also often complained of by those who suffer from conjunctivitis associated with much mucus discharge. Wiping or washing away the offending flake or layer of mucus from in front of the cornea, relieves the symptom, and shows what was responsible for it. The current explanation of this phenomenon, that the coloured rings are caused by the eye being lined by a layer of mucus leaves something to be desired, for there would seem to be no valid reason why such a lining should produce the effect in question. This reflection suggested a line of experiment to the author : If a drop of white of egg is placed between two slides and squeezed out, a clear transparent slide is produced. If, however, the two glass covers are freely rubbed on each other, the film of white of egg is broken up by a number of tiny air-bubbles, and on again looking through the contrivance, prismatic colours are seen. These attain their maximum brilliance wherever the bubbles are smallest and most numerous, and fade away where they are large and scattered, an observation which can easily be confirmed with the aid of a low-power microscope. Other viscid fluids, such as certain oils, give exactly similar results. An analogous series of experiments was made on the eye : A drop of egg albumin or oil instilled into the

conjunctival sac failed to give rise to the appearance of halos, nor was it found possible to break up the fluid sufficiently to cause this phenomenon, though it is possible that this might be done in a laboratory, with the aid of suitable apparatus. On the other hand, it seems not unlikely that the movements of the lids over the eyeballs may have precisely the same effect on the mucus lying between them as those of the glass slides have on the egg albumin. The rarity with which patients see halos through mucus suggests that the exact conditions favourable to the production of these phenomena are not often met with, but there is an interesting observation in favour of the hypothesis toward which we are leading up. In certain patients with chronic catarrh, one notices, on everting the lids, the presence of small air-bubbles in the conjunctival folds. An examination under the microscope of a drop of mucus from such an eye sometimes shows it to be full of tiny air-bubbles, closely resembling those seen in the rubbed-up white of egg film. The same thing may be observed after rubbing an ointment into the eye. Now Fraunhöfer long ago pointed out that the coloured rings we see on looking through a glass plate covered with steam or lycopodium, are diffraction phenomena produced by the globules of steam or the grains of powder, and that a necessary condition of their appearance is that the grains or globules should be of nearly uniform size (Sheard). This explains the halo seen when a drop of blood is introduced into the conjunctival sac. It also suggests an explanation of the rarity of the phenomena in connection with mucus in the sac, for it seems likely that the concatenation of circumstances (thickness of mucus, increase of lid movements, etc.), necessary to form a film of fine uniform bubbles in the conjunctival secretion, may be a comparatively rare event, but nevertheless one which may sometimes occur.

There is yet another way in which halos may be produced in an eye which is exuding an undue amount of mucus, as was proved by a recent experience of the author's. A patient, who from time to time is troubled with chronic catarrh, associated with the seeing of coloured rings, was examined on one of these occasions. The test was a little difficult, as the halos tended to pass away ; the diameter of the orange ring seen was about 25°. The secretion from his eyes revealed clumps of mucus, in which were embedded masses of leucocytes, most of which proved to be polymorpho-nuclear in type. This at once explained the origin of the coloured rings, and led to an experiment being made with a drop of blood in the conjunctival sac of an eye. Extremely vivid halos were then seen, and a measurement of the orange red gave the figure of over 19° for this circle. On a closer examination, it was found that inside the blue ring of this rainbow there was another orange red, measuring 11° 24'. Outside the main rainbow there was still another. It is possible, if not probable, that the ring measured in the catarrhal case was not that of the innermost halo. An obvious source of fallacy in the measurement of these halos is thus revealed. The fact, already mentioned, that they disappear at once on washing the eye, clears up the diagnosis without the least difficulty, and so only an academic interest attaches to the mensuration of these rings.

A last word as to the measurement of halos may not be out of place in the interests of those who are not prepared to make the comparatively simple calculation necessary for the purpose. With the light 10 feet from the observing eye, the diameters of the halos will be approximately as follows : For 4°, 8·5 ins. ; for 5°, 10·5 ins. ; for 6°, 12·5 ins. ; for 7°, 14·75 ins. ; for 8°, 17 ins. ; for 9°, 19 ins. ; for 10°, 21 ins. ; for 11°, 23·33 ins. ; for 12°, 25·35 ins.

Before leaving the subject, it is of interest to mention an unusual case recorded by von Graefe of a workman, suffering from glaucoma, who " from time to time had *blue spectra* before his eyes ; he had seen rainbows round the candle, and when he fixed an object whilst in this state, or exposed the eye to the light, the colour spectra revolved like a wheel, and the sight became so dim that he could no longer recognise even large print. After a night of good sleep, vision was always perfectly acute again." This revolution of a wheel of light before the field of vision has, in the author's experience, been observed in a patient suffering from asthenopia, with no suspicion of glaucoma. An oscillatory or rotatory movement of the scotoma is known to be a symptom, though a rare one, of eclipse cases. The question is dealt with in the author's work on *Tropical Ophthalmology*. With regard to the blue spectrum mentioned, an experiment with glass exposed to different depths of steaming will show the reader that the amount of blue in the halos produced is capable of considerable variation. Possibly the same occurs in glaucoma. An explanation of this has already been offered.

Von Graefe also speaks of a symptom, which may accompany a late stage of glaucoma, but which in his judgment should really be referred to the co-existing atrophy of the optic nerve. It consists in objects in the street appearing to the patient as though they were covered with snow. He thinks this phenomenon " should be carefully distinguished from the glaucomatous chromopsiæ."

The interest which glaucoma patients take in their halos can be turned to very valuable account. Once an intelligent person has had his attention drawn to them, he is constantly on the look out for them ; their presence or absence then constitutes a very delicate test for the onset of periodic increases of tension in the eye. The success or failure of meiotic treatment can also be controlled, and in not a few instances the recurrence of halos warns the patient of the return of tension in an eye which has been operated on by a method which has failed to give permanent relief. A patient of the author's is in the habit of looking out for a return of tension by watching the matches he uses to light his pipe. He finds that a match held out at arm's length *in the dark* constitutes a very delicate test indeed ; even in dull daylight it is no mean criterion of a rise in the level of intra-ocular pressure.

The reception of light on parts of the retina other than the macula is said to have no influence on the perception of glaucomatous halos ; nor does the state of contraction or dilatation of the pupil make any difference.

Anæsthesia of the Cornea.—If the sensitiveness of the

surface of the eye is tested during one of the congestive attacks in a case of early glaucoma, it will be found to be very distinctly diminished. When the eye resumes its normal condition and the subjective phenomena disappear, the anæsthesia to a large extent passes away, but after a number of attacks have occurred, the sensitiveness of the cornea appreciably and permanently diminishes, till in the end it is practically abolished.

Nor is the deepening anæsthesia the only sign of corneal trouble, which manifests itself as the eye passes from the early into the pronounced stage of glaucoma ; for in each congestive attack, the corneal haze becomes more marked, until finally the membrane acquires a steamy look as if it had been breathed upon ; its surface may appear distinctly rough. Moreover, in consequence of the changes which are occurring in the ciliary body, deposits may be formed (k.p.) on the back of the cornea, and can then be detected with the aid of a loupe.

Nevertheless the cornea tends to clear in the intervals between the congestive attacks, and even in a very late stage, it may be found to be quite transparent, unless some form of degeneration has taken place. In that case, hyaline deposits may be found upon its surface ; or it may present well-marked zonular opacity ; or a vesicular or bullous change may set in ; or even deep ulceration of the cornea may be met with, leading to pan-ophthalmitis and phthisis bulbi.

The Anterior Chamber.—In the early stage of glaucoma, the *anterior chamber* is always found to be *shallow* during the congestive attacks. Later in the stage of pronounced glaucoma, this shallowing becomes permanent ; but it is still more accentuated during the congestive attacks, and indeed in acute glaucoma it may be so extreme as to make the performance of an iridectomy very difficult and very hazardous. This phenomenon has been discussed at length in Chapter III., and is due in the early stages to an overdistension of the vitreous body, to a congestion of the ciliary body, or to both, and later on to an adhesion of the base of the iris to the sclera and cornea,

THE DIAGNOSIS OF GLAUCOMA 187

and to a slackening of the zonule from overdistension. In the late cases the angle of the chamber is actually obliterated, and it is of great importance that we should be able to ascertain how far forward the band of adhesion extends, for upon this point depends so much of the safety or otherwise of operative procedures undertaken for the relief of glaucoma. There are several methods of examining the angle of the chamber :

(1) Norman's method. By using a Würdemann's transilluminator and pressing it against the skin of the lower lid, or better still against the cocainised eyeball, a ring of light is seen in the normal eye surrounding the cornea immediately behind the limbus. This brightly illuminated band marks out the space all round between the angle of the chamber and the limbus. The farther forward the angle is obliterated by adhesions the narrower is this band said to become, up to the point at which its complete disappearance shows that the process of obliteration has reached the limbus itself.

(2) Salzmann's method. This takes advantage of the fact that the angle of the anterior chamber can be examined from the side by direct or indirect ophthalmoscopy. Much valuable information may thus be obtained as to the depth of the chamber, the presence of peripheral synechiæ, etc.

(3) Examination of the angle of the chamber by an electric-lit loupe or by means of a Zeiss' corneal microscope. The writer finds this the most valuable and the easiest of all the methods. The information it affords is always useful and sometimes indispensable. Messrs. Zeiss have recently constructed a set of lenses, which are to be directly applied to the eye (" eye adhesion glasses ") ; these are to be used with their corneal microscope, and it is claimed that, by their aid, the angle of the chamber is laid open for inspection. The device is too new to be profitably discussed, but those who are interested can obtain full information from the firm, or from their agents.[1]

A measurement of the depth of the anterior chamber is of much less value than an accurate estimate of the state of

[1] Messrs. Martin & Tomkins, 51 Margaret Street, Regent Street, W. 1.

closure of its angle, but still it is a factor which we cannot afford to neglect. F. Lindstedt believes that a systematic examination of the kind is likely to yield important results for the conception of the nature of different forms of glaucoma ; he has devised an instrument which allows rapid measurements of the depth of the anterior chamber to be taken, without the need of resorting to any calculations. The fact that the work has been done under the ægis of Professor Gullstrand at Upsala stamps it as being worth careful notice.

An effort in the same direction has been made by Raeder, who uses a single-tube corneal microscope, and by a suitable arrangement of prisms causes the images of the cornea and iris to fall on the same perpendicular plane and thus to be seen simultaneously by the observer. The depth of the chamber is read off directly on a scale attached to one of the prisms. Accuracy up to 1·0 mm. is claimed for the instrument. The surface of the cornea is brought into view by dusting it with finely powdered xeroform. The edge of the pupil is used as the deep point of fixation.

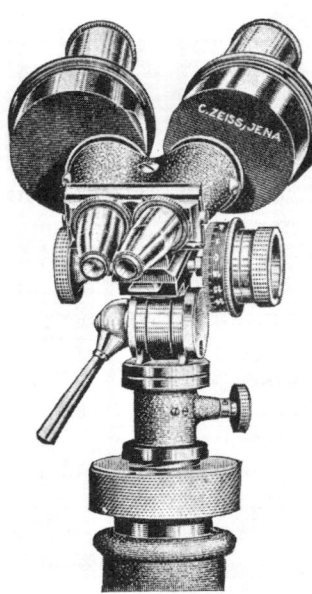

Fig. 29.—Microscope head with Dr. Ulbrich's graduated drum attached.

(About ¼ full size.)

A third device is that of Ulbrich, and consists of a graduated drum, which is attached to the Zeiss' corneal microscope, and which can be seen on the right-hand side of Fig. 29. This drum is fitted to the left-hand pinion-head, and is so graduated as to give the apparent depth of the chamber in tenths of a millimetre, whence the actual depth may be computed by a simple calculation.

It is manifest that it would be of great value to be able

to follow a suspicious, or even a certain but slowly progressive, case of glaucoma with periodical records of the depth of the chamber, and to add these to the information gained by tonometry and other methods.

During the acute and subacute exacerbations of glaucoma, the *contents of the chamber* are frequently found to be *turbid*. This is obviously the result of the condition of the ciliary body and possibly, though to a much less extent, of that of the iris. As a consequence of this turbidity, deposits may occur, as already mentioned, on the back of the cornea ; the net result is to give an impression of an alteration in the colour and pattern of the iris far in excess of that which really exists. That this is so, is sometimes very evident after emptying the chamber in the course of a paracentesis, or of an iridectomy.

The Iris.—The sign of glaucoma, which in the minds of surgeons is most closely associated with the iris, is that of *dilatation of the pupil*. This sign is a constant feature of the transient attacks met with in the early stage, and is associated in them with a sluggish reaction of the iris, whether to light or to accommodation. As the early attacks pass into those of the established stage, both the dilatation of the pupil and the sluggishness of the iris become markedly increased, until at a late stage the iris is represented merely by a thin grey band of inactive tissue, which is hardly apparent as it crouches behind the limits of the limbus. The dilatation of the pupil is not uniform the whole way round. It is often more exaggerated in the vertical than in the horizontal diameters, and in the upper rather than in the lower meridian of the eye. The result is that the enlarged pupil is frequently of an oval shape with its long axis vertical, and is not seldom eccentric and displaced upwards. But this is not the only sign we find in connection with the *iris*. If the congestive attacks are acute or subacute this membrane may become extremely *congested and distinctly altered in colour*, as well as in texture, an effect, the appearance of which is heightened by coincidental changes in the cornea and aqueous. Later, the natural colour of the membrane fades to a *greyish* hue and *atrophic patches* appear upon its surface ; these, when illuminated with the ophthalmoscope, are found to be translucent, the fundus reflex showing clearly through them. A not infrequent, and very characteristic appearance is a velvety black edge to the margin of the pupil, due to an *ectropion of the uveal pigment* at the pupillary margin, in consequence of the shrinking of the iris stroma (Fig. 30). The signs we have been describing are characteristic of

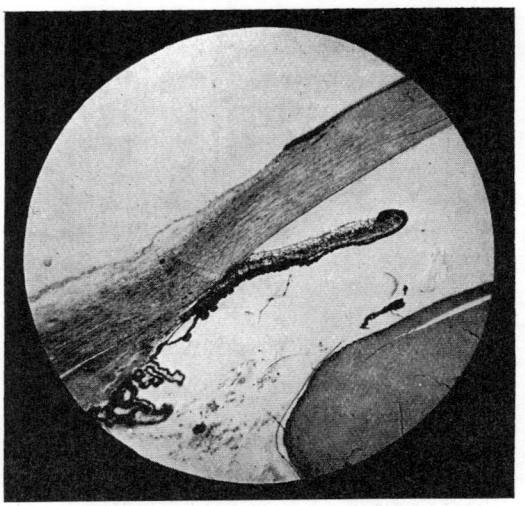

FIG. 30.—Ectropion of the uveal pigment.
(*Photograph by E. E. from specimen kindly supplied by Mr. Treacher Collins.*)

congestive glaucoma, and with the exception of dilatation of the pupil, are not found in the simple form of the disease. If the latter has run an absolutely non-congestive course, the pupil may be of moderate or even of normal size, and the iris is usually little if at all altered in colour, though its reaction to light may be almost or completely lost. Until the atrophic stage is far advanced, the pupil still responds to the action of meiotic or mydriatic drugs, even when the light reflex is feeble or absent. It is possible that exception may be taken by some to the suggestion that any colour changes are ever seen in the iris in cases of simple glaucoma. The writer has found that such changes do occur, and he attributes the uniform grey coloration then observed to a slow and partial atrophy of the iris stroma, and of its pigment. It would indeed be strange if, apart altogether from the cicatrisation following a long-standing congestive condition, one did not find evidences of atrophy in the iris, as well as in every other structure within the eye, as a result of the long continued ischæmia, to which the structures have been subjected by reason of the increased fluid pressure within the globe.

The *cause of the dilatation of the pupil in glaucoma.* It is generally assumed that this dilatation is a result of interference with the ciliary nerve trunks and with their terminals in the sphincter of the iris, as a result of the increase of the intra-ocular pressure. The objection has been raised that the dilator nerve fibres would be equally exposed, with the constrictor fibres, to the influence of increased pressure, and that the function of both would therefore be interfered with simultaneously. This argument does not seem to be a valid one, for the following reasons: The normal, comparatively small size of the pupil is presumably maintained by the excess of power of the constrictor muscle over its dilator antagonist. If the influence of both these muscles were to be simultaneously withdrawn, we should expect the result to be a marked dilatation of the pupil, in correspondence with the excess of power above indicated. Apart from this there is another factor to be reckoned with, viz., the presence of vaso-constriction of the vessels of the iris, as a result of the rise in intra-ocular pressure, for it is universally admitted that such vaso-constriction leads to dilatation of the pupil, just as vaso-dilatation does to constriction of the pupil.

It is more difficult to explain why the dilatation met with in glaucoma is not of a more regular character. Why does the pupil assume an oval shape ? And why is the dilatation so frequently found to be specially marked in an upward direction ? It has been suggested that regional differences in the degree of vascular constriction present may be the determining factor in producing these pupillary irregularities. It must, however, be freely admitted that in mentioning this explanation we are trespassing very far on the domains of hypothesis.

The Ciliary Body.—The earliest sign of glaucoma to be associated with the ciliary body is a *weakness of accommodative power*. The need of changing his glasses at an unexpectedly early date is sometimes the first thing which leads a patient to consult a medical man. The accommodative weakness is best marked during the congestive attacks, whether in the early or in the pronounced stage, but it does not completely pass away in the interval, with the result that the patient's presbyopia steadily progresses at a rate disproportionate to the advance of his age. Two causes have been assigned : (1) An interference with the function of the ciliary nerves owing to the increased pressure to which they are subjected ; and (2) a clogging of the ciliary muscle and of the suspensory ligament with the products of disturbed action of the ciliary body. The latter factor can probably act only in those cases in which an inflammatory element enters into the disease, but possibly these are not so rare as has been thought. The former is undoubtedly the more important. It probably acts in two ways : (*a*) By direct pressure upon the nerve trunks, plexuses, and branches, leading to their atrophy, and (*b*) by an interference with the normal circulation, on which the nerves and their branches are dependent for their nutrition. It is obvious that the latter of these factors is by far the more important of the two. The whole problem is identical with that which confronts us in studying the atrophy met with in the optic nerve and the retina, and its fuller consideration will be deferred until we come to deal with those structures.

Of not less importance than the failure of accommodation is a condition of congestion of the ciliary body. This is almost certainly present even in what have been usually described as prodromal attacks, though the evidence is not then so well marked as it becomes in the stage of pronounced glaucoma. We have already discussed this subject in the preceding sections and it need not be further dealt with here.

It is of interest to record that Hiere has suggested the use of fluorescein in the differential diagnosis between glaucoma and iritis. He states that when administered by the mouth, the stain fails to pass into the anterior chamber, if the ciliary body is healthy, but readily makes its appearance there, if cyclitis is present. Hamburger supports this statement, whilst Gutmann goes farther and claims to have succeeded in making the above test, by injecting fluorescein subconjunctivally; he thus avoids the bronzing which occurs after the ingestion of the drug. It hardly seems likely that surgeons will very often feel called upon to apply such means of diagnosis. In any case Hiere's method carries with it very obvious objections.

The Lens.—In connection with this structure there are three changes to be considered : (1) *Alterations in the refractive power* of the eye, (2) the appearance of *cataract*, and (3) the peculiar *green reflex*, which is so characteristic of the disease as to have given rise to the term " glaucoma."

(1) *Refractive changes.*—We have already spoken of premature presbyopia and explained its genesis. We have also stated that owing to a forward movement of the diaphragm of the eye, the anterior chamber becomes shallower than normal. It is obvious that a forward movement of the lens must result in an increase of the refractive power of the dioptric system of the eye. In other words, emmetropia will be turned into myopia, hyperopia will tend to be neutralised, and myopia will be increased. The change is not, however, sufficient to compensate for the progress of the presbyopia, which remains the dominant factor in the situation. It is probable that the displacement forward of the lens is to some extent compensated for by the increased pressure which is thus exerted upon its anterior surface, and which by flattening it, would tend to decrease its refractive power. In an adult the increased distension of the globe is probably insufficient to affect the refraction of the eye.

It is the experience of most ophthalmic surgeons that a certain number of their glaucoma patients, who complain of a recent defect in vision, prove to be hypermetropic instead of myopic. This is easily explained : The original condition in such cases was one of latent hyperopia ; this has become manifest under the paralysing influence of the increase of pressure acting upon the third nerves and their terminals in the ciliary muscle.

(2) *Cataract.*—It is necessary to distinguish sharply between three conditions which are frequently confused, viz., (*a*) cataract secondary to glaucoma, (*b*) glaucoma secondary to cataract, and (*c*) cataract occurring as an accidental complication of glaucoma. The need for a correct diagnosis is the more urgent since a decision on this point powerfully influences the line of treatment to be adopted.

(*a*) THE FORM OF CATARACT SECONDARY TO GLAUCOMA is characterised by the want of definition in its appearance. It looks more like a smoky, greenish, or bluish haze than like one of the ordinary forms of cataract. On examining an ordinary cataract through a dilated pupil, either with the electric ophthalmoscope or with a corneal microscope, the details of the opacity can be clearly and definitely seen. No better method for this purpose exists than that of placing a + 10 D. lens in the aperture of the ophthalmoscope, using a bright illumination, and employing a parallel beam of light (all of which is easily done with one of the modern self-lit ophthalmoscopes). Working at 10 to 14 inches and increasing or lessening the distance till sharp focus is obtained, a beautiful picture is seen, in which every detail of the opacity is thrown up dark against the bright background of the fundus reflex. When employing this method, it is not possible to fail to recognise a cataract if present. The dilatation of the pupil, if necessary, can be made with the assistance of euphthalmin. Should this drug fail to produce mydriasis, we can fall back on homatropin. It cannot be denied that there is always a slight element of risk in dilating the pupil of a glaucomatous patient (p. 140). It is therefore most important that we should employ a

THE DIAGNOSIS OF GLAUCOMA

meiotic afterwards, and that we should keep the patient under observation until meiosis has fully replaced mydriasis. This practice was the routine for many years in Madras without our ever having had the slightest cause for anxiety. Indeed Edward Jackson and some other American surgeons go a step farther than this, for they deliberately instil a mydriatic into an eye in which they suspect glaucoma, with a view of determining whether the tension rises in consequence. If it does, they consider the diagnosis appreciably strengthened. In certain cases the method is of undoubted value, but it is obviously one which needs to be very carefully safeguarded.

(b) GLAUCOMA SECONDARY TO CATARACT.—The appearance of the lens in these cases is characteristic of primary cataract of the intumescent variety, the history is unmistakable, and the existence of a primary and hitherto uncomplicated cataract in the opposite eye often clinches the diagnosis.

(c) CATARACT OCCURRING AS AN ACCIDENTAL COMPLICATION OF GLAUCOMA.—Any surgeon in large practice must meet with a certain number of cases in which he finds it difficult, if not impossible, to trace a definite connection between an opacity of the lens and a co-existing glaucoma. The two are obviously fortuitously combined; at any rate it is difficult to come to any other conclusion. Indeed, why should this not be the case ?

(3) *The green reflex of glaucoma.*—This is not really pathognomonic of this disease, for a very similar appearance may be seen in eyes suffering from other diseases, and even in the normal organ of an old person, provided that the pupil is dilated. The condition necessary for its production is a dilatation of the pupil, combined with some want of transparency in the aqueous humour, lens, or cornea, or in all three.

Optic Nerve and Retina.—The changes found in the optic nerve and retina are (1) pallor of the disc ; (2) depression of the floor of the disc, the so-called " cupping of the disc " ; (3) an alteration in the direction of the individual vessels as they pass from the disc on to the surrounding fundus ; (4) a dragging over of the retinal vessels in a bundle, towards the nasal side of the fundus ; (5) the presence of pulsation in the retinal vessels ; (6) a change, both actual and relative, in the size of the retinal arteries and veins. We shall take these up in turn.

(1) *Pallor of the disc.*—This is due in some measure to a constriction of the vascular supply as a result of increased intra-ocular pressure, but mainly to an atrophy of the fibres of the optic nerve. The time-honoured view is that, when the lamina cribrosa yields under pressure, the whole nerve-head is thrust bodily backwards. It is generally accepted that its fibres must thereby be subjected to injury, for they are sharply bent and at the same time stretched over the unyielding crest-like edge of the scleral foramen. The pressure to which they are exposed throughout their course, and especially at this bend, would presumably tend to cause them to atrophy. In addition to this their supply of blood is interfered with, (i.) owing to the increase of the intra-ocular pressure (we shall return to this subject presently), and (ii.) owing to the double bend introduced into their course, firstly at the margin of the floor of the disc, and secondly as they pass over the edge of the disc on to the fundus. As the nerve fibres undergo atrophy, their normal pink colour, which is due to their free blood supply, gives place to an increasing pallor. At the same time, owing to the atrophy of the nerve fibres, the lamina cribrosa becomes exposed at the bottom of the disc, and shows up as a white area, stippled with greyish dots, the latter representing the apertures in the membrane through which the nerve bundles pass.

This pallor of the optic disc is not merely a subject of academic interest. On the contrary, it is a sign of deep pathologic import, and one which often sheds a flood of light on the prognosis of the case. It is best seen in those late cases in which surgical interference has been long delayed, and its significance lies in the fact that, even though the eye may be successfully decompressed, there is a grave danger that the interference with vision, both central and peripheral, may continue until the patient loses all or nearly all his sight. The process of nerve atrophy, set in train by the pressure to which the nerve and the retina have been subjected, only too often continues up to the point of complete blindness. It is of interest to watch the two eyes of a patient, operated on at the same time for glaucoma, and with equal technical success, so far as decompression is concerned, and to observe how the

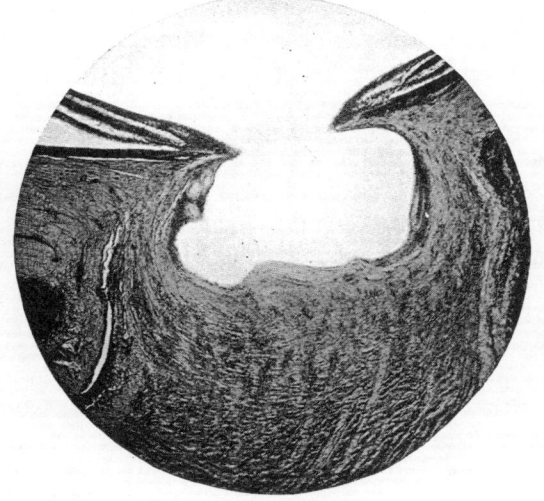

Fig. 31.—Cupping of the optic disc (glaucomatous).
Note (1) the sharp scleral spur on the right side; (2) the overhanging edges; and (3) the retinal vessels hiding under the latter. × 20.
(*Photo by Mr. W. Chesterman.*)

less pale nerve may maintain or even improve its functional activity, whilst the more atrophic one may go steadily downhill.

(2) *Cupping of the optic disc* is, next to the increase in ocular tension, the best-known sign of glaucoma (Fig. 31). It owes its origin to the fact that the foramen, through which the optic nerve enters the eye, is guarded only by the comparatively weak and thin lamina cribrosa. We have discussed the anatomical features of this part of the eye

at some length in Chapter I. Part II., and have shown that they satisfactorily account for (i.) the shape of an advanced glaucoma cup, (ii.) the overhanging edges seen in such a cup, and (iii.) the apparent interruption in the continuity of the blood vessels as they emerge from it.

It has further been shown in the same section that the strength, position, and composition of the lamina cribrosa vary very widely in different eyes, and that these variations in anatomical structure must greatly influence the ophthalmoscopic appearances presented by different cases of optic atrophy, whether the latter is associated with intra-ocular pressure or otherwise.

The view which has long been accepted by ophthalmologists is that a yielding of the lamina cribrosa—this weak spot of the scleral tunic—takes place at an early date in all glaucoma cases, and increases steadily throughout the progress of the excavation until the floor of the cup is depressed almost to the depth of the scleral wall itself.

Such an idea, like others of our misconceptions of glaucoma pathology, is probably due to the fact that the material from which our deductions are derived is, in dealing with this disease, almost invariably obtained from very late cases. Fuchs has recently made an attack on the time-honoured views which we have held so complacently and so long, and has shown that the effect on the lamina cribrosa of an increase of the intra-ocular pressure is nothing like so simple as we have hitherto supposed. In the earlier stages, the whole of this supporting framework is not affected, for it is the glial tissue which yields first to pressure and disappears, whilst the connective tissue lamellæ of mesodermal origin are still able to hold their ground. The glial fibres in the anterior part of the nerve-head are first destroyed, and their destruction, according to Fuchs, actually precedes that of the nerve fibres themselves. Later still, the glial elements of the whole framework of the intra-ocular portion of the nerve disappear. All these changes may occur *before any displacement of the lamina cribrosa* is in evidence. If, however, intra-ocular pressure is continued, the lamina yields as a whole, being pushed back into the optic nerve trunk, which is thereby proportionally shortened, and at the same time made thicker. Part of this thickening is due to changes in the nerve fibres, and to the development within the nerve of a condition which resembles a profuse œdema. Later, when atrophy is established, the nerve becomes thinner than before.

It remains to state, in support of what has been put forward above, that Fuchs has notes of four cases, in which the sectioned papillæ showed depressions of their surfaces varying from 0·45 to 0·73 mm. ; in none of these cases was the lamina markedly displaced, the cupping being due to destruction of the glial tissue and of the nerve substance. It is both noteworthy and strange that no evidence could be discovered in these cases of any increase, either in the strength or thickness of the lamina, such as might explain its remaining in position ; indeed, in some of them, it appeared to be thinner than normal.

The sequence of events would appear to be as follows : (1) The disappearance of the delicate anterior glial fibres ; (2) the disappearance of the deeper glial fibres incorporated in the lamina, or their fusion under pressure with the connective tissue lamellæ ; (3) the bending backward of the connective tissue lamellæ, which build up the lamina ; (4) the compression, sclerosis, and even thickening of the lamina, probably as a result of the load it has to bear ; and finally (5) the thinning and atrophy of the lamina as a result of continued pressure ; at this stage, not only do the individual fibres become thinned and even disappear, but also a formation of spaces occurs, the lamina being thus increasingly broken up.

Side by side with these changes in the supporting framework of the intra-ocular portion of the nerve, we have to take account of what is happening to the nerve fibres themselves. This is the more necessary because the course of events appears to differ widely in different cases, even so far as the nerve elements themselves are concerned.

Thus, we may find extensive atrophy of the nervous tissues at a stage when only the anterior glial fibres have disappeared, and when the connective tissue lamellæ, and consequently the lamina which they build up, are still in a normal position. Under such circumstances, as Fuchs points out, the picture presented might be that of an increased physiological cup with nerve atrophy. We have but to remember how deep the connective tissue lamellæ may lie from the surface of the papilla in certain cases, and to cast our minds back for a moment to Fuchs' observation of cups up to nearly 0·75 mm. in depth occurring under these conditions, to realise how difficult the ophthalmoscopic diagnosis of the exact condition present may easily become. On the other hand, in some cases, the lamina may yield at an early stage, whilst the nerve fibres are still intact. From the point of view of the symptoms presented, the cases will vary greatly. On the one hand, there may be comparatively shallow cupping with marked atrophy and early loss of vision ; on the other, deep cupping with very moderate atrophy and comparatively little impairment, either of central or peripheral sight.

If we may accept Fuchs' work—as there is every reason to believe we may, not only on account of its author's reputation, but also because it falls into line with our clinical experience of increased intra-ocular pressure, with all its variations in the signs and symptoms present—we are bound to agree with its author that the problem of glaucoma is not the simple one of the physical effects of pressure alone. No one who has studied the congeries of conditions which we classify under the term " glaucoma " can fail to be convinced of the depth of our ignorance on the subject we are discussing. This admission, however, implies neither sympathy nor agreement with the views that sometimes find expression in medical literature, to the effect that the symptoms of glaucoma are independent of a rise in intra-ocular pressure. Such an idea is little likely to be accepted by anyone, who has devoted any attention to the subject, and who takes broad, balanced views of the situation. Unfortunately, the study of glaucoma has, perhaps more than any other domain of ophthalmology, been invaded by theories which have had little to recommend them, and which have only served to add confusion to the subject. Fortunately, their influence has generally been ephemeral, though it can hardly be said to have been harmless.

The most conclusive evidence that cupping of the optic disc is present, is derived from a comparison under ophthalmoscopic examination of the floor of the disc with the general level of the fundus. Supposing that we are examining an emmetropic eye without any lens on our ophthalmoscope, we can see the details of the fundus at the margin of the disc in sharp focus, but if we shift our gaze to the floor of the disc, we notice that the vessels lying upon it present a blurred outline, and that no structure there is distinctly seen. If now we place minus lenses of increasing strength in the ophthalmoscope aperture, we are at last able to focus the previously blurred vessels sharply, and at the same time to see clearly the stippled appearance of the lamina cribrosa. The structures on the fundus level are now in their turn out of focus. On looking at the ophthalmoscope we can calculate in diopters the value of the difference between the two levels, and on the assumption that a difference of three diopters represents a depression of the disc through 1 mm., we can form a fair idea of the depth of cupping present. On this basis, Morax has estimated it as varying from 0·30 mm. to 1·60 mm. It is easier to appreciate the meaning of these figures, if we remember that the real diameter of an optic disc is about 1·5 mm. Another method of attacking the same problem would be by measurements made on the cadaver. Salzmann states that the thickness of the sclera is greatest at the posterior pole, and that according to Stilling, it varies between 0·50 mm. and 1·6 mm. If we examine the depth of the most advanced glaucoma cups taken from our anatomical material, we observe that the bottom of the cup in extreme cases lies below the level of the posterior surface of the sclera. This is in accordance with the observation common to many surgeons, that if, in excising a glaucomatous eye, we cut close to the sclera we may open the globe through the foramen opticum. The exact depth of the cup, as measured in pathological sections, is well below the true figure, owing to the shrinking of the tissues under the action of hardening reagents, but we may infer that it is sometimes well over 1·5 mm.

The *test by parallactic displacement* seems to the writer to be a survival from the days when ophthalmoscopy was in its infancy. It must, however, be admitted that it still has many advocates. It is best carried out with the aid of the indirect method. An excellent description of the method is given by Fuchs, in his text-book (p. 112), to which those who are interested are referred. Whilst not denying that the test may be of use in rare instances, its employment as a routine method seems to be an anachronism in these days of accurate direct ophthalmoscopy, conducted by means of modern self-lit instruments.

(3) An *alteration in the apparent direction of the retinal vessels*, as they pass out from the surface of the disc, over its edge to reach the fundus.—At a very early stage, the only thing one can notice is a slight *bend or kink* in both veins and arteries, just inside the edge of the disc. This is seen earlier in the former than in the latter. Sometimes this kinking is only observable in certain directions, but as time passes on it becomes more general and in the vast majority of cases involves the whole circumference of the disc evenly and regularly. Later, as the cupping deepens, the kink in the vessels becomes so pronounced, that a small portion of each artery or vein comes to be *hidden under the overhanging edge* of the cup. Later still there is an *apparent discontinuity in* the course of each *vascular trunk* when it is traced along the floor of the disc and then out on to the fundus. Indeed this may be so marked as to lead a beginner to doubt whether the vessel he sees emerging at the edge of the disc is really the same as the one he has traced out toward it. This phenomenon is so frequently mis-

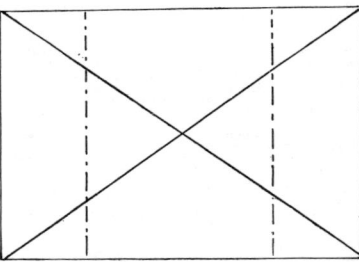

Fig. 32.—The red lines are to represent blood vessels. The dotted lines indicate where the paper is to be folded the first time.

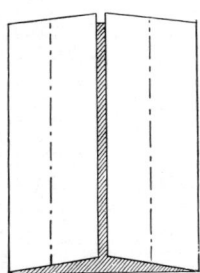

Fig. 33.—The first folding of the paper shown complete; the dotted lines show position of the second fold.

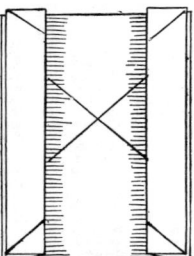

Fig. 34.—The second folding of the paper shown completed.

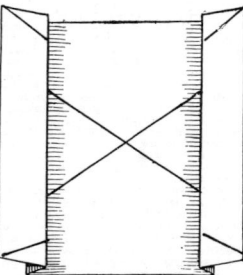

Fig. 35.—The double flaps raised in concertina fashion, to show the overhanging edge of the disc and the apparent alteration in the direction of the vessels as they emerge on the plane of the retina.

THE DIAGNOSIS OF GLAUCOMA

understood by students, and is so easily explained by the aid of a little device, which the writer used for many years in his university teaching, that he thinks it worth while to explain the method here. Take a half-sheet of note paper, 7 inches long by 4½ wide (the exact dimensions are unimportant), and join the corners by drawing two diagonal red lines (Fig. 32), thus making a multiplication sign, whose four arms are designed to represent four emerging vessels ; fold each edge of the paper forward towards the centre, so that the two edges meet each other over the centre of the multiplication sign (Fig. 33). Take each edge in turn and fold it backward to meet the first folds (Fig. 34). Then raise the two double flaps so made, forward in a concertina-like fashion and look down on the device from above (Fig. 35). The unfolded part of the paper, lying flat on the table, diagrammatically represents the floor of the disc ; from the first fold to the second on each side represents the shelving wall of the disc ; from the second fold to the free edge represents the fundus level. The apparent break in the continuity of the straight lines originally made is very striking, and aptly illustrates our point.

(4) *A dragging over of the retinal vessels in a bundle towards the nasal side of the fundus* is a not very uncommon phenomenon in late cases of glaucoma (Fig. 40). The appearance is a very striking one. In the presence of considerable opacities in the cornea and lens, the bundle of red lines running inward and the contrasting dead whiteness of the disc in every other direction, furnish a picture, which even in the absence of any other sign, and in the presence of an opacity too great to permit the cupping of the disc to be clearly seen, is nevertheless unmistakable. This dragging over of the vessels to the nasal side is, the writer believes, always associated with some measure of posterior staphyloma, and is an evidence of traction on the retina, similar to that which is seen in cases of high myopia.

(5) The next point to note is the presence or absence of *pulsation in the retinal vessels.* It will be convenient

to take arterial and venous pulsation separately, dealing first with the former.

THE ARTERIAL PULSE.—This pulse is so characteristic, that, when once seen, it can never afterwards be mistaken for anything else; it flashes out over the whole breadth of the disc, affecting every branch of the artery thereon, and even on to the fundus beyond. It is, however, best observed on the disc itself, for, in the retinal part of the optic nerve, the vessels lie wholly superficial to the nerve fibre layer. It is seen whenever the intra-ocular pressure surpasses the pressure in the arteries during the period of diastole, but is lower than the latter during the systolic period. It is an indication that the circulation through the eye is being maintained during only a part of the cardiac cycle. It is therefore quite distinct from the ordinary arterial pulse which can be observed in the healthy eye by the use of such instruments as Gullstrand's large ophthalmoscope. A diastolic pulse can be produced in any eye by the exercise of gradually increasing digital pressure, and the phenomenon can be easily watched with a self-lit ophthalmoscope. *The diagnostic point in a glaucomatous eye is that this pulse is much more readily produced than it is under normal conditions*; indeed in some cases a very light pressure will suffice to make it appear. On the other hand, *the general text-book impression that spontaneous arterial pulsation is a manifestation of glaucoma is a myth*. Such an event is extraordinarily rare, and probably can only occur under very exceptional conditions, for an intra-ocular pressure, sufficient to cause it, will raise the whole vascular pressure within the eye; needless to say the diastolic arterial pressure is included in this rise, and thus the continuance of a pulse in the arteries is automatically interfered with.

It must not be forgotten that a pulsation of the retinal arteries may be due to several different conditions :—

(i.) The arterial pulse-wave may be carried beyond its normal limits throughout the body, and the eye manifestations thereof may be merely a part of the whole.

THE DIAGNOSIS OF GLAUCOMA

Examples of this condition are to be found in aortic regurgitation and in Basedow's disease.

(ii.) The arterial pressure may fall rapidly throughout the body, *e.g.* in cholera, or syncope, or after profuse hæmorrhage, and the intra-ocular arterial pressure may for a short period be low relatively to the intra-ocular pressure.

(iii.) The fall in arterial pressure within the globe may be due to some form of localised compression of the trunk of the arteria centralis retinæ, *e.g.* that met with in optic neuritis, or in some orbital tumours. In either case—(ii.) or (iii.)—the diastolic pressure may prove insufficient to maintain a steady flow through the retinal arteries, with the result that the flow is resumed with each systole of the heart and interrupted with each act of diastole, a pulse being thus produced.

(iv.) Owing to an increase in intra-ocular pressure, the diastolic pressure in the retinal arteries may be insufficient to secure a continuous flow of blood. The result, viz., an arterial retinal pulse, is the same as that discussed in the previous paragraph, though the underlying condition is here a rise in intra-ocular pressure, and not a fall in arterial pressure.

The differential diagnosis between the pulse due to an increase in tension and that resulting from one of the conditions mentioned above need not detain us further. It is, however, of interest to remind the reader once again that the retinal arterial pulse of glaucoma is not a true pulse, but a manifestation of intermittence in the inflow of blood into the eye, and further that it is seen only in the neighbourhood of entry of the arteries, and *not* throughout the course of the vessels.

THE VENOUS PULSE.—It is generally believed that an accentuation of the venous pulse is a sign of glaucoma. Another belief has gone hand in hand with this, viz., that a similar increase in pulsation is met with after the use of mydriatic drugs. The correctness of the former assumption has recently been challenged by Bailliart, and the subject has been elsewhere discussed at some length by the author. For our present purposes it may suffice to state the case as follows : (1) A strong venous pulsation is not infrequently found in glaucomatous eyes ; (2) in such eyes, later examinations, following the successful relief of tension, have, in a number of instances, shown the disappearance of this pulse, or its very marked diminution ; (3) notwithstanding all this, marked venous pulsation is certainly not an invariable feature of the glaucomatous eye ; indeed, it may be totally absent in really hard globes.

With regard to the allied question of the influence of mydriatics, it cannot be disputed that in some cases the instillation of one of these drugs causes a very marked increase in the pulsation present, or the appearance of a pulse in veins which previously had not shown one.

The whole question of the presence of a venous pulse in the normal eye is an extremely involved one, for the phenomena observed, when a large number of healthy eyes are examined, vary to an extraordinary degree. If we know so little of the normal venous pulse, it is unsafe to formulate wide deductions on the subject of the same phenomenon under conditions of disease. The author's personal opinion is that the presence of a strong venous pulse in an eye suspected to be glaucomatous, is a contributory point in favour of the suggestion that the intra-ocular pressure is raised, but is at the same time one which can only be taken in conjunction with all the other available evidence presented by the case.

Before dismissing the subject of retinal pulsation, it is of interest to record an observation made by Foster Moore, apropos of the pulse which is often observed on the indicating needle of the tonometer, when taking a reading of ocular tension. He observed that this pulse was markedly obscured in the subjects of arterio-sclerosis, with high arterial tension, although it was well marked in very high tension eyes apart from arterio-sclerosis The plain inference is that the changes associated with arterio-sclerosis damp down and mask the pulse in the ocular arteries.

THE DIAGNOSIS OF GLAUCOMA 207

(6) *Changes in the calibre of the retinal vessels.*—The retinal vessels are exposed to the influence of increased pressure in two distinctly different ways, viz., (i.) at their points of entry into or exit from the eye, and (ii.) during their whole course within the globe. The latter factor obviously acts in the direction of diminishing the calibre of both sets of vessels, whilst the former has a different action on the arteries from that which it has on the veins. It is obvious that an increase of intra-ocular pressure, which pushes the optic nerve and the lamina cribrosa bodily backwards, must subject the nerve-head, and the vessels within it, to very distinct compression. The influence of such a compression will be less felt by the arteries than by the veins, and this for a double reason, viz., (i.) that the walls of the former are more resistant than those of the latter, and (ii.) that the pressure within the arteries is very much greater than that within the veins. Nevertheless, as a result of the pressure, the calibre of the arteries is constricted, and the volume of blood entering through them is correspondingly restricted; whilst the damming back of blood in the veins brings about a state of venous congestion. The outcome of all this, from the ophthalmoscopic point of view, is a narrowing of the retinal arteries and a dilatation of the veins; the latter vessels, as time goes on, may even show so great a degree of distension and tortuosity as to give rise to the appearance of a mass of vascular loops lying on the depressed floor of the disc, and in its immediate neighbourhood. This appearance is exaggerated if, for the want of a suitable minus glass on the ophthalmoscope, these vessels are looked at out of focus, and therefore blurred. It is obviously easy to avoid such a source of fallacy.

It would be a very great mistake to suppose that the changes we have enumerated as occurring in the optic disc and in the retinal vessels, are to be found in every case of glaucoma, or that they appear early in the course of the disease, for such is not the case. In the very early stage, the evidence on which to found a diagnosis may be of the weakest. A slight shallow cupping of the disc, a scarcely perceptible alteration in the normal size-relationship of the retinal veins and arteries, and an unusual pallor of the nerve-head, may be all there is to form an opinion on. Little by little evidence accumulates, and it cannot be too strongly emphasised that, in doubtful cases, the correct attitude is one of unwearying, wide-awake, watchful waiting. We shall return to this later, but before leaving the changes found in the disc, there are two questions that merit careful attention, viz., (i.) the differential diagnosis between the glaucomatous cup, and those conditions which may be confused with it, and (ii.) the consideration of those anomalous cases of pathologic cupping which we meet with from time to time.

The glaucomatous cup (Fig. 36) must be distinguished (*a*) from a physiological cupping (Fig. 37), (*b*) from the shallow cupping (Fig. 38) which sometimes attends an atrophy of the optic nerve, and (*c*) from a coloboma of the optic nerve (Fig. 39) or of its sheath.

We take first the features which characterise each form of cupping in its most typical manifestation, beginning with *the glaucomatous cup* (Figs. 36, 40, and 41). In this form, and in this alone, the lamina cribrosa is, at least in the later stages of the disease, thrust backwards, and consequently the depth of the cupping is then considerably in excess of what is usually met with in physiological or atrophic cases. Secondly, the cupping, as judged of by the course of the vessels, involves not only the entire circumference of the disc, but also the whole of its area. On this subject the author desires to be most emphatic. He has watched many cases of glaucoma from an early stage and has seen the whole floor of the nerve-head appear to recede from the start. This is the ordinary course of events. It is true, as will be shown later, that a physiological cup may pass over into a pathological one, and may do this so subtly that it may, for a time, be hard to say whether there is definite evidence of high tension or not ; but these cases are rare exceptions and not the rule. Thirdly, it is associated with

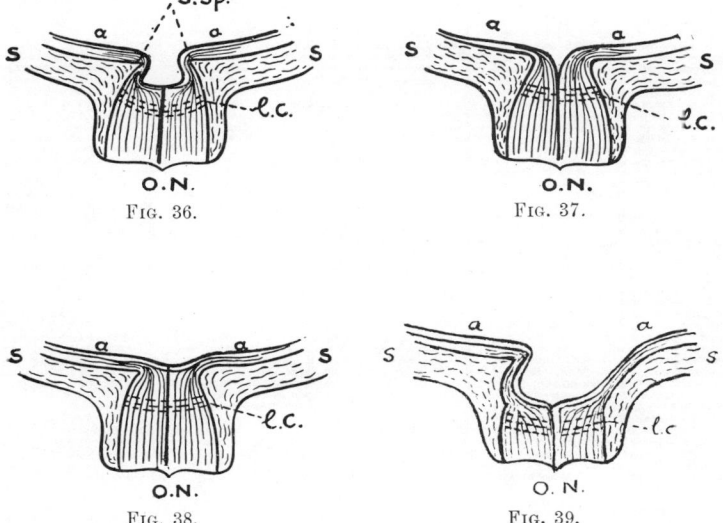

Fig. 36, glaucomatous cup; Fig. 37, physiological cup; Fig. 38, cup of optic atrophy (modified from Fuchs); Fig. 39, coloboma of the optic nerve (diagrammatic) (E. E.). O.N., optic nerve; *l.c.*, lamina cribrosa; S., sclera; S.Sp., scleral spur, which is supposed to damage the retinal fibres, as they bend over it; *a, a*, retinal artery.

THE DIAGNOSIS OF GLAUCOMA

a tendency to the appearance of abnormal pulsation of the vessels, and with an alteration in the relative calibres of the arteries and veins. Fourthly, the natural pink colour of the nerve is replaced at a late stage by a bluish or dirty greenish-white hue ; von Graefe described the appearance as " dull and waxy." Fifthly, the grey dotted markings of the lamina cribrosa are then seen over the whole of the floor of the disc.

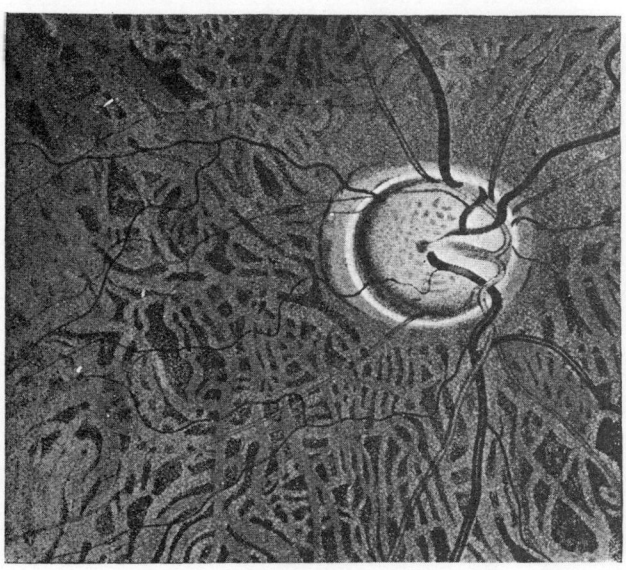

FIG. 40.—Glaucomatous cupping of optic nerve. (Oeller.)
Note the kinking of the vessels as they emerge. Note also the way in which they are drawn over in a bundle towards the nasal side.

In the *physiological cup* (Fig. 37) we notice that the depression is rarely very deep, and that it involves a part only of the disc. This is usually the outer quadrant. The vessels which pass outwards can be traced without a kink or interruption of any kind from their first appearance at the centre of the disc, right out on to the fundus. The vessels coming up on the nasal side may, however, present a very distinct bend or kink, or even an apparent interruption of their course; they are of a natural size and show no abnormal pulsation. That portion of the nerve-head, usually the outer quadrant, which is excavated by the cup, is white in colour, and shows the grey stippling characteristic of the appearance of the lamina cribrosa. The rest of the papilla has the normal pink tint.

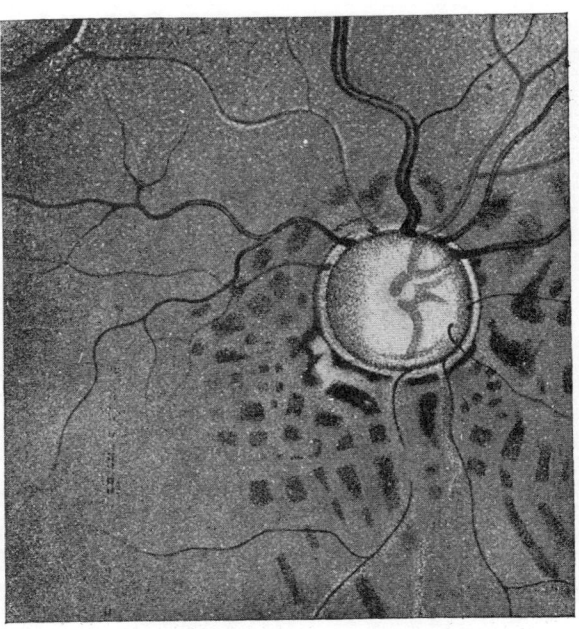

FIG. 41.—Glaucomatous cupping of the optic nerve with thickening of the coats of the vessels. (Oeller.)

Note the sharp kinking of the vessels at the edge of the optic disc. Note also the tendency to drag all the vessels over to the nasal side.

The *atrophic cup* (Fig. 38), which is met with in simple or primary optic atrophy, is usually very shallow indeed, and could consequently only be mistaken for a glaucomatous cup in the very early stage of the latter. On the other hand, by the time this form of cupping is sufficiently pronounced to be in danger of being mistaken for that due

THE DIAGNOSIS OF GLAUCOMA 211

to increased pressure, the other evidence of atrophy is so marked as to be unmistakable. The sharp definition of the disc margin, its characteristic stippled greyish-white colour, and the absence of any change in the size, etc., of the blood vessels, together with the normal appearance of the surrounding fundus, are usually sufficient to enable us to arrive at a prompt and

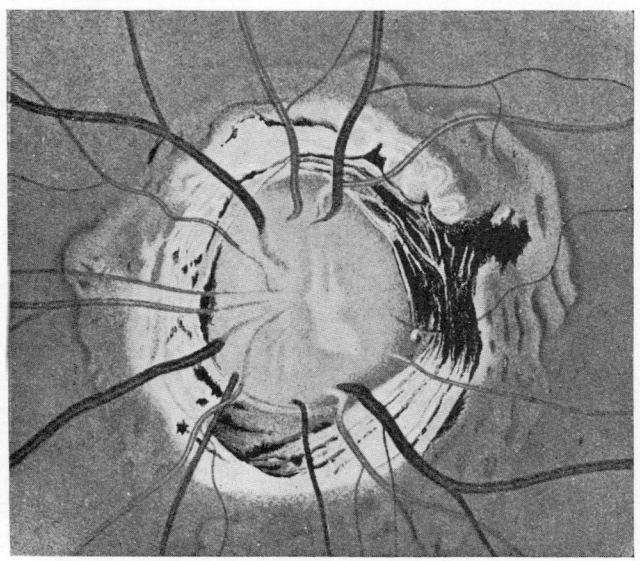

FIG. 42.—Coloboma of the optic nerve. (Oeller.)

decisive diagnosis, even before we have examined the colour fields.

Coloboma of the optic nerve (Figs. 39 and 42).—This condition is often associated with other abnormalities of the eye, and especially with coloboma of the choroid. The apparent disc is usually much enlarged, and the cup may be of great depth. If the defect is partial, it usually affects the inner or lower part of the disc. Fig. 42 is taken from Oeller. Morax considers that a coloboma of the optic nerve, such as is therein represented, may be easily mistaken for a glaucomatous cup, the diagnosis being made only by very careful attention to all the signs and symptoms presented by the patient. He lays stress on the point that the colobomatous excavation gives the impression of an irregular funnel; further, the vessels, as they emerge from the cavity, are not evenly kinked or bent. The history of the case and the symptoms present must, of course, be taken into account.

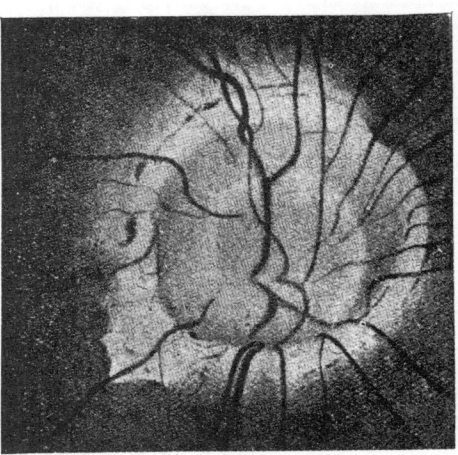

Fig. 43.—Coloboma of sheath of optic nerve. (Oeller.)
Note that the kinking of the vessels takes place well outside of the edge of the optic disc.

Coloboma of the sheath of the optic nerve.—Here again, according to Morax, the margin of the depression is found to be irregular; moreover it is situated outside the limits of the papilla at a distance of $\frac{1}{3}$rd or $\frac{1}{4}$th of a disc-diameter from the latter. The condition is even more rarely met with than coloboma of the optic nerve itself (Fig. 43).

From a consideration of typical instances of the various forms of *cupping*, we turn now to those, fortunately uncommon, *atypical cases* which present so much difficulty in diagnosis.

In very early cases of glaucoma, cupping of the disc is absent, and as time goes on, we have an opportunity of watching the evolution of this phenomenon. At first the cup is extremely shallow, suggesting in its conformation the depression met with in optic atrophy, but with this difference that the characteristic greyish-white colour of the atrophic condition is absent, the normal pink

THE DIAGNOSIS OF GLAUCOMA 213

hue of the nerve-head being seen. There are, however, cases in which a disc which is perfectly normal looks whiter than usual by contrast with a dark fundus. On the other hand, it has been pointed out that a pallor of the nerve-head may be a very early sign of glaucoma, and indeed in some cases such a pallor is quite marked. It is obvious that a doubt may sometimes arise as to whether we are dealing with an unusually pale normal disc or with one whose loss of colour is an early sign of the disease we are discussing. Our doubts in any individual case may be accentuated when we remember Fuchs' recent work on the lamina cribrosa dealt with in Chapter I. Part II. It was there pointed out that variations in the position and strength of that membrane may profoundly influence the depth of the cupping observed under various pathological conditions. The difficulty may be much accentuated should a rise of tension supervene in an eye which is the subject of a previous optic atrophy.

Then again, in most cases, the slight bend in the direction of the vessels, which indicates to us that cupping is commencing, is usually found to involve the whole periphery of the disc. Whatever vessel we trace, we find that just before it passes on to the fundus, its course shows a slight bend. This is the usual condition, but unfortunately it is not universal. The writer on one occasion had under his care a medical man, who had been kept under very close observation. At a very early stage of the disease, all the vessels, except the upper ones, passed out absolutely straight. Later a bend could be traced in every single vessel just before it arrived at the fundus. Later still, after a successful trephining, the vessels again straightened out to some extent. In this connection, it is important to remember that in not a few advanced cases of glaucoma, the excavation of the disc is noticed to be much more marked in certain meridians than in others.

A still more curious phenomenon may be met with. A well-marked glaucoma cup may be present, involving every meridian of the disc and doing so equally; but the depression may not involve the whole area of the nerve-head; a band of greater or less width of undepressed margin surrounds a central cup. As time goes on, more and more of this outside band becomes encroached upon by the excavation, till in the end the usual typical appearance of complete cupping is produced. Speaking on purely clinical grounds, the explanation seems to be obvious. Just as the lamina cribrosa is the weakest part of the ocular tunic and therefore the first to yield under pressure, so it is conceivable that in some cases its centre is weaker than its periphery, and is therefore the first part to give. The author has long advocated the view that, if these cases are examined in the pre-glaucomatous stage, they will, one and all, be found to present a central circular physiological cup. A. Hugh Thompson has recently illustrated this point by a reference to a number of specific cases. In these "flask-like cups" he has found it very difficult to draw a distinction between physiological and glaucomatous conditions. He believes that up to middle age, the cup seldom extends over more than half of the diameter of the disc surface, whereas in older patients, nearly the whole of the disc area may be involved (Fig. 44). He lays stress on the great importance of keeping all suspicious cases of this nature under careful observation, and of noting our findings in terms of the proportion of the diameter of the cup to the diameter of the disc; the extent of the uncupped margin in different meridians should also be stated. It is of interest to mention here that Gradle has recently suggested a graphic method of recording types of excavation of the optic nerve-head.

Another aberrant type of cupping of the disc is that in which a physiological excavation is closely imitated. It is a rare form, but there seems absolutely no doubt that it exists. A case in point may be quoted: Some years ago a European ophthalmic surgeon visited Madras with the request that we should trephine both his eyes. He had naturally followed the progress of his own case with the

THE DIAGNOSIS OF GLAUCOMA 215

greatest interest and accuracy. The diagnosis had been confirmed by a European colleague of his own, second to none as an authority on glaucoma. The tonometer showed a very appreciable rise in tension in both eyes, and vision was steadily failing; on ophthalmoscopic examination, the discs presented the appearance one would have expected to find in optic atrophy attacking an eye which had previously shown deep physiological excavation. The outer

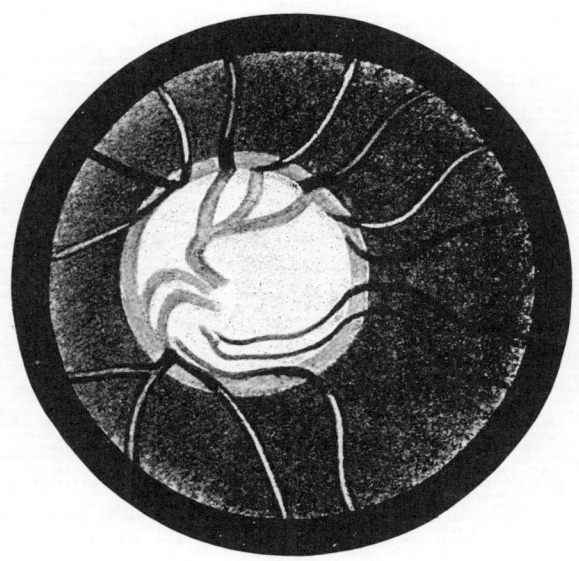

Fig. 44.—Left disc of a woman, aged 52 years, showing large intra-marginal cup, without any symptoms of glaucoma. (A. Hugh Thompson.)

third of each disc sloped steadily up to the fundus level, and vessels could be traced on it without a kink at any part of their course. Both eyes were trephined; within a fortnight, the improvement in vision and the enlargement of the visual fields were unmistakable. One could only throw out the suggestion that the deep physiological cupping, which had been seen by an expert many years before the onset of glaucoma, had influenced the appearance of the case; and indeed this explanation would appear to be the only one, which will cover other cases of the same kind.

Pickard has recently studied the size and the characters of the physiological cup as met with in different decades of life, and has shown strong reason for the inference that there is a tendency for the physiological cup to enlarge as age progresses. He thinks that small increases of pressure, acting for long periods of time on discs which are lacking in resisting power, may cause enlargement of the cups, though vision may not necessarily be interfered with. He would not, however, include such cases as glaucomatous, unless the pressure exerted proved sufficient to interfere with the function of the organ. These would appear to be valuable and suggestive findings, but the author cannot go with Pickard in his view " that the glaucoma cup is usually a simple and symmetrical enlargement of the physiological cup." It is, to say the least of it, possible that growth has as much to do as pressure with the enlargement of the physiological cup as life advances. Moreover, as Pickard admits, we must distinguish sharply between a long-continued pressure which produces anatomical changes without perceptible pathologic consequences, and the distinctly morbid increase of pressure met with in glaucoma. To the author's mind the difficulty of the position begins when a pathologic cupping is grafted on a physiologic cupping, and even then only in certain cases. Such an event is a rare one and is not either usual or common. At least, that is a probable view of the case.

Lastly, confusion may arise when a nerve-head, which is the seat of a deep physiological cup, undergoes simple atrophy. A consideration of all the features of the case will probably lead to a diagnosis, but, if not, the eye must be watched and followed until a decision can be arrived at.

The present would appear to be a very suitable occasion to emphasise two lessons : (1) A diagnosis of glaucoma should never be attempted, as is sometimes done, on the consideration of a single sign alone, be the importance of that sign what it may, but every factor which can guide our judgment should be taken into account in forming a decision; and (2) many a doubtful case will become clear to the surgeon, who will watch its progress in the light of carefully made notes. It is true that glaucoma is a disease, in which to delay is dangerous, but there are times when watchful waiting is the only policy to pursue. Once it has led to a diagnosis, we can assume the offensive and act with decision, whereas a premature interference entails disadvantages, which it is needless to specify.

Retina.—We have already been considering the retina under the previous section, but it is now necessary to devote a little of our attention exclusively to that membrane. Under the conditions of a rise in intra-ocular pressure, the retina is exposed to (1) compression, (2) stretching, (3) anæmia, and (4) congestion.

The thrusting back of the nerve-head obviously involves some stretching of the retina. A like effect is probably produced, though usually only to a very slight extent, by the distension of the globe. Throughout its course from the optic disc to the ora serrata, the retinal cup is exposed to steady compression whenever the ocular tension rises, for it lies between the contents of the eye which are at an increased pressure and the unyielding scleral tunic. The compression to which the central retinal artery is subjected, as it lies in the nerve-head before its emergence, and that to which all its branches are exposed from their point of emergence onward, lessens the volume of blood flowing through its channels and thus establishes a condition of anæmia. On the other hand, the obstacle to the outflow of blood through the retinal veins, interposed by the same pressure at the nerve-head, dams back the venous blood and tends to establish an unhealthy condition of venous congestion, which must interfere with healthy metabolism. We thus find at work those deleterious influences which spring from a defect in the quantity of blood supplied, and from an obstruction to the removal of waste products. Lastly, another element of compression comes in, and that too of a very dangerous nature; for as the nerve fibres curl over the edge of the optic foramen they are, as we have previously shown, exposed, if the intra-ocular pressure rises, to injury against the sharp edge of the sclera, which bounds the anterior outlet of the foramen. This point will be better appreciated after a study of Fig. 31.

The Choroid.—There can be no doubt that during acute and subacute attacks of glaucoma the choroid shares with the ciliary body its state of congestion. There is evidence of this in the venous condition of the globe and especially in the distension of the vasa vorticosa. As the disease goes on, the choroidal coat tends to atrophy under the influence of steady pressure. Under these circumstances the part most affected will obviously be the inner coat, with its fine capillary vessels. To see this change in its most marked form, and at its earliest onset, we must examine those regions where the choroid is most firmly attached to the investing coat of the eye, viz., at the margin of the optic disc and at the points where the vorticose veins pierce the scleral coat. In each of these neighbourhoods we find a ring of choroidal atrophy, the evidence of which is to be sought in the appearance of a white or yellowish areola. This is the explanation of the ill-defined band of discoloration so commonly seen surrounding the cupped disc of a late glaucoma and known to surgeons as the " glaucomatous halo." The phenomenon is due to the white sclerotic coat being seen through the atrophied choroid. In time the whole surface of the choroid becomes affected. Its capillary stratum disappears, together with the layer of the retinal pigment, and in this way the deeper vessels of the choroid are exposed, giving the fundus the characteristic tessellated appearance which we commonly associate with a late stage of glaucoma or of myopia. It is needless to say that the nerve-elements of the retina, which are dependent for their nutrition upon the choroidal circulation, share in the prevailing atrophy A further point of interest, and one to which we shall have occasion to return later, is that the effect of an evenly distributed increase of intra-ocular pressure will be most felt by those vessels which are situate farthest from the heart. It would therefore be only what we should have expected, were we to find that the structures, nourished by the choroidal circulation (the deeper layers of the retina), suffer first at the periphery of the eye, and later towards its centre. To this subject we shall have occasion to return later on.

Koeppe's Sign.—Koeppe has claimed that glaucoma can be recognised in what he has termed a pre-glaucomatous stage, by the aid of the Gullstrand slit-lamp, and this months or even a year before any other sign of the disease has appeared. He supports his claim with observations on eight cases in which he watched the development of the disease, commencing at periods when, in the absence of this sign, the patients would have been said to be absolutely free from glaucoma. The pathological side of the question has been mentioned in Chapter III. Part III., and we shall here confine ourselves to the clinical aspect of the case : The pigment granules, which are presumed to be set free by the morbid change present, wander free in the form of a fine dust and find their way into the iris stroma, where they become visible as a powdery deposit on the anterior limiting layer of the iris. The latter presents a peculiar dense appearance, which suggests that it is covered by a very fine membrane. The pigment dust can also be seen in the aqueous, on the posterior surface of the cornea, and on the anterior and posterior capsules of the lens. It is presumed that it is also present in the angle of the chamber. Schieck has confirmed these findings, and so, up to a certain point, has Gradle, who writes : " Further investigation and time will prove whether or no this finding (of Koeppe's) is pathognomonic of glaucoma ; but certain it is that in every case of glaucoma, which I have examined with the slit-lamp, the iris has been peppered with discrete pigment granules. These are brown or black, and are so small that they can just be seen plainly with a medium magnification (20 diameters). They lie on the surface of the iris, apparently covered with endothelium, and they extend into the depths of the iris crypts. The peripheral area of the iris contains these granules in the greatest profusion, and here they have the appearance of having been sprinkled on to the surface from a fine pepper pot. Koeppe's contention as to their diagnostic value remains

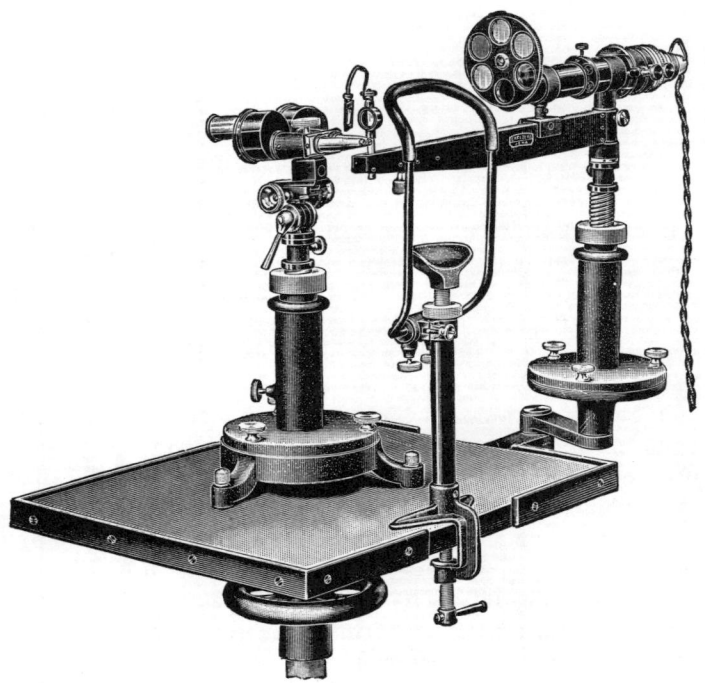

Fig. 45.—Zeiss' corneal microscope, standing on glass table to left of figure. Movable arm carrying Gullstrand's slit-lamp, revolving disc of glasses and lens for focussing the light on the eye to right of figure. Between the microscope and the movable arm is seen the head-rest. The author prefers the large lens to that here shown at the left end of the arm.

to be proved, but the presence of the granules cannot be disputed."

The author, too, has been able to see these granules in some, but not in all of his glaucoma cases; he feels that, whatever may be the final verdict of ophthalmology as to the value of the sign, we clearly have to do with a very

THE DIAGNOSIS OF GLAUCOMA 221

interesting phenomenon, and with one whose presence should be sought for in every doubtful case of glaucoma, the progress of this sign being watched with the aid of precise and careful periodical notes. The slit-lamp has therefore a new value to the surgeon who deals with glaucoma cases (Fig. 45).

It must be obvious that if we can really make sure by such observations that a subject, otherwise apparently well, is heading toward disaster, a prophylactic operation (trephining or other form of sclerectomy) will be placed on an entirely different footing from that which it now occupies. This will be illustrated from the following experience : Quite recently, the author saw in a single week two cases of acute glaucoma. Both were very intelligent people, and had been under periodic observation by able surgeons, and yet both were allowed to run into a condition of acute congestive glaucoma with total blindness of the affected eyes before being submitted to operation. The fact that both of them did excellently after trephining is immaterial to the present contention, which is that surgical interference should, *if possible*, have anticipated the onset of the acute condition, and so have been undertaken at a time when it would have been easy, safe, and free of anxiety, instead of in all the stress, danger, and uncertainty of a surgical emergency. Everything turns on the words " if possible," and the further investigation of Koeppe's sign may prove whether it is so or not. The matter is worthy of our very serious attention.

The Size of the Globe.—Priestley Smith has shown that, on the average, the diameter of the cornea is less in glaucomatous eyes than it is in those of people who do not suffer from this disease. He found that the average horizontal corneal diameter of glaucomatous eyes was 11·1 mm. against 11·6 mm. in healthy globes. He also ascertained that small corneas belong as a rule to small globes, and was therefore able to assert that small eyes are more liable to suffer from primary glaucoma than large ones are.

There is another item of clinical evidence which points

in the same direction : The operating surgeon looks down on an eye with the patient lying flat on his back, and with the lids widely separated from each other. Under these conditions the eye tends to fall back as far as possible within the orbit. Anyone who has a large surgical practice cannot, under these conditions, fail to be struck with the difference between the glaucomatous globe and an average non-glaucomatous organ. He notices that the latter tends to fill up the front of the orbit, thus bringing the plane of the ocular conjunctiva not far behind that of the face. In the glaucomatous eye on the contrary, the scleral wall, as it leaves the cornea, tends to follow a plane passing back at an angle to that of the face ; the consequence is that one can see far back into the orbit between the globe and the orbital walls. In other words, the eye gives one the impression that whatever may be its length antero-posteriorly, it is smaller than natural in its other diameters, and is in fact too small for its socket.

The above remarks were largely founded on Madras experience. An interesting confirmation of them has come from others who are likewise working in the tropics : In the course of a discussion during the 1917 meeting of the Ophthalmological Society of Egypt, Fischer drew attention to the frequent occurrence of non-congestive glaucoma in that country. A number of speakers attributed this, in part at least, to the small diameters of the corneæ, so often met with in the natives.

The author has long felt very much dissatisfied with the available apparatus for the measurement of the diameter of the cornea, and this after trying the various methods which have been recommended. The requisites for a perfect instrument of the kind are as follows : (1) The patient's head must be absolutely steady ; for this purpose a chin-rest and forehead-band are required. (2) The instrument itself must be rigidly fixed on a firm stand. (3) The patient's eye must have a definite point of fixation, to ensure that it does not move during the momentary period, whilst the observer is shifting his gaze from one end of the scale to the other. (4) The scale and eye must be sufficiently magnified to enable the observer to measure accurately in tenths, and preferably in twentieths of a millimetre. Messrs. Zeiss are constructing especially for the author such an instrument which will give a magnification of 8 diameters. It can be substituted in a few seconds for their corneal microscope, and slips on to the (standard adjustment) stand of that instrument ; it is focussed by a rack-and-pinion movement.[1]

REFERENCES

BAILLIART, P.—*Ann. d'ocul.*, vols. cliv. and clv.
CARTER, R. BRUDENELL.—" Appearance of Colour Spectra to the Aged," *Nature*, Nov. 8, 1917.
CHANCE, J. BURTON.—*Oph'h. Year Book*, 1918, vol. xiv. p. 150.
DRUAULT.—*Arch. d'ophtal.*, March 1898 ; and Communication to Congress of Utrecht, 1899.
ELLIOT, R. H.—*Tropical Ophthalmology*, London, Oxford Medical Publications, 1920 ; " The Yielding of the Optic Nerve-head in Glaucoma," *Brit. Journ. of Ophth.*, 1921, vol. v. p. 307 ; " The Retinal Pulse," *ibid.*, Nov. 1921, vol. v. ; "The Halos of Glaucoma," *ibid.*, Nov. 1921, vol. v.
FUCHS, E.—" On the Lamina Cribrosa," *Arch. f. Ophth.*, 1916, vol. xci. part iii. ; *Textbook of Ophthalmology* (Duane), 6th edition, Philadelphia and London, 1919.
FUMIATZEW, *Arch. d'ophtal.*, Jan.–Feb. 1915.
GRADLE, H.—*Amer. Journ. of Ophth.*, 1921, vol. iv. pp. 428 and 672.
KOEPPE, L.—*Heidelberger Ophth. Gesell.*, July 31 and Aug. 1, 1916 (abs *Arch. of Ophth.*, 1918, vol. xlvii. p. 106); *Zeit. f. Augenh.*, vol. xl. p. 138; and *Münch. med. Woch.*, 1917, vol. lxiv. p. 1113.
LINDSTEDT, FOLKE.—*Arch. f. Augenh.*, vol. lxxx. p. 104 ; and *Ophthalmology*, July 1916, p. 734.
MOORE, R. F.—*R.L.O.H. Reports*, 1915, vol. xx.
MORAX, V.—*Glaucome et Glaucomateux*, Librairie Octave Doin, Paris, 1921.
PICKARD, R.—*Proc. Roy. Soc. of Med.*, April 1921, vol. xiv. No. 6, p. 31.
RAEDER, G.—*Amer. Journ. Ophth.*, 1919, vol. ii. p. 292.
SALZMANN, M.—*Anatomy and Histology of the Human Eyeball*, translated by Dr. E. V. L. Brown, Univ. of Chicago Press, Chicago, 1912.
SCHIECK.—*Klin. M. f. Augenh.*, 1918, vol. lxi. p. 332 ; and *Bericht der Ophth. Gesell.*, Heidelberg, 1918.
SCHIÖTZ, H.—*Om. Nogle optiske equeskaber ved. cornea*, Christiania, 1882 (quoted by Sheard).

---

[1] *Vide* Appendix, p. 639.

SHEARD, C.—" Diffraction in the Human Eye and the Phenomena of Coloured Rings," *Amer. Journ. Ophth.*, 1919, vol. ii. pp. 185 to 195; and " Physiological Optics," *Amer. Encyclopedia of Ophth.*, vol. xiii. pp. 966–8.

THOMPSON, A. H.—*Trans. O.S. of U.K.*, 1920, vol. xl. p. 334.

VON GRAEFE.—" Iridectomy in Glaucoma," *New Sydenham Society*, 1859.

PART III

The Diagnosis of Glaucoma (*continued*)— Subjective Phenomena

SUMMARY :—Pain.
          Lachrymation.
          Nausea and Vomiting.
          Photopsiæ.
          Rainbows round Lights.
          A Diminution of Visual Acuity.
              Of Medial Origin.
              Of Neuro-retinal Origin.

We have taken the anatomical structures of the eye in turn and have considered the signs and symptoms of glaucoma, which are referable to changes in each of them. There are certain subjective phenomena, which for convenience' sake it is better to discuss separately, although they may have been already touched upon under the previous headings. These will next be taken up *seriatim*.

Pain.—This varies enormously in different cases. Speaking broadly, it is here as elsewhere a measure of the congestion present. A simple glaucoma may run its course without the patient ever having experienced a moment's pain in the eye. Even in the case of subacute glaucoma, the early mild attacks may be accompanied only by a feeling of weight, discomfort, or pressure in the globe. These sensations may occur periodically, and may not last long on each occasion (Morax). On the other hand an acute congestive attack is always marked by great suffering. Neuralgic pain is felt, not only in the eyes, but in the head, ears, teeth, and neck. Indeed in not a few cases the pain is principally referred to one of these other parts, and the patient seeks relief at the hands of a specialist in the dental, aural, or nasal surgery, instead of consulting an ophthalmologist. What is more, his own medical man often falls into the same error, with disastrous results for sight. The agony may be so great as to lead to vomiting and pyrexia. The attack sounds, as it were, the whole riotous gamut of trigeminal suffering. In yet another case there is constant, wearying headache, never absent for weeks at a time, and subject to occasional exacerbations. Pain in the eye and tenderness of the globe are, as a rule, concomitant symptoms. Many of the patients have learnt that sleep will greatly lessen, or even do away with their symptoms. A meal frequently has the same effect, as also has the administration of a free purgative. A strong point in confirmation of the diagnosis is the early relief conferred by the use of meiotics. On the other hand, drugs like phenacetin and antipyrin are quite useless in these cases.

In seeking an explanation for the sufferings of the glaucoma patient, we must remember (1) the long and exposed course of the ciliary nerves, as they lie between the distended contents of the eye and the unyielding sclera, (2) the existence of the rich ciliary nerve plexus, (3) the abundant distribution of sensory nerve fibres to different parts of the eye, and (4) the very varying degrees of engorgement met with in all parts of the eye, and especially in the highly vascular ciliary processes. When we do so, we cannot wonder, that an increase in the pressure to which the parts are subjected, should lead to pain, which may be very severe and even paroxysmal in character. Another factor, which perhaps we should not forget, is the overstretching of the tunic of the eye, for it is quite conceivable, that this of itself may be productive of pain.

Lachrymation.—According to Morax, various reflex troubles may be very suggestive of the commencement of glaucoma; the most suspicious of these is lachrymation occurring by fits and starts, and not connected with wind or other outside influences.

Nausea and Vomiting.—These symptoms deserve especial notice, if only for the fact that they sometimes are so prominent as to absorb the attention of the surgeon and of the patient, to the exclusion of the far more important ocular evidence of the disease. Morax states that, even if the condition is untreated, the actual vomiting subsides within 24 or at most 48 hours, whilst the sensation of nausea may persist for 2 or 3 weeks longer. He has met with patients suffering from subacute attacks, in whom the feeling of nausea was the only warning sign of a fresh rise in intra-ocular pressure.

The centripetal nerves in this reflex disturbance of the gastro-intestinal system, are the ciliary branches of the first division of the 5th; these convey the afferent impulses to the medulla, from which efferent impulses pass out along the pneumogastric nerves to the stomach, along the phrenic nerves to the diaphragm, and along the spinal nerves to the abdominal muscles.

Photopsiæ, or subjective sensations of light, are not unknown in the early stages of congestive glaucoma. It is possible that they are more frequently met with in Eastern than in Western practice. They take many forms, one or more of which may be described by the same patient. Thus we hear (1) of flashes of light, compared sometimes to summer lightning, or in the tropics to dancing fireflies; (2) of a ball of fire, that rolls across the field of vision from side to side; (3) of sudden, sharp, flash-like spots of light which appear for an instant, and then are lost; and (4) of a continuous luminous glow, which may last for seconds, or minutes, or even longer. The patient may volunteer the information that he sees these phenomena most when he is tired. They would appear to be specially common when he is getting into bed, or has just turned out the light, or soon after he has lain down to sleep. They are most troublesome when the eyes are shut, but not infrequently appear when they are open.

Photopsiæ are also seen under many other conditions, *e.g.*, in exudative choroiditis, in the early stages of detachment of the retina, in blows on the eye, and though rarely, in the course of retinal hæmorrhages ; in fact, they are likely to appear whenever the retina is irritated, dragged upon, or otherwise interfered with. Nor must we forget that very similar phenomena, but of central origin, are met with in neurasthenic patients suffering from errors of refraction, in some of those, who are subject to megrim and other nervous affections, and in the course of fainting attacks. The bearing of these remarks on a differential diagnosis is obvious. It is said that photopsiæ of retinal origin tend to be relieved by rest, and therefore to cease as the night progresses ; whilst those of cerebral origin are often most troublesome at night, and at other like times, when the eyes are not actively stimulated from the ordinary sources of visual impressions.

Rainbows round lights.—This subject has already been so fully dealt with in previous sections, that a mere mention suffices for it now.

A **diminution of visual acuity** is a frequent if not a constant sign of glaucoma. It may be due to a number of different causes, all of which admit of a classification under one of two headings, (1) medial, and (2) neuro-retinal.

(1) *Medial.*—Anything which interferes with the clearness of the dioptric media of the eye will lessen the acuity of vision, and in glaucoma there are quite a number of factors of this nature. All of these have been dealt with in the previous pages, and it will be sufficient now merely to enumerate them : (i.) Interference with the refractile power of the cornea, owing to overstretching of that membrane ; (ii.) corneal œdema ; (iii.) deposits of various kinds on the posterior surface of the cornea ; (iv.) permanent alterations in the structure of the cornea, due to degenerative changes, ulceration, etc. (these are late manifestations) ; (v.) turbidity of the aqueous ; (vi.) opacities in the lens, whether secondary to glaucoma or otherwise ; (vii.) deposits of various kinds on the surface of the lens capsule ; and (viii.) (rarely) vitreous opacities, due to trouble in the ciliary body and choroid.

(2) *Neuro-retinal.*—The neuro-retinal causes of diminu-

tion of the central visual acuity must be considered together with those, which lead to one or another of the alterations in the visual field; for, from the ætiologic standpoint the two conditions are inseparable. The subject is too big to be dealt with here, but will be discussed at length in the two following parts (Parts IV. and V.) of this chapter.

REFERENCE

Morax, V.—*Glaucome et Glaucomateux*, Librairie Octave Doin, Paris, 1921.

Part IV

The Diagnosis of Glaucoma (*continued*)— The Visual Field

Summary :—The nature of the Changes met with in the Visual Field.
    Small and Large Object Perimetry.
    Self-lit and Reflected-light Instruments.
    The Anatomical Distribution of the Nerve-fibre Bundles in the Retina.
    Perimetry with Large Objects; the Findings in Glaucoma.
        Restriction of the Nasal Field.
        Concentric Shrinking of the Field
        Roenne's Nasal Step.
        The Colour Fields.
    Perimetry with Small Objects.
        The Principles on which it depends.
        The Findings characteristic of Glaucoma.
        Bjerrum's Method, and its modifications by others
        The Author's Scotometer.
        Bjerrum's Sign.
        Seidel's Sign.
        The Author's Sign.
          The Normal Blind Spot.
          The Value of the Sign in the Positive Diagnosis of Glaucoma.
          The Value of the Sign in Revealing Important Alterations in the Field either as the Result of Treatment or Otherwise.
          The Value of the Method in Proving the Absence of Glaucoma.

The Explanation of Detached Areas of Paracentral
Defect.
Invasions of the Central Area of the Field.
The Development of a Glaucoma Field.
Central Scotomata.
Their Rarity, and Late Appearance.
Their great Importance, when present.
The Variety in the Shapes assumed by Glaucoma Fields.

The nature of the changes met with in the visual field as a result of chronic glaucoma.—These changes are so characteristic as to be of the greatest value, not only in the diagnosis of doubtful and difficult cases, but also in any estimation of the progress the disease is making. For their clear comprehension, it is advisable that two methods of perimetry should be employed, viz., (1) that with (comparatively) large objects, and (2) that with small objects. Before proceeding to discuss these in turn, a few general remarks will be pertinent.

Small and large object perimetry.—In all perimetric work, it is necessary to state (i.) the size of the object used, (ii.) the distance of the eye from that object, and (iii.) the illumination and colour of the object. Be the distance worked at what it may, a full normal field for a white object can be obtained from a healthy eye, if we use that object of such a size that its diameter subtends an angle of half a degree at the nodal point. This, when working with a daylight perimeter of 330 mm. radius, requires the object to be between 2·6 and 2·8 mm. (at least 2·59) in diameter. To use larger objects is of no advantage, since it does not increase the size of the field, whilst it lessens the accuracy of the observations made. If, on the other hand, we *reduce* the dimensions of the object used, we find that even in normal subjects, the size of the field obtained is considerably decreased, till when we come to work with a 1 mm. object at a distance of 2 m., the field has been found to be practically circular, and to extend to about 26 degrees all round. Features of great value may be learnt from such a chart which do not appear if we work with larger objects.

A. H. H. Sinclair has recorded on a single chart the

visual fields obtained by working with objects of different sizes at different distances. Figs. 46 and 47 show composite charts constructed on these lines. Another suggestion of value made by the same writer and shown in the legends of the figures, is that of stating the size of the object used as the numerator of a fraction, whilst the denominator denotes the distance of the eye from the perimeter; both are expressed in millimetres. This method will be used throughout this volume. It is in line

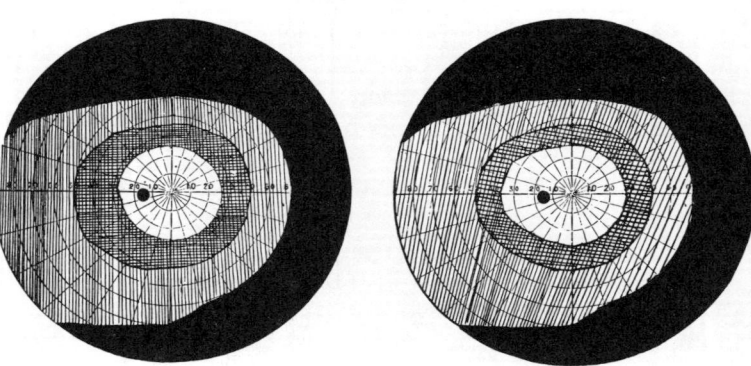

Fig. 46.   Fig. 47.

Fig. 46.—L. E. Diagrammatic representation of average normal visual fields obtained by tests—$\frac{1}{2000}$, $\frac{6}{2000}$, and $\frac{10}{300}$. (Modified from Dr. A. H. H. Sinclair.)

The numerator gives the diameter of the object in mm.; the denominator gives the distance of working—*i.e.*, the radius of the perimeter arc in mm. The fields are enumerated from within outwards.

Fig. 47.—L. E. Diagrammatic representation of average normal visual fields, constructed from Bjerrum's estimates.

The fields from within out are for $\frac{3}{2000}$, $\frac{6}{2000}$, and $\frac{10}{300}$ tests.

with our usual practice in the measurement of the visual acuity.

Any who are interested in the methods of perimetry in glaucoma cases, will be well repaid by reading the papers on the subject by Willbrand, Sym, Sinclair, Traquair, Walker, and others.

Self-lit and reflected-light instruments.—It must never be forgotten that the retina of a glaucomatous patient is very easily fatigued. It is consequently of advantage to estimate his field in a subdued light, by the aid of self-lit objects. Willbrand pointed this out about twenty years ago, and put it into practical use by working in a cellar with a large perimeter. Fuchs, guided by the same principle, some fifteen years ago, had a self-lit device made (by a London firm of instrument makers) which was capable of being fitted on to the arm of an ordinary perimeter. This product of his ingenuity is of considerable interest, as it is the obvious prototype of the large number of similar pieces of apparatus, which are now to be found in different parts of the world, bearing the names of various surgeons. Probably the best of these is the de Zeng perimeter (of 33 cm. radius) placed on the market some years back. Not the least of the advantages of self-lit perimetry lies in the perfect control of the intensity of the illumination obtained ; and that too by purely mechanical and readily adjustable means. We are independent of variations in daylight, and can vary our light from dulness to brilliancy at will. Moreover, we are not troubled by shadows thrown by the patient's head or body ; and we can, if we choose, work in a half-light or in the dark. The importance of this last fact justifies its reiteration, since it is sometimes possible to obtain satisfactory results, when working in a subdued light with a glaucomatous patient, whose daylight answers are unreliable. On the other hand, it is not recommended that one should do perimetry in actual darkness, for under these conditions the spot of light, however small, is seen even by a much damaged part of the retina, and the delicacy of the test is much reduced in consequence. An extraordinarily large and full field may be recorded, when in reality considerable defects are present, both in the periphery and also in the paracentral region.

The same source of confusion is introduced if, in practising perimetry, we employ too brightly illuminated an object. The danger of doing this is decidedly greater when we are working with self-lit instruments, than it is with reflected light. The activity of the retinal stimulation by means of even the smallest apertures, transilluminated with electric light, is extraordinary. The surgeon must be on his guard against this source of fallacy, and must keep his lights dull. There is still another objection to brightly illuminated objects, viz., that they readily over-stimulate the retinal elements, and so introduce fatigue phenomena.

There are other drawbacks to self-lit perimetry, which must be stated : The instruments are more expensive than ordinary perimeters ; they also require a certain amount of attention, and of practical knowledge of electricity. Moreover allowance must be made for the adaptation of the eye to the subdued illumination used, and the conditions of the examination must be kept as constant as possible. Given the desire to work under the best possible conditions, and the willingness to overcome the initial difficulties, none of these objections really carries much weight ; but they obviously concern matters of personal environment, as to which each surgeon must judge for himself.

The medical man is ever an individualist, and it is in the last degree unlikely that the methods of perimetry will ever be really standardised. What it is really important to realise is that although, in the present state of affairs, the results obtained by different workers may not be comparable with each other, yet any intelligent and painstaking surgeon can evolve a system which will in his own work yield strictly comparable and practically consistent results.

Whatever instrument a surgeon decides to work with, it is essential that he should accustom himself to it, and " learn " it ; and inasmuch as the ordinary daylight perimeter is at present far the most widely used, the electric instrument starts at a disadvantage, which it will take years to nullify, even under the most favourable conditions. To sum up, it is not contended that most excellent work cannot be done with the ordinary perimeters, but rather that, given patience, application, and determination, the best results may possibly be secured in the end,

THE DIAGNOSIS OF GLAUCOMA 233

by the adoption of the electric-lit instruments. This is, however, admittedly, a matter of opinion.

The anatomical distribution of the nerve-fibre bundles in the retina.—In discussing the changes found in the visual field in glaucoma, one stereotyped method has hitherto been adopted. The curtailments of the field,

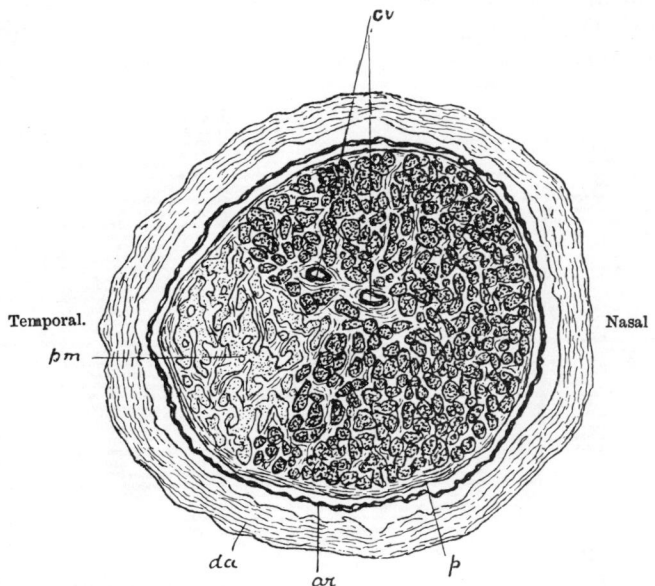

FIG. 48.—Cross-section of the optic nerve with atrophy of papillo-macular bundle. (Section made 4 mm. behind eyeball.)

At the temporal side, a wedge-shaped segment, pm, is distinguished from the rest of the cross-section by its paler colour; du, dural sheath; ar, arachnoid sheath; p, pial sheath; cv, central vessels of the retina. (After Fuchs.)

whether central, paracentral, or peripheral, are first described, and each is then explained in turn by a reference to the anatomical distribution of the nerve fibres. It appears more rational to reverse the procedure, and to precede our consideration of the whole subject by a clear résumé of what anatomy can teach us. This line is therefore now deliberately adopted.

If we consider a cross-section, made close to the globe, of an optic nerve suffering from atrophy of the papillo-macular bundle (Fig. 48), we observe on the temporal side a wedge-shaped segment distinguished from the rest by its paler colour. This segment represents the atrophied bundle, and occupies roughly one-third of the whole cross-section of the nerve and of its periphery. The distribution of this bundle in the normal eye is to the macular region and to the area lying between that and the temporal

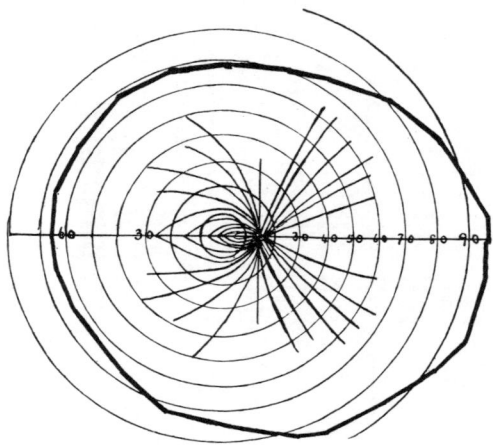

Fig. 49.—Diagram R. E. visual field (after Baas) to show the distribution of the nerve fibres in the retina, especially those on the nasal side, whose arcuate course explains the nature of the Bjerrum scotoma and the Roenne nasal step. (Seen from in front.)

edge of the papilla, whilst the remaining two-thirds of the nerve supply the whole of the rest of the retina. The outstanding feature of this arrangement obviously lies in the disparity between the small size of the retinal area represented, and the large bulk of the nerve allocated to a special purpose. The great importance of the macular area is sufficient to explain this apparent anomaly. It is usually believed that in the macular region, each of the cones is connected with a separate nerve fibre, in order that every stimulus of the element shall be separately conveyed to the brain, whereas in the more peripheral parts of the retina, one nerve fibre probably serves as the transmitting line for the impulses of a number of nerve elements.

The bundles of fibres found in the remaining two-thirds of the cross-section of the nerve supply the whole of the rest of the retina. Their distribution will be made more clear by a reference to Figs. 49 to 52. In Fig. 49, taken from Baas, a comprehensive view is shown of the whole area of the seeing retina, and the course of the optic nerve fibres is indicated in each and every direction. Fig. 50 shows the same features much more elegantly, though the field covered is not so large. Fig 51 is more diagrammatic, but it is hoped that it may prove helpful. In Fig. 52, the more central parts of the fundus are shown on a still larger scale, and the optic disc is divided into four quadrants. We can dismiss the nasal half of the disc in a very few words since the whole of the fibres which emerge from it fan out evenly to supply the same half of the retina; these, of course, correspond with the temporal half of the field.

Let us return now to the temporal half of the papilla, and divide it hypothetically into six parts, each of which corresponds to one-twelfth of the whole circumference of the disc. As we have already shown, the inner four-twelfths (*i.e.*, one-third of the whole periphery) are taken up by the emergence of the papillo-macular bundle. There remain two twelfths adjoining the vertical meridian, one above and one below. We may call these the supero-temporal and infero-temporal bundles of the optic nerve fibres. If we study these in the two diagrams, we will see certain features of their distribution:

(1) The most temporally situated fibres, both above and below, sweep round the macular area to meet each other along the temporal horizontal raphé.

(2) Along their line of meeting they do not communicate with each other. There is a sharp boundary between them along the horizontal raphé as definite as a clean parting in a head of hair.

(3) As we follow the bundle up from its temporal border towards the vertical meridian (whether above or below), we find that the more temporal fibres take the same arcuate course as do those which skirt the central region of the retina. We likewise find that they too meet each other without decussating along the whole of the temporal raphé of the retina.

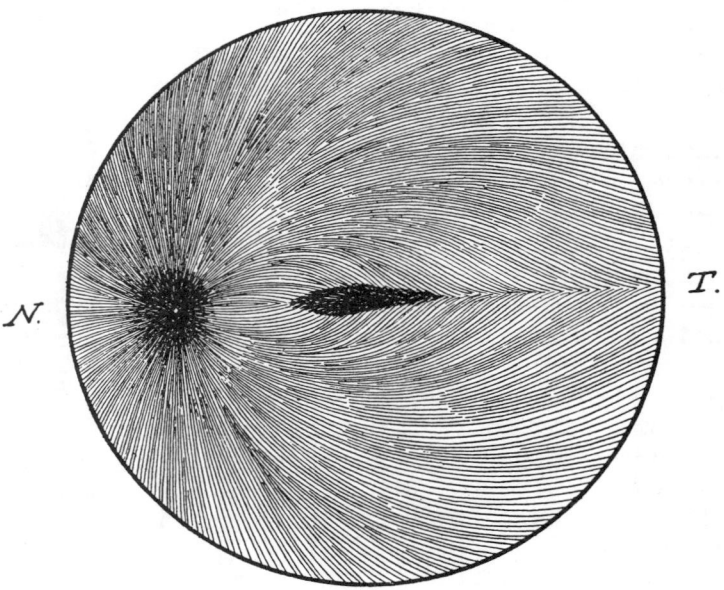

FIG. 50.—The distribution of the retinal nerve fibres. (Luther C. Peter.)

(4) Lastly we come to those fibres which fan out to fill in the rest of the retina.

(5) Inasmuch as these supero-temporal and infero-temporal bundles of fibres supply the whole of the temporal half of the retina, with the exception of the comparatively small area supplied by the papillo-macular bundle, and inasmuch as they pass over a very narrow portion of the disc edge to do so, it is obvious that they must be considerably heaped up on each other along the line of their emergence from the papilla.

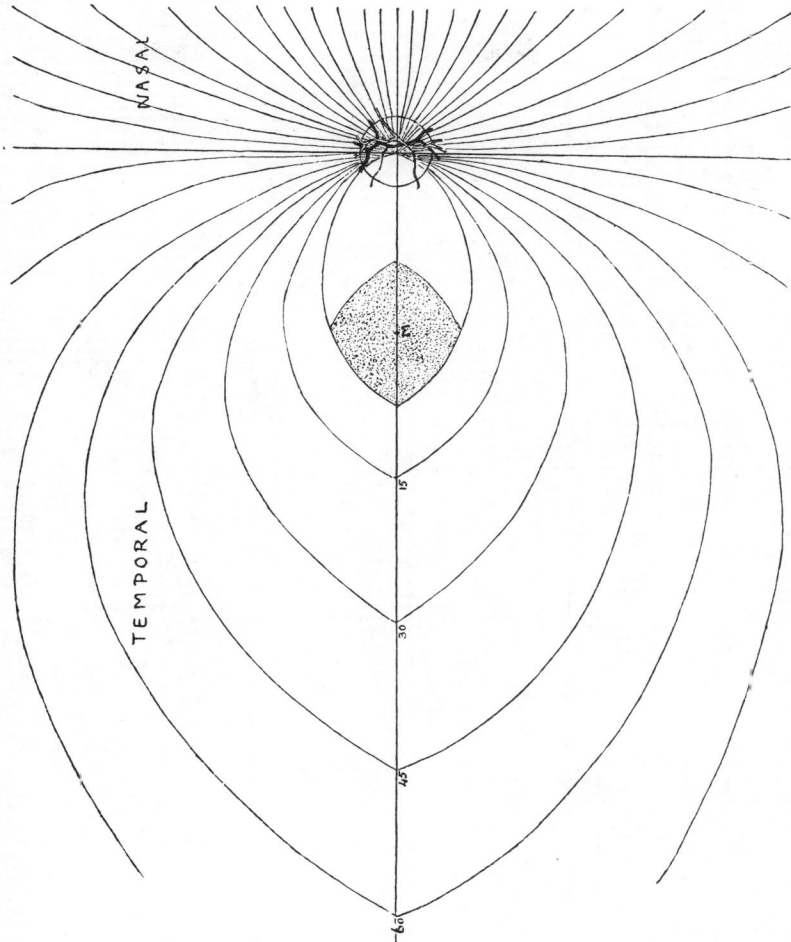

Fig. 51.—Diagram to show the distribution of the nerve fibres on the retina, L. E.

The arrangement is deduced from a study of the phenomena found in examinations of morbid visual fields. Notice (1) the large area of disc occupied by the central bundle of fibres; (2) the relatively small size of the macular area; (3) the manner in which the fibres from above and below meet cn the horizontal raphé up to the 60° limit, and fan out beyond it; (4) the bow-shaped curve of the bundles in the inner area.

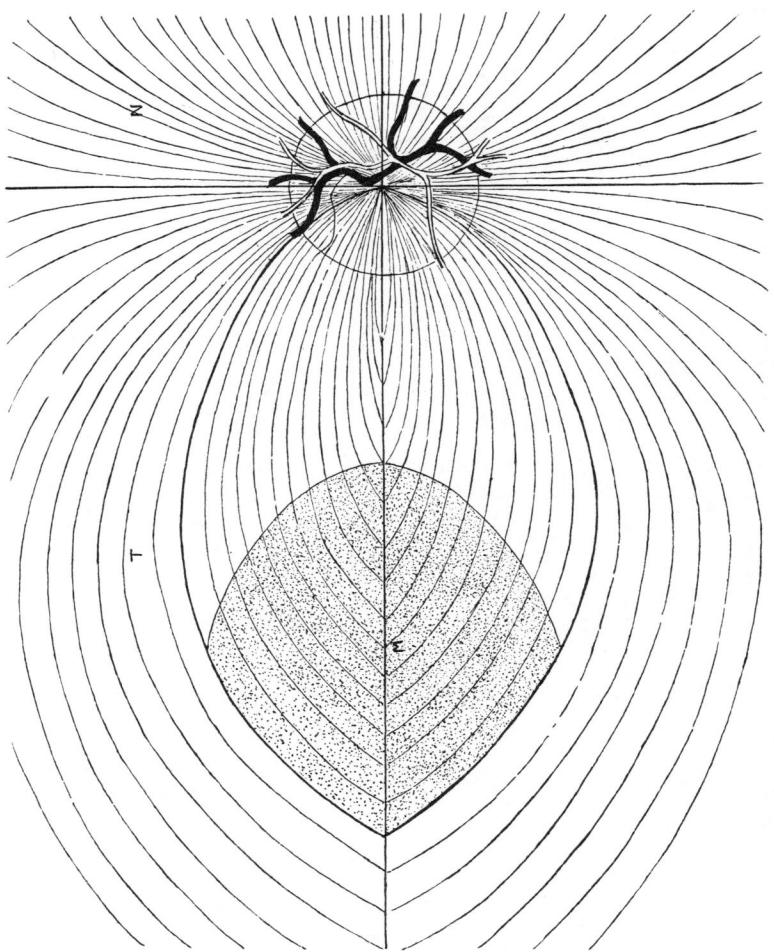

Fig. 52.—Diagram showing the central parts of Fig. 51, on a larger scale, L. E. Notice the very small circumference of the disc allotted to the emergence of the upper and lower bundles of fibres, which supply by far the greatest part of the temporal retina. The vessels will be observed to lie almost wholly on the nasal half of the optic disc. The other features of the diagram should be taken in connection with the legend of the previous figure.

THE DIAGNOSIS OF GLAUCOMA 239

A striking confirmation of our views as to the distribution on the retina of the fibres of the optic nerve has been furnished by work recently carried out with the red-free light of Vogt. Under this illumination the retinal nerve fibres are plainly visible and their course can be easily followed. "The central fibres are directly horizontal.

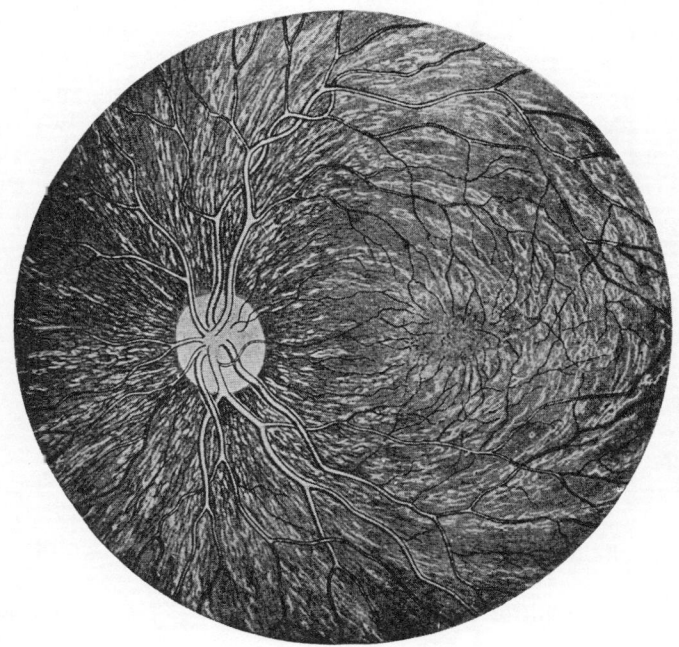

FIG. 53.—The fundus seen by red-free light. (Affolter.)
(*Amer. Journ. Ophth.*)

Above and below these are bundles that surround the foveal zone in a close sweeping arc at its temporal border. These are bounded by circular enveloping fibre-bundles which meet and interweave in a zone temporal to the macula. At first they meet at an obtuse angle which becomes more and more acute as we recede from the macular zone" (Von der Heydt). Some of the points thus made are illustrated for us in Fig. 53.

PERIMETRY WITH LARGE OBJECTS

It has already been stated that when we speak of perimetry with large objects, we mean that the latter are not less than 2·6 mm. to 2·9 mm. in diameter on an ordinary daylight perimeter with a radius of from 30 to 33 cm. Many surgeons, however, employ unnecessarily large discs, those of 5 mm. and even of 10 mm. being in constant use. This is an error in most cases, since it detracts from the accuracy of the results obtained. It is only in patients with very deficient visual power that any advantage can be obtained from such a course. Those who work with electric perimeters will find it of advantage to use even smaller diameters, a self-lit aperture of 1 mm. furnishing at 33 cm. a very full field. Much valuable information can be obtained from large object perimetry, for there are certain outstanding features of a typical chart of the kind made from a glaucoma patient. These are : (1) That the nasal field is first affected ; (2) that at a later stage there is a strong tendency for the field to undergo uniform concentric contraction ; (3) that a large percentage of the records, if carefully taken, show the sign known as Roenne's step ; and (4) that the colour fields are extraordinarily little affected, shrinking *pari passu* with the contraction of the field for white. We shall take up these points in turn.

(1) **Restriction of the nasal field.**—The perimetric change, which is usually regarded as being characteristic of chronic glaucoma, begins as a restriction of the nasal field (Fig. 54A). This fact has been a prominent feature of the statistics of all those who have examined a large number of cases of glaucoma, although there has been a wide difference of opinion as to the exact frequency of the phenomenon. Thus, Schmidt-Rimpler estimated that the shrinkage began on the nasal side in more than 50 per cent. of all cases. Treitel believed that this was far too low an estimate, and considered that if the cases were only seen early enough, nasal shrinkage would be found to be almost constantly present. Baas has discussed this

THE DIAGNOSIS OF GLAUCOMA

question in an able and practical manner, and seems disposed to think that the truth lies midway between these two extreme views. The difficulty of obtaining large statistics on the subject at a very early stage of the disease is practically insuperable; whilst those secured at a later period are obviously open to fallacy. Though it may not be permissible to commit oneself to definite figures, it may unhesitatingly be said, that the percentage of early cases in which the nasal field of vision is first

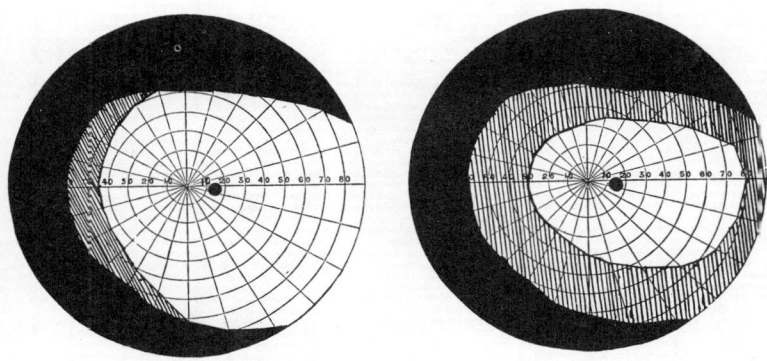

Fig. 54A. Fig. 54B.

Fig. 54A.—Early shrinkage of the nasal field, R. E., in chronic glaucoma. The shrunken portion is shown shaded. ($\frac{3}{330}$.)

Fig. 54B.—A later stage of Fig. 54A.
Concentric contraction is in progress; it will be observed that the nasal field continues to suffer more than the temporal, and its lower portion more than its upper. ($\frac{3}{330}$).

affected is so high as to give a strong diagnostic significance to this form of retraction of the field.

In rare cases the defect has been observed to start on the temporal side. More frequently it does so in either the upper or the lower quadrant. Even when the nasal sector is the first to be attacked, it by no means follows that it is so to an equal extent on both sides of the horizontal meridian; indeed, if the perimetric observation is carefully conducted, it will very often be found that either the upper or the lower quadrant bears the brunt of the assault (Fig. 62). This will be better understood, when we come to speak of Roenne's sign. Meanwhile it is of interest to ask whether the upper or the lower quadrant is more frequently affected. The evidence of large statistics is not in favour of a definite answer being given to this question. There does not seem to be any preference shown.

(2) As the disease progresses, the **contraction of the visual field** becomes more marked, its peripheral limits gradually receding all round from its boundary towards its centre (Fig. 54B). The upper and lower quadrants usually suffer more extensively than the outer, but the tide of blindness rolls in steadily, if slowly, from every direction, until finally the area, in which perception is left, is reduced to a small oval, irregular, or slit-like field, which may include within its limits both the centre of vision and the blind spot (Fig. 55). At this stage, and indeed for some time before it, the patient suffers severely from what may be spoken of as " tube vision "[1] (*i.e.*, he sees as a normal sighted person would see if he were looking down a narrow tube). Unfortunately this is not all; the next thing to go is central vision, which is swept away before the rising tide of blindness, leaving the patient only a small eccentric area of vision (Fig. 56), which may maintain its contact with the blind spot to the last. Finally, even this remnant of sight is snatched from the unfortunate sufferer, and life-long darkness overwhelms the eye.

Though the above description outlines the usual course of the disease, many atypical forms are encountered. Sometimes the restriction of a part or of the whole of the nasal field progresses at a rate out of proportion to that which holds in any other quadrant. Or, the upper or lower field, or both, may be affected simultaneously with the nasal, the only available area left being that which is on

---

[1] This is usually, but very incorrectly referred to as " telescopic vision "; such a term is obviously objectionable, as there is no magnification whatever of the image perceived. Hence the desirability of adopting the more accurately descriptive term " tube vision."

THE DIAGNOSIS OF GLAUCOMA

the temporal side. In yet other cases the loss may be at the expense of either the upper or lower quadrant. It does not at all follow that the two glaucomatous eyes of a single patient will necessarily be similarly affected. The writer had under his care a case in which one eye had only the upper temporal field left and the other only the lower temporal (Figs. 57 and 58), with the somewhat curious result that the patient was able to walk comparatively

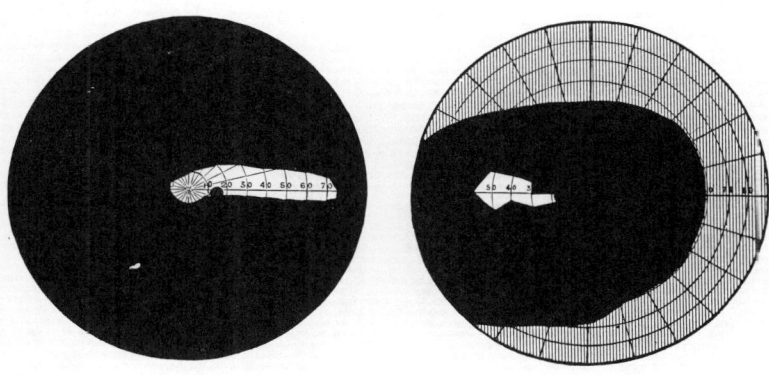

Fig. 55. Fig. 56.

Fig. 55.—Late case of chronic glaucoma, visual field, R. E. Only a narrow field is left on the temporal side, and including the centre of vision; V.A. still good; tube vision present.

Fig. 56.—Small eccentric area of vision left in a case of long-standing chronic glaucoma, L. E.
Notice the Roenne's step above the horizontal meridian.

boldly in a room full of furniture, in spite of the fact that he had lost central vision in both eyes.

As a rule the absence of sectoring is a prominent feature of glaucoma fields, but exceptions to this rule may be met with, as is to be seen in Fig. 59, taken from Baas. That writer states that when marked sectors are found in the field, the colour sense is apt to be early lost over large areas. In such cases it would appear that there is an element of disease present, which is quite distinct from glaucoma, and which is more nearly related to primary atrophy of the optic nerve. The interest of this observation centres round those cases in which the failure of vision continues to progress after the relief of pathologic tension by a perfectly successful operation. It is possible that the primary optic atrophy and the glaucomatous changes are co-incidental in some cases. Again, the damaging effect of pressure may predispose the nerve to the influence of any of those morbid changes which are known to be liable to result in atrophy. Lastly, we cannot altogether exclude the possibility that there is

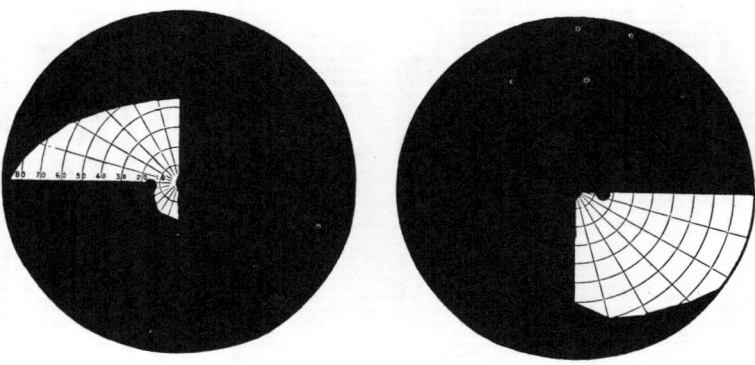

FIG. 57.—L. E. $\frac{10}{300}$.   FIG. 58.—R. E. $\frac{10}{300}$.

The above are visual fields of a patient in a late stage of chronic glaucoma. He could steer himself with comparative ease even in a room full of furniture. The disease was diagnosed twenty years earlier. Trephining resulted in an improvement in the fields.

in some cases a specific form of glaucoma closely associated with progressive atrophic degeneration of the nerve.

It has already been said that the last remnant of vision is usually to be discovered over a narrow horizontal area on the temporal side, but one sometimes finds that instead of this being horizontal, it is situated towards the upper outer, or lower outer quadrant of the field (Fig. 60).

Although it may, strictly speaking, be out of place in

THE DIAGNOSIS OF GLAUCOMA

a discussion on diagnosis, it is difficult to refrain from mentioning the widely accepted view that it is dangerous to operate, when the restriction of the field has reached close up to the centre of vision. The writer has trephined many cases of this kind with the happiest results, and he can only recall very few operations which were followed by a decrease in the existing area of the visual field, whilst, in a large number of cases the fields distinctly enlarged after the operation. This subject will

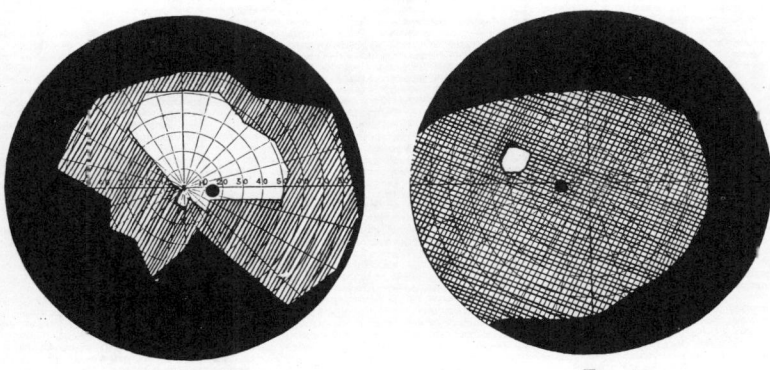

FIG. 59.   FIG. 60.

FIG. 59.—R. E.—Chronic glaucoma.

The white area shows the field three months later than the shaded portion. The sectored nature of the defect is very unusual. Taken by large-object perimetry. (Baas.)

FIG. 60.—Visual field of L. E., represented by a limited patch on the temporal side, in which colour vision was retained. The rest of the field had quite gone.

again be taken up later on, in connection with van der Hoeve's work.

(3) **Roenne's nasal step.**—This sign will be spoken of at much greater length after we have dealt with the subject of Bjerrum's scotoma. Indeed, it was a consideration of the latter phenomenon that led Roenne to anticipate the presence of his nasal step in glaucoma fields. For the present we must confine ourselves to a short statement of the leading points in connection with it :

(a) It has already been said that the constriction of the

246 GLAUCOMA

nasal field may from an early date predominantly affect either the lower or the upper part of the area. This is due to the fact that the optic nerve fibres radiating to that area are more seriously damaged than are those to the opposite segment. A reference to Figs. 49 to 52 will

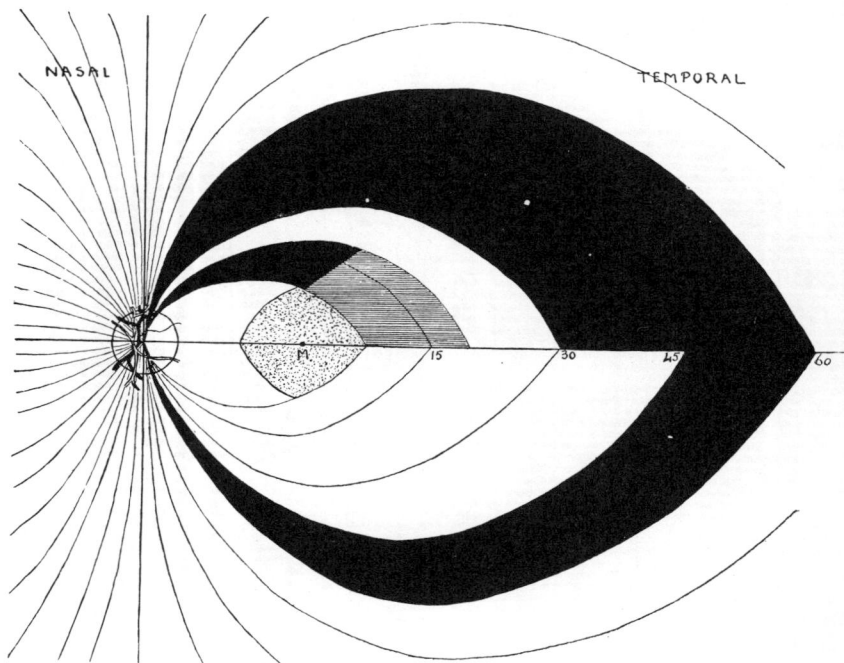

Fig. 61.

The diagram shows roughly the defects in the nerve bundles of the retina, which would correspond with the visual field defects shown in Fig. 62. It is to be remembered that the illustration is diagrammatic and only approximate.

remind us that the fibres, which sweep round to meet (but not to interdigitate) on the horizontal raphé, do so in arcuate curves, each of which is larger than that within it.

(b) If these arching fibres, as they proceed to the temporal extremity of the retina, are equally damaged, both

THE DIAGNOSIS OF GLAUCOMA

at the upper and at the lower margin of the disc, the result will be an even impairment of the nasal side of the field.

(c) If, on the other hand, either the upper or the lower fibres are most damaged, the field supplied by these will show a corresponding restriction. This is diagrammatically illustrated in Fig. 61.

(d) The result of this unevenness of lesion is manifest on a carefully made perimetric chart, and constitutes Roenne's nasal step, which is well shown in Fig. 62 and in a number of the other illustrations. On following the horizontal meridian from the blind spot toward the nasal margin, it will be observed that the limits of the field no longer correspond above and below that meridian. To take Fig. 62 as an example: Whereas the field above the nasal meridian extends out nearly to the 50° circle, that below it is much more extensively curtailed, stopping short of the 30° line; the point on the horizontal meridian, at which in this instance the curtailment of the field begins below, is seen to be sharply marked out in a step-like manner.

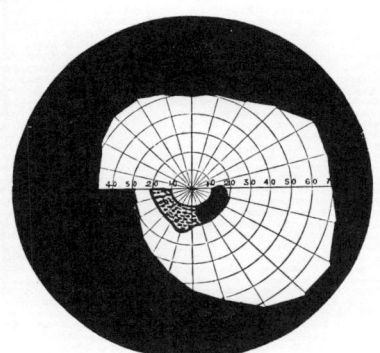

FIG. 62.—Chart from R. E., with chronic glaucoma.

Bjerrum's sign is well shown. So also is Roenne's step. The lesion to the bundles of optic nerve fibres lies at the upper temporal edge of the disc, as shown in Fig. 61. Over the dotted area vision is indistinct.

It is important to bear in mind that Roenne's step can be more easily shown with large-object perimetry than with small. It is *very frequently present*, and the only reason that it is not more often discovered is that many surgeons are in the habit of moving their test object along a few only of the radial diameters. To elicit this sign we must first carefully examine the radial meridians of the field on either side of the horizontal nasal meridian; and then, we must move our test object in successive concentric arcs across the length of this line for a short distance above and below it. If we do so, we shall find a sharp step emerge on our chart in place of what under the ordinary methods only appears as a gradual sloping away of the field at this part.

(4) **The colour fields are but little affected in glaucoma,** and though they shrink *pari passu* with the contraction of

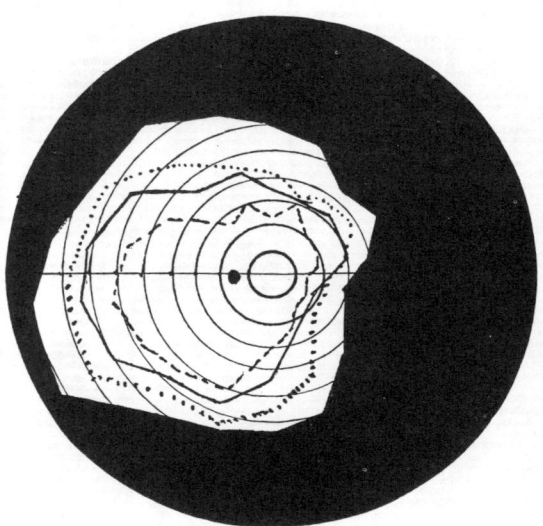

Fig. 63.—Visual field of L. E. (Baas) showing the colour fields remaining large and closely following the shrinkage of the white field.
The changes are due to glaucoma. The inner lines, from without in, are for blue, red, and green.

the white field (Fig. 63), they may retain their relationship to that area and to each other until the very end. Indeed, colour perception may be retained even in that eccentric area of the visual field, which is the last to suffer extinction (Fig. 60). This observation is of great importance in view of the profound changes which the colour fields are known to undergo in cases of optic atrophy. Its significance from a diagnostic point of view does not need to be emphasised. When, in a case of glaucoma, the colour fields are found to be markedly affected, we may unhesitatingly assume that another factor besides that of chronic glaucoma has entered into the case. This matter will be again dealt with at a later stage.

Perimetry with Small Objects

It will probably be acknowledged by all those who have taken any interest in the subject, that the value of Bjerrum's work has not even yet been fully appreciated by the profession at large, or indeed by the great majority of ophthalmologists. The very principles on which it is founded appear to be sometimes misapprehended. It is therefore necessary to explain them, even if doing so involves some small amount of repetition.

In testing the central visual acuity, we take account of the distance at which the examination is being made, and of the size of the smallest object which the patient can definitely see at that distance. The reasons which govern us in so doing are too well known to require mention. Likewise, in dealing with the field of vision, we find that as we pass from the centre of the retina to its periphery, there is a very definite fall in visual acuity, so that an object below a certain size, which is clearly seen at the centre, ceases to be visible when carried out some distance toward the periphery. Within certain limits, the smaller the size of the object, the sooner is it thus lost to view. We can map out the normal visual field for an object of any definite size. In doing so, we find that the smaller the object we use, the more contracted is the field, until finally, when dealing (by daylight) with a 1 mm. object at a distance of 2 m. (probably the limit for convenient working), the visual field of a normal person is discovered, as we have already shown, to be included in an area, which roughly corresponds with the 26 degree circle of a perimeter chart (Fig. 46).

Under pathological conditions, the visual fields taken with small objects are found to show further modifications. In glaucoma, the chart so obtained presents characteristic features, and may thus be of great value in enabling us to

250 GLAUCOMA

arrive at a correct diagnosis. These features are (1) that the area over which the field (as shown by the small object test) is lost, is always continuous with the blind spot over a larger or smaller extent of the latter's periphery, and (2) that that portion of the field of vision which still remains (under the small object test), however small it may have become, is usually continuous with that spot.

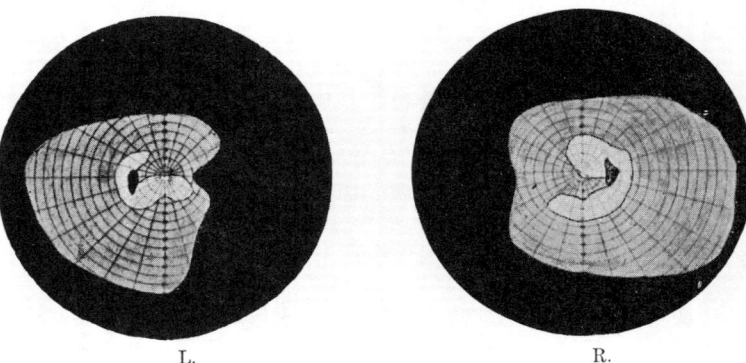

L.   R.

Fig. 64.

The charts (right $V. = \frac{6}{6}$ p., and left $V. = \frac{6}{18}$) are from a case of chronic glaucoma, and show Bjerrum's glaucoma symptom. The area of the most fully preserved vision, indicated in white, is seen in contact with the blind spot of Mariotte, while the area of relative defect, shaded in grey, is also in contact with the blind spot. Note the characteristic curved or horn-shaped projection of the area of most fully preserved vision passing round the temporal side of the blind spot. The charts also show clearly the relative scotoma, or area of relative defect, passing in close relationship to the fixation point, and thus giving an important indication as to treatment. The tests used were right eye, $\frac{3}{250}$ and $\frac{1}{2000}$; left eye, $\frac{3}{250}$ and $\frac{3}{3000}$. (Dr. A. H. H. Sinclair.)

These two points are beautifully illustrated in Figs. 64, 65 and 66, which are reproduced here by the kindness of Dr. A. H. H. Sinclair. They are worthy of study from other points of view as well. Fig. 67 by the same author shows in marked contrast the condition met with in optic atrophy, where the area of most fully preserved vision is in both charts widely separated from the blind spot, which in its turn is wholly surrounded by the region of relative defect.

THE DIAGNOSIS OF GLAUCOMA

Sinclair has put the matter very clearly and concisely thus : " The area of relative defect can always be traced up to the blind spot, provided a sufficiently small test-object be employed, and the area of most fully preserved vision is always in contact with, *but does not surround*, the blind spot." These points will be made clear by a study of Figs. 64 to 66.

Sym, in his *Diseases and Injuries of the Eye*, has expressed

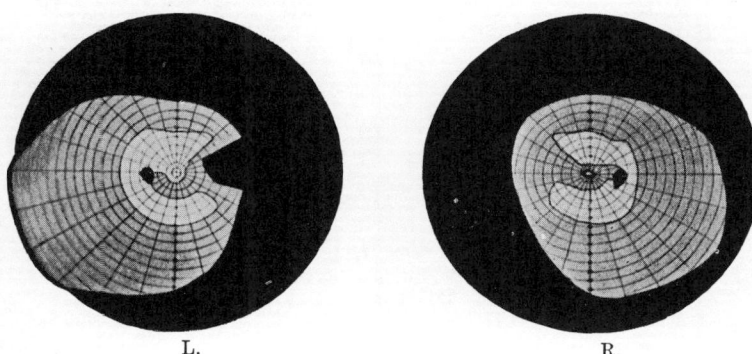

L. R.

FIG. 65.

These charts are from a case of chronic glaucoma showing typical fields. In the right eye, in which V. $=\frac{6}{36}$, a small islet of well-preserved vision remains at the fixation point, while the relative scotoma surrounding this islet passes from the nasal side of the field to the blind spot of Mariotte. In the left eye, in which vision $=\frac{6}{24}$, the relative scotoma passes to the blind spot also from the nasal side of the field, forming an arc with its concavity towards the fixation point. The tests used were right eye, $\frac{1.0}{300}$ and $\frac{2}{2000}$; left eye, $\frac{1.0}{300}$ and $\frac{2}{2000}$. The area indicated in white shows the part of the field in each eye over which a $\frac{2}{2000}$ test was seen. (Dr. A. H. H. Sinclair.)

the same facts graphically, and in an unusual manner in the following words : " The characteristic feature is shown in this, that the blind spot is no longer *an island in a sea of vision*, but the tide has at one part or another receded, so that the 'island' is in continuity somewhere with the shore " (of lost sight).

Before proceeding any farther with this subject, we must stop to describe the method of carrying out the necessary examination.

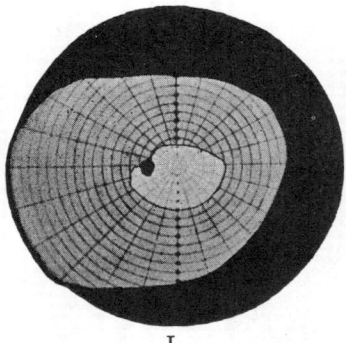

L.   R.

Fig. 66.

Charts from an example of chronic glaucoma occurring in a man of over seventy-five years of age. The right eye, in which $V.=\frac{6}{18}$, showed, in addition to Bjerrum's symptom, the usual evidences of well-marked glaucoma, with a history of gradual failure of central vision. The left eye, in which $V.=\frac{6}{8}$, was regarded by the patient as free from defect. Central vision was full, and the outer limits of the field were of normal extent. The only evidence of glaucoma was Bjerrum's symptom, which was quite definite, and is well seen on the chart. The tests used were right eye, $\frac{\pi \cdot 5}{250}$, $\frac{6}{2000}$, and $\frac{2}{2000}$; left eye, $\frac{2}{250}$ and $\frac{1}{2000}$. (Dr. A. H. H. Sinclair.)

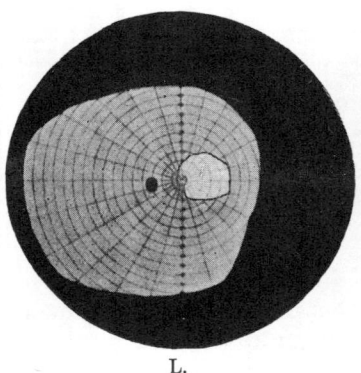 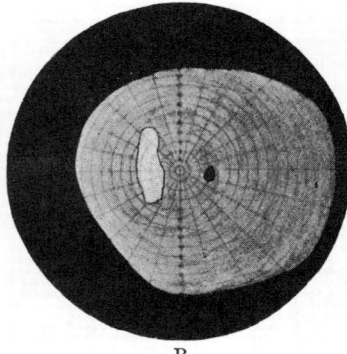

L.   R.

Fig. 67.

Charts from a case of double optic atrophy, showing how the area of most fully preserved vision, indicated in white, is separated from the blind spot of Mariotte, and how the area of relative defect surrounds the whole blind spot. Contrast this with one of the glaucoma charts. The tests used were in each eye $\frac{10}{300}$ and $\frac{2}{2000}$. (Dr. A. H. H. Sinclair.)

THE DIAGNOSIS OF GLAUCOMA

Bjerrum's Method.—During the years 1889 to 1892, Professor J. Bjerrum published accounts of his new method of examination of the visual field by means of small objects. He worked with his patient 2 metres distant from a large screen, 2 metres square, and used small dull white objects of various sizes, his choice resting on those of 6 mm. and 3 mm. in diameter. The screen was of dull black cloth so mounted that black-headed pins could be stuck into it to mark the boundaries of the field under examination. We have already shown what Bjerrum considered to be the normal fields for 6 mm. and 3 mm. objects respectively at a distance of 2 metres. Bjerrum transferred the fields which he obtained on his screen, to ordinary perimeter charts, in the way usually employed when working with non-self-registering instruments. A large number of efforts have been made to save labour in this respect. Some employ white chalk to mark out the field boundaries, and photograph the results.

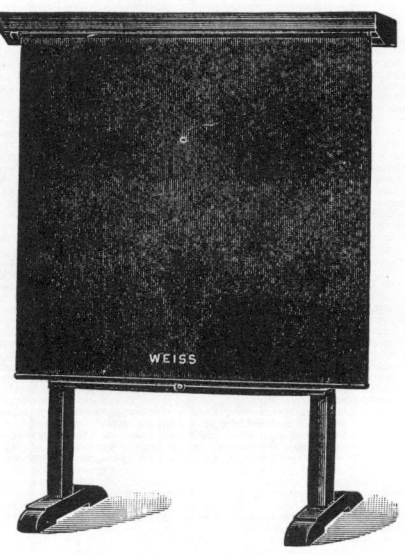

FIG. 68.—Bjerrum's screen in black velvet, 1 metre square, on portable stand. (Edinburgh model.)

Others use a camera lucida, and transfer the findings to specially designed charts. Marx uses coloured steel balls, moved round the face of a black cloth screen, by means of a magnet held behind it, and charts his findings on the back of the cloth. The Edinburgh school follows Sinclair in employing a special tangent rule for the same purpose in combination with a very handy form of Bjerrum screen (Figs. 68 and 69). E. O. Marks, of Brisbane, has devised a very ingenious apparatus whereby the observations made on the Bjerrum screen are automatically recorded on a chart. Fig. 70 shows the general appearance of the appliance. Full details can be obtained through the reference provided at the end of the chapter.

Priestley Smith long ago devised a handy daylight scotometer for the rapid and easy examination by the circular method of the central area of the visual field. The test is a rough one, but it takes little time and is therefore of value. The inventor's dictum is, that "it is necessary to explore the 10 degree circle as well as the 25 degree circle, in order to exclude Bjerrum's sign. If there is no defect in either," he considers "there is no glaucoma." The fact that he and others have recommended working from and round the blind spot, has led some to speak of "enlargement of the blind spot" as a sign of glaucoma. The expression is unfortunate. It is not that the physiolgical blind spot is enlarged in the sense that its area of absolute blindness is increased, but rather that it becomes merged in the characteristic Seidel or Bjerrum scotoma.

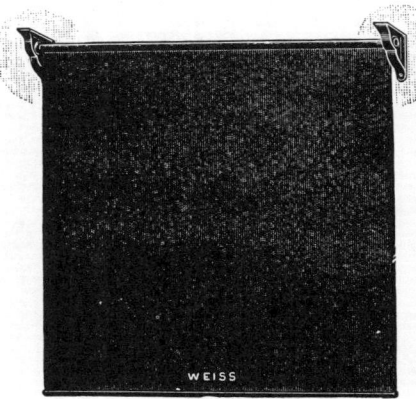

Fig. 69.—Bjerrum's screen as in Fig. 68, but mounted on spring roller and fixed to the wall by brackets.

L. C. Peter and others agree with Priestley Smith in preferring to do their scotometry at the usual perimeter distance of 33 cm. Not a few observers avoid the circular method of examination, working radially to start with, and then across the length of the scotoma or in various other directions. They think that they get better results thereby. In such matters great latitude must be allowed for personal opinions. On quite a different footing, from the point of view of criticism, is the widely prevalent and slovenly practice of constructing a chart on the strength of a very limited number of observations.

For a good many years the writer had been endeavouring to measure, with some degree of accuracy, the normal blind spot, and that met with in glaucomatous subjects. The publication of Seidel's paper served as an added

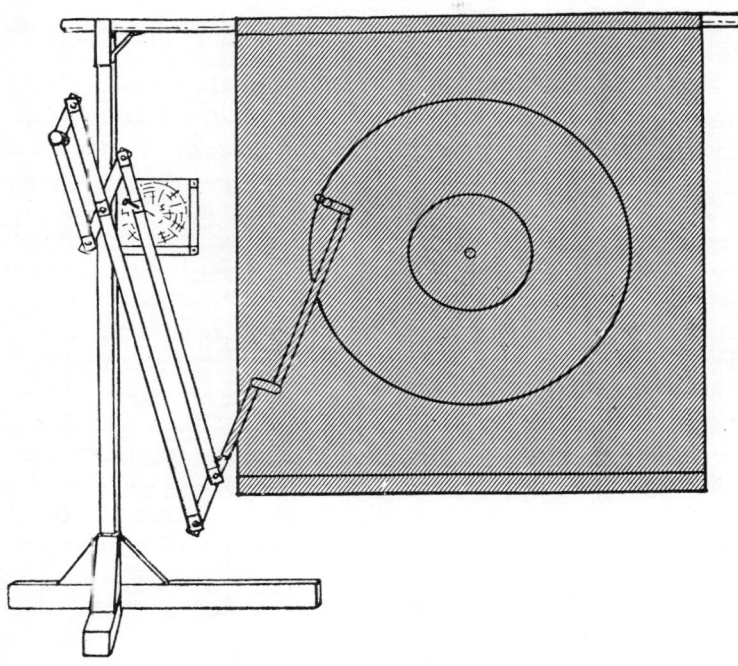

Fig. 70.—E. O. Marks' recording scotometer.
This consists of an attachment to the Bjerrum screen, which enables the results to be automatically recorded on a graduated chart.

stimulus to this research, which was conducted largely with the aid of Bjerrum's screen. The results, however, failed to give full satisfaction, and it was this sense of failure which led to the introduction of a new instrument, designed to carry out in practice three principles which, at least to the author's mind, it is of great importance to conserve and combine, if rapid, accurate, and reliable

clinical results are to be obtained. These principles are :
(1) That of circular instead of radial examination of the
field of vision (Priestley Smith), (2) that of the examination
of the field at intervals of 1° (author), instead of at those of
5° or even 10°, as is so often done ; and (3) that of the
magnification of the scale on which the phenomena are
observed, making the scotomata easier to detect, and more
striking to the examined eye (Bjerrum). It will be of
interest to discuss these points in turn.

(1) *The circular method* of examination has special
advantages in glaucoma cases : It will be remembered
that the fibres emerging from the optic disc sweep in curves
around the central area of vision to reach the horizontal
raphé (*vide* Figs. 49 to 52). Now we believe that the
paracentral scotomata of glaucoma are due to injury
suffered by the bundles of nerve fibres as they cross the
edge of the disc ; it is only reasonable to suppose that
such scotomata will take their form from and follow
the direction of the damaged bundles ; indeed we know
that they tend to be arcuate. It is always much easier,
both for the surgeon and for the patient, if, in mapping a
scotoma, we pass through its longest and not through its
shortest axis. Moreover in the author's experience, a
scotoma will be carried farther if we pass from the blind
into the seeing area instead of in the opposite direction.
It has been pointed out by the advocates of other methods
of glaucoma perimetry that they do not find the sign
which the author has described in connection with his
scotometer, and which has been recorded also by many
others who have used the instrument ; it has consequently been suggested that this points to it being an
artefact. It seems much more reasonable in view of the
constancy with which other observers have obtained the
sign, to attribute the failure of other methods to yield
it, to their technical inability to demonstrate it. Lastly,
we must not forget that in order to map out any area
accurately, there is no method equal to that of doing it in
circles, and this for mechanical reasons which are self-
obvious.

THE DIAGNOSIS OF GLAUCOMA

(2) One can explore the whole field out to the 26° circle at 1° intervals by means of 26 circles easily, accurately, and mechanically traced for us by a rotating disc, whereas to do this at the same intervals working radially from the centre would demand 360 observations and would hopelessly tire the patient. Moreover, the closely set radial lines would for the first 10° or 15° be practically impossible to dissociate from each other. This comes back to the statement with which the last paragraph closed, viz., that to obtain accuracy we must use the circular method.

(3) Whatever may be the verdict of other surgeons, nothing would shake the author's conviction that the magnification of scotomata, whether these be physiological or pathological, makes the patient's task enormously more easy, and the surgeon's results much more accurate. We cannot therefore afford to give up the Bjerrum method. To do so would be a retrograde step. Such, at least, is the author's strong opinion.

The Author's Scotometer (Fig. 71) consists of a circular disc, a little over one metre in diameter, covered with black cloth, and rotating on a central axis. At the centre is a small fixation object, and there is an arrangement to keep the patient at the correct distance of one metre from the screen. From the centre to the periphery along one radius, or if preferred, across the whole diameter, the wheel is marked out by longer and shorter stitches of black silk into 5° and 1° spaces. The rotating objects consisted originally of 1 or 2 mm. discs of white blotting paper, which readily adhere to the cloth, and can easily be moved from one degree mark to another, as in Priestley Smith's scotometer. It has, however, been found quicker and more convenient to substitute a white bead for these discs. This is threaded on a length of black silk which runs from the centre to the periphery of the rotating screen, on the marked meridian, along which it can thus be easily and quickly moved. The arrangement for reading off the meridian of observation is also borrowed from the Priestley Smith instrument; it consists of a cardboard disc fixed to the centre of the back of the screen, and graduated from 0° round to 360°, the figures reading clockwise. A black band on this disc denotes the line along which degrees of measurement are marked on the face of the cloth. The whole is mounted upon an adjustable metal stand, to the top of which is fixed a stationary

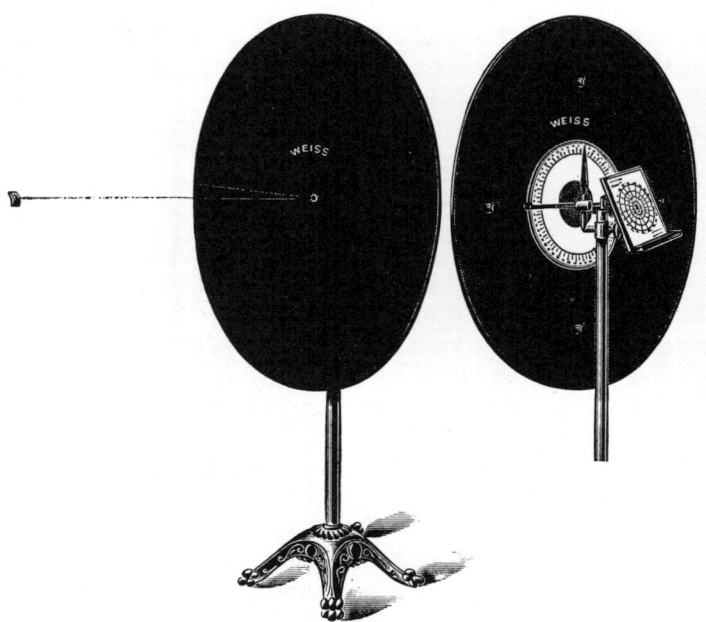

FIG. 71.—Author's scotometer.

The front view is shown to the left, the back to the right. In the latter one of the charts is seen on the desk, for direct registration of the readings, if required. The author prefers to take the first readings on the form shown in Fig. 74, and to transfer these subsequently to a chart.

perimeter-pointer and a desk for carrying the sheet of paper on which the observations are recorded. Four white hand-knobs on the back of the disc make its rotation easy to accomplish.

If the discs of blotting-paper are used, they can be readily cut with an old trephine blade of suitable size; a large stock can thus be made in a few minutes.

THE DIAGNOSIS OF GLAUCOMA

A head-rest, to secure the fixation of the eye in one position throughout the examination, has been provided (Fig. 72). In order to make sure that the centre point of the screen is exactly on a level with the eye, the surgeon uses a special pointer (Fig. 73). With this he measures the height of the eye from the ground after the patient's head has been fixed in the rest; the pointer is then turned on to the face of the screen, which is raised or lowered until the level is correct, before the examination is commenced.

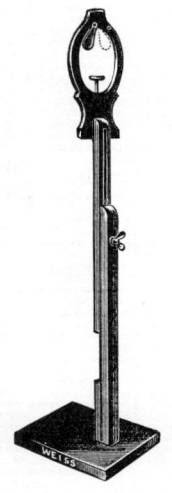

FIG. 72.—Author's head-rest for scotometer.

Method of working.—This varies a little according to whether the surgeon makes use of an assistant or not; the author invariably does so. He stands behind the perimeter and makes notes of the observations on the form shown in Fig. 74. The 5° and 10° circles are first explored, and then he works outward at intervals of 1°, till he passes beyond the limits of the blind spot, or till he reaches the periphery. If there is the slightest doubt, he should work right out to the boundary of the perimeter (26°), and should also work inwards to the centre; in doing so, it is sometimes advisable to take the readings at intervals of 2° instead of 1°, if the patient is easily fatigued. Whichever eye is being examined, each observation starts at 0°, and the wheel is rotated counter-clockwise (as seen

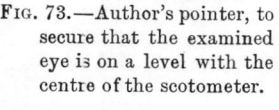

FIG. 73.—Author's pointer, to secure that the examined eye is on a level with the centre of the scotometer.

260   GLAUCOMA

from behind) from 0° to 360°, just as in Priestley Smith's method. The degrees at which the disc is

Degrees Measured Radially from the Centre of the Screen.	For the Registration of the Readings obtained round each Circle.									
1										
2										
3										
4										
5										
6										
7										
8										
9										
10										
11										
12										
13										
14										
15	⑯⓪	18⓪	②①⓪	240						
16										
17										
18										
19										
20										
21										
22										
23										
24										
25										
26										
27										

FIG. 74.

Side of eye..
Size of test object..
Colour of test object.........................: ....

When the test object is visible, mark the degrees (circularly) in ordinary pencil writing; when it is dimly seen, place a ring round each entry; when it is lost to view, underline the figures. This system is illustrated opposite degree No. 15; the meaning of the record there given is that the test object was seen dimly from 160° to 180°, was lost from 180° to 210°, was again seen dimly from 210° to 240°, and was then clearly seen from 240° right round the circle to 160°.

Any other system of marking can be used, provided it is adhered to throughout.

lost, found, lost again, and so on, are noted on each rotation of the disc, and are subsequently transferred to a special chart. Examples of such charts are seen in

THE DIAGNOSIS OF GLAUCOMA

Figs. 75 and 76. This work is greatly facilitated by the use of a pair of compasses armed with a lead pencil. Pads of charts are supplied with the instrument, each chart measuring 8 in. by 10 in.

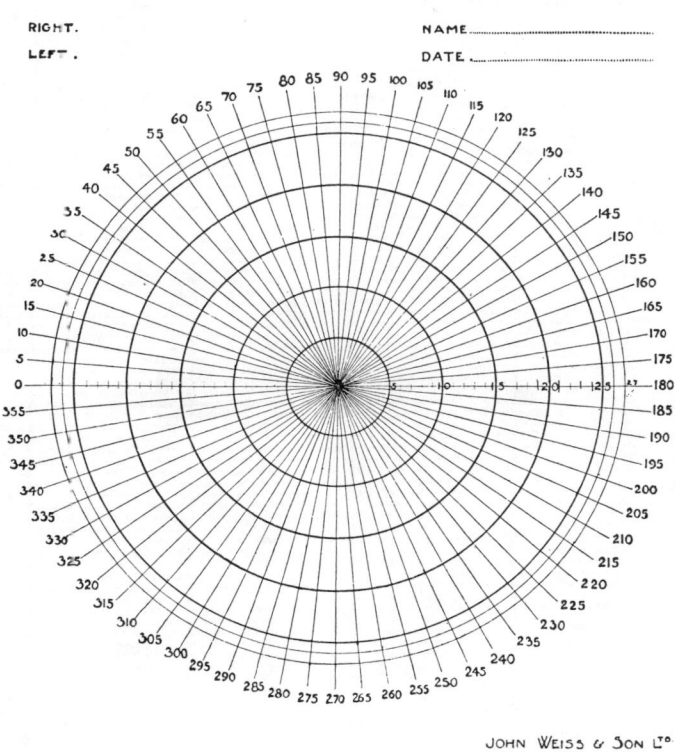

FIG. 75.—Special chart for use with the scotometer.

The assistant, standing beside the patient, (1) takes care that the eye does not deviate from the fixation spot; (2) watches that the patient does not alter the distance of the eye from the screen; and (3) moves the white object along the face of the instrument as directed.

262 GLAUCOMA

A full examination of the central field from 0° to 26° (each degree circle being examined in turn) takes from a quarter to half an hour with an intelligent patient. To map out the blind spot alone takes from five to ten minutes.

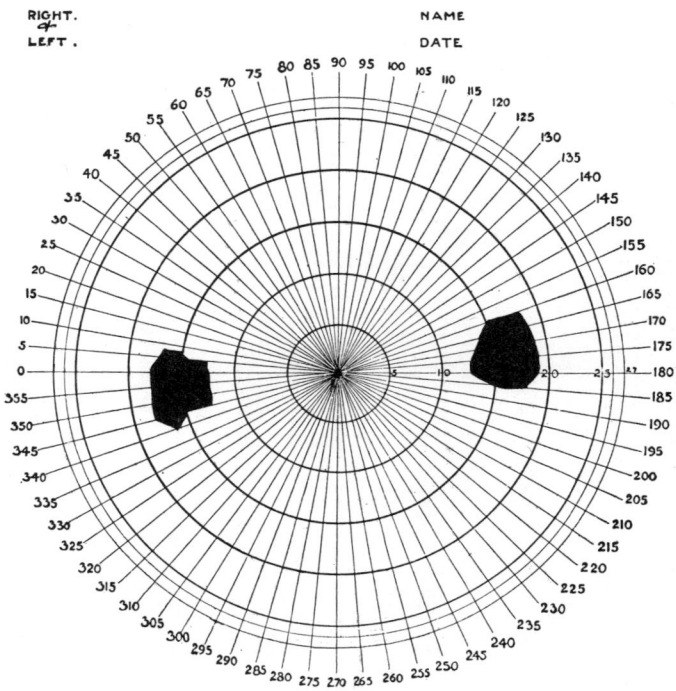

Fig. 76.—The normal blind spots, charted on one of the special charts.

It has been mentioned that there are a number of electric-lit instruments before the profession for the performance of small-object perimetry. Most of these consist of a device mounted on a long black handle, and bearing a little bulb, in front of which rotate two discs carrying

THE DIAGNOSIS OF GLAUCOMA

coloured glasses, and diaphragms respectively (Fig. 77). They are worked in connection with some form of Bjerrum screen. The credit for the original idea belongs, as has already been said, to Fuchs. A. C. Hudson has devised a light spot perimeter with a quadrant arc of 1 metre radius, provided with an ingenious arrangement for automatic registration. The author, dissatisfied with the limitations imposed by the flat screen, had specially built for his use a perimeter of 1 metre radius, adapted to work either in the dark or by reflected light (Fig. 78). It consisted of the usual rotating quadrant arm, very strongly built, and rigidly fixed to the dark room wall. A device

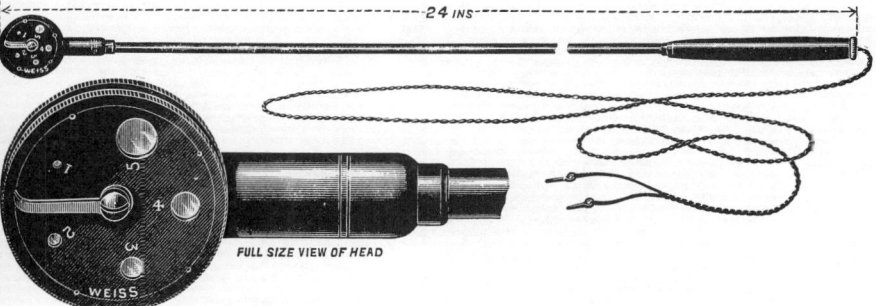

Fig. 77.—A scotometer, intended for use in the dark, with a Bjerrum screen, but now superseded by the rotating disc.

travelled along the arm, and was capable of transmitting white or coloured light through apertures of various sizes from 0·5 mm. upwards, whilst the central fixation object was also self-luminous. A very simple arrangement permitted of the instrument being used by the aid of reflected, instead of transmitted light. In practice, however, the apparatus proved disappointing, and since the advent of the author's new scotometer just described, it has been dismantled, and definitely discarded. Indeed the general tendency among those who have tried the self-lit instrument seems to be in the direction of reverting to daylight, at least so far as the large-arc perimeters are concerned. The 33 cm.-arc de Zeng instrument is, however,

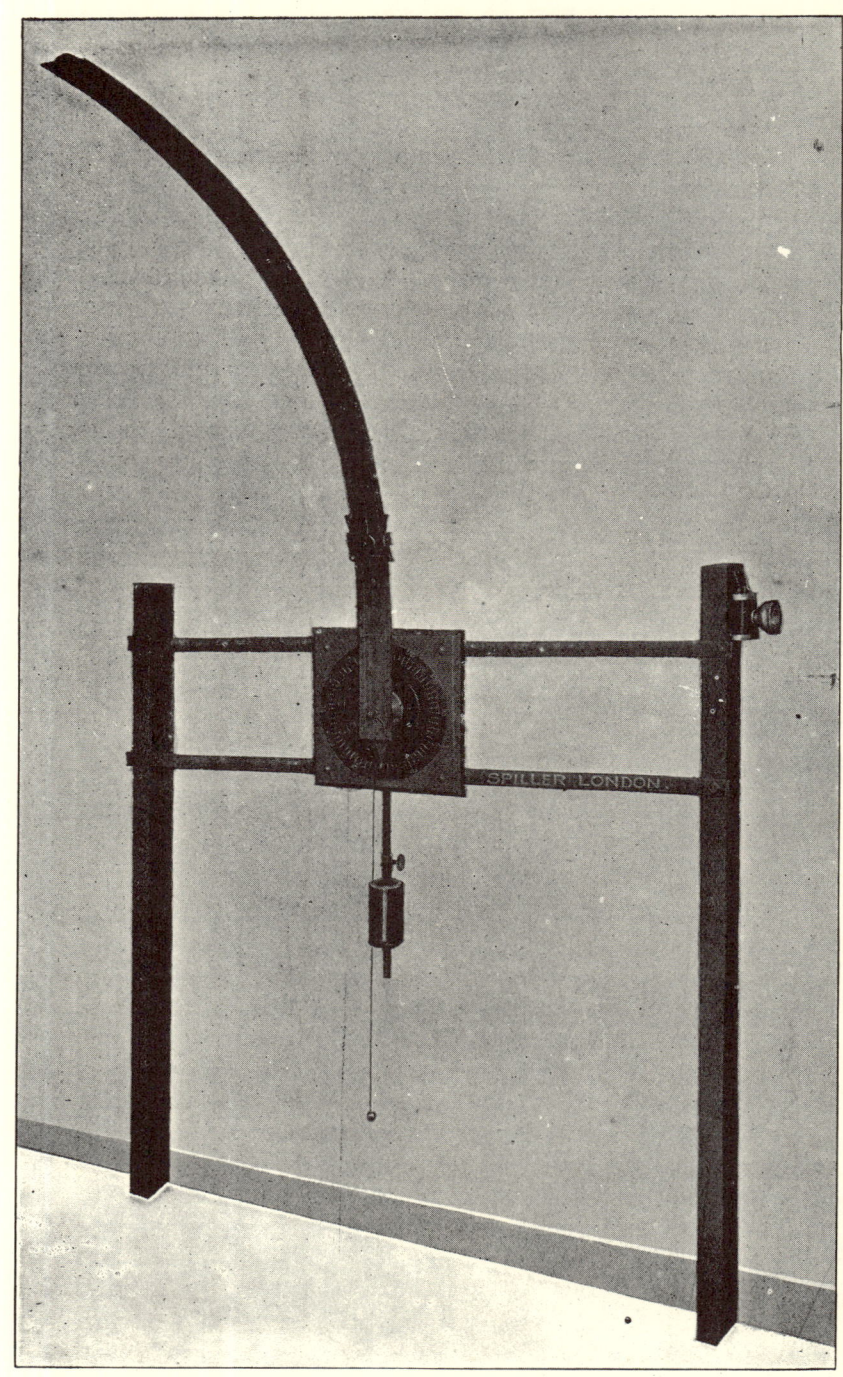

Fig. 78.—The author's large-arc perimeter.

THE DIAGNOSIS OF GLAUCOMA

on a different footing and is a valuable possession in the dark room.

It will be observed that in a large number of the charts illustrated, the results of large, and those of small object perimetry are recorded together. This is done for convenience' sake and has much to recommend it, always

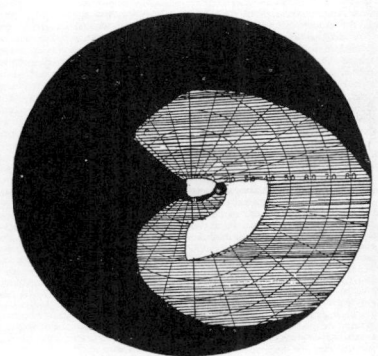

FIG. 79. 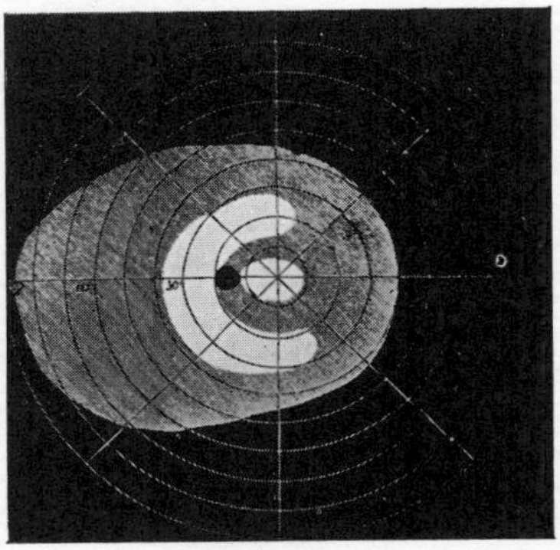   FIG. 80.

FIG. 79.—(Bjerrum.) Chronic glaucoma, R. E.

Fields for $\frac{10}{300}$ and $\frac{4}{2000}$. The latter field is divided into two parts, a central zone and a peripheral bow-shaped zone. Note that the blind spot is continuous with the relative defect both above and below and also with the field for small objects. Part of the arched Bjerrum scotoma is absolute, and reaches out from the blind spot to the area of absolutely lost peripheral vision.

FIG. 80.—(Bjerrum.) L. E.

A double arcuate scotoma surrounds the central visual area. The blind spot lies in contact with the relative scotomata, and with the two areas in which the small object can still be distinguished. The larger one of these by its horseshoe form indicates its connection with the distribution of bundles of nerve fibres.

provided that those who read the charts clearly understand their composite character.

A word as to the most favourable working distance for small-object perimetry :—The author's preference is for 1 metre. This makes it possible to keep within convenient dimensions a screen which will work out to beyond the 25° circle. It is also the limit of convenience for the size of a rotating quadrant arc.

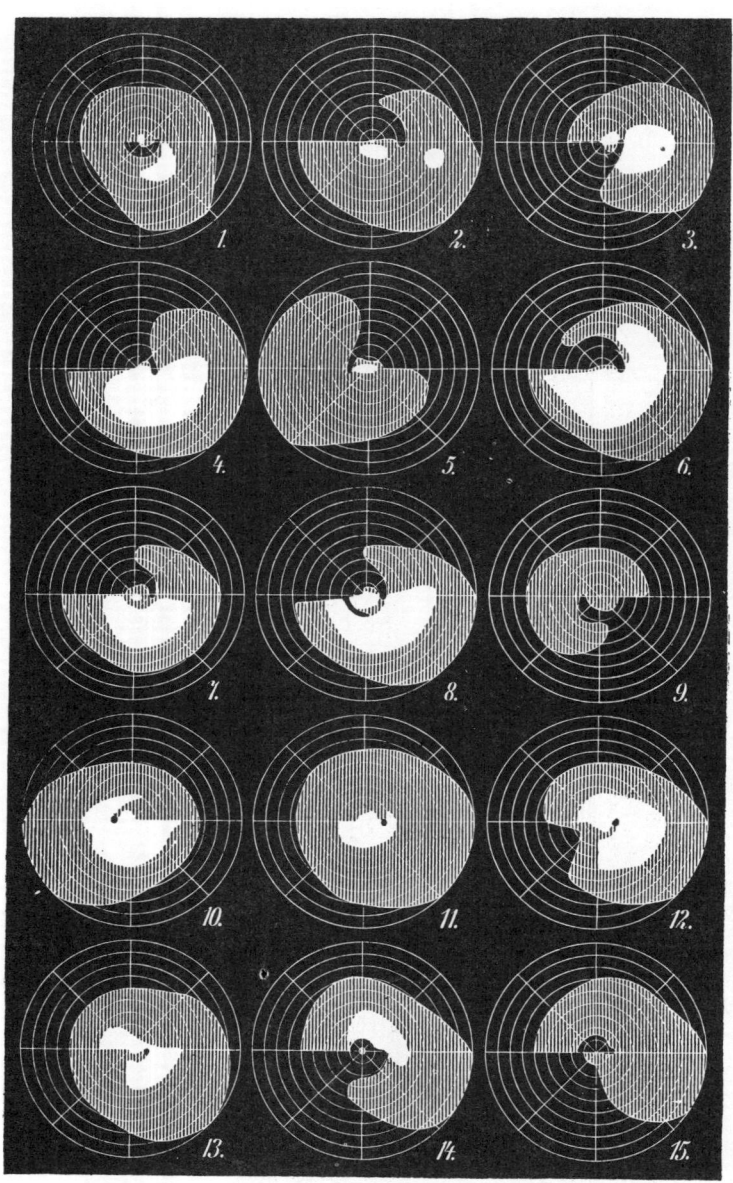

Fig. 81.—(Reproduced by kind permission of Professor Roenne.)
For description of charts see opposite page.

Bjerrum's Sign.—Before the Tenth International Congress of Medicine, in 1890, Bjerrum described a defect in the visual field, which he had discovered by means of small-object perimetry, and which he regarded as strongly suggestive of the presence of glaucoma. This consisted of an arcuate or of an annular scotoma, which started from the blind spot and swept round either above the central area of fixation or below it, or both (Figs. 79 and 80). He laid special stress on the fact that the starting-place of these curved defects was invariably the blind spot; from this and from their shape he asserted that they must be due to the destruction of a limited bundle, or of limited bundles, of nerve fibres, the injury to which lay either at the margin of the papilla or in its near neighbourhood. The bundles in question emerged from the upper or from the lower margin of the papilla on its temporal side (Figs. 51 and 52). No other theory would explain the fact that the defects found correspond strictly with the distribution of such nerve bundles. Bjerrum argued that if the lesion were at the upper margin of the disc, the curving scotoma would sweep round the lower border of the central area of vision; if it were at the lower margin, it would pass above it; whilst if it were dual in nature, an annular scotoma would result.

Roenne's Step.—It has already been pointed out that Roenne carried Bjerrum's work a step farther, when he argued that, assuming the correctness of the anatomical

---

Chart 1 is a typical glaucoma field; there is a small bow-shaped Bjerrum's scotoma, proceeding from the blind spot and terminating on the nasal horizontal meridian by a sharp boundary-line. Charts 2 to 9 show wide defects, each of which passes from the blind spot to become continuous with the boundary of the field in one nasal quadrant, whilst the opposite nasal quadrant is wholly or almost wholly preserved. The boundary-line between the preserved part and the defect runs along the nasal horizontal meridian for a shorter or longer extent. Charts 10 to 13 resemble the above, except that in them the defects are relative and can therefore only be shown by the Bjerrum method. The examination with large objects merely shows a normal field, or at the most a peripheral indentation of that field. Charts 14 and 15 show the reverse condition, the preserved part of the visual field being demonstrated by its boundary in the horizontal meridian, thanks to the activity of a still functional retinal nerve bundle. (Condensed from Roenne's description of the charts.)

data put forward by the latter writer, the scotomata produced must show characteristic features at still another point, viz., in the horizontal meridian of the visual field to the nasal side of the centre of vision. This argument will be easily followed by anyone who has studied the remarks made a few pages back on the anatomical distribution of the nerve fibre bundles in the retina. As has already been said, it explains the valuable sign known as Roenne's step (Fig. 62). The mass of work, on which Roenne's deductions rest, will be better appreciated by anyone who will study the two beautiful plates reproduced in Figs. 81 and 82 from that writer's original work, and by his kind permission. It is surprising how little attention these valuable studies have attracted. Taking up several of the leading text-books in the English language, one does not even find Roenne's name in their indexes, and yet it is safe to predict that posterity will grant that name a very special niche in the temple of glaucoma fame.

Neither Bjerrum, nor those who have followed him, have been under any misapprehension as to the pathognomonic significance of the field defects he described, for they have recognised that closely similar defects may be found (a) in any pathologic condition, which interferes with the integrity of definite nerve bundles on the disc, or in its neighbourhood, *e.g.*, retrobulbar affections of the optic nerve, hæmorrhagic papillo-retinitis, and retino-choroiditis juxtapapillaris, and even in (b) embolism of the central artery of the retina. In the last-named condition (Bjerrum) it was shown that the distribution of the retinal vessels closely corresponded to that of the nerve fibres.

Seidel's Sign.—Before we continue our study of Bjerrum's scotomata, it will be convenient, in the first place, to refer to the work that has been done on the same subject by another of his pupils, viz., Seidel. This writer has found that very early in glaucoma, a characteristic change can be found in the blind spot. This consists of wing-like extensions of that spot either upwards or downwards, or in both directions. The small scotomata so produced present a curved contour, whose concavity always faces the fixation

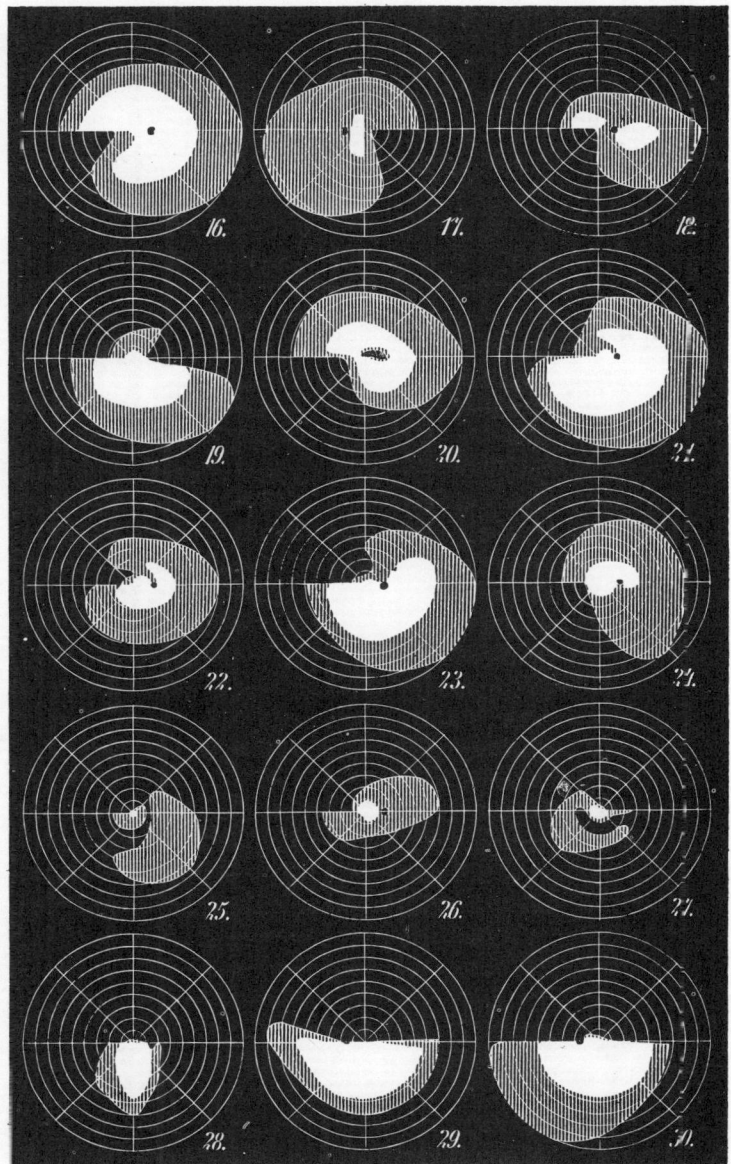

Fig. 82.—(Reproduced by kind permission of Professor Roenne.)
Charts 16 to 24 show the nasal step as the only characteristic sign of glaucoma in the field, but in the last four of them small-object perimetry indicates the true nature of the case. Charts 25 to 28 show that even small fields may prominently demonstrate a distinct nasal step. Charts 29 and 30 show horizontal hemianopsia in glaucoma; looking back at some of the earlier fields, it will be seen that slight indications of this form of defect occur in them.

point. They differ from those described by Bjerrum and his school in their size, being much smaller and therefore easily overlooked. From the first they are continuous with the blind spot ; their opposite extremities taper, sometimes even to a point.

Seidel claims that these scotomata may be found in the apparently perfectly healthy eyes of patients, whose opposite globes have already shown signs of glaucoma, and he believes that a diagnosis can sometimes be made in this way, at a time when there is no other sign pointing to even the faintest suspicion of the disease. A little later when the scotomata are better marked, but before pathological cupping of the disc can be seen, he has found a pallor of the papilla, which he considers to be an evidence of the early advance of glaucoma.

Should the condition of increased intra-ocular pressure continue, Seidel's sign will pass on into Bjerrum's sign. On the other hand, should it be relieved, a Bjerrum's scotoma may undergo retrogression, thus passing back into a Seidel's scotoma ; and again, a Seidel's scotoma may greatly diminish in size, or may totally disappear, leaving the blind spot normal once more. From all this it is clear that these scotomata are merely a transition form in the development of the field defects described by Bjerrum. Fig. 83 shows some characteristic forms which Seidel's sign may take. These are from his original drawings. It should be especially noticed that he never figured them except as continuous with the blind spot from the first, whereas Bjerrum and others, who have followed in his footsteps, have depicted the characteristic Bjerrum's scotoma as sometimes making its first appearance at some little distance from the blind spot, and later becoming continuous with it. This is probably largely a question of the time at which the observation is made and of the accuracy with which the examination is conducted. The resemblance in general configuration between the scotomata depicted by Seidel and by Bjerrum is sufficiently striking to attract the attention even of the least observant.

The Author's Sign.—The author in his study of Seidel's

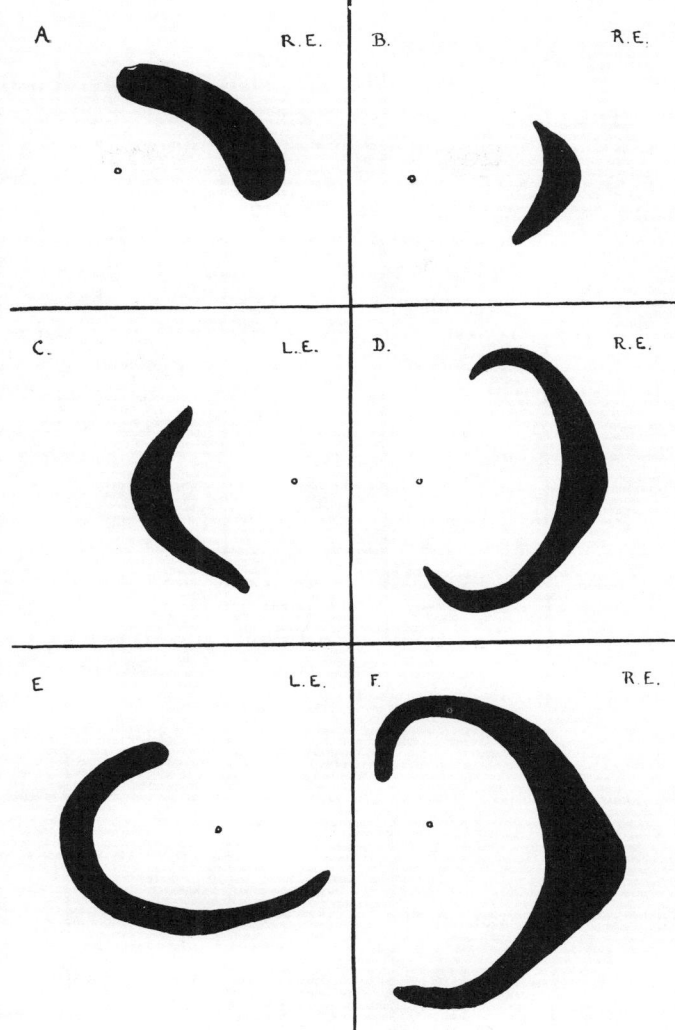

Fig. 83.—Seidel's paracentral scotomata, as mapped out by Sattler and himself, in early cases of glaucoma.

The circular dot represents the fixation point of the visual field in each case. The side of the eye is indicated by the letters R. E. or L. E., as the case may be. In A, the scotoma lies above the horizontal meridian. In B, it lies mostly below it. In C, D, E, and F, it stretches both above and below it; the later illustrations show progressively better marked and larger scotomata.

All the figures were taken with a 3 mm. object at a distance of 1 m. from the screen, and then photographed. They are only a few of the most typical ones of a large number published by Seidel.

sign had from the very first considered it extraordinary that this scotoma should have been invariably figured and described as having pointed or rounded undivided extremities (Fig. 83) ; this was not what might have been expected, on the assumption that the phenomenon is due to an injury to the fibres of the optic nerve, either on the disc or at its edge. Looking at the way in which the fibres emerge from the disc, it has always seemed more likely that, if the scotoma were charted with sufficient accuracy, its upper and lower limits would present more or less ragged edges, instead of ending in points as described by Seidel. In other words, instead of one point at each end, we should expect to find a number of points corresponding to the numerous bundles of nerve fibres damaged at the edge of the disc. From the time that he first read Seidel's work in 1914, the writer, struck with the possibilities it presented, had been endeavouring to follow it up in his glaucoma material, but, as already stated, it was not until he obtained the new scotometer that he was able to take accurate readings all round the circle at each degree from the centre out to 26°. Previous to doing this, and when working by the radial method, he obtained unsatisfactory charts, representing scotomata resembling those described by Seidel. At the same time he was often puzzled by relative scotomata, which were very hard to map out, and which occurred at a distance from the blind spot defect. As soon, however, as the new instrument was installed, it was found easy to make accurate, consistent, and self-explanatory charts. The ragged pointed ends of the scotoma which had been expected as the outcome of reasoning, materialised as a constant factor of the glaucoma chart. The paracentral scotomata found above or below the centre of vision or in other regions, and separated from the blind spot defect by an area of acutely seeing retina, were quickly recognised for what they are. These points will be better realised by a reference to the chart shown in Fig. 84, and also to a number of the charts which follow it. Before turning to study them, however, it is very important to make it clear that the new and somewhat startling features they present

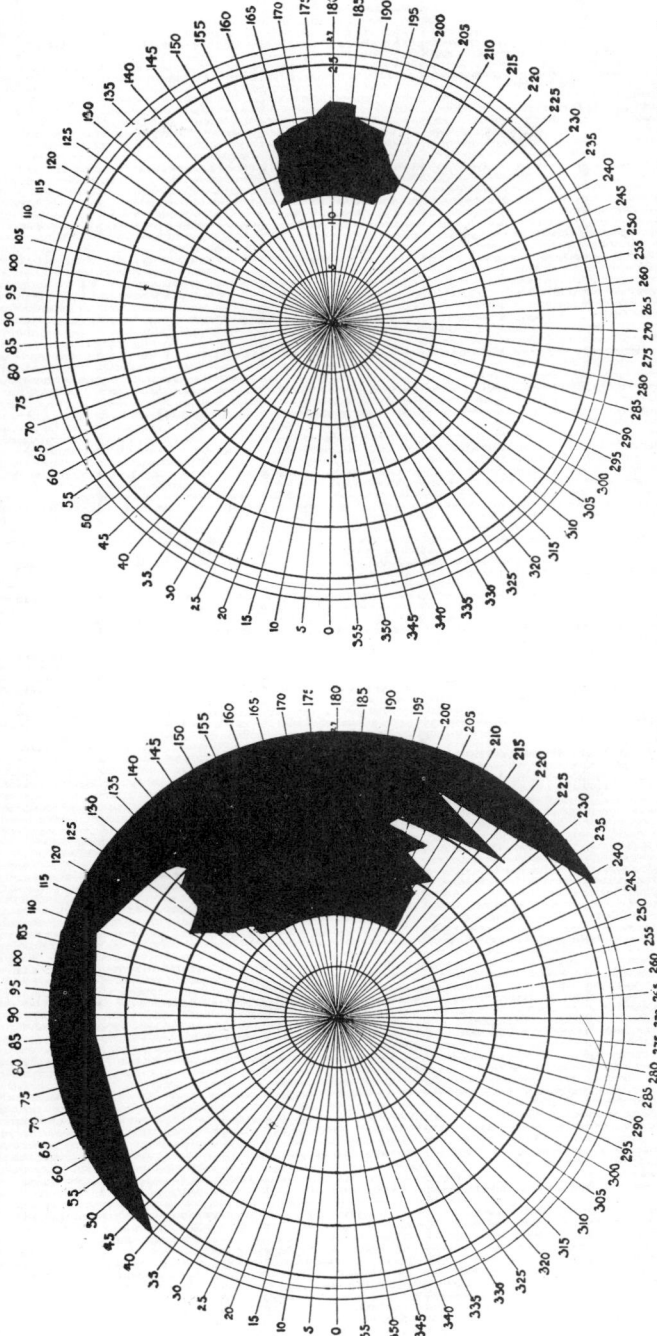

FIG. 84.—Defect mapped out by author's scotometer in an early case of glaucoma a few days before operation.

Note the irregularity of the endings of the upward and downward extensions of the scotoma; these show a number of points, which presumably represent lesions of small bundles of fibres.

The test object in both examinations was a 2 mm. disc of white blotting paper. Each circle represents 5°.

P.S.—A third test was made six weeks after the operation, and the blind spot was then found to be practically normal, having undergone a considerable further contraction.

FIG. 85.—Defect in the same case as above, ten days after relief of tension by a successful trephining.

The pointed peculiarity can still be traced in this scotoma.

are not—as has been suggested by some who possibly have not had the advantage of a practical experience of the use of the instrument—the products of errors in a method of subjective examination. They occur again and again in cases of glaucoma, though less marked in some than in others. A repetition of the observation on the same patient reproduces them in just the same form. An intelligent patient's answers are clear, confident, and consistent, for the moving spot can be charted almost to a degree. It goes out and reappears so sharply that after taking a reading the observer can reverse the rôle, and, going over the same circle, can tell the patient exactly when it is lost or comes again into sight. Moreover, any surgeon who uses a scotometer with ordinary care will get the same results as the writer, as has been proved by the experience of a number, who have been kind enough to communicate with him on the subject.

THE NORMAL BLIND SPOT.—The normal scotomata, as mapped out by the new instrument, are usually absolute throughout their extent, but sometimes reveal an area of relative defect around their edges. They are often pointed; at times more, and at others less so (Fig. 86); the points may occur both above and below, or in only one of these neighbourhoods; rarely two points are seen below, and still more rarely above. An effort has been made to ascertain whether there is any connection between these points and the emergence-areas of the retinal vessels, but no success in this direction can be claimed. The shapes of the blind spots vary greatly, as also do their dimensions. Though there is usually a rough resemblance between the blind spots of the two eyes, they may vary considerably in shape, and to a lesser extent in dimensions. The average lateral measurement of a number of blind spots was 5·48°, and the average vertical measurement 8·15°. The maxima and minima recorded were laterally 7° and 4°, and vertically 10·5° and 6·25°. The findings are, therefore, generally in accord with those of other instruments used for the same purpose. In no case has the blind spot of a normal eye shown any resemblance whatever to the defect so regularly found in eyes affected with high tension. In myopia, and in all the other conditions which give rise to an enlargement of the blind spot similar to that met with in glaucoma, there should be no difficulty in assigning a definite cause for the phenomenon.

THE VALUE OF THE SIGN IN THE POSITIVE DIAGNOSIS OF GLAUCOMA.—It is imperative to recognise from the first that the sign now under consideration is not pathognomonic of glaucoma; it enables us to recognise a lesion, or lesions,

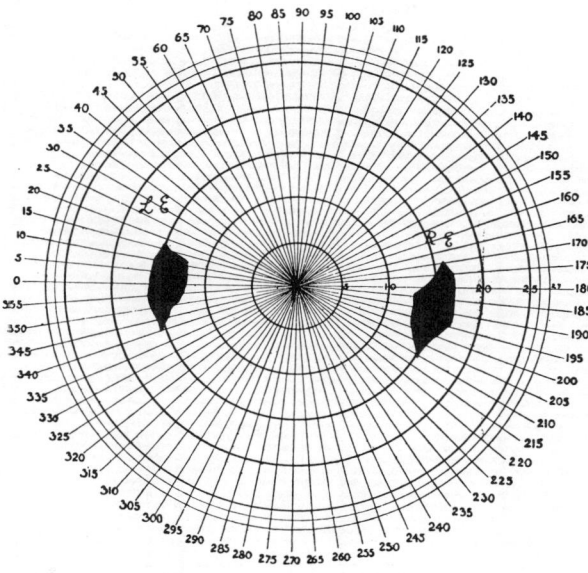

FIG. 86.—Right and left.
Miss F. S.—22nd September 1917.

of a number of bundles of nerve fibres, either on the optic disc or at its edge; but it does not indicate the specific nature of that lesion. When we meet with ophthalmoscopic or other evidence which leads us to suspect the presence of glaucoma, our diagnosis is very greatly strengthened, and may even be confirmed, if a chart of the paracentral field shows the new sign. Our greatest difficulties occur either in very early, or in very slowly progressive cases of glaucoma, and in both instances the new scotometer comes to our aid in a very practical manner. Fig. 84 is illustrative of this point; so also is Fig. 87, which was charted from a case sent to the writer by an ophthalmic surgeon, who was in difficulties, because, whilst he felt sure that the right eye was glaucomatous, he was in grave doubt about the condition of the left, in which the signs of high tension were all very feebly

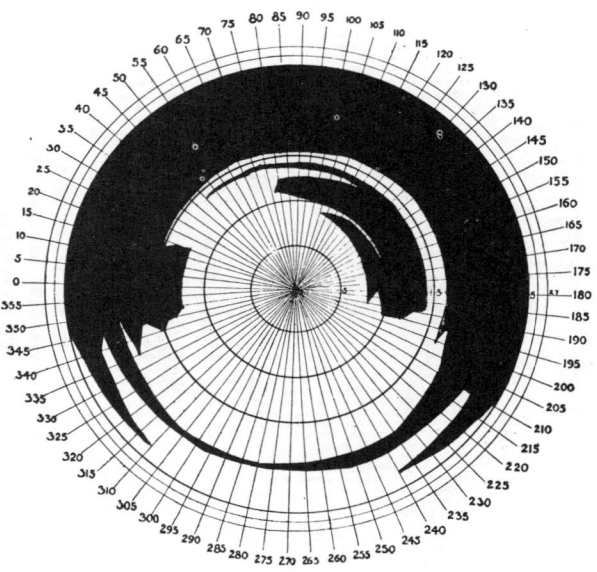

Fig. 87.—Left.
Mrs. J.—5th March 1918. Juv. glaucoma.

marked; the cupping was doubtful, the central visual acuity was normal, and the visual fields were not contracted. The examination of the central and paracentral field left no doubt as to the diagnosis. Both eyes were trephined, and the correctness of the conclusion was confirmed by the extraordinary change which took place in the paracentral scotoma, and which may be seen in Fig. 88. A comparison of the two figures shows the ease with which the results of treatment can be

THE DIAGNOSIS OF GLAUCOMA 277

followed up, but this is a point which will be dealt with later.

Fig. 89 was from a suspected case of very early glaucoma in which the other evidence was of the slenderest, and meiotic treatment proved sufficient to keep the eye in *statu quo* for the time at least. It will be observed that there is comparatively little increase of the area of absolute

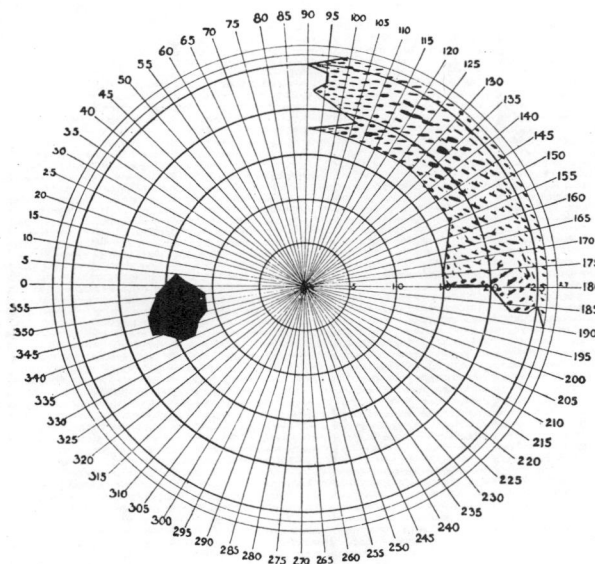

FIG. 88.—Left.
Mrs. J.—Eleventh day after operation, 19th March 1918; trephined, 7th March 1918.

scotoma, whilst the relative area is so much enlarged as almost to constitute Bjerrum's sign. In addition to this, the detached areas of paracentral defect are to be noticed in this figure as also in the preceding ones (Figs. 87 and 88), and in some of those which follow. We shall discuss these detached scotomata later on. They are phenomena of great clinical interest.

There is another important point which is well brought out by Fig. 89, viz., that the increase in the size of the blind spot may be mainly confined to its upper and lower limits, whilst its breadth is relatively much less affected. Priestley Smith's dictum was that " it is necessary to explore the 10° circle as well as the 25° circle in order to exclude Bjerrum's sign "; and his opinion formerly was that " if there is no defect in either, there is no glaucoma." A case to which his attention was subsequently drawn

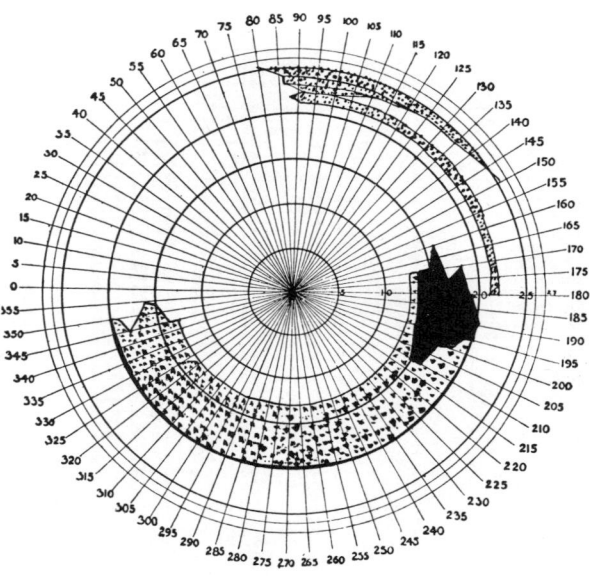

Fig. 89.—Right.
Mrs. L.—18th October 1917.

somewhat shook his faith in these beliefs. It is submitted that the present work explains the difficulty. If we pinned our faith to Priestley Smith's earlier rule, and if we worked only along the horizontal meridian or close to it, we should have diagnosed an absence of glaucoma in the case from which the chart in Fig. 89 was taken, whereas a fuller examination of the field showed at once the grave suspicion attaching to this case. Other interesting examples of the same kind of thing are to be found in many

THE DIAGNOSIS OF GLAUCOMA

of our charts, but it is not possible to reproduce them for want of space.

THE VALUE OF THE SIGN IN REVEALING IMPORTANT ALTERATIONS IN THE CENTRAL AND PARACENTRAL FIELD, EITHER AS THE RESULT OF TREATMENT OR OTHERWISE. —Several illustrations have already been given of the improvement of the central and paracentral fields as the result of operative interference (see Figs. 84 and 85, and 87

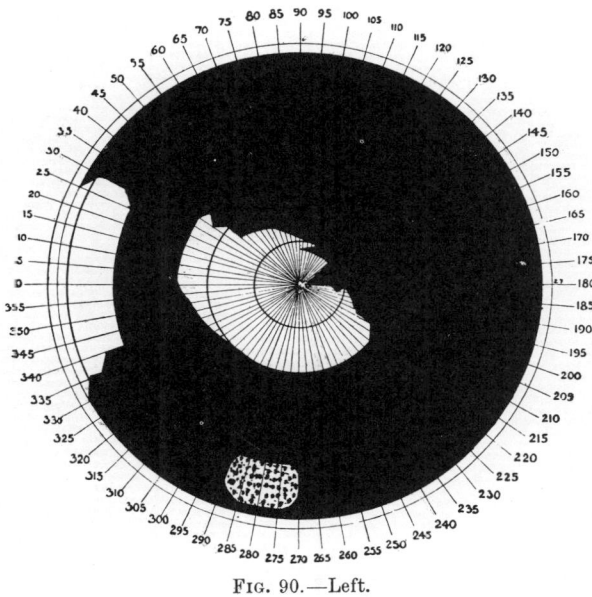

FIG. 90.—Left.
Mr. C.—26th October 1917.

and 88). Figs. 90 and 91 make an instructive addition. The scotomata had approached so close to the centre of vision that the question had been raised whether operation was justifiable. The risks were pointed out to the patient, and though nearly eighty years of age, he was so convinced from his own observation that he was going steadily downhill towards blindness, that he had no hesitation in staking all on a single throw. The left eye was the worse. Fig. 90 was its field taken just before the operation, and Fig. 91

six weeks later. It is instructive to observe (1) the way in which the small relative scotoma below broke through, and (2) the other evidence of improvement in the available area of vision.

Figs. 92 and 93 have quite a different interest; they show the paracentral scotomata before and after operation, and it will be observed that, though a successful and uneventful trephining completely reduced the rise in intra-

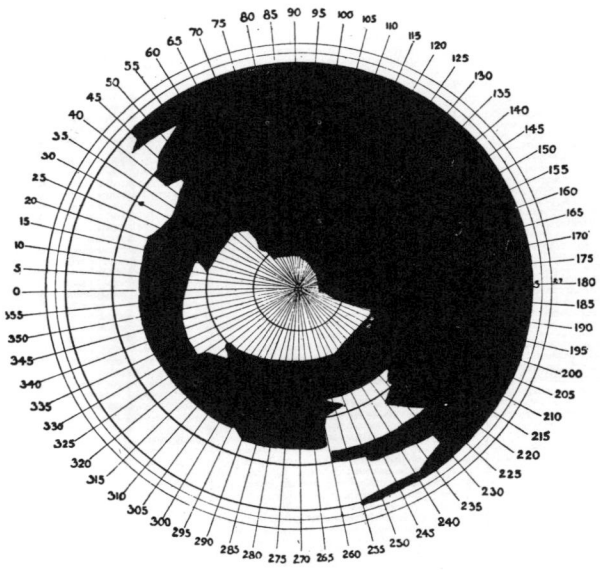

Fig. 91.—Left.
Mr. C.—14th December 1917.

ocular pressure which accompanied an attack of secondary glaucoma, nevertheless, the area of defect showed a marked increase, a fact of which the patient was fully aware. It is consoling to be able to add that he has for nearly four years maintained useful vision despite the somewhat alarming increase of his scotoma which followed hard on his operation.

From the foregoing observations and illustrations it is clear that we have here a means whereby we can easily and accurately measure the defects in the paracentral areas of the fields of vision, and can take note of the changes which occur in them from time to time as the result of operative or other treatment, or of the progress of the disease apart from any interference. Many statements made by patients, which at first sight appear contradictory, are shown to be quite consistent, in the light of

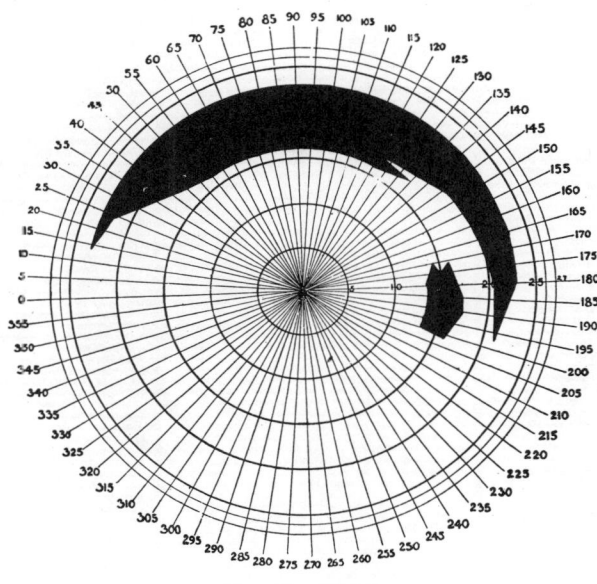

Fig. 92.—Right.
The Rev. J. B——.—7th February 1918.
R.E.V.c̄ + 1·0 sph. = + 3·0 ↷ = $\tfrac{5}{6}\tfrac{15}{6}$ ±.

the evidence obtained from these charts. For instance, it may be found that after operation central visual acuity is unchanged and the visual field, taken with an ordinary perimeter, remains full, and yet the patient may assert in the most positive manner that he sees worse or better than he did before. The changes revealed by the new scotometer will clear up the mystery.

THE VALUE OF THE METHOD IN PROVING THE ABSENCE OF GLAUCOMA.—This point was well illustrated by the following case : The patient, whose father had been successfully trephined for glaucoma, consulted an ophthalmic surgeon, who told him that he had suspicious cupping of the optic discs. In view of his family history, this opinion caused him some alarm. The cupping did not appear to the writer to be of the glaucomatous type, nor could any other signs of a pathological rise in tension be elicited, even after a

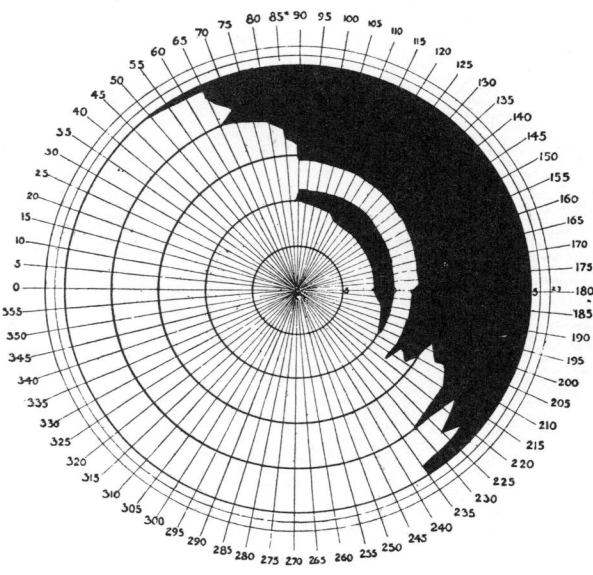

Fig. 93.—Right.

The Rev. J. B—. —21st February 1918. Showing large increase of scotoma following operative release of tension (fourteen days after trephining).

thorough and routine examination. The blind spots were accordingly mapped out and proved to lie well within normal limits, thus definitely settling the question ; for, to the writer's mind, the absence of changes in the blind spot and in the paracentral area is conclusive against the diagnosis of glaucoma. A measurement of the patient's corneal diameters showed that these were above the average, and it was therefore possible to assure him not only that he had not got glaucoma, but also that he was unlikely to develop it in the future. The passage of nearly four years has abundantly confirmed the correctness of this opinion.

THE EXPLANATION OF DETACHED AREAS OF PARACENTRAL DEFECT.—The anatomical distribution of the nerve fibres in the retina has not been worked out with absolute certainty, but it is generally accepted that those fibres which lie nearest the periphery of the nerve, supply the juxta-papillary areas of the retina, whilst the fibres at the centre of the nerve pass out to the retinal periphery (Fig. 101). This arrangement suggests an obvious explanation of the spread of the blind spot outward in different directions in glaucomatous eyes, for, as has been pointed out by Collins and Mayou, the most peripheral fibres are the most likely to be injured by pressure against the edge of the sclerotic as they pass out of the glaucomatous cup. How sharp the ring-edge of such a cup may be can be gathered from an anatomical examination of eyes which have long been subject to high tension. How, then, can we explain the not infrequent presence of detached areas of scotoma in the paracentral fields of glaucomatous subjects ? (1) It may be that we are here dealing with variations in the anatomical arrangements of the nerve fibres ? (2) Again, it is possible that the answer is to be sought and found in lesions to the nerve fibres on the disc itself, and not at its edge. From close examination of a glaucomatous cup, it seems clear that the fibres which originally passed down close to the centre of the papilla must have undergone much more stretching in order to occupy their new positions than did those which from the first ran in their natural course along the shelving side of the scleral foramen. Possibly it is to some factor in connection with the paths of the different bundles of fibres that we are to ascribe the causation of the phenomena of detached paracentral scotomata seen in a number of these figures.

(3) Lastly, we must in no case lose sight of the anatomical variations met with in the supporting framework of the optic nerve-head, and of the great probability that, in consequence of those variations, the nerve-head yields

differently in different eyes, and unevenly even in the same eye. We are, therefore, justified in expecting that the injury inflicted will fall on different bundles of fibres in different cases, and so materially influence the signs of disease present in the perimetric picture.

INVASIONS OF THE CENTRAL AREA OF THE FIELD.—It has long been known that, although in the vast majority of cases it is the rule that glaucoma spares the centre of the field of vision, very marked exceptions to this rule occur. It would take us too far were we to attempt to argue why the papillo-macular bundle should so often escape injury, and should at times be so definitely overwhelmed by it, but the clinical significance of invasions of the central area is such as to demand very careful study.

The new scotometer has—in the author's experience at least—given precision to the investigation of the subject, and has made it possible to formulate certain statements thereon :

(1) Invasions of the central field within the 13° circle are much more common than is generally supposed. A systematic examination of the central area will convince anyone, who sees many cases of glaucoma, of this fact.

(2) Such invasions tend to move steadily onward towards the obliteration of the upper, or of the lower central field, or of both. Two distinct clinical types may thus present themselves :

(i.) When the scotoma is confined to either the upper or the lower field, the condition may amount to a nearly complete central hemianopia, before the patient is aware of the serious defect in his sight. Such can only be the case when the opposite eye is comparatively normal, and when the patient does not happen to have tested the two eyes separately. The hemianopia is always superior or inferior, and never nasal or temporal, and this for obvious reasons.

(ii.) When the invasion of the central field takes place simultaneously above and below the horizontal meridian, the patient is more likely to detect it at an early date. If he is now examined at intervals, the progress of the formation of a ring scotoma can be watched through all its stages.

In the earliest of these, comparatively thin arcs of scotoma may be seen to be thrown out from the blind spot above and below till they meet on the horizontal meridian at the opposite side of the chart to form a ring ; other similar arcs inside or outside the first ones can be traced later on ; these fuse in time with the early arcs, and so form heavy scotomatous rings, which blot out a large part of the paracentral field (Figs. 87 and 91). It does not necessarily follow that each of these arms of damaged field extends from the first in an unbroken course from the blind spot to its meeting-place with its fellow. On the contrary one or both may at first be separated from the more or less enlarged blind spot, in the form of detached scotomata ; or again one or both may fail to reach right round to the horizontal raphé on the opposite side, but in time, the patches of active field so left behind become included in the progress of the scotomata, and a complete ring is thus formed.

(3) It has been suggested that the cases in which the central area becomes abolished after a decompression operation are those where a ring scotoma is present, and further that an urgent hint of the inadvisability of operative interference is thus furnished by the scotometric field. The author is convinced that this is a fallacy : In one of the very few cases in which the central field was lost in his practice after a trephining, an inferior arc-scotoma—and that not a very wide one—was alone present, the upper paracentral portion of the field being absolutely clear. On the other hand, he has operated successfully on a number of cases of ring scotoma without any complication ensuing. Figs. 87 and 88, and 90 and 91 illustrate this point. These and numerous other charts in the author's possession show that a central scotoma, even though it be ring-shaped, may reach within a very few degrees of the centre of vision, and yet be safely and successfully submitted to trephining. It will be found on p. 290 that this is also in accordance with van der Hoeve's findings.

Before leaving the subject of this new sign of the presence of glaucoma, it is imperative to reiterate that no claim is made that it has a pathognomonic significance. Such is far from being the case. On the contrary it is but a link—albeit a very valuable one—in the chain of evidence on which our diagnosis hangs. This principle was clearly recognised by Bjerrum and his followers in all their work, for they knew that defects closely similar to those they described could be found in *any* pathologic condition which interfered with the integrity of definite nerve bundles either on the disc or in its neighbourhood.

The Development of a Glaucoma Field.—Much of the ambiguity which clouds our comprehension of the nature of glaucoma fields will be removed if we understand clearly that a great deal depends (1) on the stage of the disease at which the field is taken, and (2) on the exact technique adopted. There is, however, a third factor running through all glaucoma cases which it is intensely important we should understand and allow for : (3) We believe that the changes in the visual field are simply a manifestation of damage inflicted on the fibre-bundles of the optic nerve, as a result of pressure and of the consequent interference with the blood supply. To this topic we shall have to return later. Our present point is that the nerve bundles affected are very different in different cases—more especially when we are dealing with early phases of the disease. This is readily explained by our knowledge of the variations in anatomical structure met with in the supporting framework of different optic nerve-heads (*vide* pp. 16 and 198). What is more, the intensity of the affection of the fibres varies enormously according to the nature and acuteness of the disease.

Let us assume that in the examination of each suspected eye the surgeon makes two sets of observations (1) with an ordinary 33 cm.-arc perimeter with the use of objects calculated to give a full field (*vide* p. 229), and (2) with some form of Bjerrum screen (the author prefers his own scotometer for the purpose). Let us at the same time confine ourselves to the consideration of cases in which the congestive element is not markedly in evidence, in other words to the so-called chronic cases, or those with, at the worst, slightly marked, subacute intervals of exacerbation.

THE DIAGNOSIS OF GLAUCOMA 287

In a considerable number of such cases—and probably in the great majority of them—the first discoverable sign of glaucoma will be either (i.) an enlargement of the blind spot, or (ii.) the presence of one or more detached, paracentral scotomata, somewhere around the periphery of the circles between 10° and 25°. These manifestations of nerve-damage—whether, from the first, they are in continuity with the blind spot or otherwise—may be relative or absolute. As the disease progresses, they increase in length and in breadth, and tend (i.) to become absolute throughout their whole extent, and (ii.) to join up with the scotoma spreading out from the blind spot, even if at first they are detached from it. At the same time—always provided that the author's scotometer is used—they show more and more clearly the jagged features associated with the sign which has already been described. Very soon the arc-like form, originally described by Bjerrum, can be clearly traced, and it is observed that the scotoma now has the characteristics with which that surgeon's work has made us familiar, viz., (1) it begins at the blind spot, (2) it sweeps in a curve round the fixation area to reach the nasal portion of the horizontal raphé, and (3) it gradually melts into, and becomes continuous with the areas of defect in the periphery of the field.

In the meantime, changes have been in progress in the charts taken with the 33 cm.-arc perimeter. In the earliest stage of all it may be difficult, if not impossible, to satisfy oneself that the field is not fully normal. The changes in the blind spot are too vague and too slight to be registered by this instrument; but, as time passes on, it may be observed that this spot is larger and more easily mapped out than it is under normal conditions; it may show an increase in breadth, but much more frequently, the increment is either in the upward or downward direction, or in both. Vague, relative, paracentral scotomata may also make their appearance. Later still, a distinct arcuate Bjerrum scotoma may sometimes be easily traced even on the charts made from the small perimeter.

Much more noticeable phenomena have, however, been

288 GLAUCOMA

manifesting themselves at the periphery of the field. These, which have been already dealt with, consist in a contraction of the visual field and in the appearance of Roenne's step. Repetition on this subject is unnecessary.

Lastly, whilst the field is shrinking from without and being invaded from within, a third change is going on within it, viz., the gradual shrinkage from without inward of the area throughout which a small object can be seen at a relatively large distance, when the examinations are con-

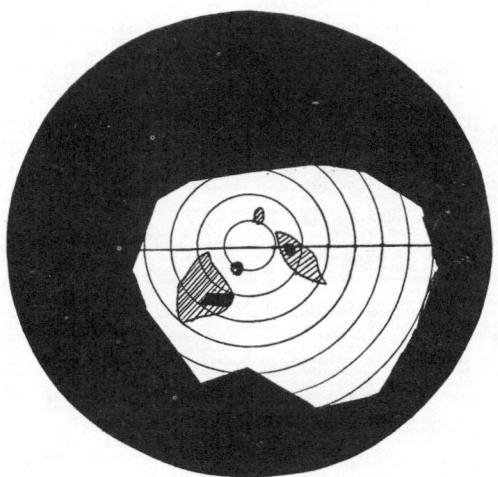

FIG. 94.—(After Baas.) Field of R. E. showing paracental scotomata, some of which are separated from the blind spot. From a case of chronic glaucoma.

ducted on the Bjerrum principle. For the sake of clearness, we may put the matter in slightly different words, trusting that the importance of the subject will be more than sufficient excuse for a repetition of the lessons to be learnt : In the development of a glaucoma field, there are three great changes in progress :—(1) a steady contraction of the periphery of the whole field as measured by large object perimetry. This replaces the normal peripheral area of the field by an increasing zone of absolute blindness. (2) A similar contraction of the peripheral portion of the smaller field, as mapped out by small-object perimetry.

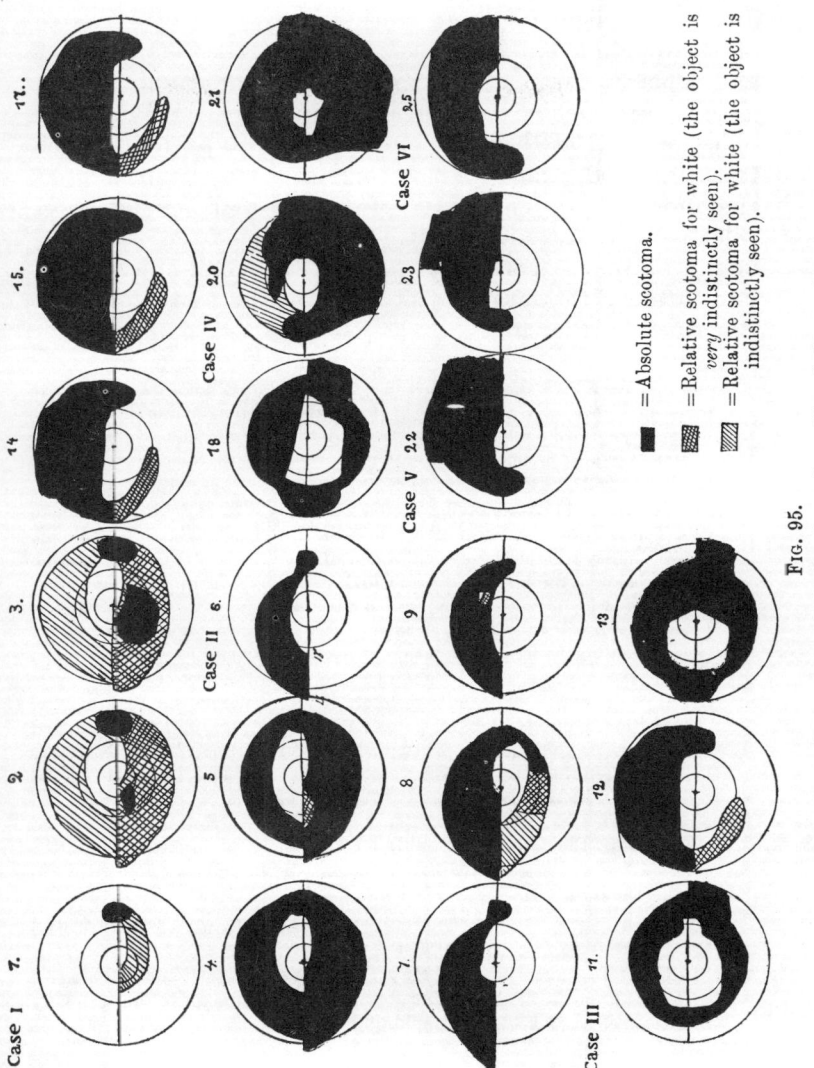

FIG. 95.—Charts showing the progress of central scotomata by van der Hoeve. In Case I., the increase in the scotoma was slow; it was much more rapid in Case II. Chart 6 was taken on 7th June 1915. The scotoma was then 13° from the fixation point. Operation was refused and pilocarpine was employed. On 17th June Chart 7 shows the scotoma 5° from the fixation point; on the 21st (Chart 8) it was 2° from the fixation point, and a bow-shaped scotoma had begun below, which was absolute at the blind spot,

Just as the field for large objects is invaded by the area of surrounding blindness, so also it, in its turn, invades and replaces the periphery of the field for small objects. There is, in fact, a concentric shrinkage of the total field of vision, and at the same time of the two parts of which it is composed, which we may somewhat loosely speak of as the inner or absolute area of vision, and the outer or relative area of vision. (3) The invasion from the blind spot toward the periphery, first of the small-object field, and later of the large-object field, by the scotomata first described by Bjerrum.

and relative a little distance from it. On the 22nd Elliot's trephining was performed, the scotoma being 1° from the fixation point; the lower scotoma vanished and the upper receded to 13° from the fixation point (Chart 9), whilst a small relative island appeared in the scotoma. Van der Hoeve believes that in this case central vision was saved by trephining.

In Case III., Chart 11 shows a ring scotoma in the L. E. and continuation of this defect into the lower nasal loss of the visual field. The R. E. showed a large absolute scotoma above (Chart 12), 4·5 from the fixation point; below is a relative scotoma which does not join up with the blind spot, but which reaches the horizontal meridian. Operation refused, pilocarpine instilled. One week later (Chart 13) the scotoma in the left eye is approaching the fixation point on three sides, and is only 4° from it on the nasal side, whilst in the right eye (Chart 14) the scotoma is 2·5° from the fixation point. Sixteen days later, R. E., scotoma was within 1° of the fixation point (Chart 15); L. E. (seen in Fig. 96), the field had shrunk nearer the fixation point, and showed Roenne's step. Next day Elliot's trephining was performed on left eye, and at a later date on the right eye. The improvement in the left eye, which encouraged trephining of the right eye, is shown in Chart 18. Van der Hoeve draws special attention to the fact that trephining was safely performed though the scotoma was within 1° of the fixation point in the left eye and within 3° of it in the right eye.

Case IV., L. E., shows an increasing scotoma making its way over the central area; sclerotomy failed to arrest it.

Case V., Chart 22, taken on 28th May 1914, shows the scotoma reaching to within 2° from the fixation point above; it broke through to the periphery in the upper nasal field. A trephining on 3rd June arrested its progress (*vide* Chart 23).

Case VI., Chart 25, is another instance of a central scotoma invading the central area.

Van der Hoeve published these charts to "show that in scotomata up to less than 1° from the fixation point, Elliot's trephining does not cause involvement of the macular area. Meiotics and sclerotomy failed, and iridectomy was contra-indicated owing to its dangers."

THE DIAGNOSIS OF GLAUCOMA

The invasion of the central area of the visual field by scotomata has been discussed in connection with the author's scotometer. We return to the subject for a short space to refer to the work of various other surgeons.

Central scotomata.—It is characteristic of glaucoma that whilst it greatly restricts the limits of the field of peripheral vision, it tends to spare the centre almost to the last. We may thus find a vision of $\frac{6}{6}$ in a patient whose fields are so restricted that he can no longer find his way about alone. Such a condition is, however, only met with in cases in which a congestive element has been wholly or almost wholly absent. Perimetry will then often show the central visual area to be intact or nearly so.

Exceptions to this rule occur, and their importance is out of all proportion to their frequency, for very obvious reasons. The central area may be curtailed by defects which spread inward from its upper or lower margin, or from both (Figs. 95 and 96); or again, the whole of the central field, or its upper or lower half, may be impaired or lost at a comparatively early period of the disease,

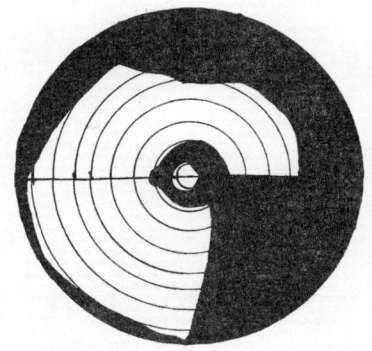

FIG. 96.—(Van der Hoeve.) Glaucomatous field, L. E., showing ring scotoma, invasion of the central area of vision, and Roenne's nasal step.

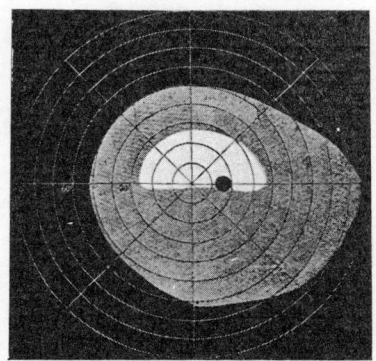

FIG. 97.—(Bjerrum.) R. E. The small-object field is completely lost below the horizontal meridian. The central field has gone with the rest. ($\frac{10}{300}$ and $\frac{4}{2000}$.)

though this is rare (Figs. 97, 98 and 99 ; see also Figs. 81 and 82). When the central defect is hemianopic, it is often in association with a corresponding impairment of the whole field of vision. Defects in the central field, limited more or less strictly to one or other of the nasal quadrants, are also met with ; their genesis will best be understood by studying Roenne's charts found in Figs. 81 and 82. Fig. 100 should also be examined in this connection.

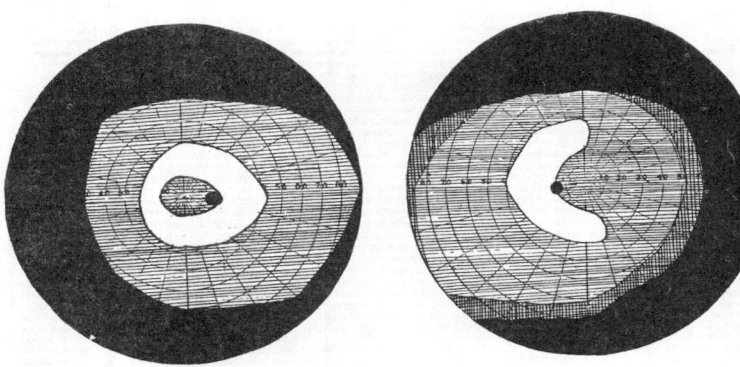

FIG. 98.   FIG. 99.

FIG. 98.—(Bjerrum.) R. E.

The white area is ring-shaped, surrounding a central relative scotoma; the blind spot lies at the temporal end of this scotoma. White field $=\frac{4}{2000}$; shaded field $=\frac{10}{300}$.

FIG. 99.—(Bjerrum.) L. E.

From the same patient as Fig. 98. The white field ($\frac{4}{2000}$) is a large, peripheral, bow-shaped area, touching the blind spot round the outer half of its circumference ; shaded field $=\frac{10}{300}$.

Van der Hoeve has drawn special attention in a very valuable paper to the importance of the early recognition of the cases in which paracentral scotomata tend to invade the centre of vision (Fig. 95). This matter will again be referred to under Treatment, but the importance of the subject is so great, that its main points may be mentioned here. They are : (1) That the patient's only safety lies in immediate operation ; and (2) that iridectomy and all operations which open the eye widely are very dangerous, whilst sclero-corneal trephining saves central vision.

If we turn back to Fig. 52, and to what has been written on the anatomical distribution of the nerve fibre bundles in the retina (see p. 235), we shall see that the expression " the spread of a paracentral scotoma to the central region " is liable to lead to confusion in the reader's mind, for he may interpret it wrongly. On the perimeter chart it is true that the one scotoma appears to flow over into the other, but if we look for the underlying causes of the change, we must probably do so, *not in the field*, but at the edge of the disc. When we turn our attention to this region, the wonder arises, not that central scotomata should occur, but that they should be so uncommon as they are. We must, however, leave this attractive problem till we come to deal as a whole with the explanation of the various phenomena which characterise glaucomatous fields.

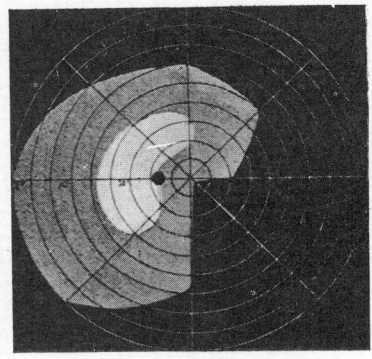

FIG. 100.—(Bjerrum.) L. E.

There is a large absolute quadrantic defect downward and inward reaching up to the fixation point. The small-object reaches the blind spot. The small-object field is bow-shaped; it lies to the outer side of and in contact with the blind spot.

The variety in the shapes assumed by glaucoma fields. — The attentive reader of the preceding pages cannot fail to have been struck by the large number of factors which enter into the formation of a glaucoma field, by the varying intensity of action of each such factor in different cases, and by the consequent extraordinary and endless variety of field forms encountered. The beautiful plates, which have been reproduced from the works of Bjerrum, Roenne, Sinclair, and others, will afford the student an opportunity of accustoming his mind to this diversity of detail, which is, however, associated with a close similarity in the broad features of all the charts. Instances will be seen of hemianopia, of ring scotoma, and of many other uncommon types of visual field. It is hoped that the genesis of each of these will become nore obvious after a study of the next part of this chapter.

REFERENCES

BAAS, K.—*Das Gesichtsfeld*, Stuttgart, 1896.
BJERRUM, J.—*Tenth International Congress of Medicine*, Berlin, 1890.
ELLIOT, R. H.—" On a New Form of Scotometer, and a Sign elicited by its Use," *Trans. O.S. of U.K.*, 1918, vol. xxxviii. p. 185.
HUDSON, A. C.—*Proc. Roy. Soc. Med.*, Section on Ophthal., 1917.
MARKS, E. O.—Section in Ophth. of Australian Med. Congress, Brisbane. Instrument made by A. H. Field, Central Buildings, Edward Street, Brisbane.
MARX, E.—*Brit. Journ. Ophth.*, Oct. 1920, vol. iv. p. 459.
PETER, L. C.—*Principles and Practice of Perimetry*, Lea & Febiger, Philadelphia and New York, 1916.
ROENNE, H.—*Archiv f. O.*, 1909, vol. lxxi. pt. i. p. 52
SEIDEL, E.—Von Graefe's *Archiv f. O.*, 1914, vol. lxxxviii. p. 102.
SINCLAIR, A. H. H.—*Trans. O.S. of U.K.*, 1905, vol. xxv. p. 384.
SINCLAIR, A. H. H.—*Trans. Edin. Med. Clin. Soc.*, 1906, vol. xxv. p. 249.
SINCLAIR, A. H. H.—*Ophth. Rev.*, 1914, p. 80.
SYM, W. G.—*Diseases and Injuries of the Eye.*
TRAQUAIR, H. M.—*Ophth. Rev.*, 1914, p. 65.
VAN DER HOEVE, J.—*Zeit. f. Augenh.*, 1915, vol. xxxiv., parts 4 to 6.
VON DER HEYDT, R.—*Amer. Journ. Ophth.*, 1919, vol. ii. p. 123.
WALKER, C. B.—Knapp's *Arch. Ophth.*, 1913, vol. xlii. p. 577.
WILLBRAND, H.—*Perimetry and its Clinical Value*; translated by Pooley; Norris and Oliver, vol. ii. p. 189.

PART V

The Diagnosis of Glaucoma (*continued*)

SUMMARY :—Explanation of the Genesis of the Characteristic Phenomena found in the Visual Fields in Chronic Glaucoma.
    (1) The Lesions Responsible for the Field Defects in Chronic Glaucoma.
        (I.) Those referable to the area of the cupped disc or to its edge.
        (II.) Those which come into operation outside the area of the disc.

(2) The Factors which determine the Wide Variations found in the Visual Fields of different glaucoma patients.

The Characteristic Concentric Contraction of the Visual Field in Glaucoma.

(1) Anatomical Considerations.
(2) Interference with the Retino-choroidal Circulation.
(3) Direct Injury to Retinal Structures.

The Early Restriction of the Nasal Portion of the Visual Field in Chronic Glaucoma.

The Consideration of a few Remaining Points.

Explanation of the Genesis of the Characteristic Phenomena, found in the Visual Fields in Chronic Glaucoma

We have reached a stage in our study of the subject, when we naturally pause to ask ourselves, what are the anatomical, physiological, and pathological factors which underlie and determine the characteristic features of the visual fields in glaucoma. Unfortunately the information at our disposal is neither so abundant nor so accurate as we could desire. The field opened up for original research is both fruitful and immense, although much spade-work will have to be done before we can hope to reach accurate conclusions. The student of ophthalmology, who is looking out for lines on which to conduct research, will find all he needs here. The work will repay his toil, and should lead to definite results; it does not demand an elaborate outfit, and it calls for little save the expenditure of time, care, and patience. For the present, we must be content to review the facts in our possession, and to advance as far as they permit us to do. In so doing, we are confronted with two questions of outstanding interest:

1. What are the lesions, which produce the various field defects we have been discussing ? and

2. Why do their results vary so widely in different cases ?

We shall take these subjects in turn :

(1) **The lesions responsible for the field defects in chronic glaucoma.**—The suggestions under this heading have been numerous, and have varied considerably in value. We shall endeavour to classify and discuss them :

I. *Those which are referable to the area of the cupped disc or to its edge.*

A. Mechanical injury to the nerve fibres,

(i.) by pressure against the sharp edge of the unyielding margin of the foramen scleræ ;

(ii.) by overstretching of the fibres in the segment of the nerve affected by the glaucomatous cupping, in order that they may take up the new positions which they are forced to assume in the cup ; and

(iii.) by the trauma inflicted as a result of the increased pulsation in the vessels commonly associated with a rise in intra-ocular pressure.

This last suggestion, despite the authority from which it emanates, appears fantastic. Apart from this there is another strong objection to it. The vessels lie mainly in the nasal half of the disc, whose fibres are represented on the temporal side of the field, and this is precisely the area in which defects usually appear least and latest.

B. Localised inflammatory action involving the nerve (Roenne). The author is unaware that such a suggestion has any support from anatomical findings.

C. Pressure on the nerve fibres due to the local extravasation of fluid. This possibility would appear to receive some support from the recent work by Fuchs, which has already been discussed.

D. Interference with the central retinal vessels, as they lie within the nerve-head, or on the surface of the disc,

(i.) due to kinking, as the result of the double-bend imposed on each of them by its altered course round the walls of the cupped disc ;

(ii.) due to the increase of the intra-ocular pressure, which (*a*) cuts down the supply of arterial blood to the retina, and (*b*) impedes the normal escape of venous blood from it ; and

(iii.) due to actual injuries sustained by the vessels, as a result, in one way or another, of the increased pressure present. Here again the objection holds that there is no evidence of the existence of such injuries, and we may therefore throw out an idea founded on so doubtful an hypothesis.

We come next to

II. *Those factors which come into operation outside the area of the disc :*

A. Compression of the retina itself (in all its layers), under the increased pressure of the intra-ocular contents against the unyielding scleral coat ;

B. Compression of the vessels, which nourish the retina, throughout their course against that coat. It is obvious that this will act more powerfully on the veins and capillaries than on the arteries, and that it will probably be most felt by those of them which are situated most peripherally ; this fact deserves to be very carefully borne in mind. The above remarks apply with equal force to the branches of the retinal and chorio-capillary circulatory systems. The result of pressure will be that the retinal tissues will suffer from a deficiency in the supply of arterial blood and a difficulty in the removal of waste products. It matters little, from the point of view of our present argument, whether these vessels are for the nourishment of the retinal elements themselves, or of the conducting nerve-fibres. In either case, their functional activity will in the first instance be damaged, owing to defective nutrition, whilst later on degenerative changes will supervene.

C. Obstruction of the retinal lymph circulation. Edridge Green has maintained that throughout life there is an intermittent, but frequently repeated flow of fluid from the periphery of the retina to the optic nerve neighbourhood. This fluid is presumed to be secreted by the chorio-capillary circulation, and to traverse the space between the retina and its pigment layer. The fact that this space corresponds to the remains of the cavity of the primary optic vesicle makes it possible, if not probable, that such a circulation of lymph may take place in it. According to Green, it bathes the free extremities of the rods and cones, and obtains from the former the photo-chemical substance, which we speak of as visual purple, and on which, as he maintains, the cones depend for their functional activity. It is stated that any factor which unfavourably influences the production of the visual purple, acts deleteriously on the patient's light sense. An increase of intra-ocular pressure is such a factor, and, if we were to presume that Green is correct, it would not be difficult to see how it might act ; for, both by obstructing the outflow in the neighbourhood of the optic nerve, and also by tending to close the space, throughout its whole area, it would slow down the flow of photo-chemical fluid, and so impair the activity of the percipient elements, and reduce the strength of normal stimulations of the retinal elements to a subnormal level. It must be admitted that, in the present state of our knowledge, the above reasoning can only be accepted with reservation and caution.

(2) **The wide variations found in the visual fields of different glaucomatous patients.**—The factors which determine these variations are :

I. The form of glaucoma present.

II. The period of the disease at which the examination is made.

III. The entry into the individual case of the various factors which determine the exact lesion present ; these factors have been indicated in answering our previous question.

IV. The presence of anatomical variations (a) in the supporting framework of the optic nerve-head ; (b) in the way in which the nerve-fibre bundles are arranged as they leave the disc ; and (c) in the support which those bundles receive from the sheaths of the vessels which accompany them. Of these three factors, by far the most important is the first ; it has already been discussed at some length in our earlier pages The remaining two are much more hypothetical.

I. *The form of glaucoma present.*—In all forms of glaucoma the visual functions are profoundly disturbed, but the exact nature of the disturbance varies greatly according to the clinical type of the affection. Thus, it has been stated that an attack of glaucoma fulminans may within a few hours produce absolute and permanent blindness and

THE DIAGNOSIS OF GLAUCOMA 299

that, following such an attack, not a vestige of sight may remain whether central or peripheral. Again, an acute attack of glaucoma of much less severity than the preceding may very greatly reduce both central and peripheral vision, though, under favourable circumstances, a very large measure of recovery will take place, if the increase of pressure is not maintained for too long a period. A similar result is said to be obtained by exerting firm and continuous digital pressure on the eyeball; it is alleged that, as a result of such pressure, the functions of the retina are found to be temporarily abrogated. It may be questioned whether this is altogether a safe experiment to make.

We are probably justified in assuming that in acute and subacute glaucoma, the general blurring of the perimetric picture is due to interference with the vascular and lymphatic circulations, and possibly also to mechanical injury to the retina, and especially to its ganglionic and terminal elements.

In chronic glaucoma we find a widely different state of affairs. The central vision may for a long time remain little if at all affected, whilst, as has already been pointed out, the following phenomena are observed:

(a) A steady concentric contraction of the whole field of vision;

(b) a characteristic early restriction of the nasal portion of the field;

(c) Roenne's step;

(d) the appearance of paracentral scotomata; and at a late period

(e) the invasion of the central area of the retina by scotomatous defects.

II. It is obvious that *the period of the disease* at which the examination is made must exercise a very great influence on the perimetric findings. The student of the subject will better appreciate this point, if he will carefully study the charts of the visual fields which have been reproduced in the previous part of this chapter from the works of Bjerrum, Roenne and others.

With regard to our headings (III.) and (IV.), it has been

decided, after careful consideration, that it will make for clearness in the conception of our subject, if, instead of pursuing it by discussing those headings at length, we turn to consider in detail the phenomena we have just named. Our object in doing so will be to seek the nature of the lesion which accounts for each of them, and to endeavour to evolve some semblance of order from the many conflicting data before us.

The Characteristic Concentric Contraction of the Visual Field in Chronic Glaucoma

(1) **Anatomical considerations.**—In endeavouring to explain this phenomenon we must first seek to get at certain anatomical facts, the consideration of which has been deliberately left over to the present occasion: The fibres of the optic nerve expand to form the retina by an anatomical arrangement, which may be compared to the stem and bowl of a wine-glass. The stem represents the nerve, the bowl the expanded retina ; the latter is thickest near the nerve and gradually thins, so far as its nerve layer is concerned, as we pass forward. The obvious reason for this thinning is that nerve fibres are constantly being dropped to form connections with the corresponding retinal elements. It could not fail to be of great interest, if we could lay claim to have such a knowledge of the anatomical distribution of the fibres of the optic nerve to definite areas of the retina, as would furnish a reliable explanation of the type of retraction of the visual field commonly met with in glaucoma. Would such a claim be justified by facts ?

Fuchs states dogmatically that "those fibres which come from the peripheral portions of the retina lie in the centre of the optic nerve, while those which rise from the central regions of the retina lie along the margin of the nerve." Gradle takes the same view. If we were to found our arguments on the doctrine of probabilities (possibly a dangerous thing to do), the arrangement above described would be that which we should expect to find, for it would seem unreasonable that each successive ring of nerve fibres, as it drops to make a communication with its appropriate circle of retinal elements, should have to find its way through a maximum thickness of those nerve fibres, which are passing on to a more peripheral destination. It would appear more natural that the fibres, dropped for each successive circle, should be those which have just been uncovered by the passage outward to their nerve elements of those other fibres, which immediately covered them up to that point. This is illustrated by Fig. 101. Writing on this subject Berry says: "There is much to be said, too, in favour of Bunge's views as to the position in the nerve of the fibres passing to other parts of the retina, viz., that the more centrally situated fibres supply the more peripheral portions of the retina."

Collins and Mayou on the other hand, write as follows: "The nerve fibres destined for the periphery of the retina, which lie on the outer portion of the optic nerve, are more liable to be exposed to pressure against the sclerotic as they enter the eye than those destined for the central region." They go on to say that this "explains the manner in which vision fails in glaucomatous cases, in which the process begins at the periphery of the retina, thus producing a contraction of the field of vision."

We are thus confronted with two opposite statements of the existing anatomical conditions. At first sight the explanation offered by Collins and Mayou appears very attractive, especially if we examine a section of a glaucomatous cup under the microscope, and observe the sharply projecting scleral edge seen on each side of such a specimen. Unfortunately, however, it is difficult to accept it, ingenious and attractive as it appears, for it seems certain that the view adopted by Fuchs is the right one. We are therefore driven to ask what is the element in the case which favours a lesion of those fibres of the optic nerve, which lie at its centre as compared with those at its periphery. The subject is one of considerable difficulty, but an answer is suggested by a careful examination of specimens of deeply cupped nerve-heads, such as the one

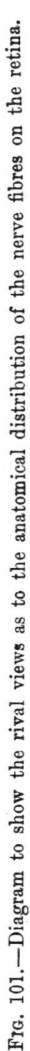

FIG. 101.—Diagram to show the rival views as to the anatomical distribution of the nerve fibres on the retina.

For the sake of clearness it is made extremely diagrammatic. The optic nerve is seen entering through the sclera, which latter is marked in heavy black. Next to the sclera are shown the retinal elements, and then the nerve-fibre layer of the retina. All other parts are omitted. To the left is shown the distribution of the nerve fibres according to Fuchs. It will be observed that those fibres which come from the peripheral portion of the retina lie in the centre of the optic nerve, whilst those which rise from the central regions of the retina lie along the margin of the nerve. To the right we see the distribution according to Collins and Mayou. Here the nerve fibres from the periphery lie on the outer side of the nerve, whilst those from the peripapillary region lie at its centre. It will be observed that, under such an arrangement, each fibre, as it sinks to its retinal element, has to traverse a maximum thickness of the nerve-fibre layer of the retina. Such an arrangement would *a priori* be most unlikely.

depicted in Fig. 31. It seems clear that the fibres which originally passed down close to the centre of the papilla must have undergone considerably more stretching in order to occupy their new position than did those, which from the first ran in their natural course along the shelving side of the scleral foramen (Fig. 5). The former are profoundly displaced, whilst the latter are scarcely so at all. If then we may argue that the nearer the fibres are to the axis of the nerve, the more liable they are to overstretching, whilst the nearer they are to the periphery, the less they are stretched, we find one possible explanation at least of the concentric contraction of the visual field which is so typical of glaucoma ; for the central fibres in the optic nerve-head would be damaged earliest and most profoundly whilst the peripheral ones would escape the longest.

It was Roenne who first pointed out that what appears, under large-object perimetry, as a mere sloping defect in the visual field, stands revealed by Bjerrum's method as a well-marked step, and therefore as the result of a lesion of the nerve bundles on the disc or at its edge. Many of the contractions of the visual field, with which we are familiar when using the ordinary method of perimetry, are therefore to be ascribed to such nerve bundle lesions, either at the upper part of the disc, or at the lower part, or at both. We have already alluded to this in the preceding part of this chapter. Important as these considerations are, there are two other factors in the case which must not be overlooked, and which now demand our attention. We shall take them in turn.

(2) **An interference with the retino-choroidal circulation.**—It is commonly argued that since the vascular pressure is lowest at the periphery of the retina, the nutritional supply to that area will fail first under the adverse influence of an increase in the intra-ocular pressure. This statement has been made as though it furnished a complete explanation of the shrinkage of the glaucoma field from without toward the centre. It is, however, to be remembered that in other conditions in which pressure is absent, *e.g.*, in

optic atrophy, the same phenomenon (concentric contraction) presents itself. Furthermore, in retinitis pigmentosa, the changes begin, not at the extreme limit of the visual field, but as an annular scotoma lying within a peripheral circle of field, which obviously corresponds with a belt of still actively functional retina. It has been suggested that this phenomenon indicates that the area of lowest nutritional activity lies, *not* at the ora serrata, but in the neighbourhood of the equator. In this instance (retinitis pigmentosa), there is no question of a rise in intra-ocular pressure ; it is, therefore, significant that cases are on record in which the performance of sclero-corneal trephining has improved and extended the shrunken visual field. The obvious explanation is that the operative lowering of the intra-ocular pressure increases the vascular supply of the periphery of the retina, and thereby improves its nutrition. This observation casts a sidelight on the subject we are discussing. It must, however, be admitted that the whole question is veiled in difficulty and uncertainty. We would, nevertheless, seem to be justified in supposing that any factor, which interferes (as increase of pressure undoubtedly does) with the freedom of the ocular circulation, will at least help to cause a shrinkage of the field from without inwards. In the early stages nutrition will be impaired ; later, if the unfavourable conditions continue to prevail, the onset of atrophy will be favoured. It must be obvious that if there is an injury to the nerve fibres of the retina, such as we believe is often, if not always, present in glaucoma, any factor which damages the nutrition of those fibres, or of the terminal elements and ganglion cells which are connected with them, must exaggerate the effect of the adverse influences present. It is the story of an army which, while it is attacked from in front, has its communications interfered with behind the fighting line. Such interference will not directly cause a defeat of the soldiery, but it will intensify the weight of the hostile blows, and aggravate the misfortunes of the troops attacked.

(3) **Injury to, and consequent degeneration of the terminal elements and ganglion cells of the retina.**—It

THE DIAGNOSIS OF GLAUCOMA

has been pointed out in the previous paragraph how circulatory disturbances affect these important structures. Altogether apart from this, however, there is another element present, viz., that of direct trauma, for these delicate parts are exposed over long periods to the crushing weight of an increase in the intra-ocular pressure, and the results of this influence are to be seen in degeneration of the ganglion cells, and in both degeneration and displacement (squashing down laterally) of the rods and cones. We know that, even under favourable circumstances, the percipient elements are more active towards the centre of the retina than towards the periphery. We also know that the cones become fewer and more primitive as we pass out from the fovea towards the ora serrata ; indeed, Green states that they are fifteen times as large in the former area as they are in the latter. Whether a receiving instrument be mechanical or vital, its power of transmitting an impulse depends not merely on the intensity of the stimulation it receives, but also on its own power of receptivity. If we take a number of instruments of the same kind, all of which can transmit a stimulus of a certain intensity, and if we reduce the sensitiveness of all alike by a definite ratio, the messages will drop out first from those instruments which were originally least sensitive. But there is another way in which the feebler messages may be cut out, viz., by increasing the resistance of the fibres which carry them. Such an increase must occur in glaucoma, when the nerve bundles are injured on the disc or at its edge. Moreover, the resistance to the passage of a message along a fibre increases with the length of that fibre, even under normal conditions, and probably still more so under abnormal ones. There is thus every reason, looking at the question from the electrical point of view, for the failure of the peripheral field at an earlier date than the central.

We have, then, to take into account (1) the original sensitivity of the percipient elements, which varies according to their position on the retina ; (2) the damage those elements have sustained, whether by reason of nutritional changes, which are due to alterations in their circulation, or by direct trauma, such as may follow an increase of intra-ocular pressure ; and (3) the interference with the conductivity of the nerve fibres concerned, as a result of injury or of impairment of their nutrition.

It might have been thought that a careful study of the morbid phenomena, which accompany an attack of simple glaucoma, would yield indications whereby we might be able to form an opinion as to the relative influence of the various factors we have been discussing. The early interference with the light sense, the late retention of perception of colours in the visual field, and the peculiar vagaries in the shapes of the field in different cases, all seem features of promise. It must, however, be confessed that an analysis of the evidence is both disappointing and conflicting. Speaking broadly, however, we may say this much : The great underlying factor in chronic glaucoma is an interference with the nerve bundles, either on the optic disc or as they emerge from it. Other factors are probably only contributory. The various shapes of fields we meet with are we think to be explained by differences in the anatomical arrangements, which attend the passage of the optic nerve through the scleral foramen. This subject will be again referred to shortly, when we come to speak of those phenomena (*e.g.*, Bjerrum's sign), which are unquestionably and wholly due to an interference with definite bundles of nerves.

The condition we have been discussing differs very widely from that which we meet with in acute cases, where the crushing out of all vision, both central and peripheral, not merely betokens a profound interference with the circulation of the eye—an interference so great that it may actually bring about complete stasis—but probably also indicates a severe mechanical crushing of those delicate and important structures (especially the terminal elements and the ganglion cells), on the integrity of which the perception and conduction of the visual impulses depend.

At the same time, we must remember that very few cases, if any, of glaucoma are absolutely innocent of a congestive element throughout their course. Such an element may be in abeyance over long periods, and may be but feebly marked, in which case the field phenomena are practically those of the simple condition. On the other hand, there are not a few cases which some surgeons will pass as simple, which they would regard with an element of suspicion if they made a practice of testing the ocular tension at different times of the day and night. It would come to many of them as a surprise under these circumstances to find the rise that sometimes follows sleep. It has already been pointed out that such a rise is easily explained by the absence during sleeping hours of the muscular pump-action described by Arthur Thomson. The result is an accumulation of an excess of fluid within the eye, and a consequent rise in intra-ocular pressure. That such a rise must be attended by some obstruction to the escape of blood from the eye is practically certain. Here we have the shadow of congestive glaucoma thrown across the picture. Who shall say how great the cumulative effect of such a factor may in time become ? The author believes that it is written on many fields of vision plain for the discriminating observer to read.

The Restriction of the Nasal Portion of the Field of Vision in Chronic Glaucoma

The next question for which we seek an answer in anatomical and pathological facts is : **Why is the nasal portion of the visual field commonly affected earlier than the temporal in cases of chronic glaucoma ?** The usually accepted explanation is that, inasmuch as the optic papilla is situate to the inner side of the macula lutea (which latter is the centre of vision, and which lies in the visual axis of the eye), the fibres passing on to the temporal side have a longer course to pursue than those passing to the nasal ; the extremities of the former are consequently more peripheral than those of the latter, the blood-pressure in their vessels is therefore lower, and the resistance these offer to an increase of intra-ocular pressure is correspondingly less. And since it is the fibres of the

GLAUCOMA

temporal side of the eye which are connected with the nasal field of vision, and *vice versa*, it is the nasal field which is first affected under the pressure of glaucoma.

This argument is so patently unsound, that the wonder is, not merely that it has endured so long, but that it was ever entertained for a moment. Let us consider the question : In correspondence with the configuration of the face, the nasal field of vision only reaches out to the

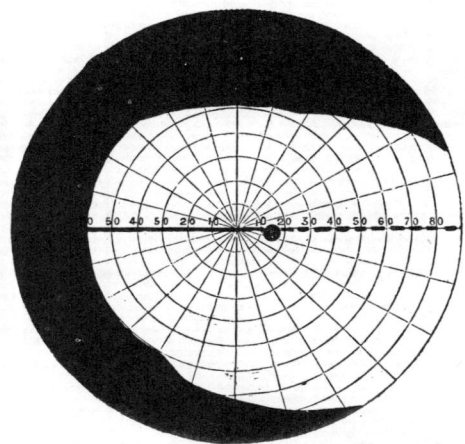

FIG. 102.—Diagrammatic representation of field of vision to be studied in connection with the schematic section of right eye.

The lengths of field, marked in strong and broken lines respectively, correspond to the distribution of the nerve fibres on the temporal and nasal sides of the optic disc, and therefore also to the length of retinal vessel on the temporal and nasal sides of the point of emergence of the vasa centralia retinæ. Compare with Fig. 103.

60° limit, from the fixation point ; whereas the temporal field passes out to the 90° circle (Fig. 102). The centre of the blind spot lies 15° to the outer side of the fixation point (which latter corresponds on the perimeter chart to the position of the centre of the macula lutea on the retina), and therefore 75° (blind spot to centre = 15° + centre to nasal limit of field = 60° ; total = 75°) from the nasal limit of the field. It likewise lies about the same distance, *i.e.*, 75°, from the temporal boundary of the field

THE DIAGNOSIS OF GLAUCOMA 309

(from centre of vision to temporal limit of field = 90°, minus distance from blind spot to centre, represented by 15° = 75°). The assumption that a measurement of degrees

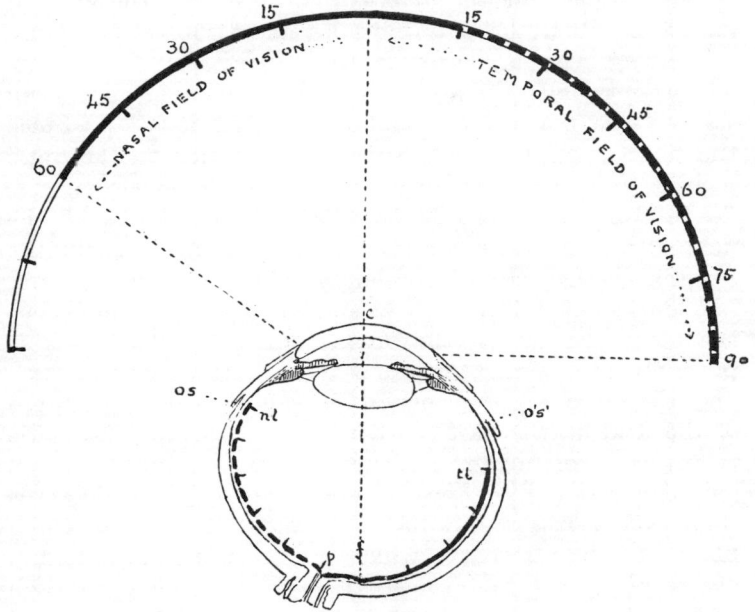

Fig. 103.—Schematic section of right eye, in horizontal plane.

p, papilla ; *f*, fovea ; *tl*, most anterior part of temporal retina, corresponding to the nasal limit of the visual field ; *nl*, most anterior part of nasal retina corresponding to the temporal limit of the visual field ; *os* and *o′s′*, ora serrata. From *p* to *f* comprises an area corresponding to 15° on the visual field. Note that this area is on the nasal side of the visual axis *cf* ; it is therefore represented on the temporal side of a chart of the field, of which it furnishes the medial segment. For diagrammatic purposes, the remainder of the retina has been divided up into areas, each of which corresponds to 15° on a chart. It will be observed that from *p* to *nl* there are five of these divisions, representing therefore 75°, whilst from *p* to *tl* the distance is exactly the same. The blood-pressure in the terminal arteries at *nl* and *tl*, must therefore be the same; whilst that in the vessels at *o′s′*, on the temporal side, will obviously be lower than that at *cs*, on the nasal side. The retina on the nasal side of the papilla is marked by a broken line, as is also that part of the field which corresponds to it ; whilst the retina on the temporal side of the papilla and its corresponding field are shown by a thick continuous line. The blind spot is situate at the point where the broken and continuous lines meet on the field of vision.

along the perimetric field can be interpreted as distances on the retina is sufficiently accurate for our present purposes. Also, what applies to the retinal vessels can be equally argued for the arteries which supply the choroid (and through it the outermost layers of the retina), since the ciliary vessels perforate the scleral coat in a ring, which surrounds the optic nerve. From what has been said we may now make the following deductions : (1) Since the blind spot (Fig. 103) (which corresponds to the optic papilla, from the centre of which the retinal vessels emerge) lies midway between the two lateral boundaries of the field of vision, there can be no serious difference in the lengths of the arterial trunks supplying the two lateral boundaries of the field ; (2) under these circumstances the blood-pressure of the vessels supplying the retina is probably practically the same at both these boundaries ; and therefore (3) the current explanation of the failure of the field on the nasal earlier than on the temporal side is unworthy of further credence, and must be abandoned. One suggestion has, however, been made which deserves some consideration. It has been pointed out that those fibres of the optic nerve which pass to the nasal side, fan out regularly and take the shortest possible course to reach their destinations ; whilst those which pass to the temporal side (and which correspond in function with the nasal half of the visual field), have to curve round the papillo-macular area on the way to their distribution. The suggestion made is that, in consequence of this deflection from what would have been their course had it not been for the intervention of the papillo-macular bundle, the length of the nerve fibres, and consequently of their accompanying vessels must be materially increased. To this the reply may be made : (1) That the size of the papillo-macular area is relatively small, and that all things considered it is unlikely that this factor is very important ; (2) that the retinal vessels are very far from slavishly following the course of the nerves ; and (3) that the choroidal circulation is independent of the anatomical arrangements of the nerve fibres.

In criticism of what has been written above, the following argument may be put forward : (*a*) The temporal branches of the retinal vessels are decidedly larger than the nasal ; (*b*) this points to their having a longer course, and argues that the peripheral extremities of their capillary circulation are farther removed from the optic papilla than are those of the nasal vessels ; (*c*) the above points being granted, it may be assumed that the blood-pressure in the vessels at the temporal extremity of the retina must be lower than that at the nasal extremity. This is probably correct ; indeed, it seems to be a logical consequence of the fact that the optic papilla, which is the emergence point of the retinal vessels, lies internal to the retinal centre of vision. If Fig. 103 be referred to, this point will be made clear ; it simply means that the distance p.os. (from the optic papilla to the nasal ora serrata) is less than the distance p.o's'. (from the optic papilla to the temporal ora serrata). It has, however, no bearing on the point at issue. What really interests us just now is a comparison between the distances, p.nl. and p.tl., *i.e.*, the distances from the optic papilla to the nasal and temporal boundaries of the *actively functional* retina. That area of retina, which lies beyond the point tl., has nothing to do with the visual field as we know and map it. Our concern is with those areas of retina *which correspond to the boundaries of the visual field on our charts*, and we are interested in the blood-pressures at these extreme limits but not outside them.

Another, but widely different suggestion, which has been made is that inasmuch as the temporal branches of the retinal artery are larger than the nasal ones, the blood-pressure in the former should be higher than that in the latter, if comparisons are made at equal distances from the point of bifurcation of the main trunk. The argument *taken for what it is worth*, tells against the currently accepted theory we are discussing ; for the presence of a higher blood-pressure in the temporal vessels would be all in favour of a later, rather than of an earlier loss of the nasal side of the visual field.

Examined in the cold light of anatomical facts, the

currently accepted explanation of the early failure of the nasal field in chronic glaucoma breaks down hopelessly, as we have already said ; nor does an examination of the question from a pathological standpoint yield it any support ; for how are we to explain the following unquestionable facts ?—(1) It is not always necessarily the strictly nasal field which goes first, it may be the upper nasal field, or it may be the lower nasal field, or, though much more rarely, it may be the temporal field ; (2) one may sometimes see the nasal field, not only first affected but practically wiped out, almost if not quite up to the fixation point, whilst a large, and even a very large, temporal field still remains. It must be quite obvious that in such a case the relative lengths of the blood vessels supplying the two areas cannot be the determining factor.

Having failed to find the explanation of the early shrinkage of the nasal portion of the field, or of the later concentric contraction of its boundaries, in the circulatory theory, we turn to consider what can be said in favour of the phenomena being due to trauma inflicted on the nerves in the glaucoma cup, or at its edge.

In speaking of Roenne's step, we have shown that the curtailment of the nasal portion of the field, or of the upper or lower nasal portions, or indeed of any other part thereof, may be easily explained by a reference to the method of distribution of the fibres of the optic nerve to the retina. So far as the anatomical possibilities of the case are concerned, we are on firm ground here ; but it is when we seek to explain why certain masses of nerve fibres should be affected earlier than others, that our difficulties begin. It has been shown that the fibres which pass out to the greater portion of the temporal side of the retina (*i.e.*, exclusive of the macular area), lie in the supero-temporal and infero-temporal bundles, each of which occupies about one-twelfth of the circumference of the optic disc (Figs. 51 and 52). Now, it is these very fibres which are most prone to be damaged in chronic glaucoma. Can we find any anatomical reason why this should be so ?

It has been pointed out that there is reason to believe

THE DIAGNOSIS OF GLAUCOMA 313

that stretching of the fibres would fall most severely on those which are most central in the nerve, and would thus attack the peripheral area of supply of the retina sooner than the central ; but this is not all. It is a familiar observation that the area of greatest contraction of the visual field can often be correlated with the site of the maximum cupping of the optic disc. Where the cup is most overhanging, one finds that the field corresponding to the fibres of that part is most damaged. On the other hand, where there is no preponderance of local cupping, the shrinkage of the field tends to be concentric ; this is especially seen in the pathologic cupping of a disc, which has from birth shown deep central physiologic cupping. It has also been stated (Dr. Alan Greenwood) that in those cases in which the vessels lie on the temporal, instead of on the nasal side of the disc, the shrinkage observed from chronic glaucoma is on the temporal instead of on the nasal side of the field. The suggestion is that the vessels, or the connective tissue which supports them, lend an element of resistance to the nasal half of the disc through which they usually emerge, and so protect the surrounding nerve fibres from excessive stretching, with the result that the corresponding temporal field is spared. To test this point, the author has examined a number of sections of cupped optic discs, and the evidence so obtained has seemed to support the view that the vessels and their surrounding connective tissue, oppose an obstacle to the displacement of the nerves in their neighbourhood, as compared with that of those at the opposite side of the disc, which are not similarly supported. Attractive as such an hypothesis is, it cannot be adopted without further investigation. There is one difficulty in accepting it, viz., that the bundle for the macular area, which lies between the two bundles (supero-temporal and infero-temporal) which we are now discussing, appears to escape injury up to a very late stage in the disease. This certainly cannot be a question of support derived from the vessels.

There is another solution of the difficulty, which was suggested with some diffidence in the first edition of this work, and which has received important anatomical confirmation from the recent work by Fuchs, dealt with on pp. 14 to 17 and 198 of the present book. It is that the supporting framework of the optic nerve-head varies greatly in different eyes, and that this determines to a very great extent the area over which yielding takes place earliest and most extensively. The obvious inference is that those nerve-fibre bundles will be most damaged which lie in the neighbourhood of the greatest yielding and *vice versa*. This explanation would appear to be the most mechanical, the simplest, and the most satisfying of all those which have hitherto been offered. It may, however, be open to question whether it covers the whole ground. On that subject it would indeed be rash to dogmatise.

The Consideration of a few Remaining Points

There are still a few points, which deserve further consideration in connection with those phenomena (Roenne's step, and Seidel's, Bjerrum's, and the author's signs), which are admittedly due to damage to the bundles of nerve fibres on the disc or at its edge. A number of questions arise to which it is quite certain that we cannot return dogmatic answers. In one form or another they have cropped up at intervals in the preceding pages, and have there been dealt with as far as circumstances have permitted. We return to them now simply with a desire to avoid leaving more ragged edges to the discussion than we can help, and we ask ourselves :

1. Why should the bundles of fibres which immediately adjoin the area of central vision be the first to be attacked ?

2. Why should these nerve-bundle-injury phenomena start, as in the majority of instances they undoubtedly do, in the neighbourhood of the disc, and work outwards ?

3. Why, again, should one sometimes find that the scotomata in question begin far away from the blind spot (even at the horizontal raphé where the fibres end), and later work their way into it ?

4. How are we to explain the undoubted fact that,

whereas central scotomata are rare in chronic glaucoma, they may not only occur comparatively early in the disease, but may definitely affect either the upper or the lower half of the central field, thus proving that the phenomenon is a result of definite nerve-bundle injury, and not of general pressure or interference with the circulatory mechanism ?

(1) The selection of the bundles, which immediately adjoin the macular area of the retina, for early injury presents us with a very knotty problem. The anatomical features of the question have already been discussed, and we have also pointed out the objections to the suggestion, that certain fibres are longer spared because of the support they receive from the connective tissue surrounding the retinal vessels. There remains the presumption that the cause of the lesion is a mechanical one, which is most intense at the spot where the particular fasciculus concerned in Bjerrum's scotoma crosses the disc or emerges from its border. If we accept this as the true explanation, we must likewise apply it in our search for an answer to certain other mysterious phenomena. We have often asked ourselves : Why should the arcuate scotoma of Bjerrum lie sometimes above the area of central vision, sometimes below it, and sometimes in both positions at once ? Why again should a field defect, which begins as a very indefinite scotoma spread and spread till at first a large area and later the whole of the visual field is involved and finally blotted out ? Why should the quadrant first affected and the progress of the defect vary from case to case ? As has already been indicated, the most hopeful answer would seem to be that the lesion to the nerve-fibre bundles, as they fan out to their distribution on the retina, is determined by an anatomical and variable factor, connected with the yielding of the lamina cribrosa under pressure. Where there is most yielding there will be most lesion, and *vice versa*. The area which yields first is likely to be that which will yield most quickly and most severely, whilst the converse will apply to the parts that in the early stage proved most resistant. The varying nature, strength, and arrangement of the connective tissue lamellæ and

bundles which build up the supporting framework of the optic nerve-head, supply the key to the mystery of the very variable symptomatology of glaucoma. That, at least, is the author's view.

(2) With regard to our second question asked above: The fact that, as a rule, the scotoma begins from the upper or lower edge of the disc and works peripherally away from it (as we showed it does, when we were dealing with Seidel's sign) would appear to indicate that it is the nerve fibres, which are connected with the retinal elements lying in the near neighbourhood of the disc, that are first affected. If the reader will turn back to what has been said on this subject on p. 301, he will find that we there accepted Fuchs' view that those fibres " which rise from the central regions of the retina, lie along the (peripheral) margin of the nerve." It will be remembered that Collins and Mayou suggested that the peripheral nerve fibres are " more liable to be exposed to pressure against the sclerotic as they enter the eye, than are those " which lie at the centre of the nerve. Whilst there is a strong reason, which we have already given, against accepting their ingenious suggestion as an explanation of the concentric contraction of the visual field, there would seem to be valid grounds for adopting it to interpret the cause of the phenomenon we are now discussing.

(3) What then is the meaning of the scotomata, which begin at a distance from the blind spot and work back to it ? We have already suggested the possibility that this aberration from what is usually found has its cause in an abnormal peculiarity in the distribution of the nerve fibres affected, whereby those which pass out to become connected with nerve elements at some little distance from the disc, are situate more peripherally in the nerve-head than are those which supply the parts in the immediate peripapillary area. It must be confessed that this is little more than a guess. No one who will carefully examine a section of a deeply cupped optic nerve, such as is depicted in Fig. 31, can fail to be struck with the sharp edge presented to the nerve fibres by the inner border of the scleral ring. It is to be remembered that

THE DIAGNOSIS OF GLAUCOMA

under the conditions of high tension prevailing in the eye, such a ring would present considerable rigidity. Its possibilities for the infliction of injury on the delicate structures which curl over it, are too obvious to need further comment.

(4) Lastly with regard to central scotomata as met with in chronic glaucoma, we need only point out that the manner in which a part of, or even a complete half of the central field may be wiped out, whilst the rest of the area remains as functional as ever, points clearly to the phenomenon being a result of an injury to definite nerve bundles, and not a consequence of general pressure or of interference with the circulatory mechanism ; for in the latter case, the whole central field would be damaged simultaneously, as it is in attacks of acute glaucoma.

There are large gaps in our knowledge, and we must wait for further data before we can attempt to fill them in. It would be unscientific to adopt any other course.

REFERENCES

BERRY, SIR G.—*Textbook of Ophthalmology.*
COLLINS, E. T. AND MAYOU, M. S.—*System of Ophthalmic Practice,* "Pathology," Rebman Ltd., London, 1911, p. 226.
FUCHS, E.—*Archiv f. O.*, 1916, vol. xci. part iii.
GRADLE, H. S.—*Ann. Ophth.*, Oct. 1915, p. 641.
ROENNE, H.—*Archiv f. O.*, 1909, vol. lxxi. p. 52.

PART VI

The Diagnosis of Glaucoma (*continued*)

SUMMARY :—Tonometry.
        The Schiötz Tonometer and its Modifications.
        The Limitations in the Clinical Usefulness of Tonometry.
        Method of using a Tonometer.
        The Schiötz Tonometer Readings.
        The McLean Tonometer Readings.
    The Examination of the Light Sense in Glaucoma.

TONOMETRY.

Ophthalmic surgeons have long been profoundly dissatisfied with the results of digital tonometry ; this has been clearly shown by the large number of efforts which have been made to devise a satisfactory instrument wherewith to estimate the ocular tension. The finger-tip method is but a rough and ready means towards the attainment of our purpose. Apart from the fact that it is both inaccurate and uncertain, it has the great disadvantage that the observer is apt to be biased in his estimate of the condition present by his personal hopes and fears.

For many years past surgeons have desired to obtain, and have striven to construct a mechanical appliance which should be sensitive to small changes in pressure, and accurate in recording them, whilst, at the same time eliminating all elements of personal prejudice from the records obtained. In so doing, they have devised instruments working on two distinct principles, (1) that of applanation, and (2) that of impression. The Maklakoff instrument is an example of the former class ; it recorded the amount of flattening undergone by various eyeballs under the influence of a known pressure, viz., that of the weight of the instrument, and was a distinct advance on anything that had preceded it, but it suffered from the great disadvantage that it was only capable of giving a very limited number of different readings, and that its accuracy left a good deal to be desired. The impression tonometer works on a different principle ; its object is to furnish a record of the amount of indentation or dimpling which a given eye undergoes under the influence of a known pressure, mechanically applied by the instrument (Fig. 104). This principle has appealed to a large number of workers, but the mechanical difficulties have been so great that model after model failed to command the confidence of ophthalmologists, until, in 1910, Professor Schiötz introduced the tonometer, which has so justly made his name famous. Other modifications of this instrument have since appeared, and some of these will be dealt with presently, but nothing that has been done or that ever will be done, can dim the lustre of Schiötz's great achievement. No paper on glaucoma that ignores modern scientific tonometry is in the least likely to command respectful attention either now or in the future. The time is long past when to possess and to use a Schiötz tonometer was a mark of originality or peculiarity, or when the merits and demerits of mechanical tonometry could be seriously discussed. After years of long waiting, the Schiötz tonometer has come into its own, and there must be very few ophthalmic surgeons who do not possess one, who do not employ it constantly, and who have not formed very definite ideas

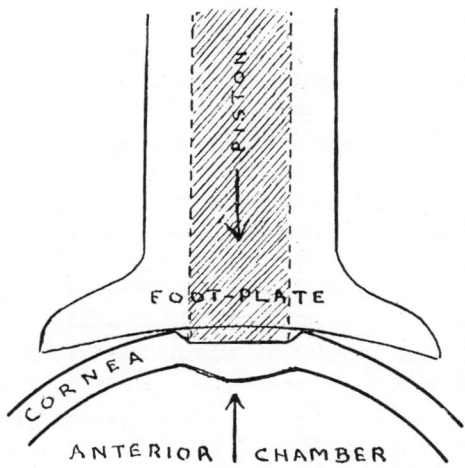

Fig. 104.—To explain the principle of the Schiötz tonometer. A section showing the depression of the cornea under the influence of a fixed weight. (Morax.)

as to its value. The student of to-day is trained in its use, just as naturally as he is in that of the thermometer or of the binaural stethoscope. If he is not, he certainly should be. These remarks in no way imply a criticism of those who would discuss the limitations of the modern tonometer, and the varying value of its records in different cases. What they do imply, and what the author believes all scientific workers will accept, is that the tonometer has come to stay, and to form an essential part of the ophthalmologist's equipment for his daily work.

GLAUCOMA

The Schiötz Tonometer.—The original model of this instrument is shown in Fig. 105A. The footplate, *f*, rests on the eye, whilst the rod, *a*, carrying the weight, *l*, dimples the eyeball by virtue of the pressure it exerts. The harder the ball, the less the dimpling, and *vice versa*; the amount of the dimpling is transmitted to the lever and shown on the scale. By means of a graph or table the readings so obtained can be translated *approximately* into intra-ocular pressure in mm. of Hg. Valuable as this instrument unquestionably is, it has certain mechanical disadvantages which have led other observers to endeavour to modify it. Most marked of these has been the difficulty—not a very serious one, but still somewhat annoying — in changing the various weights attached to the rod when measuring different degrees of hardness of the eye. To remedy this, Gradle devised an instrument (Fig. 106) whereby the weight could be altered by merely dropping flat metal discs over a stylet. There were other small mechanical alterations, which Gradle considered made the instrument easier to use. There can be no question that many ophthalmologists welcomed an easy method of changing the weight employed.

A much more serious modification of the instrument is the very beautiful model devised, and originally made with his own hands by McLean. There were several respects in which McLean thought that the Schiötz tono-

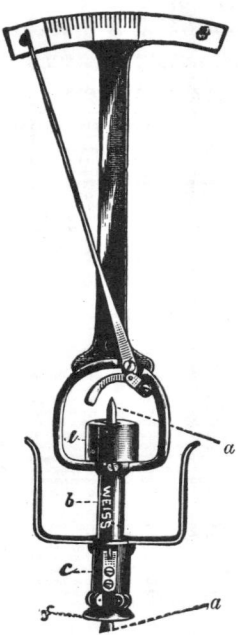

FIG. 105A.—Schiötz tonometer, original model.

aa, sliding rod on which *l*, the weight, is fixed; *b*, a hollow cylinder in which *a* slides; *c*, the collar on which *a* moves by wheel bearings; *f*, foot-plate which rests on the eye. The rod *a* actuates the lever above it, and so records on the scale on the arc.

THE DIAGNOSIS OF GLAUCOMA

meter could be improved upon : (1) The reading scale of the instrument is too far away from the eye under examination ; (2) the necessary translation of the reading into mm. of Hg. is cumbrous ; (3) the chart supplied is a trying one to decipher ; (4) the method of changing

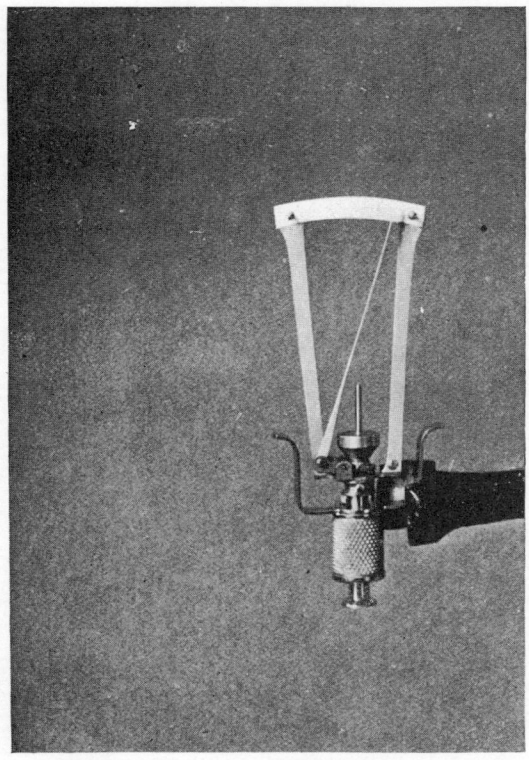

FIG. 105B.—Schiötz tonometer, new model (shown held in a clamp).

weights is difficult and time-consuming ; (5) the plunger fits the footplate barrel so closely that capillary attraction may impair the accuracy of the reading. The McLean tonometer (Fig. 107) was made with the view of doing away with these diasabilities.

Schiötz's reply to these criticisms will now be given.

The author's commentary is embodied with them, in order to save repetition : (1) The distance between the reading scale and the eye matters but little. The author's opinion, after using both instruments, is that McLean's innovation is in this respect a distinct advance. (2) Tonometer readings cannot be accurately translated into intra-ocular pressure in mm. of Hg., and it is preferable to state the weight used, the reading obtained, and the pressure inferred in the following form : $\frac{5\cdot5}{5}$ 16·75 mm. Hg. or $\frac{7\cdot5}{8\cdot5}$ 14·7 mm. Hg. The numerator of the fraction is the weight used, the denominator the lever-deflection observed, and the following figure the pressure deduced.

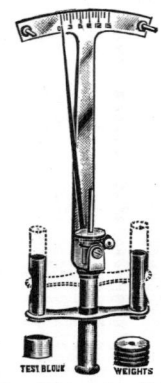

FIG. 106.—Gradle's tonometer.

To the author's mind the introduction of such a fraction is confusing, if not misleading, and he much prefers the method which he has himself adopted for years of stating the three readings in a line, viz., first, the weight used, second, the reading obtained, and last, the deduced pressure. McLean short-cuts the calculations and arrives directly at the deduced pressure. Putting aside for the moment the question as to which of the two observers is correct in his estimate of the intra-ocular pressure, and assuming that neither of them asserts that his method gives mathematical accuracy in the reading deduced, it would seem to be of comparatively little importance which method of stating the results obtained we

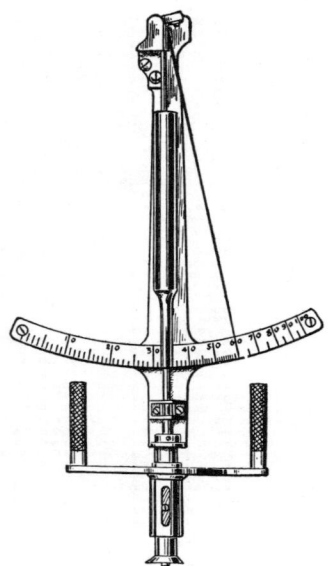

FIG. 107.—The McLean tonometer.

adopt, always provided that the system employed is clearly stated. (3) Schiötz suggests that the chart can easily be enlarged. Another alternative is the adoption of a table for the chart, as suggested by Ellett. (4) Schiötz considers that it is a disadvantage to employ a constant weight, and believes that much more reliable indications are obtained by varying this factor according to the needs of the individual case. He defends this thesis in some detail and with arguments which seem to carry weight. (5) Schiötz is sceptical as to the influence of capillary action ; he thinks that this factor may be considered to be negligible. The author has strong practical reasons for believing this opinion to be correct.

That Schiötz is fully alive to the possibilities of improving his tonometer is evident from the fact that he has recently constructed a new model (Fig. 105B) in which the plungers and weight form one piece, which is put into the cylinder from above. If a heavier load is needed, another weight may be placed on top of the first one. It is hoped that this instrument may be obtainable before long at Jacobsen's Electriske Verksted, Christiania. It is quite certain that the instrument will be accorded a prompt and widespread welcome. The author has used both Schiötz's and McLean's tonometers, and he is confident that either of them will prove invaluable to the surgeon who accustoms himself to its use.

It is important to draw a sharp distinction between two quite different purposes for which a tonometer may be employed : (1) The scientific, and (2) the clinical. Before going any farther, we must clearly understand the nature of the information which we obtain from a tonometer. This instrument gives us a measure of the depth to which the coat of the eyeball is indented under the influence of a known pressure ; the more tense the eyeball, the less this indentation, and *vice versa*. We are thus able to infer the measure of the tension of the tunic of the eye from the amount of the deviation which the lever of the instrument records in use. Now the tension of the ocular tunic is in its turn largely dependent upon the pressure exerted upon it from within by the fluids of the eye, in other words, upon the intra-ocular pressure. It must therefore be obvious that every time we take a tonometer reading of an eye and translate that reading in terms of intra-ocular pressure, we are acting on data furnished by a series of deductions.

The conditions under which the tonometer and thermometer are used are, to some extent, comparable. The only known method of scientifically testing intra-ocular pressure is by means of a manometer, whose needle is introduced into the eye (Fig. 10). To do so clinically is as impossible as it is to place a thermometer directly in the blood-stream; consequently in both cases we have to do with inferences when making our readings. On the other hand, the thermometer is probably capable of much more accurate calibration than the tonometer has been hitherto, for it actually measures temperature, while the tonometer only infers pressure (intra-ocular). A tonometer must be calibrated by the aid of manometer readings on living or dead human or animal eyes, or on artificial eye-drums of suitable make. There is, however, unfortunately a further possible source of error; for all eyes, with the same intra-ocular pressure, do not necessarily give the same tonometer reading. The radius of curvature of the globe has to be taken into account; a tonometer, calibrated for an eye of one radius, will give lower readings of intra-ocular pressure with an eye of a larger radius, and higher readings with one of a smaller radius. On this point all, who have carefully worked on the subject, appear to be unanimous. Then again, the rigidity or elasticity of the tunic of the globe will theoretically affect the readings profoundly. This was shown by Priestley Smith when he experimented on formalin-hardened globes. It is obvious that the more rigid the globe, the less impressible will it be, and *vice versa*. Where, however, authorities differ, is in the matter of the extent to which this factor influences the readings obtained. Some observers think it to be of such great importance that it invalidates their scientific accuracy. McLean, on the other hand, whose admirable work on a large number of living eyes entitles his opinion to the greatest respect, does not agree with this assumption, and believes that, provided we have to do with a living eye, the overwhelming factor in the determination of the tonometer reading is the intra-ocular pressure, the condition of the tunic being comparatively unimportant. Obviously gross pathological change, such as calcification of the tunic, is excluded.

From the experimental and purely scientific point of view, we cannot unhesitatingly assume that the readings given us by any tonometer with which we are acquainted can be relied on as presenting us with the accurate intra-ocular pressure of an eye. This, however, from the practical point of view, is a matter of comparatively little importance. What the present tonometers do for us may be here shortly stated : (1) They give us an approximate reading of the intra-ocular pressure, provided that the globe measured is neither microphthalmic, nor unduly distended, and that the tunic does not show marked pathological alterations. (2) They enable us, in the light of these readings, to say whether the intra-ocular pressure observed in any case comes within the normal range for the particular instrument in use, or whether it is above or below that range, thus indicating normal tension, hypertonus, or hypotonus. (3) They enable us to compare the two eyes of the same patient, and to take note of any differences between them. (4) They also enable us to trace the variations in intra-ocular pressure which any one eye undergoes from time to time.

In the first edition of this work, the author stated with some diffidence his personal conviction that the relative readings of tonometry are of much greater practical importance than the absolute ones. The years that have passed since then have served to lessen the diffidence, and to strengthen the emphasis with which he reaffirms this proposition.

Be it clearly understood, that what has been said above is in no sense meant in depreciation of the efforts to place tonometry on a scientific and accurate basis, or to perfect the calibration of the instrument in such a way that the figures obtained by workers in different parts of the world may be strictly comparable with each other. Their object has simply been to show how far we have progressed, and what results we may fairly claim to have attained—this and nothing more. There remains one point of very practical interest to which attention should be drawn. It is probable that in most instances, a surgeon will get the best value out of tonometry in his daily work if he takes up one model, and uses it uniformly in his practice. He will learn its indications and estimate their value far better than if he chops and changes. It is the old lesson, which we have all learnt with the racquet, the billiard cue, and the gun, that we are best served by the instrument to which constant use has accustomed us.

The limitations in the clinical usefulness of tonometry.—When speaking of the limitations of tonometry, writers have in the past been primarily concerned with the fact, which we have already discussed, that the deduction of intra-ocular pressure from a tonometer reading is largely inferential. The subject which concerns us at present has a much deeper and more significant interest for the ophthalmic surgeon. It is that of the limits of the usefulness of the instrument to us in our daily practice. Some little repetition will be necessary, but it is hoped that the great importance of the subject will serve as a sufficient apology.

It has already been pointed out that extreme variations in the radius of curvature of the cornea and of that of the globe may materially influence the deviation-readings of the tonometer and may consequently give an erroneous impression of the intra-ocular pressure present. Schiötz cites very thinly-walled buphthalmic eyes, and large globes with high myopia, as illustrative of this point. The deviation reading obtained may lead us to infer a normal intra-ocular pressure, although the true condition may be one of hypertonus. Again he cites very small eyes, which have small corneæ with small spherical radii; in these the foot of the tonometer fails to be in contact with the cornea to its full extent. "The results will be the same as if the foot were smaller; the deflections will be smaller and the pressure will appear greater than it really is." It is obvious also that cases of conical cornea, or of a cornea unduly flattened by scarring will be unsuitable for the use of an ordinary tonometer.

There is a strong tendency at the present time to draw a distinction between hypertension and glaucoma, and to use the term " glaucoma " as if it applied to the primary form of the disease alone. No stronger evidence of this could be given than the fact that one of the most able, experienced, and far-seeing writers of the present day has recently stated that " the most important limitation of the practical value of the tonometer is that it gives readings from which high intra-ocular tension and glaucoma would be inferred, when the disease glaucoma, or any special tendency to it, is entirely absent, as in the rise of tension following discission of a crystalline lens, or that following the operation for secondary cataract " (Jackson). Another, taking as his text the distinction between primary and secondary glaucoma, emphasises the importance of distinguishing between hypertension and glaucoma (Uribe-Troncosco). Yet other writers have spoken of a rise in intra-ocular pressure as being but one of the signs of glaucoma, albeit an important one. The author would be far from wishing to set his opinions in opposition to these and other writers of eminence, but rightly or wrongly this is the way the question presents itself to him : (i.) The term " glaucoma " has come to be widely accepted as the equivalent of a hypertension of the eye leading to the production of morbid phenomena, and it seems a pity to depart from this custom, if only for the reason that great confusion will result from doing so. (ii.) An increase of intra-ocular pressure does not necessarily bring about the appearance of these morbid phenomena, but it is the central factor of glaucoma, and all the signs and symptoms of the disease can be traced back to it. (iii.) The causes of glaucoma are protean, and its manifestations are numerous and widely various, but the one factor, common to all cases of the condition, is a rise in the intra-ocular pressure. (iv.) The tonometer will, under suitable conditions, not merely indicate the presence of such a rise, but will provide us with data which enable us to infer the amount of the rise, and so to judge of the probability or otherwise of the appearance of signs and symptoms of glaucoma; it must, however, be clearly understood that the height of the rise in pressure is not the only factor in the determination of the onset of glaucoma; and on the remaining factors the tonometer indications shed no light whatever. (v.) Moreover, the instrument will give us no indication whatever of the underlying causes, which have been responsible for the hypertonus.

We none of us believe that hypertension can exist indefinitely without the appearance of glaucomatous signs and symptoms. Take the instance above cited of the swollen, wounded lens: We watch the eye, and refrain the while from premature interference, because we know it to have been healthy before the injury, and we believe and hope that, if we give it time, its own natural powers of excretion will eliminate the swollen cortical matter, which is blocking up the excretory channels, and so lead to a fall in tension. In addition to this, we have sufficient confidence in the activity of the retinal and choroidal circulatory systems of such an eye, to believe that no great harm will accrue to the nerve elements during the passing period of stress. We would not trust an eye predisposed to glaucoma under similar conditions. In all our cases of hypertonus, we take into careful account the many other factors which enter into the case, and we never think of forming an opinion as to diagnosis, prognosis, or treatment on any one sign or symptom alone, even though that one be so important and significant as a rise in the intra-ocular pressure.

If, in some directions, the clinical usefulness of the tonometer is limited, we must gratefully acknowledge that in many ways this instrument has widened our horizon and increased the precision of our diagnosis: Marbaix has called attention to cases in which the use of the tonometer cleared up an otherwise difficult diagnosis: A rise of tension led to the recognition of a previously undetected mild cyclitis. In a case of parenchymatous keratitis, a reading of 70 mm. Hg. led to the substitution of pilocarpine for the mydriatic previously used, and reduced the tension to normal. Peripheral choroiditis was likewise revealed by an increase of intra-ocular pressure. In high myopia, an unsuspected glaucomatous complication was discovered. In a diabetic with impaired vision, the recognition of high tension led to the employment of pilocarpine, with the result that the intra-ocular pressure was reduced, and the patient was brought into a better condition for operation. Uribe-Troncosco dilates on the value of the tonometer as a means for the detection of glaucoma at a much earlier stage than would otherwise be possible. Morax, in his recent valuable book, states that the use of the tonometer has reached such a point as to make the instrument as indispensable as the ophthalmoscope or the trial case, and he urges every ophthalmologist to see to it that he does not fail to make full use of an instrument, which enables us to diagnose hypertension at an early stage, and so adds greatly to the efficiency with which we are able to treat our patients. He would have the ophthalmic surgeon live with the tonometer at his elbow, for by thus doing, he will diagnose many cases at a much earlier stage than he otherwise would, and will find a dangerous rise in tension present in many eyes in which he would not otherwise have suspected it. It would not be difficult to quote yet other writers who hold similar opinions. The author need hardly say that he agrees cordially with them.

Method of using a Tonometer.—The patient should be examined in the recumbent or semi-recumbent position ; it does not matter much which, so long as he is made quite comfortable, and is so placed that he can easily and naturally raise his chin sufficiently to ensure that the plane of the face is kept horizontal (Figs. 108 and 109). It is quite impossible to do reliable tonometry with the chin continually dropping, and the head tending to assume an oblique or even a vertical position, for the examiner is then continually being worried as to the source of error thus introduced, and consequently cannot give his whole attention, as he undoubtedly should do, to the work in hand. For this reason the writer prefers to measure tensions with the patient lying flat on a bed, or on a comfortable couch, and in such a position that it is difficult, if not impossible, for him to drop the chin. It is argued that to make the patient lie down flat frightens him, and that it is therefore preferable to place him in a chair.

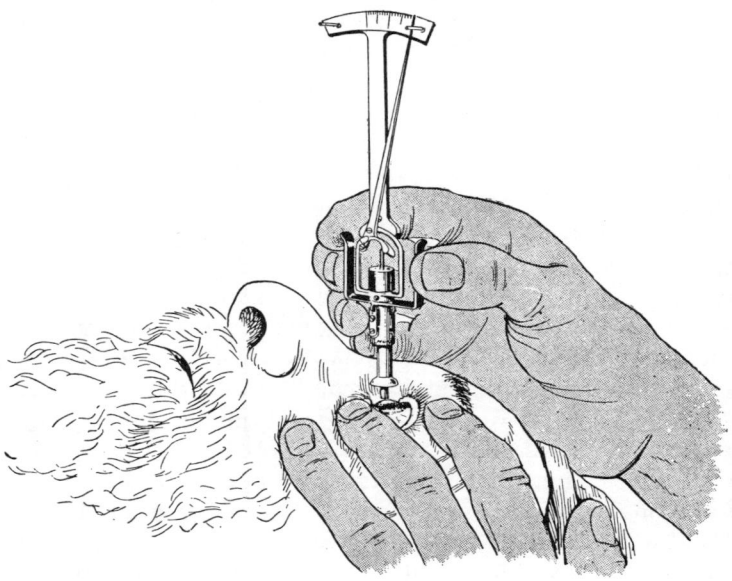

Fig. 108.—The Schiötz tonometer being gently lowered on to the eye under examination whilst the fingers of the left hand separate the lids.

The question involves one of those subtle psychological problems, which each surgeon must solve for himself. In doing so, be his decision what it may, he will show whether he has, or has not, the power, whilst carrying out his purpose, to dominate his patient's imagination. The essential point, which must not be lost sight of, is that the position adopted should be that which makes a reliable examination of the eye as certain as possible.

On each occasion, before estimating a tension, the

THE DIAGNOSIS OF GLAUCOMA 331

observer should test the instrument on the artificial cornea supplied, in order to make sure that the needle-indicator points towards the zero of the scale.

The footplate of the tonometer should be sterilised by immersion in absolute alcohol and then dipped in warm, recently boiled water before application; this latter has the double advantage of removing all spirit, which would

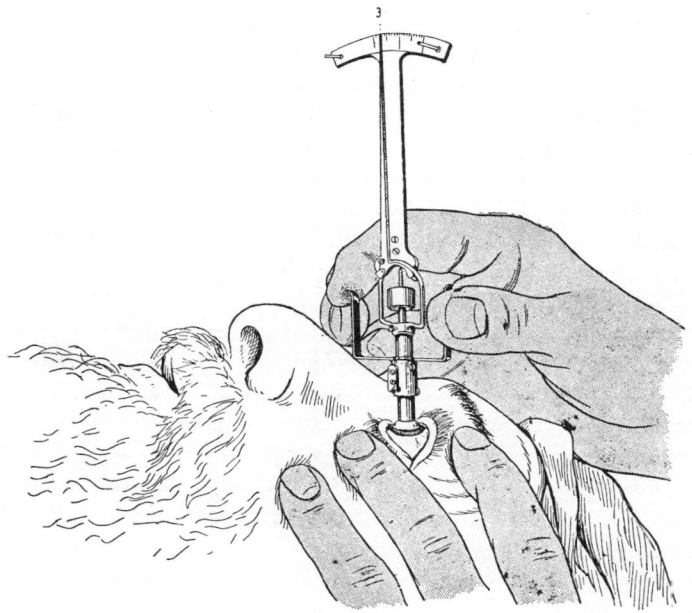

Fig. 109.—The footplate on the tonometer is resting on the cornea and the needle of the instrument is giving a reading.

be injurious to the eye, and as suggested by F. Moore, of lessening the shock of the application. If the surgeon fears that the fluid sucked up between the plunger and the barrel may influence the reading (as suggested by McLean), he may be content with warming the footplate of the instrument by holding it at a little distance above a spirit fame. The spirit will be effectually evaporated at the same time. It is not well to burn it off, as doing so will in time affect the plating of the tonometer. In many old-standing cases of glaucoma, the tension can be taken without anæsthetising the eye, but in case of doubt, and always in nervous patients, it is well to instil a drop of a 2 per cent. solution of holocaine beforehand. To avoid the danger of corneal abrasion, a drop of sterilised liquid paraffin should be instilled into the eye, just before taking the reading, or better still, the footplate may be just moistened with the lubricant by allowing the central rod to dip lightly into a small quantity of it on a sterile watch-glass. This is a measure of some importance, as the state of the corneal epithelium in late glaucoma is such as to demand considerable care in the manipulations used, and especially so after cocaine has been instilled. Indeed, in doubtful cases, it is better to postpone a tonometric examination until the patient is either in a home or in a hospital, or else to do it in his own house. Much undeserved discredit might attach to the surgeon, were the patient to suffer from even a simple and transient corneal ulceration after a tonometry; and the incident might be magnified by foolish or unscrupulous persons to the material detriment of one who was greatly in advance of his detractors. In saying this much, it is important to insist that there is absolutely no danger in the manipulation we are describing. All that is involved is a need for the exercise of that measure of care which the wise surgeon can never afford to dispense with, in the practice of a profession, which is beset with pitfalls.

It is most important that the eye should be looking straight upwards, for readings taken on the periphery of the cornea are unreliable. It is therefore a good plan to arrange the patient so that his eye comes immediately beneath a mark, or better still a light on the ceiling. *Faute de mieux*, the object can be hung above the couch or chair by any convenient means. The subject is asked to fix this object with the eye not under examination. This is greatly superior to the method of asking the patient to "look straight up," in which case the eye often wanders round a comparatively large perimeter. If the fellow eye is blind, the patient's hand should be placed in the desired position, and he should be asked to fix it; he will then usually look steadily in the correct direction. There is one small objection to this, which has been pointed out by M. L. Hine, viz., that the act of convergence is associated with a slight increase of intra-ocular pressure, the mean average excess being 4·9 mm. Hg. As, however, the method advocated is probably the only one by which reliable indications can be obtained in certain cases, the obvious thing to do is to make a small tentative deduction in the reading, in all eyes in which the tension recorded lies in the doubtful zone. The practice of introducing a speculum during tonometry is unnecessary; moreover the pressure of this instrument may easily complicate the examination by increasing the intra-ocular pressure. A nurse or an assistant should hold the lower lid down out of the way, whilst the examiner controls the upper one with his left hand, and applies the tonometer with his right. This latter manoeuvre should be slowly and steadily performed, avoiding any sudden or unexpected movement. It is well to explain beforehand to the patient what is about to be done, and to emphasise that the procedure is painless, and devoid of any real inconvenience, but that it requires intelligent co-operation on his part. A few preliminary trials with the lids held open, and the instrument brought down, but not applied, sometimes prove of considerable value.

The advice usually given is that three estimations of the tension should be made, and that the average of these should then be taken. If care be exercised to perform the tonometry as above described, it is not often necessary to make more than one application of the instrument. For one thing, the tension tends to fall appreciably under repeated examinations, and for another the danger of corneal abrasion is considerably increased thereby. In quite a large percentage of cases, the indicator of the tonometer shows a distinct pulse (evidently the arterial pulse of the eye). If this phenomenon be obtained, one may probably rest assured that the tension has been correctly recorded, and that further applications are unnecessary, for it will rarely, if ever, be seen unless the eye is in a correct position and all avoidable sources of friction in the instrument barrel are excluded. It is essential that the instrument itself should be applied vertically, and that its footplate should rest as nearly as possible on the centre of the cornea. The skilful use of a tonometer undoubtedly requires care and practice, but the difficulties of obtaining a good technique are certainly not great.

The Schiötz Tonometer Readings.—With a little experience the surgeon will usually be able to decide which weight should be used on the tonometer. If the tension is approximately normal, the 5·5 gm. weight should be first placed in position. A reading of from three to six divisions on the scale will show that the intra-ocular pressure is not raised, whilst one of less than three calls for the use of the next weight (7·5 gm.). The most reliable results with the 7·5 gm., 10 gm., and 15 gm. weights are obtained with a deflection of between one and five divisions of the scale. When the deflection is greater than five, the next lower weight must be used; when it is less than two, the next higher is needed.

Cridland has discussed at some length the question of the limits of the normal intra-ocular pressure as given by the Schiötz tonometer. From the work of previous observers he finds that the average normal reading stands at 19·1 mm. Hg., whilst the limits of normal tension are from 12·3 to 36·1 mm. Hg. Schiötz's original findings were that normal intra-ocular pressure varies from 15 to 25 mm. Hg. Cridland gives his own results from the examination of 1001 presumably normal eyes. "The average of the whole is 20·06 mm. Hg. The lowest recorded result was 11·5 mm. Hg., and it was observed in two eyes of different patients. In 1·7 per cent. only was the tension under 15. The highest record was 30 mm. Hg. in four eyes in three patients; and the percentage of cases with a pressure of over 25 was 3·4." Adding his own figures to those of other observers, he states the average normal reading as 19·58 mm. Hg., and its limits as from 11·9 to 28·5 mm. Hg. But in view of the small number of cases below the 15 or above the 25 mark, he appears to endorse Schiötz's original findings, which for all practical purposes may we think be accepted in clinical work.

The McLean Tonometer Readings. — These are uniformly higher than those obtained by Schiötz, for McLean considers that the Schiötz readings are far too low to be accurate. This subject has already been discussed in a previous chapter, and need not detain us further. The intra-ocular pressure is read directly on the scale of the instrument—a procedure, the objections to which have already been discussed—and any pressure between 22 and 40 mm. Hg. is assumed to lie within normal limits. McLean has fixed 40 as the upper limit of safety, because he has never found a normal eye, which registered above 40, although he has found a number of such eyes which did register as high. On the other hand, he has found a few that registered 36 mm. Hg. with the McLean tonometer, and 22 with the Schiötz, in which symptoms of glaucoma were present. In normal young adults—not above 25 years of age—he has frequently found intra-ocular pressures of between 35 and 40 mm. Hg., while in those of more advanced years—above 60—who did not present symptoms of glaucoma, it has not been infrequent to register readings of below 30 mm. Hg.

Schiötz has criticised the McLean instrument on the ground of its *high fixed* weight, but McLean's experiments on living human eyes would seem to show that it is a very accurate instrument in high-pressure eyes, whatever it may be in normal ones. It only remains to add that clinical experience with the instrument serves to prove that its indications in normal cases can be safely relied on, for they are consistent with the other features present.

McLean asserts that a tonometry can be performed with his instrument "as a routine step of the ophthalmologist's examination, without adding more than three minutes to the time allotted to each patient." He is of opinion that " one good reading with the tonometer, placed squarely on the centre of the cornea, is to be preferred to an average of three or four possibly faulty readings, especially if there is a regular oscillation of the needle of from 1 to 6 mm. Where an oscillation occurs, the lower limit of that oscillation is to be considered as the intra-ocular pressure of that eye."

Butler's Tonometer Charts.—Harrison Butler has sug-

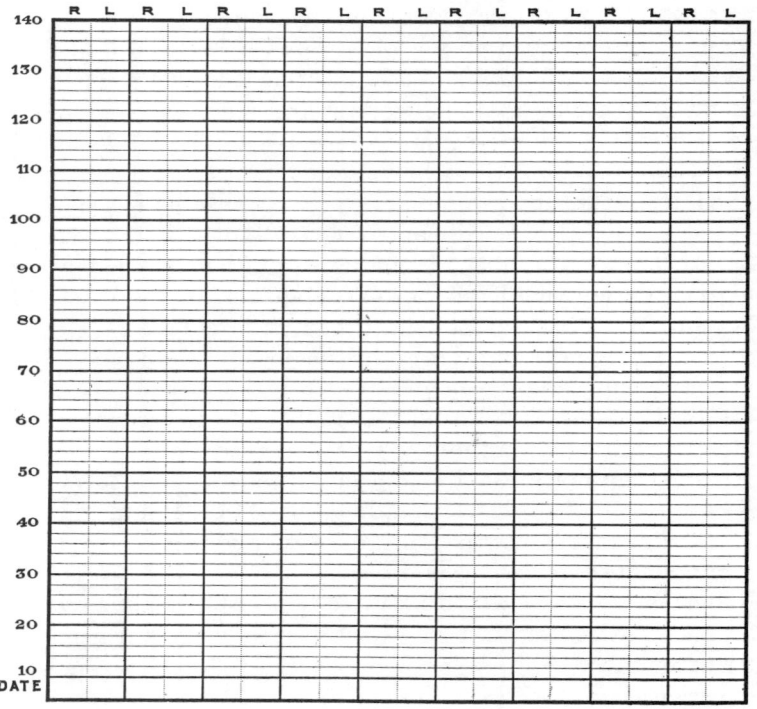

Fig. 110.

gested the plotting of the tonometric readings of any one patient upon a chart, which he has had made for him by Messrs. Charlton & Co. of Birmingham, and which he finds effects a great saving of time. He writes: "Mere inspection shows the progress of the case and the effect

THE DIAGNOSIS OF GLAUCOMA

of any operation which has been performed. I plot the right-eye tensions in red ink, the left in black. The charts may be obtained from Messrs. Weiss." One of them is shown in Fig. 110.

In closing this section there is one point, often emphasised in this volume, on which we would again lay the utmost stress : Our real safeguard lies in remembering that, in a doubtful case of glaucoma, we must go by *no one sign*, but must take into account every possible factor that may help us in forming an opinion. If still in doubt, we must suspend judgment and watch the march of events.

The writer holds more strongly than ever before that the most important rôle played by the tonometer, is not so much as an aid to diagnosis, though even here its value is very great, but rather as a means of watching the progress

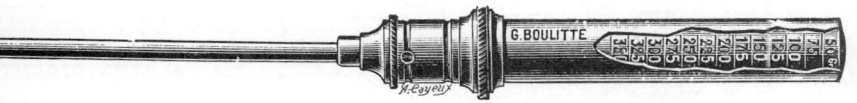

FIG. 111.—Bailliart's ophthalmo-dynamometer.

of a case, and of controlling our estimates of the value of the means we employ to combat the rise of intra-ocular pressure.

BAILLIART'S OPHTHALMO-DYNAMOMETER (Fig. 111).—This instrument is intended to measure the diastolic and systolic blood-pressures in the retinal artery. It acts by means of a spiral spring, being in fact a delicate spring-balance. The button end is applied to the region between the upper and outer recti muscles, either through the eyelid or straight on to the globe. Pressure is made toward the centre of the eye, and the amount of force employed in any given experiment can be read off in grammes by the scale shown on the side of the instrument. With the dynamometer in one hand and the electric ophthalmoscope in the other, the observer watches the effect of the applied pressure on the retinal artery. When pulsation commences in this vessel, the diastolic pressure is read off, and when it again ceases, under an increase of the pressure applied, the systolic pressure is noted. A calculation, which is not altogether above criticism, is involved.

From the clinical point of view the chief value that can be claimed for this instrument would seem to be that it enables us to ascertain the retinal arterial pressure (both systolic and diastolic) of any suspected eye, and so to institute a comparison between this and the intra-ocular pressure, as found by a tonometer. So far the method has not been widely practised clinically, and very few opinions have been expressed on the subject. Those who are interested are advised to study Bailliart's papers and the reviews of them in the *British Journal of Ophthalmology*.

It will be remembered that T. Henderson showed a similar instrument before the Ophthalmological Society in 1914.

The Examination of the Light Sense

There can be no question that the light sense is profoundly affected in glaucoma. We know this well from the bitter complaints of those of our patients who are suffering from the disease. They frequently tell us of their difficulties when they pass from a brightly lighted room into the dark of the night, or even into a poorly illuminated passage. Similarly, when they come into a bright light out of darkness or comparative darkness, they are obliged to stand still for a while until they become adapted to the new conditions. Nor is this all, for very bright days dazzle them all the time, whilst in dull, cloudy weather, or in the twilight, they are keenly conscious of a difficulty in finding their way about.

A considerable interest attaches to changes in the light sense as furnishing diagnostic evidence of the early stages of the disease. Beauvieux and Delorme maintained that the differential light sense is the first to be attacked, and this too at a period when the other evidence of glaucoma is still scanty. According to their findings, the minimum light sense (*i.e.* the perception of a minimum or threshold stimulus) is only diminished when optic atrophy is present.

These changes are independent of any diminution either in the central visual acuity or in the peripheral vision.

The experience of British observers appears to be widely different from this. Wallace Henry has experimented on glaucomatous patients with a photometer, and has found "that in the earliest stages of glaucoma there is a rapid reduction in the light minimum sense, but only a very slight reduction in the light difference sense, whilst in incipient atrophy the reverse is the case." A. S. Percival's findings agree with Henry's. He says: "I have always found light minimum much more diminished than light difference in glaucoma, and I always rely on this test for distinguishing between an eye with physiologic high tension, and one with pathologic high tension, in the absence of other signs. I have notes of two or three cases in which I have found the light minimum sense diminished, and which I saw some years after with obvious glaucoma." For a test of light difference, he uses white rotating discs, with black sectors on them, and for light minimum he employs black discs with similar but smaller white sectors. These are similar in principle to Young's Threshold Test Rings. The latter observer has worked mainly with his threshold-test cards, and his findings in glaucoma are certainly suggestive, in spite of the fact that his cases are not very numerous. W. W. Sinclair, working with Young's cards, obtained similar results, but points out that his records too are few in number. The reader is referred to their writings.

The author has been not a little troubled by the fact that, when working with white rings on a black ground, and black rings on a white ground, he has not by any means found evidence of failure in light sense as an invariable occurrence in cases of glaucoma, even when the disease has been pronounced, always provided that the correction of any error of refraction has been carefully attended to, and that central visual acuity, as tested by the Snellen types, was normal. He is far from wishing to challenge the correctness of the observations made by the above-named workers, and is fully conscious that the difference in the results obtained may admit of a simple explanation, but of the fact he has stated above he is quite sure. Several of the patients were extraordinarily intelligent men. One of them was but a few years ago the leading authority in Great Britain on his own medical speciality. His case had been diagnosed without hesitation by a colleague, and he simply came to the author for a confirmation of the opinion that an operation should be performed. There was no doubt or hesitation about this, and yet he could count every one of the rings on a Young's card, either black on white or white on black.

A second case was equally arresting : The patient is a High Court judge. He was first operated on for glaucoma by a colleague in November 1913. He came under the writer's care in 1916. The right eye was then practically blind ; the left had good vision, but typical glaucomatous field changes with an inferred intra-ocular pressure of 45 mm. Hg. in R. E. and 32 mm. Hg. in L. E. (Schiötz). Both eyes were trephined, and the tension remained low for nearly four years. On 26th July 1921 there was a typical return of glaucoma with an inferred pressure of 30 mm. Hg. in the R. E. and 40 mm. Hg. in L. E. He was again trephined, and has made a very satisfactory recovery, with relief of pressure and general improvement, though the damage to his field is much greater than it was a year ago. In spite of the fact that he had great difficulty in adapting himself to bright sunlight, or to darkness, or to twilight, and that he was then beginning to show a fresh return of pressure in the eyes, his seeing (left) eye could pass a full normal test by the Young's dot cards at the close of 1920. On the 9th November 1921, although his difficulties of light adaptation were even worse than before, he counted 8 out of 9 black rings on a white card, and 9 white rings on a black card, rotated on Young's instrument.

The above two cases are merely illustrative, and similar instances could easily be multiplied. It suggested itself that the method of examination might be responsible for the discordance between the author's findings and those of others, although this was extremely unlikely. Recourse was then had to the author's photometer, and to

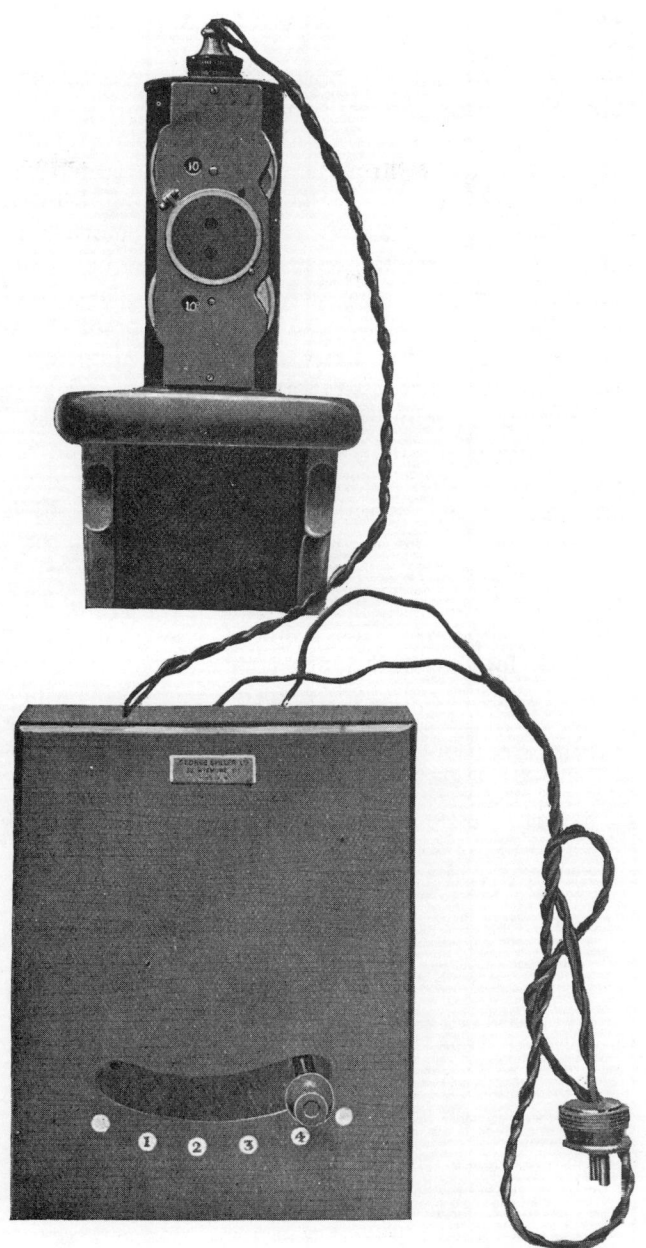

Fig. 112.—The author's light sense apparatus.
See note on next page.

the Zeiss instrument—both of which are described below—but the results were still the same.

When one comes to think the matter over, these findings of acute central light perception, associated with a difficulty experienced by the patient in orienting himself in dim illumination, are really in accord with the other phenomena of glaucoma : We know that, if the case has been a simple one, the central visual acuity for form may remain very high indeed, whilst the perceptive power of the peripheral field may greatly diminish. Again, deterioration may occur in the paracentral area of vision, which may lead the patient to complain of an increasing difficulty in moving about amongst obstacles, at a time when he can readily read $\frac{6}{6}$ in a good light, and when he may show no constriction of the boundaries of the visual field under the rougher perimetric tests. If this is true of the acuity of vision for form, it is surely only to be expected that it may be equally true of that for light perception. Looking at the question from this point of view, we may anticipate that so long as the congestive element is absent from a case, the central light perceptive power—whether for light

---

The apparatus consists of (1) a vertical lantern which acts as the light source, and of (2) an electrical resistance which controls the intensity of illumination. The lantern encases a tubular frosted lamp of eight candle-power placed centrally within, the only egress for light being through two apertures placed close together on the outer casing. On the front of the lantern two pairs of circular discs are arranged, containing respectively a series of apertures 1, 2, 5 and 10 mm. in diameter and a series of neutral tinted lenses of standardised densities, ranging from 1 to 7. Both the apertures and neutral tinted lenses can be introduced immediately before the two apertures in the casing already described. Spring catches working into grooves on the edges of these discs determine the correct positions before the apertures. The values of the tints and the sizes of the disc apertures being registered in small openings, are conveniently read from the front of the instrument. An additional circular disc containing a No. 20 neutral tint glass can be superimposed over the two apertures through which light appears. The resistance is wound with a standard resistance wire of unvarying efficiency. Five contact points can be covered by a moving switch arm to obtain varying degrees of illumination, from the maximum brilliancy to a dull red glow, the contact points being numbered on the wooden casing which encloses the resistance. With this instrument, it is possible to measure, with great accuracy, both the threshold light stimulus and the differential light sense.

minimum or for light difference—will be but little damaged; the changes will probably start from the periphery of the field, or from the paracentral area, or from both, and will only attack the centre at a late stage of the disease. Once, however, that the acute or subacute interferences with circulation, which characterise the congestive form of the disease, make their appearance, we may expect the centre to suffer early and severely in its powers of light perception, just as it does in its acuity of vision for form.

Probably the most satisfactory method of testing the light sense in the glaucomatous is by some form of photometer. Percival has found Chibret's Chromatoptometer and Photometer a handy and speedy instrument to use. Others used Förster's instrument. The author had an apparatus made for his use by Messrs. Spiller (Fig. 112). In mechanical details, this left something to be desired. Since its appearance, Messrs. Zeiss have adopted the three principles on which the instrument was made—the use of an electric bulb, of different depths of neutral tint glass, and of diaphragms of varying apertures—and have recently constructed a small and very compact photometer (Figs. 113 and 114), with which the author is now working.

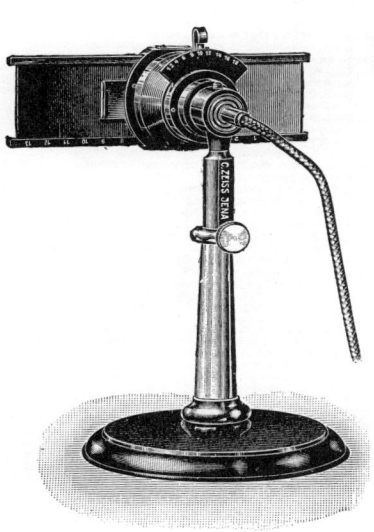

FIG. 113.—Zeiss' visual photometer, mounted on a round foot, with small lamp and cable, with five-point diaphragm, iris diaphragm and Goldberg wedge.

Where all these instruments break down, however, is in standardisation. We shall never make real progress until we get a photometer which can be relied upon to give the same readings wherever and whenever it is used. For this reason, J. W. Downey's new instrument seems worthy of a trial. It contains a series of discs of a radio-active substance, sold under the trade name of Marvelite, which consists of sulphate of zinc impregnated by radium. These are substituted for the lights of a photometer, and are damped down by being covered with varying numbers of layers of celluloid. They are put up in a suitable instrument, the details of which appear to be well worked out.

It is to be most sincerely hoped that the subject of the

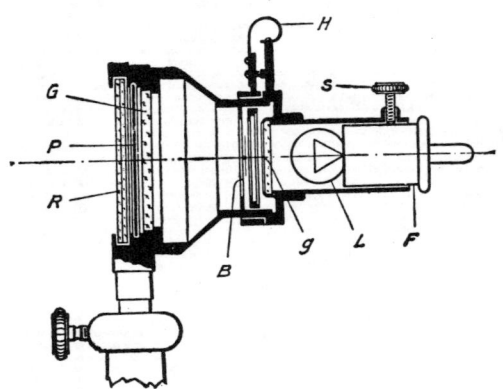

Fig. 114.—Zeiss' photometer on section.

Cross-sectional elevation of the lamp casing of the visual photometer; F, lamp holder; L, frosted incandescent lamp bulb; s, clamping screw; g, opal glass plate; B, iris diaphragm; H, regulating lever; G, opal glass plate; P, five-point diaphragm; R, Goldberg wedge.

failure of the light sense in glaucoma will receive a very large amount of attention in the near future. It is one which will well repay the work spent on it, and which, apart from its scientific interest, may lead to important, practical results from the clinical standpoint.

REFERENCES

Bailliart, P.—*Ann. d'ocul.*, 1917, vol. cliv. p. 257; and *Brit. Journ. Ophth.*, 1818, vol. ii. p. 487.

Bailliart, P.—*Ibid.*, 1919, vol. clvi. p. 672; and *Brit. Journ. Ophth.*, 1921, vol. v. p. 71.

BEAUVIEUX AND DELORME.—*Arch. d'opht.*, vol. xxxiii. p. 93.
BUTLER, T. HARRISON.—" A Tonometric Chart," *Brit. Journ. Ophth.*, 1920, vol. iv. p. 279.
CRIDLAND, B.—*Ibid.*, 1917, vol. i. p. 352.
DOWNEY, J. W.—*Amer. Journ. Ophth.*, 1919, vol. ii. p. 13.
ELLETT, E. C.—*Ophth. Rec.*, 1914, vol. xxiii. p. 97.
ELLIOT, R. H.—" Tonometric Values," *Brit. Journ. Ophth.*, 1919, vol. iii. p. 426.
GRADLE, H. S.—" Tonometry, with a Description of a Tonometer," *Ophth. Rec.*, Sept. 1912.
HENRY, WALLACE.—*Brit. Med. Journ.*, July 24, 1920, p. 111.
HINE, M. L.—*Trans. O.S. of U.K.*, 1916, vol. xxxvi. p. 226.
JACKSON, E.—*Trans. Amer. Acad. Ophth. and Oto-Laryng.*, 1916; and *Ophth. Year Book*, 1918, vol. xiv. p. 81.
MCLEAN, W.—" Experimental Studies in Intra-ocular Pressure and Tonometry," *Arch. Ophth.*, 1919, vol. xlviii. p. 23.
MCLEAN, W.—" The Tonometry of Glaucoma," *Arch. Ophth.*, 1920, vol. xlix. p. 301.
MCLEAN, W.—" Further Experimental Studies in Intra-ocular Pressure and Tonometry," *Brit. Journ. Ophth.*, 1919, vol. iii. p. 385.
MORAX, V.—*Glaucome et Glaucomateux*, Librairie Octave Doin, Paris, 1921.
PERCIVAL, A. S.—Personal communication.
SCHIÖTZ, H.—*Arch. f. Augenh.*, vol. lxviii. part i. p. 77.
SCHIÖTZ, H.—*Brit. Journ. Ophth.*, 1920, vol. iv. pp. 201 and 249.
SINCLAIR, W. W.—*Ibid.*, 1918, vol. ii. p. 386.
URIBE-TRONCOSCO, M.—*Amer. Journ. Ophth.*, vol. i. p. 799.
YOUNG, GEORGE.—*Brit. Journ. Ophth.*, 1918, vol. ii. p. 384.

CHAPTER V

SECONDARY GLAUCOMA

SUMMARY

PART I
INTRODUCTORY.

PART II
ÆTIOLOGY.
- (1) Perforation of the Cornea with Entanglement of the Iris.
    Perforating Wounds of the Cornea, associated with Anterior Synechia.
    Ulceration of the Cornea, with Perforation and Prolapse of the Iris
    The Results of Fistula of the Cornea.
- (2) Annular Posterior Synechia.
- (3) Dislocation of the Lens—
    Anteriorly,
    Laterally,
    Posteriorly.
- (4) Wounds of the Lens—
    Accidental,
    Surgical.
- (5) Intumescent Cataract.
- (6) The Absorption of Crystalline Lens matter in the Eye affected with Cataract
- (7) Following Cataract Extraction.
- (8) Following Iridectomy.
- (9) Aniridia.
- (10) Intra-ocular Tumours—
    of the Iris,
    of the Ciliary body,
    of the Choroid,
    of the Retina.
- (11) Detachment of the Retina.
- (12) Thrombosis of the Central Retinal Vein.
- (13) Intra-ocular Hæmorrhage.
- (14) Irido-cyclitis.

PART III
TREATMENT.

Part I

It is necessary to preface this chapter with the remark that there is no *essential* difference between primary and secondary glaucoma. If a pathologic rise of intra-ocular pressure can be traced to the action of some local antecedent disease, we speak of the case as one of *secondary* glaucoma; failing this we term it *primary*. There are strong links connecting the two groups, and it is possible, if not probable, that a fuller knowledge of the pathology of some of the cases, which we now classify as primary, would enable us to relegate them to the secondary group.

The study of secondary glaucoma is of great importance to the surgeon for three reasons :

(1) It throws a valuable light on the ætiology of the primary form of the disease.

(2) It shows the need for early and careful diagnosis in every case of glaucoma which presents itself.

(3) It lays emphasis on the fact that in our treatment of cases of glaucoma, we must not be content merely to strike at the rise in intra-ocular pressure, but must also, and in the first instance, direct our attention to the discovery of any causative condition which may be present, and to the removal of such a factor if possible.

Part II

Ætiology

The causes of secondary glaucoma may be broadly divided into two groups :

(1) Those which act by bringing about a closure of the anterior chamber, and thus shutting off the stream of fluid from the excretory outlet in this neighbourhood, and

(2) those which owe their influence to a change in the constitution of the intra-ocular fluid. Such a change may be due, either to an alteration in the composition of the fluid (*e.g.*, from the presence of albuminous matter

in solution therein) or to the suspension in the fluid of solid particles of various kinds (epithelial cells, pigment masses, lens or vitreous debris, etc.). Both these changes tend to block the excretory channels mechanically, and so to impede the outflow of the aqueous current through them.

It would be a reasonable plan to pursue our study of secondary glaucoma by taking up in turn these two great groups of ætiological factors ; but, as a matter of convenience, the scheme adopted by Priestley Smith in his classic article, which has been the foundation of all subsequent work on the subject, is preferable. It is to review in turn the various morbid conditions which may give rise to secondary glaucoma, pointing out the method of action of each. We shall accordingly adopt this plan, and shall take structure by structure, starting from the cornea and working backwards.

(1) **Perforation of the Cornea with Entanglement of Iris in the Opening.**—When " the anterior chamber is opened by a wound or ulcer, the aqueous escapes, the iris applies itself to the cornea and prolapses through, or adheres to the margins of the wound. So long as the aperture remains open, the aqueous drains away and the eye remains soft ; when it closes, it becomes hard, for the aqueous has now insufficient access, or no access to the filtration angle " (Priestley Smith). Before discussing the various conditions which fall under this heading, there is one primary point to make : They one and all depend on a wide obstruction of the filtration angle by an interference with the iris, which results in the adhesion of its base to the adjacent part of the cornea.

(A) *Perforating wounds of the cornea associated with anterior synechia.*—These represent the simplest possible condition met with under our first heading. It frequently happens that during the withdrawal of the instrument which has inflicted the injury, a gush of escaping aqueous carries the iris into the lips of the wound, which are then plugged and closed, at the expense of the entanglement of the uveal membrane in their embrace ; or, again, when the corneal wound is large and irregular, not only may the iris become entangled in it, but the chamber may continue to leak, thus allowing the neighbouring structures of the eye, inclusive of the capsule of the lens, the ciliary body, and even the vitreous, to come into contact with, and later to become matted to the corneal wound. It is obvious that the more anterior the wound, the greater is the probability that the angle of the chamber will be effectively and widely interfered with, by the enforced apposition of the iris base to the corneal periphery. In the first instance, it is a question of mechanical obstruction,

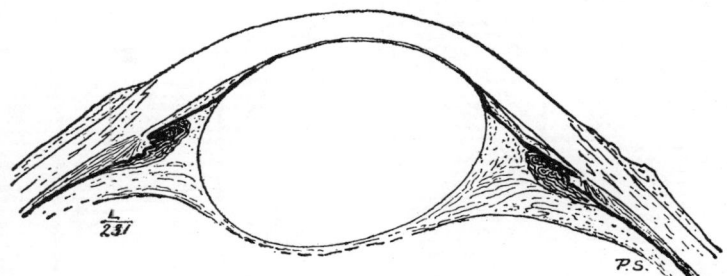

Fig. 115.—From an eye blinded by secondary glaucoma, following wound of the cornea. (Priestley Smith.)

The section does not pass through the wound. Permanent abolition of anterior chamber; access of fluid to filtration angle permanently cut off.

due to the mere apposition of the parts; later, if the conditions are favourable, as they so often are, to the spread of septic action, the opposing surfaces become fixed to each other over a wider and wider area; the shallowing of the anterior chamber and the obliteration of the filtering angle are thus made permanent, and can only be dealt with by the establishment of a fresh channel for the excretion of fluid, in other words, by a fistulising operation, if indeed by that (Fig. 115).

(B) *Ulceration of the cornea resulting in perforation and associated with prolapse of the iris.*—The history in such cases is frequently one of neglected purulent or phlyctenular ophthalmia, or of septic ulceration following a corneal injury. The condition is especially common in

Oriental countries, where disease is too often allowed to run its course unchecked. The great extent of destruction of the cornea which often takes place, together with the dangerously septic condition of the parts, favours the formation of wide adhesions between the wound edges and the deeper structures (Fig. 116). Though the method of perforation is different from that of the cases discussed in the previous section, the subsequent development of the condition is practically the same. It is, however, especially in these latter eyes that we meet with staphyloma of the cornea. The pre-existing ulceration leads to weak-

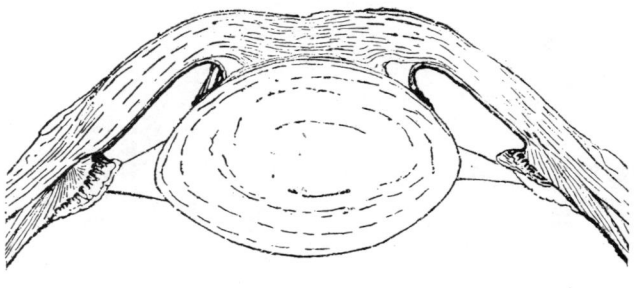

Fig. 116.—From an eye blinded by secondary glaucoma, following central perforating ulcer of cornea. (Priestley Smith.)

Permanent abolition of anterior chamber; access of fluid to filtration angle completely cut off.

ness of that membrane; the widespread inflammatory matting between it and the iris makes it softer and more liable to yield under pressure. When the wound in the cornea closes, the pressure within the eye rises, for the normal excretory channels have been effectually blocked by the adhesion between the iris base and the corneal periphery. The result is the formation of a staphyloma which may attain very large proportions. Such a condition is very commonly met with in tropical countries, and especially in the Orient, where it is often a result of improper native medical interference. Figs. 117 and 118 illustrate the point admirably. The former shows one of these enormous unsightly eyes in a negro; the latter was taken

SECONDARY GLAUCOMA

from a section of a staphylomatous globe removed in the Government Ophthalmic Hospital, Madras.

(C) *The results of fistula of the cornea.*—This condition has really been dealt with under the two previous headings, but possibly requires a little further explanation, and may therefore be shortly considered again at this stage. If the cornea is perforated, whether by a wound or as a result of

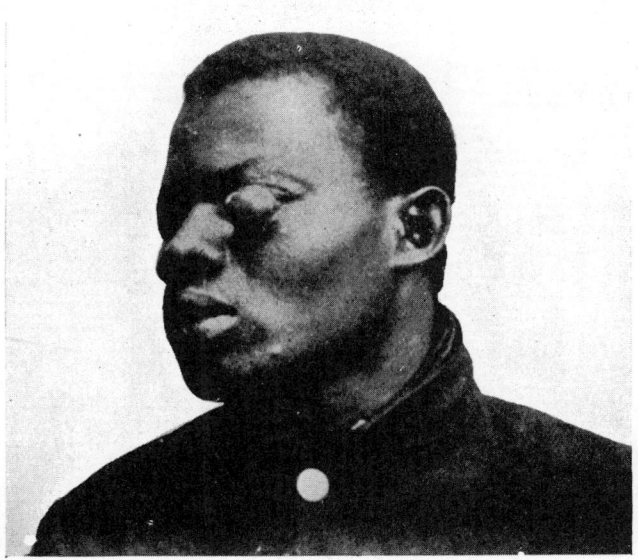

FIG. 117.—Large staphyloma of the cornea in a negro.
(*Photo kindly supplied by Mr. Edgar Stevenson.*)

disease, the aqueous escapes; whether the iris becomes entangled in the wound depends, amongst other things, on the site of the perforation; the more central the latter is, the less the likelihood of entanglement. If no entanglement takes place, the probability that leakage will endure for a longer period becomes greater. Such leakage involves an empty chamber, and a close apposition between the iris and the cornea. The longer this lasts, and the more active the septic element present, the greater is the probability of widespread and extensive adhesion between the two membranes. Such adhesions may form even apart from entanglement of the iris in the wound. With the abatement of septic action, the fistula may close, and if it does so, a rise in intra-ocular pressure will at once take place by the method already described. This is usually associated with staphyloma. The condition may again be spontaneously relieved by the reopening of the fistula under pressure. (Figs. 119 and 120.)

(2) **Annular Posterior Synechia.**—This condition, when

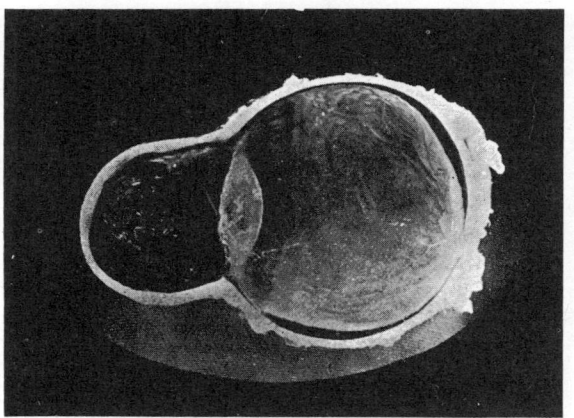

FIG. 118.—Staphyloma of the cornea: an extreme case.
(*Photo by Mr. C. J. Taylor.*)

complete, establishes an obstacle to the flow of fluid from the posterior to the anterior division of the aqueous chamber. It is usually the outcome of repeated attacks of iritis, in the course of which the pupillary edge of the iris is more and more extensively bound down to the subjacent capsule of the lens, until at last the pupil is closed throughout its entire circumference. When this stage is reached, the normal flow of aqueous through the pupil is definitely stopped; an accumulation of fluid then takes place in the posterior chamber, with the result that the iris is bulged forward like a bellying sail, the condition of

SECONDARY GLAUCOMA

l'iris bombé being thus established. The mischief already present is thereby exaggerated, for the periphery of the

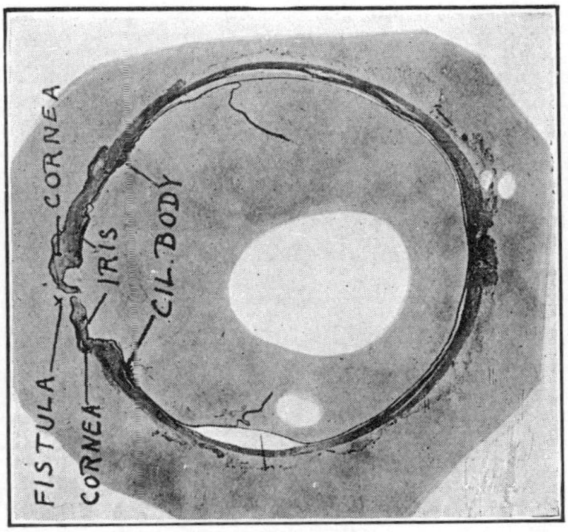

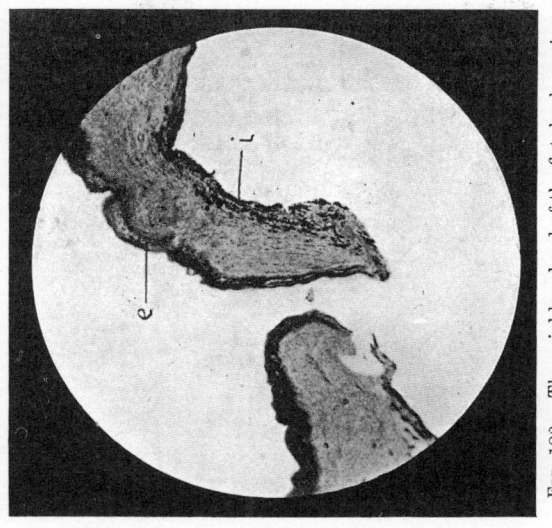

FIG. 120.—The neighbourhood of the fistula shown in Fig. 119 under high magnification.

Notice the adhesion of the iris to the back of the cornea, and the degeneration of the corneal epithelium. *i*, iris; *e*, corneal epithelium.

(*Photo by E. E.*)

FIG. 119.—Whole section of an eye, showing a corneal fistula, the formation of which relieved a staphylomatous condition, which was the consequence of a secondary glaucoma.

The anterior chamber is obliterated, the iris being adherent to the back of the cornea.

(*Photo by E. E.*)

bulging iris comes into contact with a broad zone of the corneal periphery, and thus closes the filtration angle.

354   GLAUCOMA

Such a closure is at first mechanical, but later adhesions occur with permanent obliteration of the sinus of the chamber (Fig. 121). A similar condition of *l'iris bombé* may be brought about even in the absence of the lens, the margins of the pupil then adhering to the remains of the lens capsule with which the anterior hyaloid membrane is sometimes matted. This state of affairs is found in some of

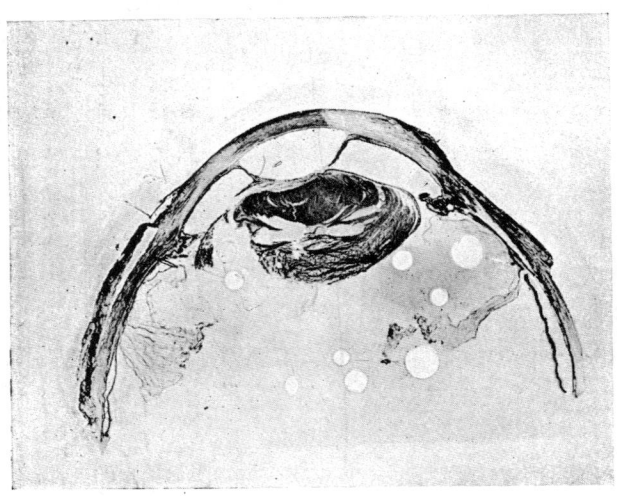

Fig. 121.—Section of the anterior part of an eyeball, showing annular posterior synechia.

The iris is extensively adherent to the back of the cornea; the pupillary area is tied down to the anterior capsule of the lens.

(*Photo by E. E. of specimen kindly lent by Mr. Treacher Collins.*)

the cases of secondary glaucoma which follow couching for cataract by Indian practitioners, and is well illustrated in Figs. 122 and 123. It may also occur after extraction of the lens; this matter will be dealt with later on in the chapter.

When posterior annular synechia is met with, without secondary glaucoma resulting, the explanation of the absence of increased intra-ocular pressure is to be sought in one of two directions: Either (i.) the ring of synechia is not complete, or (ii.) the normal secretory activity of the ciliary body is impaired.

(3) **Dislocations of Lens.**

(A) into anterior chamber,
(B) laterally,
(C) posteriorly.

(A) *Anterior dislocation of lens.*—This may either be (i.) spontaneous, or (ii.) traumatic.

(i.) *The spontaneous dislocation* of a lens into the anterior chamber usually occurs with great suddenness. In a case observed by the writer it happened to a young Eurasian boy whilst he was having a bath. Priestley Smith describes it, in a case of his, as occurring whilst the patient was stooping over a wash-hand basin. In all such instances it may be assumed that the suspensory ligament was defective beforehand. Not uncommonly the displaced lens is found to be a shrunken one. The glaucomatous condition may be spontaneously relieved by the

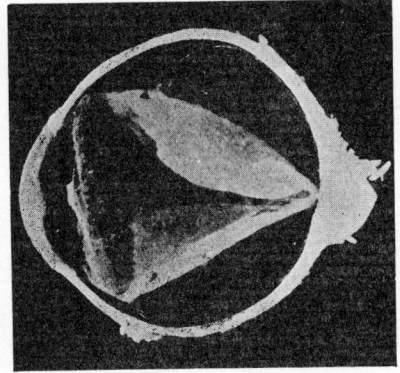

FIG. 122.—The anterior chamber is much shallowed by the bulging forward of the iris (*l'iris bombé*).

The pupil is blocked, and its edges are adherent to a layer composed of the lens capsule and the anterior layer of the hyaloid, which are inflamed and matted together; the retina is detached, and the choroid partly so. A cataract has been couched in this eye.

(*Photo by E. E.*)

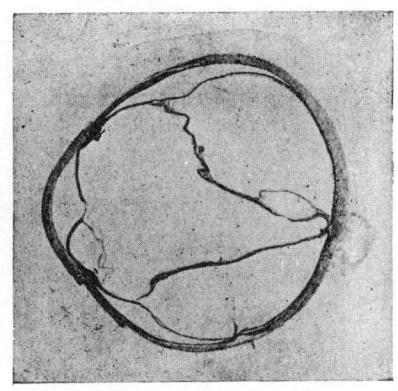

FIG. 123.—The same eye as in Fig. 122 shown cut in whole section.

(*Photo by E. E.*)

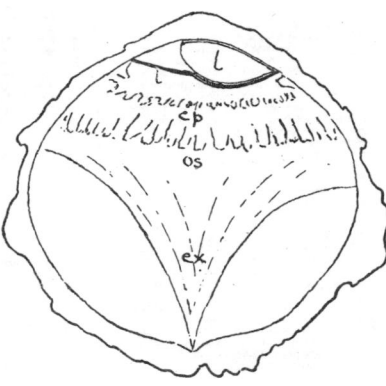

Fig. 124.—Anterior dislocation of lens.

A line drawing by E. E. from a photograph of a couched eye. *l*, lens; *i*, iris; *cp*, ciliary processes; *os*, ora serrata; *ex*, detached vitreous body.

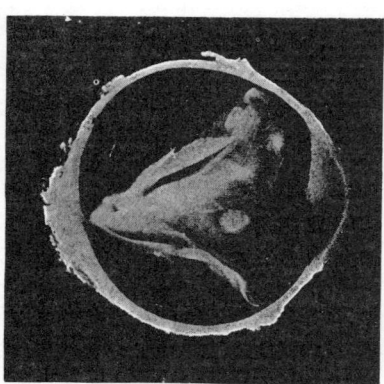

Fig. 125.—Section of an eye in which the lens had been couched.

The nucleus can be seen floating in the vitreous chamber; it passed freely between this and the aqueous chamber; retina detached.

(Photo by E. E.)

lens slipping back through the pupil of its own accord. Indeed, the same sequence of events may be repeated on a number of occasions, high tension manifesting itself each time the lens passes forwards, and being quickly reduced as soon as it slips back again. Priestley Smith has called attention to the fact that an anterior dislocation of a lens may take place without producing glaucoma; in such cases, it is clear (1) that a passage must be left through which the fluid can still make its way from the posterior into the anterior chamber around some part of the margin of the lens, and (2) that a sufficient extent of the filtration angle must still remain open to satisfy the needs of the normal excretion of fluid from the eye. He cites the case of an eye in which no rise of tension occurred until, by the use of eserin, the iris was contracted and tightened up against the posterior surface of the lens; then an acute glaucoma at once supervened.

(ii.) *Traumatic dislocation* of the lens forward may either be due to indirect violence, or may be the result of a penetrating injury. The commonest form of the latter is that met with in the East after couching for cataract; the whole lens may then be found displaced in its capsule (Fig. 124), or the latter membrane may be ruptured and the nucleus alone may escape into the anterior chamber,

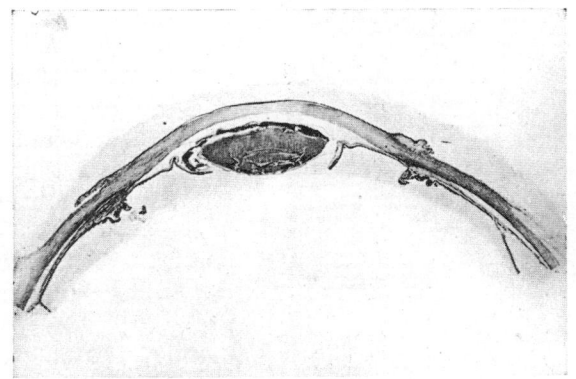

FIG. 126.—Section of the front part of an eye blinded by secondary glaucoma, owing to the lens being dislocated into the anterior chamber.

The iris was tightly wrapped round its posterior surface, and was in close contact with the posterior surface of the cornea peripherally. It has become separated from the lens and cornea during preparation.

(*Photo by E. E. from specimen kindly lent by Mr. Treacher Collins.*)

from which it may pass freely back and forth between the aqueous and vitreous chambers of the eye. Fig. 125 shows a photograph of an eye in which this happened during life.

Whether the anterior dislocation is spontaneous or traumatic, the onset of glaucoma depends largely on two factors, viz., the size of the dislocated lens mass, and the amount of irritation set up. This is well illustrated by the two figures just quoted; a small freely movable lens may pass backward and forward through the pupil without necessarily giving rise to any increase of intra-ocular tension (Fig. 125), whilst a bulky one will widely occlude the angle of the chamber, interfere with excretion and cause a rise in pressure (Figs. 124 and 126). Inflammatory action may tie the lens down in the angle of the chamber, and thus block a large segment of this excretory area (Fig. 127). Priestley Smith has called attention to the manner in which the iris may be wrapped round the posterior surface of an anteriorly dislocated lens. He writes: " No sooner is the relation of the iris and lens reversed, than the stream which previously kept the passage (from the posterior to the anterior chamber) open, closes it with a constantly increasing pressure. The iris is firmly applied to the posterior surface of the lens ; its periphery, where not supported by the lens, is driven forward against the cornea (Fig. 126). The great force exercised by the fluid in such cases is shown by the remarkable moulding of the lens to the curvature of the cornea."

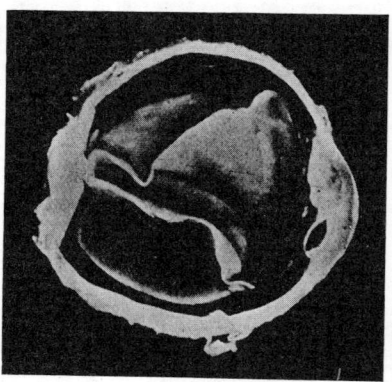

Fig. 127.—From a couched eye.

A small dark Morgagnian nucleus lies impacted in the lower angle of the anterior chamber, being fixed in position by inflammatory exudate, and thereby blocking a large part of the filtration area of the eye.

(*Photo by E. E.*)

(B) *Lateral dislocation of the lens.*—In these cases the dislocation is often partial, the lens remaining in the pupil but being pushed over to the periphery in one direction or another. The displacement is usually the result of a severe blow, but may follow some form of operative procedure. The alteration in refraction greatly impairs vision ; the pupil is irregularly dilated, being more contracted in the direction in which the lens is dislocated and

SECONDARY GLAUCOMA

more dilated in the opposite quadrant; at the same time the pressure of the lens in the former direction shallows the anterior chamber there. It is often quite easy to see the margin of the dislocated lens in the area of a dilated pupil. (Figs. 128 and 129.)

Priestley Smith has pointed out that such an accident as the above tends to close the angle of the chamber in two

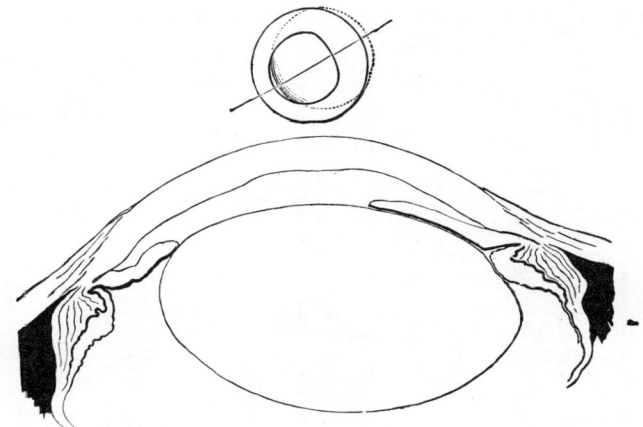

Fig. 128.—From an eye blinded by secondary glaucoma following lateral dislocation of the lens by a blow. (Priestley Smith.)

The smaller figure shows diagrammatically the direction of the dislocation, the displacement of the pupil, and the direction in which the globe was bisected. Filtration angle completely closed at the one side of the circle by direct pressure of lens against ciliary process and iris; at other parts of the circle it has probably been more or less compressed by displaced vitreous. In the larger figure the specimen corresponds as regards right and left with the smaller figure.

ways—(i.) by direct pressure of the lens on the iris and ciliary body on the side towards which dislocation has taken place, and (ii.) by a displacement of the consistent vitreous body, owing to the change in position of the lens, that body being driven forward in other directions and so indirectly effecting a closure of a wide area of angle. Bowman has recorded a case in which glaucoma complicated the presence of a congenitally displaced lens.

(C) *Posterior dislocation of the lens.*—What has been

said of lateral dislocation applies with even more force to those posterior displacements of the lens which are so commonly met with in Eastern countries as the result of the operation of couching. This subject has been dealt with at some length by the author, in his book on *The Indian Operation of Couching for Cataract*, and only a brief reference is permissible here. Glaucoma accounted for the failure of 11·05 per cent. of the total number of couched eyes (780) under review in that work. In a large number of the cases the secondary rise in tension could be traced to the influence of other injuries inflicted at the time of operation, *e.g.*, anterior synechia of the iris or capsule, and in

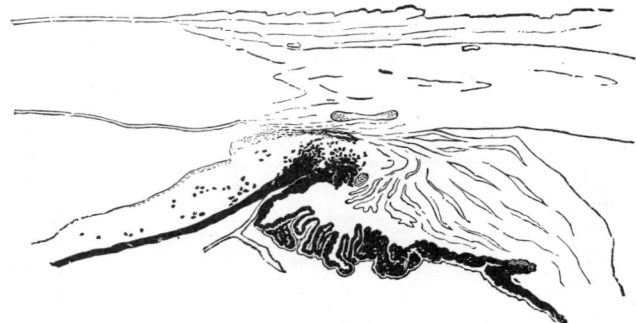

Fig. 129.—From the same eye as Fig. 128 : section through ciliary region enlarged. (Priestley Smith.)

one case, of the retina ; entanglement of the ciliary body in the scar ; blockage of the pupil and *l'iris bombé* ; the formation of a dense diaphragm across the eye, composed of the inflamed and matted anterior layer of the hyaloid, or of the capsule of the lens, or of both. In a further number, the cataract, which had been dislocated backward either into the vitreous chamber or into a space opened up between its own capsule and the anterior hyaloid membrane, had become imbedded in a firm exudate, which bound it closely to the ciliary body and the base of the iris, thereby obstructing the filtration angle over a large area (Fig. 130). In yet other cases the lens, thrust back at an angle to its normal position, was found tightly wedged between the base of the iris and the anterior hyaloid membrane; Fig. 131 shows very beautifully how such a dislocation may produce direct pressure on the iris base in one segment of the eye, whilst, indirectly, it may cause the fluid contents of the globe to bulge forward and thus close the filtration angle over a wide area in the opposite meridian. It is true that in this particular specimen the fluid bulged forward was a subretinal exudate, but none the less the mechanism of the action is well shown. Finally, it has been pointed out by A. C. Hudson that when a lens is dislocated backward into the vitreous, or when in any way the integrity of the latter is sacrificed, that body may bulge forward into the anterior chamber and produce obstruction of the filtration angle in any one of the four following ways: (1) By blockage of the channels of exudate by streamers of vitreous, or by altered vitreous cells; (2) by direct forward

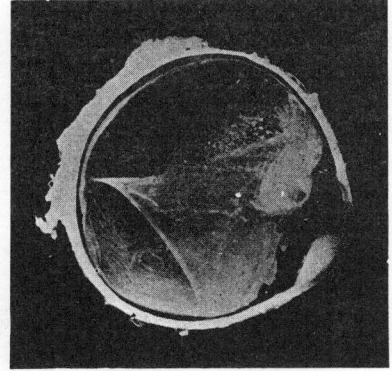

FIG. 130.—From a couched eye.
The dislocated lens is tied to the back of the iris and ciliary body by firm exudate, which is continuous with and part of the cone of inflammatory material representing the shrunken vitreous. The pressure of the lens on the iris base obliterated a large area of the filtration angle.
(*Photo by E. E.*)

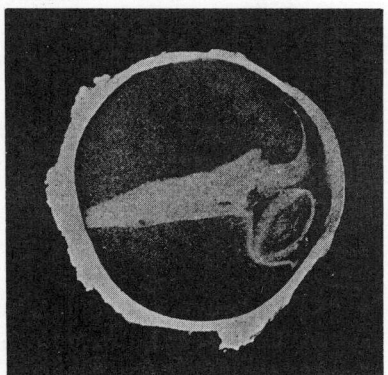

FIG. 131.—From a couched eye.
The lens has been reclined backward. It makes direct pressure on the iris base below, thereby closing the angle; it also displaces the fluid contents of the eye, and causes them to bulge forward above, thus indirectly blocking the angle of the chamber in that neighbourhood.
(*Photo by E. E.*)

362 GLAUCOMA

pressure of the advanced front part of the vitreous body on the base of the iris from behind; (3) by an accentuation of such forward movement of the iris by an overdistension of the posterior chamber, as the result of ballooning of vitreous through the pupil, and the consequent interference with the perfectly free passage of fluid from the posterior to the anterior chamber; and

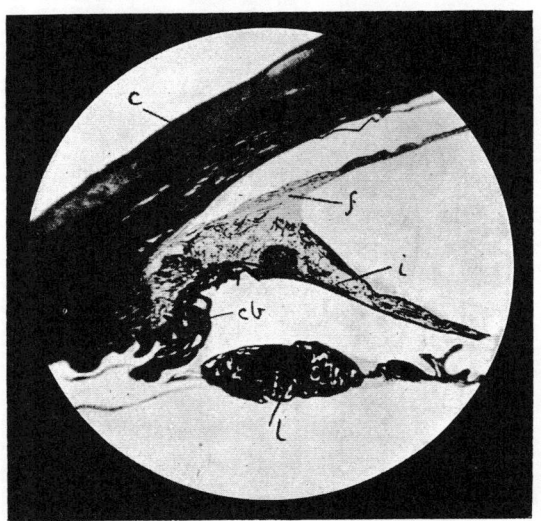

FIG. 132.

The angle of the chamber has been blocked by a new formation, possibly the result of the vitreous which had passed into the anterior chamber affording a scaffolding for the growth of endothelium of the ligamentum pectinatum, and the subsequent deposition of hyaline membranes, which obstruct the passage of aqueous to the ligamentum pectinatum. *c*, cornea; *i*, iris; *cb*, ciliary body; *l*, lens masses; *f*, new formation blocking chamber.

(*Photo by E. E.*)

(4) as the result of vitreous which has passed into the anterior chamber affording a scaffolding for the growth of the endothelium of the ligamentum pectinatum, and the subsequent deposition of impervious hyaline membranes, which obstruct the passage of aqueous to the spaces of the ligamentum pectinatum (Fig. 132). Hudson's own description has been closely followed in the above.

It remains to mention the recent work of C. A. Hegner, carried out in the University of Jena. He found that the majority of traumatic dislocations of the lens occurred in elderly people as a result of the loss in elasticity, and of the general atrophy of the zonular fibres. Secondary glaucoma proved the most frequent and the most dangerous complication of partial dislocation, occurring in 83·3 per cent. of his cases ; in some it was manifest within forty-eight hours of the injury. On the other hand, a secondary rise in tension was only observed in two out of eleven cases (18·18 per cent.) in which the lens was totally dislocated into the vitreous. There is one important difference between his cases and those which the author observed after the performance of the couching operation, viz., that the element of sepsis was largely absent from the former ; hence the vitreous remained free from inflammatory exudate and the lens did not become bound down against the base of the iris. This is in full accord with the author's experience that in those cases of couching, which escaped septic infection, and in which the lens was completely dislocated, a favourable result might last for years.

It has been suggested (Gifford) that the glaucoma and irido-cyclitis, which follow couching of the lens, may be due to the absorption of cataractous lens matter. One objection to this view is, that when a lens is dislocated into the vitreous, little or no such absorption takes place, and yet glaucoma may come on. Moreover, cases of couching, *which escape inflammatory complications*, may retain useful vision for many years. Whilst not denying that the absorption of lens matter may possibly be a factor in some cases, it does not seem at all likely that it deserves to have much importance attached to it, especially in view of the fact that a simple explanation, based on physical and pathological data, is forthcoming in the great majority of the cases.

(4) **Wounds of the Lens.**—The lens may be wounded in a number of different ways :

(A) *By accident totally independent of surgical interference.*—Such an injury may be (i.) the result of the *penetra-*

tion of the globe by an instrument or weapon, which pierces the capsule of the lens in such a way as to provide a path for the access of the aqueous fluid into the substance of the lens fibres. As a result of the imbibition of fluid the fibres swell up, and masses of disintegrated lens substance may find their way into the anterior chamber, and tend mechanically to block the filtration angle of the eye. Apart from this, the swelling of the lens is prone to cause undue pressure behind the iris, thrusting the base of that membrane forward against the cornea and so directly closing the sinus of the chamber. It is to be carefully noted that a lens dislocated into the vitreous, or one whose capsule is even widely opened on its posterior surface, shows no tendency to swell up and so to give rise to glaucoma; the access of aqueous to the wound in the lens is an essential factor in the case.

It is to be borne in mind that penetrating injuries of the globe are frequently complicated by synechia of the iris or of the capsule, either of which conditions may of itself lead to the onset of secondary glaucoma.

The bulging of lens matter through the pupil is a prominent feature in some cases, and may alone suffice, as Priestley Smith has suggested, to dam back the normal current of fluid through that aperture. At a later stage, the bulging mass may contract inflammatory adhesions to the pupillary margins of the iris, leading to the formation of a total posterior synechia, whilst the organised exudate closes the aperture in the capsule; thus a permanent blockage of the pupil may take place.

There is another way in which accidental trauma may give rise to glaucoma, viz., (ii.) when, as a result of a *blow with a blunt instrument*, the anterior capsule of the lens is indirectly ruptured. The same chain of events, which we traced in the previous instance, is again found here. Such a form of injury is, however, luckily rare.

(B) *As a direct result of some form of operative procedure.*—The infliction of such an injury may be (i.) absolutely accidental, or (ii.) a deliberate part of the method adopted. We shall take these in turn:

(i.) The *accidental wounding* of a lens in the course of an operation is by no means so rare as one could wish. It is most apt to happen in those operations in which a sharp instrument—*e.g.*, a keratome—is introduced into the anterior chamber, and the danger is greatly enhanced when that chamber is abnormally shallow, as is the case in certain diseases, and especially in glaucoma. This fact is to be carefully borne in mind, when weighing up the advantages and disadvantages of any individual operation for the latter condition. The observation applies not only to von Graefe's iridectomy, but also to Holth's punch operation and other similar procedures. An injury to the lens has occurred to some operators during a sclero-corneal trephining, but the author cannot help feeling, that with even moderate technical ability, such an accident should not occur during the course of that procedure.

(ii.) There are certain *operations* which are *undertaken with the deliberate intention of admitting the aqueous fluid into contact with the lens fibres*, viz., (*a*) the discission of a soft lens, and (*b*) Foerster's operation to hasten the maturation of a cataract. There is a close similarity between these two procedures and the two forms of purely accidental injury, which we discussed under heading (A). The discission wound closely resembles that inflicted by a fortuitous penetration of the eye ; whilst Foerster's operation almost certainly depends for its success on tiny indirect lacerations of the anterior capsule, which admit a very moderate amount of aqueous fluid into the lens mass. In both operations the effect may easily be overdone, with the result that a swelling of the lens takes place which is in danger of getting out of control, and producing a condition of congestive glaucoma, which may be very hard to treat. The author speaks of Foerster's operation, after having performed it several hundred times, and having then given it up in disappointment.

(5) **Intumescent Cataract.**—The references to this condition are comparatively scanty in European literature. It is quite otherwise in countries like India, for the simple reason that patients do not there resort to surgical aid so

freely as they do in lands where the standard of education is higher. The records of the Madras Out-Patient Room show the occurrence of this complication in nearly fifty cases yearly ; what is more, the author has seen it come on in a number of cases which were actually under his care at the time. The glaucoma is often of a very acute type. It is more than half as common again in females as it is in males. The period the cataract has lasted, before high tension supervenes, is always a protracted one, the condition resulting from continued neglect on the part of the patient to call in surgical aid until long after the lens has become fit for extraction. The patients are usually those who have contracted cataract at a comparatively early age ; this observation is in accordance with our experience that the type of cataract, which gives rise to the trouble we are discussing, is the intumescent one, which presents a pearly sectored appearance ; for this form is usually found in comparatively young patients. The appearance of the lens in these cases is characteristic of primary cataract, the history is unmistakable, and the presence of a primary and hitherto uncomplicated cataract in the opposite eye often clinches the diagnosis.

It is of interest, in connection with this tropical experience, to recall that of five cases of glaucoma, secondary to swelling of the lens in senile cataract, which were seen in the Prague clinic, three of the patients were glass-blowers and one a stoker (R. Salus). Tacke saw six cases of the same complication during forty-five years of practice, and in four of them the patients were myopes.

(6) **Glaucoma following the Spontaneous Absorption of Senile Cataract.**—For our knowledge of this condition we are especially indebted to Gifford, who holds that the spontaneous cure of senile cataract is far from being so rare as might be inferred from the statement by Hess in the last edition of the *Saemisch Handbook,* to the effect that the cases reported to date number a little over sixty. The association of glaucoma with the absorption of hypermature cataracts has been noticed, at one time or another, by Mitvalsky, Reuss, Verrey, Feingold, Jackson, Black, Straub,

and Schwenk, but the tendency in the earlier communications was to attribute the disappearance of the opaque lens to the influence of the rise in tension, or of some coincidental inflammatory condition. Gifford holds that this is a confusion of cause and effect, and believes that "the spontaneous absorption of the cortex of a senile cataract produces, in many cases, an increase of tension, which may be temporary or unnoticed, or which may lead to complete blindness." In the latter case, "the absorption of the lens is commonly attributed to the influence of the glaucoma." In support of his position he points out that he has been able to follow cases of this kind for many years without meeting with the appearance of any sign of glaucoma in the opposite eye, even though that too became cataractous, provided always that there was no undue delay in removing the cataract when it became ripe for extraction.

In the more favourable cases, the course of events would appear to be as follows : The retention for long periods of a hypermature cataract ; the sudden onset of tension with inflammatory symptoms ; the appearance in the anterior chamber of a grey deposit, which subsequently disappears, with the restoration of useful vision ; this disappearance may either be spontaneous or may occur as the result of operative interference. In some cases the absorption of the cortex does not seem to give rise to any increase in intra-ocular pressure. It must, however, be borne in mind that when the process of absorption is a gradual one, the slight rises in pressure which occur are apt to be overlooked, and their influence on the failure of vision is likely to be obscured by the blindness of the eye due to the cataract, and by the total absence of pain. If the escape of the cortex into the chamber occurs more rapidly, it may give rise to chemotaxis, and signs of irido-cyclitis. Gifford believes that the cortex, when seen in the anterior chamber, is sometimes mistaken for inflammatory exudate. According to him, the drainage areas of the eye may be blocked, (1) mechanically by the sticky cortex, (2) as a result of chemotaxis, and (3) by both the above influences acting in concert. To attribute the absorption of the cataract to the inflammatory condition is, he thinks, to put the cart before the horse; he holds that such a view is "based upon a misinterpretation of the congestive symptoms which accompany the absorption of the cortex," and that it "is as erroneous as the belief that the absorption depends upon the occurrence of glaucoma."

An eye which has successfully passed the first danger of glaucoma from the spontaneous cure of cataract, is still open to the further peril of high tension from dislocation of the loose nucleus into the anterior chamber. There is also the question as to whether the gradual breaking down and absorption of the nucleus may not lead to the same form of trouble as we have been studying in connection with the absorption of cortex.

Gifford believes that the greater danger of glaucoma from the absorption of lens material in hypermature cataract in adults, as compared with that met with in soft cataract, is to be explained by an appeal to the mechanical and chemical peculiarities of the former. In support of this suggestion, he instances the glaucoma which accompanies essential atrophy of the iris, and which he believes to be due to the product of iris disintegration.

(7) **Post-operative Glaucoma, following the Extraction of Cataract or the Needling of an After-cataract.**—It has been known since the days of Bowman and von Graefe that there is a danger of glaucoma after the successful extraction of a lens, and a still greater one after the needling of a capsule, left at the first operation. No known method of procedure ensures an immunity from this dangerous complication. For our recent knowledge of the subject we are indebted to Priestley Smith, to Natanson, to Treacher Collins, and to many others.

A number of different conditions may give rise to the form of glaucoma which we are discussing. We shall take these in turn:

(i.) That in which a *down-growth of epithelium* takes place *along the track of the wound* (Meller and Fuchs), *into the anterior chamber, which it eventually lines completely*, thus opposing a strong obstruction to the escape of fluid

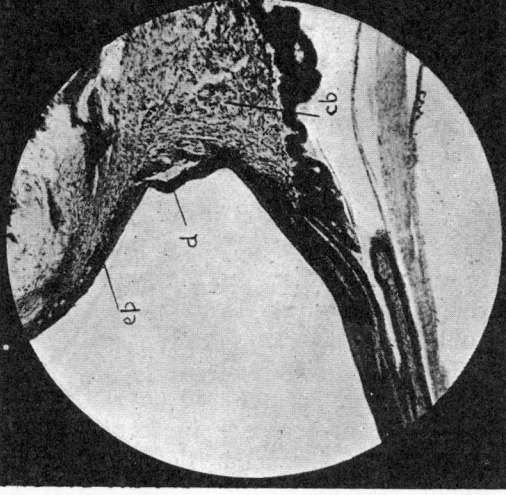

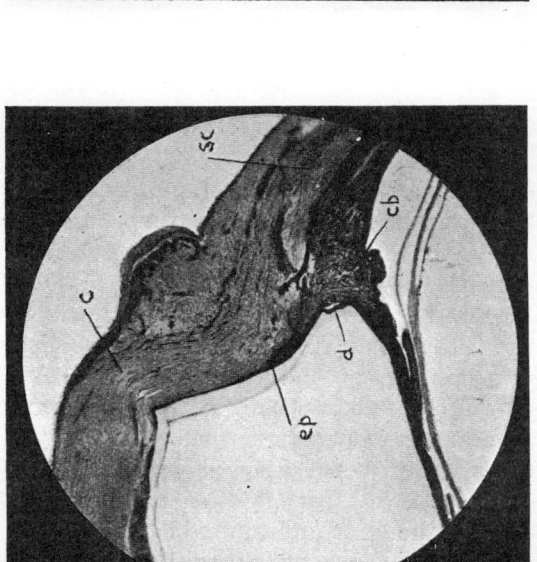

FIG. 133.—Epithelial cyst of anterior chamber.

The epithelial layer is shown as a dark band all round the chamber.

The epithelial layer is detached over a small area (*d*) in the angle itself; *c*, cornea; *sc*, sclera; *cb*, ciliary body; *ep*, lining layer of epithelial cells.

FIG. 134.—Shows the angle of the chamber more highly magnified.

The nuclei of the epithelial cells can be distinctly seen.

(Photos by E. E. from specimen kindly lent by Mr. Treacher Collins.)

through the filtration angle and through the crypts of the iris (Figs. 133, 134 and 135). Collins, who was the first to describe these cases, says of them : " The increased tension to which the cyst gives rise does not make its appearance until some months after the operation ; there may be for a time good vision, so that the operation appears to have been a success. Then slowly the glaucoma manifests itself with superficial œdema and haze of the cornea. The anterior chamber will in one part appear exceedingly shallow, where the iris is pressed foward by fluid unable to pass into it, and in another part, where the cyst is situated, very deep." A diagnosis of the existence of such a cyst can sometimes be made clinically.

(ii.) *The condition in which the angle of the anterior chamber remains widely open*, and in which the presence of irido-cyclitis accounts for the rise in tension, by (*a*) altering the character of the aqueous fluid present, and so making it less fit for escape through the meshes of the pectinate ligament, and (*b*) furnishing the fluid with cells of inflammatory origin, which tend mechanically to block the open spaces of the filtration area.

(iii.) *The condition in which the angle of the anterior chamber is largely or completely closed by the contact of the root of the iris with the periphery of the cornea.*—The most important factor in the causation of this condition is undoubtedly (*a*) the entanglement in the wound-scar of a portion of the iris or of the capsule, or (*b*) the adhesion of one or both of these parts to the posterior surface of the incision (Fig. 136). Whilst accepting this as beyond controversy, it is necessary to point out that slight adhesions of the iris or of the capsule, to the scar are so common after successful cataract extraction that they may be described as the rule rather than the exception. Becker found them in two-thirds of thirty-eight cases he examined anatomically, though he was quite unable to recognise some of the slighter synechiæ clinically. It is, therefore, obvious that it is not the synechia itself that is responsible for the glaucoma, but that it in some way brings the latter condition about. The investigations of Treacher Collins

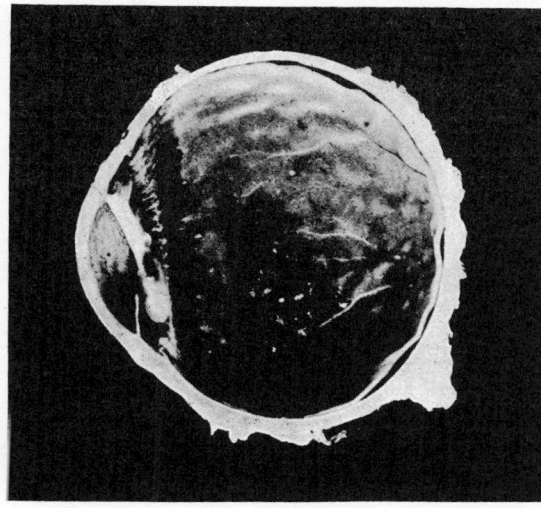

FIG. 136.—Half-section of an eye removed for secondary glaucoma, due to a capsular synechia, which followed the extraction of a cataract.

The closure of the angle in the neighbourhood of the synechia is well shown.

(Photo by E. E. of specimen kindly lent by Mr. Treacher Collins.)

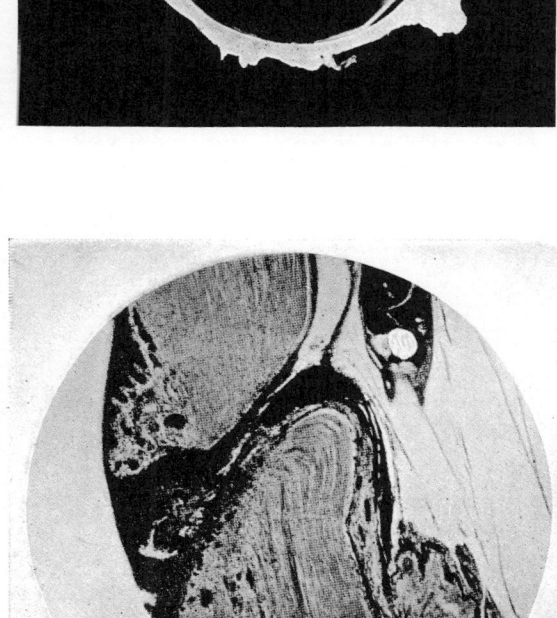

FIG. 135.—Shows an extension down of the surface epithelium along the lips of an extraction wound.

It passed into, and completely lined the anterior chamber. The condition resulted in glaucoma, which necessitated the removal of the eye.

(Photo by Mr. E. Collier Green, kindly lent by Mr. E. Treacher Collins.)

have shown its *modus agendi*, which we shall now discuss.

To commence with, we must again draw attention to the distinction between the incarceration of iris, or lens capsule, or both in the operation wound, and the adhesion of those structures to the posterior lips of the wound. It is generally accepted that their incarceration leads to a weakening of the scar, which may provide a ready path along which pathogenic organisms can find their way through an abrasion of the cornea into the interior of the eye. Irido-cyclitis may thus be readily set up. It is also generally assumed that there is another danger inherent in the imprisonment of tags of capsule in the scar, for as cicatrisation proceeds, such tags may drag on the ciliary processes; it is said that the constant movements of the iris and ciliary muscle accentuate this drag and set up a condition of ciliary irritation, which under suitable conditions, may easily be transformed into irido-cyclitis.

Agglutination of the capsule to the posterior surface of the cornea does not interfere with the healing of the wound, but it does provide the mechanism for a drag on the ciliary body; moreover, it has this in common with incarceration, that they both draw forward not only the capsule but also the iris lying in front of it, and thus tend to close the angle of the chamber. The farther forward the point of adhesion of the capsule to the cornea is, the greater is the advancement of the membranes likely to be, and the more acute the consequent closure of the angle of the chamber. Collins has laid special stress on this in connection with certain cataract cases in which a rise of tension in an operated eye does not occur until after needling, and he has suggested that the explanation is that the needle, being introduced too far forward, enables a fresh adhesion of the capsule to take place in advance of its previous attachment, with the result that an attack of glaucoma is precipitated. He has therefore advised that the needle should be introduced as far back as possible, *i.e.*, as near the iris plane as is consistent with safety. Kirkpatrick, on the other hand, introduces his needle well forward at a point midway between the limbus and the centre of the cornea. In this way he avoids the risk of impaction of the iris or capsule in his wound.

After the usual operation for cataract, it may be found that one or both lips of the tear in the capsule are caught in the depth of the incision wound; or again, the posterior capsule may bulge between the lips of the aperture in the anterior capsule and so may itself be imprisoned. In the so-called intracapsular operation for the extraction of a cataract, in which the lens is removed entire in its capsule, the anterior layers of the hyaloid body may become impacted in the incision. All such entanglements and adhesions are much more likely to occur whenever, owing to a delay in the re-formation of the chamber, the deeper structures lie long in contact with the wound.

When a combined extraction has been performed, the capsule is for obvious reasons more easily entangled in the wound than it is after the simple operation; but the latter procedure does not confer absolute immunity from capsular entanglement, whilst it heightens the danger of the iridic complication. On the other hand, the performance of an iridectomy does not necessarily prevent the impaction of the uveal tissue in the wound, for one or both of the pillars of the coloboma, or the stump of iris left, or even the anterior portion of the ciliary body may become impacted in the scar.

It remains to say a further word on the causes of the glaucoma which may follow the needling of an after-cataract. It has been pointed out above that if the needle is introduced into the eye far forward in the cornea, it may furnish a still more anterior attachment to an adherent capsule than the one it previously possessed, and so may predispose to a mechanical blocking of the angle of the chamber. In connection with dislocations of the lens backwards into the vitreous chamber, A. C. Hudson's work on the subject has been mentioned. The explanation there given of the methods, whereby filtration is apt to be obstructed, when the integrity of the vitreous body is interfered with, may be equally applied to the present case.

There are therefore two possible elements in the causation of a secondary glaucoma due to anterior synechia following the extraction of a cataract. One is the shallowing of the angle due to mechanical factors, and the other is the incidence of irido-cyclitis, which may act, not only by helping to weld together the opposing surfaces of iris and cornea, but also by the means set forth under heading (ii.) above.

(iv.) The condition in which an *annular posterior synechia* leads to glaucoma *after the extraction of a cataract,* now demands our attention. Essentially the problem is identical with that of annular posterior synechia, as met with altogether apart from the presence of cataract (see p. 352). An iritis or an irido-cyclitis is responsible for the adhesion of the pupillary edge of the iris to the subjacent tissue, which may consist of lens capsule, of anterior hyaloid membrane, or of both together. These underlying tissues are themselves infiltrated with and strengthened by the presence of an organised inflammatory exudate. The anatomical appearances present are well illustrated by Figs. 122 and 123, the only difference being that in the eye from which these photographs were taken the lens had been couched, not extracted. The leading features are the same in all cases, and include the imprisonment of fluid behind the iris, the presence of *l'iris bombé*, and the consequent closure of the angle of the chamber.

(v.) A rare condition is met with in which "the iris and posterior capsule being united and coated by inflammatory exudation, appear to *form an impermeable, or insufficiently permeable diaphragm across the eye,* which checks the passage of fluid from the ciliary processes into the aqueous chamber. An excess of fluid becomes imprisoned behind this diaphragm" (Priestley Smith). The difference between this condition and that dealt with in the previous heading, is that here the obstruction lies between the vitreous and aqueous chambers, instead of between the posterior and anterior divisions of the aqueous chamber. Priestley Smith considers that the diaphragms abovementioned may become less permeable as time goes on, or possibly that a change in the intra-ocular fluid may render the latter less capable of passage across the membrane.

(8) **Post-operative Glaucoma following Iridectomy.**—This subject has been more than once alluded to in the present chapter, and the following remarks therefore involve some measure of repetition, for which indulgence is craved, in view of the importance of making the matter perfectly clear. Little more than a classification is required. The cases may be divided into (i.) those which follow iridectomy for conditions other than glaucoma, and (ii.) those which follow this procedure when deliberately undertaken for the relief of high tension. In both (a) the lens may be wounded, (b) the pupil may become occluded as a result of iritis or of irido-cyclitis, (c) the stump of iris left may get caught in the wound, entailing all the disastrous results which may follow such a complication, or (d) the persistence of a shallow chamber may result in the adhesion of the lens capsule, the neighbouring iris, or the ciliary body to the lips of the wound. So far as our class (ii.) is concerned there remains another point to be mentioned. Iridectomy can only relieve glaucoma if the angle of the chamber is open at the site of the coloboma, or if a filtering cicatrix is accidentally established by the operation. Failing either of these conditions, the recurrence of glaucoma may be confidently expected.

(9) **Aniridia** may be (i.) traumatic or (ii.) congenital.

(i.) Traumatic aniridia may be operative or accidental. The author has three times seen the whole of the iris removed in the grip of the forceps during an iridectomy. In each case it happened to a different operator, all three of whom were men of skill and experience. Treacher Collins has shown in two cases of traumatic aniridia that a broad adhesion of the lens capsule to the wound had resulted, that the anterior part of the ciliary body had been drawn forward, and that the capsular synechia had fixed this body in its advanced position, in contact with the ligamentum pectinatum.

(ii.) With regard to congenital aniridia, a stump of iris is always present and is often adherent to the sclera at the

GLAUCOMA

extreme limit of the anterior chamber for a considerable part of the circumference; the development of the ligamentum pectinatum is faulty; part of the angle is usually open, and through this precarious filtration is carried on, until some accident reduces the available area for filtration below the necessary minimum, and so precipitates an attack of high tension (J. H. Parsons). Such cases are obviously more closely allied to buphthalmos than to secondary glaucoma in the ordinary acceptation of the term.

(10) **Intra-ocular Tumours.**—We shall take these regionally.

(i.) *Tumours of the iris* may cause secondary glaucoma

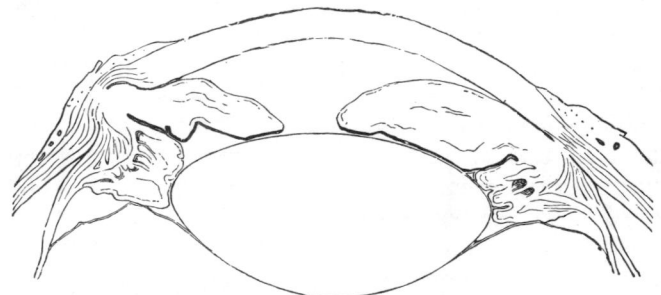

FIG. 137.—Tumour of iris and ciliary body. (Priestley Smith.)
Secondary glaucoma. Filtration angle closed.

in one of two ways: (*a*) owing to their increased bulk they may effectually close the filtration angle (Fig. 137) in a purely mechanical way; (*b*) masses of cells may be carried from the growth by the current of aqueous into the angle of the chamber, and find their way into the spaces of the pectinate ligament and the canal of Schlemm. Here again the first effect is a mechanical obstruction to the filtration of fluid through these important spaces; this action is soon greatly intensified by the proliferation of the tumour cells thus arrested (Fig. 138).

(ii.) *Tumours of the ciliary body.*—These act in the main similarly to the iris growths; but they are less favourably situated for causing direct obstruction, and consequently the onset of glaucoma is delayed. Like the choroidal

SECONDARY GLAUCOMA

tumours, they give rise to retinal detachment, but this too tends to be late in appearance.

(iii.) *Tumours of the choroid.*—Priestley Smith has laid down the following rules : " Eyes which contain tumours usually become glaucomatous if excision be long delayed. If the eye be excised while the tension is still normal, the filtration angle will be found open. If it be excised after high tension has come on, the filtration angle will be found closed. I have found no exception to this rule." Brailey's experience has confirmed this finding. The onset of the

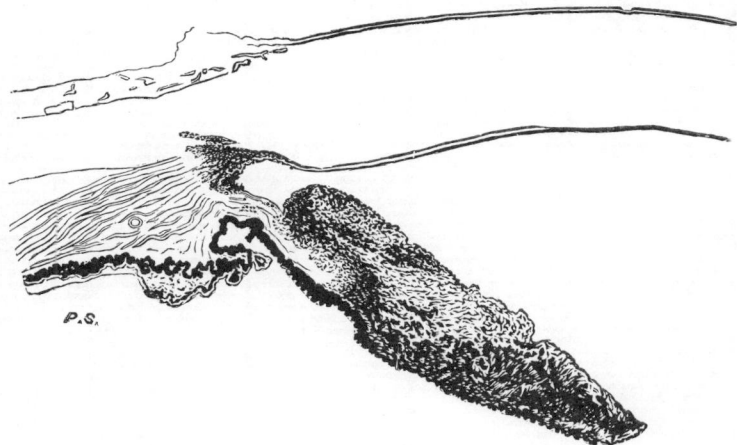

FIG. 138.—Tumour of iris. (Priestley Smith.)
No glaucoma. Filtration angle open, but infiltrated with cells from tumour.

increase of tension is contemporaneous with the displacement of the lens and iris towards the cornea. This is not due to the push of the tumour, for it may occur whilst the growth is still limited to the back of the eye (Fig. 139). It is really caused by a general overfulness of the posterior segment of the globe. The growth of the tumour gives rise to the pouring out of fluid serum from the choroid, either by compressing the choroidal veins, or in some other ill-understood way. The retina is consequently detached, but so long as any of the vitreous fluid remains, the space taken up by the growth and by the subretinal fluid is

378 GLAUCOMA

compensated for by the loss of a corresponding amount of this fluid from the vitreous body. When the retina has become totally detached and folded tightly on itself, this

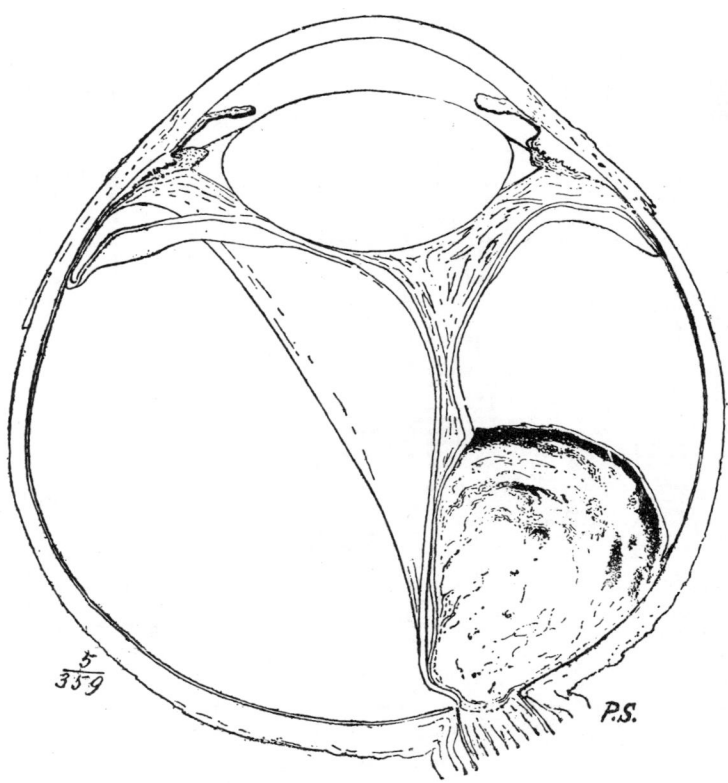

FIG. 139.—Sarcoma of choroid. (Priestley Smith.)

Secondary glaucoma. Filtration angle closed. Tumour limited to posterior half of eye. Retina totally detached. Vitreous only represented by its fibrous stroma. First diagnosed as simple detachment of retina. Acute glaucoma with very shallow anterior chamber seventeen months later. Excised on the eighth day.

means of compensation is lost, since no vitreous fluid now remains. Any further increase of the volume in the posterior segment of the eye can now only take place by the pushing forward of the diaphragm composed of ciliary body, suspensory ligament, lens, and iris. The anterior chamber is thus shallowed, the filtration angle is closed, and the reign of secondary glaucoma begins. Some pathologists have laid stress on the rôle of the deposit of leucocytes, pigment, etc. in the angle of the chamber in these cases ; others are doubtful whether this fact is of any importance ; amongst such is Weidler, who also hesitates to accept pressure on the vasa vorticosa as a factor in the production of glaucoma. Both he and Greeves have independently suggested that the closure of the filtration angle found in some cases of intra-ocular growth may be due to an inflammatory action. The latter writer suggests that possibly the inflammation is set up by some mildly toxic substances secreted by the growing organisms.

The increase of tension associated with sarcoma of the uveal tract may be so great as to give rise to a central rupture of the cornea, accompanied by free hæmorrhage ; the tumour may then easily be overlooked, the case being taken for one of hæmorrhagic glaucoma.

(iv.) *Glioma of the retina* acts in the same way as sarcoma of the choroid, so far as the production of secondary glaucoma is concerned. " Additional factors are found in the greater concentration of the aqueous, the presence of glioma cells in the angle, involvement of the iris," etc. (Parsons.)

(11) **Detachment of the Retina.**—This condition is usually associated with hypotony, but hypertony in its stead may be encountered. E. Nordensen found it in 6 out of 126 eyes suffering from spontaneous detachment of the membrane. In one case there was *l'iris bombé* ; in 3 irido-cyclitis with a deep anterior chamber ; and in 2 the cause was not stated. Priestley Smith says that the onset of glaucoma in such cases is associated with an extension of inflammation from the choroid to the anterior part of the uveal tract, and adds that the onset of secondary glaucoma is determined by the formation of posterior synechia, or by a change in the constitution of the aqueous, whereby it becomes unduly albuminous. The association of secondary glaucoma with detachment of the retina should

always raise a strong suspicion of the presence of intraocular new-growth. N. C. Keukenschryver maintains that high tension following idiopathic detachment of the retina is not so rare as it is usually thought to be, and reports five cases from Straub's clinic in support of this contention. Some of the detachments followed high myopia. In all, the detachment of the retina was complete and the angle of the chamber was closed. He believes that the retinal degeneration sets free irritant substances, which give rise to chronic inflammation in various parts of the eye, and amongst others in the structures surrounding the angle of the chamber; there is thus caused an obstruction to the free escape of fluid from the globe. The analogy between these observations and those of Greeves and Weidler, discussed under the subject of tumours of the choroid, is suggestive and merits attention. The writer has within the last few years been forced to enucleate two eyeballs under circumstances closely similar to those described by Keukenschryver, in old people with high myopia. No evidence whatever of new-growth was found either clinically or anatomically.

(12) **Thrombosis of the Central Retinal Vein.**—For most of our knowledge on this subject, we are indebted to George Coats. He pointed out that the glaucoma, which follows obstruction of the central vein, cannot be due merely to heightened intravenous pressure, or to the pouring out of a large and abnormal exudate into the vitreous, as a consequence of venous obstruction; for it does not commence to manifest itself, until from seven to nine weeks after the blockage has taken place. He thought, with Inouye, that the gradual disintegration of the blood at the back of the globe gives rise to the formation of low-grade toxins, which accumulate at the angle of the chamber, and on the surface of the iris, and there produce a quiet inflammation, which seals up the excretory channels of the eye. It would appear then that the thrombotic type of glaucoma possesses a very distinct inflammatory element; it thus comes into line with the hypertonus which we find secondary to detachment of the retina, or to intra-

ocular tumours, and which we have already dealt with. Indeed, thrombosis cases present an almost unique combination of profuse hæmorrhage, imperfect drainage, and liability to recurrences over a long period. In connection with this subject, it is of interest to recall L. Schreiber's observation that the injection of blood into the vitreous of rabbits produces remarkable changes, associated with the growth of a new formation of connective tissue ; he speaks of " the toxic action of hæmoglobin iron."

Parsons states that the presence of blood in the vitreous increases the tendency to the onset of secondary glaucoma, but that the complication may certainly occur without any trace of vitreous hæmorrhage being discoverable.

From the clinical point of view, it is well to remember that the instillation of atropin is dangerous in these cases, and that it has been followed immediately by the onset of hypertonus.

Kuemmell, from the statistics of 113 cases, found that the second eye became involved in 20 per cent. of them. This fact should make one hesitate to propose enucleation, so long as any sight whatever remains to the eye.

Mayou has drawn attention to " the occurrence of new vessels on the iris in cases of thrombosis of the central vein." He considers that " the importance of these vessels from a clinical point of view is that when associated with glaucoma, they are pathognomonic of this condition. In no case of thrombosis without some increase of tension, have new vessels been noted on the iris, and the earliest period at which new vessels were present after the onset of glaucoma was three days." On the other hand, he has found the vessels very constantly when the two conditions have been associated. Holmes Spicer noted such vessels many years previously, but was inclined to attribute them in part to the action of the eserin used to reduce the tension.

Mayou notes that the following conditions have been found associated with this form of glaucoma : old injury, uveitis, albuminuria, and detachment of the retina. He states that " the onset of glaucoma after thrombosis varied between five days and one year " in the cases of which he had notes ; and further, that " sub-choroidal hæmorrhage frequently followed iridectomy, and in the cases which were trephined, the trephine hole became subsequently blocked by exudation."

(13) **Intra-ocular Hæmorrhage.**—This may come from the retinal vessels and be poured into the vitreous ; it is then usually venous, and need not necessarily give rise to glaucoma, although there is always the danger that it may do so. More commonly the hæmorrhage is sub-choroidal, and in that case the retina and choroid are pushed forwards in front of the effusion of blood. The consequences of this are twofold : (1) The intra-ocular pressure is rapidly raised by the sudden increase of the ocular contents, which there is no time to make accommodation for by absorption of vitreous fluid, and (2) the angle of the anterior chamber is directly closed by the pressure from behind. Filtration is abruptly stopped and acute glaucoma supervenes. A blow, and not necessarily a very severe one, on an old blind eye may give rise to such a hæmorrhage, the source of which is arterial. The eye, which beforehand was probably quite soft, quickly becomes very hard and extremely painful, and owing to the excretory channels having long before become blocked, there is little chance of things righting themselves, except after a long and painful delay.

(14) **Irido-cyclitis.**—We have had occasion under some of our previous headings to refer to the influence of inflammation of the iris and ciliary body in producing a secondary rise in intra-ocular pressure, and have taken the opportunity to point out that two factors are probably operative in such an action, viz., (*a*) an alteration in the character of the aqueous, and (*b*) the blockage of the filtering angle by inflammatory cells, and other debris. We pointed out that, under such conditions, the irido-cyclitis may be, and often is, only a subsidiary factor. On the other hand, cases are met with in which this inflammation is, as far as can be seen, the one and only cause of the secondary glaucoma. Nay, more ! the irido-cyclitis

may sometimes be so ill-marked that the glaucoma may erroneously be thought to be of primary origin. Indeed some of these cases form the most subtle connecting links between primary and secondary glaucoma, and force on our minds the suggestion that much of what we accept as of the former kind may in reality be of the latter. Priestley Smith has put forward the view that, in some of these cases, the first event is a choroiditis, which gradually spreads forwards to the anterior part of the uveal tract, the exudation from the inflamed choroid into the vitreous acting as the intermediate step in the process.

The discussion on this subject would be very incomplete without a reference to the form of glaucoma which we meet with in connection with influenza, herpes zoster ophthalmicus, and other diseases which are the results of germ invasions. This subject has already been discussed in Chapter III. Part IV., and it has there been pointed out that the most probable explanation is that a low-grade irido-cyclitis is responsible for the glaucoma. Lloyd and other American surgeons have suggested that syphilis gives rise to a similar condition. This, according to them, would likewise account for those cases in which—usually in young adults—an at first apparently successful trephining ends in failure, owing to the slow closing up of the trephine hole. They urge that iodine should be freely exhibited in such patients. The author believes their contention to be correct, always with the proviso, which they themselves would freely admit, that syphilis is only one of the possible causes of this fortunately rare complication in the convalescence of our trephine cases. Tubercle, gonorrhœa, dental sepsis, or any other form of auto-intoxication may have an exactly similar effect.

This question of self-poisoning has come up in other chapters of this book. Theoretically we understand it well enough, but clinically and practically we are often at sea in the application of the principles involved to the treatment of the individual patient.

Nor do the mysteries which enwrap these cases cease with the consideration of their pathology, for, as we shall see when we come to the section on treatment, there is no class of glaucomatous eyes which calls for more individualism, more judgment, and more experience in their handling than do these.

REFERENCES

BLACK, M.—*Amer. Journ. Ophth.*, 1918, vol. i. p. 87.
BRAILEY, W. H.—*R.L.O.H. Reports*, vol. x. p. 281.
BOWMAN, SIR W.—*Ibid.*, 1865.
COATS, GEORGE—*Ibid.*, vol. xix. p. 45.
COLLINS, E. T.—*Ibid.*, 1888, vol. xii.; 1905, vol. xvi.; *Trans. O.S. of U.K.*, 1890, vol. x.; 1914, vol. xxxiv.; *Researches*, London, 1896.
ELLIOT, R. H.—*The Indian Operation of Couching for Cataract*, H. K. Lewis & Co. Ltd., London, 1917.
FEINGOLD, M.—*Amer. Journ. Ophth.*, 1918, vol. i. p. 87.
GIFFORD, H.—*Ibid.*, October 1900, and 1918, vol. i. pp. 83 and 86.
GREEVES, A.—*Roy. Soc. Med.* (Section on Ophth.), May 8, 1914.
HEGNER, C. A.—*Klin. Monatsbl. f. Augenh.*, vol. lv.
HUDSON, A. C.—*R.L.O.H. Reports*, vol. xviii. part ii.
JACKSON, ED.—*Amer. Journ. Ophth.*, 1918, vol. i.
KEUKENSCHRYVER, N. C.—" Doctorate Thesis," *Ophthalmology*, Amsterdam, April 1916, p. 533.
KIRKPATRICK, H.—Personal communication.
KUEMMELL, R.—Graefe's *Archiv f. O.*, 1909, vol. lxxii. p. 86.
MAYOU, M. S.—*Brit. Journ. Ophth.*, 1918, vol. ii. p. 521.
MELLER AND FUCHS.—*Archiv f. O.*, 1901, vol. li. part iii.
MINOR, J. J.—*New York Med. Journ.*, 1881, p. 194.
MITVALSKY.—*Centrbl. f. p. Augenh.*, October 1892, p. 297.
NATANSON, A. N.—*Ueber Glaucom in Aphakischen Augen*, Dorpat, 1889.
NORDENSEN, E.—*Die Netzhautablosung*, Wiesbaden.
PARSONS, J. H.—*Pathology of the Eye*, vol. iii. p. 1087.
REUSS—*Centrbl. f. p. Augenh.*, February 1900, p. 39.
SALUS, R.—*Klin. Monatsbl. f. Augenh.*, August 1910, p. 167.
SCHREIBER, L.—*Thirty-ninth Ophth. Congress*, Heidelberg, p. 348.
SCHWENK, P. N. K.—*Ophth. Rec.*, 1917, vol. xxvi., No. 9, p. 465.
SMITH, PRIESTLEY.—*Glaucoma*, J. & A. Churchill, London, 1891.
SPICER, W. T. H.—*Trans. O.S. of U.K.*, 1902, vol. xxii. p. 306.
STRAUB, M.—*Brit. Journ. Ophth.*, 1920, vol. iv. p. 195.
TACKE, D.—*Bull. de la Soc. Belge d'opht.*, No. 29, p. 193.
VERREY, L.—*La Clinique d'ophtal.*, April 1916; and *Annals of Ophth.*, October 1916, p. 802.

Part III

The Treatment of Secondary Glaucoma

In all cases of secondary glaucoma, in which the causative or primary disease can be recognised, it is of the first importance to attack the latter with energy and judgment. Whilst we must not lose sight of the need for symptomatic treatment, we must, above all else, focus our attention on the root-cause of the condition. For the sake of simplicity, we shall take in turn the various conditions which we have discussed in the preceding part of this chapter, and point out the main indications for the treatment of each.

Perforation of the Cornea with Entanglement of the Iris in the Scar :—*Prophylaxis.*—Much can be done in the early stages to prevent the impaction of the iris in such wounds. Still later, the performance of an iridectomy may be of great service by lessening the drag on the imprisoned iris. Sometimes the division of the synechia, followed by the energetic use of a meiotic or mydriatic, according to the exigencies of the individual case, may prove beneficial. It must, however, be borne in mind that the synechial attachments are very prone to re-form, and the operation may leave the patient worse than before. This danger is intensified, if in the first instance the impaction of the iris was accompanied by the manifestations of septic infection ; the relighting of such sepsis by surgical interference is very likely to occur.

The treatment of established glaucoma.—In these cases the hypertension is commonly associated with evidence of ocular congestion. The latter should be energetically combated by the aid of the usual means which will be discussed more fully under the heading of " irido-cyclitis." At the same time the question of performing an iridectomy or a filtering operation should be considered. If it is thought that the drag on the iris is of such a nature that it can be relieved by the former operation, a large piece of iris should be removed. If a trephining or other filtration-scar operation is undertaken, it must be borne in mind that it may have to be repeated more than once before a final satisfactory result is gained, a little progress being made each time.

Annular Posterior Synechia.—In these cases there are two objects before the surgeon, viz., (i.) the relief of tension, and (ii.) the provision of an artificial pupil for visual purposes. For the former purpose only a very small iridectomy is required; indeed an iridotomy will often suffice, for if it is performed aseptically, and does not light up old mischief, the slit or puncture in the iris, bathed by sterile aqueous fluid, may remain indefinitely unhealed, and so provide the necessary channel of communication between the posterior and anterior divisions of the aqueous chamber, which had become blocked by the closure of the pupil. For visual purposes a free portion of iris requires removal, and the most favourable direction must be selected, regard being had not merely to the direction in which we should ordinarily prefer to make our coloboma, but also to the nature and direction of the adhesions present. The object the surgeon keeps before him is, of course, to relieve tension and, at the same time, to save some remnant of vision. The acuteness of central vision and the projection of light before operation will advertise him of the amount he may expect from his procedure. It will sometimes happen that after operation a permanent lowering of intra-ocular pressure takes place, showing that the ciliary body is no longer normally active; in such cases the retina may be found to be detached.

Dislocation of the Lens into the Anterior Chamber.—The advisability of undertaking to extract the lens depends very largely on the exact conditions present. Small lenses or lens nuclei, which readily pass backwards and forwards through the pupil, are best left alone, unless by their impaction in the angle of the chamber they have definitely set up glaucoma. The reason for this advice is that such masses slip back very readily into the posterior chamber of the eye, when the patient is lying on his back, and especially under manipulative interference. If it is thought necessary to remove them, eserin solution should be instilled beforehand, and, as a first step, a needle should be thrust through the limbus to impale and fix the lens during the operation. Larger lenses should usually be removed; for, apart from the danger of secondary glaucoma, they interfere greatly with vision. Strong meiosis should be produced beforehand, and a vectis should be kept ready to scoop out the mass, should it fall back into the hyaloid cavity. It is important to delay the action of the meiotic until just before the operation, as the tightening up of the iris behind the lens has been known to precipitate an attack of glaucoma in an eye which, up to that time, had shown no sign of hypertension. It is to be borne in mind that the removal of a dislocated lens is always a hazardous procedure. Hegner relates that in Stock's clinic, extraction was attempted in 13 out of 16 cases of anterior dislocation. The eye was lost in 5, and useful vision attained only in 3; in one an expulsive hæmorrhage occurred; the principal danger lay " in the almost certain loss of vitreous." The author's experience of removal of anteriorly dislocated lenses has been decidedly less unfavourable than this, but he agrees with the main proposition that the operation is fraught with danger, and should not be lightly undertaken.

Lateral Dislocation of the Lens.—A lens, dislocated laterally, should very rarely be interfered with, save for the relief of secondary glaucoma. In Hegner's experience, the extraction of partially dislocated lenses is very dangerous, and in many cases entails the complete loss of the eye. Only in one out of eight extractions did he find good vision obtained; he ascribes the prevalence of failure to the damage done to the vitreous body and to the suspensory ligament at the time of the dislocation. His dictum will be widely endorsed. Trephining probably offers the best chance of arresting the glaucomatous condition, once it declares itself.

Posterior Dislocation of the Lens.—What has been said of lateral dislocation is even truer of posterior dislocation. Interference with the lens whilst it is floating freely in the vitreous is very hazardous. On the other hand, provided that there is no external wound, or that such wound as there was has remained sterile, the danger of secondary glaucoma is not great at all. It is the tied down lenses that produce secondary glaucoma, and these are the products of septic action ; to interfere in such cases is to ask for trouble, whether we do so whilst the lens is still floating, or after it has become fixed. Enucleation is then probably the only sound course open to us. To establish a satisfactory filtration scar, when the aqueous and vitreous chambers are practically one, is in most cases an impossibility.

Wounds of the Lens.—It has been pointed out that wounds of the lens may bring about secondary glaucoma in two distinct ways : (i.) Disintegrated lens masses may find their way into the anterior chamber and mechanically block the filtration angle of the eye ; and (ii.) the swelling of the lens may thrust the iris base forward and so directly close the sinus of the chamber. It matters not whether one, or both of these conditions is present, the indication for the removal of the lens is plain. The exact method adopted will depend on the age of the patient and on the idiosyncrasies of the surgeon.

When the secondary glaucoma is due to occlusion of the pupil by lens matter an iridectomy should be performed without delay, the lens being evacuated, if necessary.

Intumescent Cataract.—The author can claim to have had some experience of the treatment of this form of glaucoma, having operated for it on several hundred occasions, and having tried many procedures for its relief. He found that the best method of treatment was to perform a preliminary iridectomy, and to delay the extraction of the cataract until the eye had quieted down. These cases are so acute that it is not justifiable to put off the preliminary operation, but any necessary period, which the patient spends in hospital before he can be brought on the table, may be profitably spent in producing firm meiosis, in leeching the margins of the orbit, in purgation, and in the exhibition of morphia. Should the chamber prove to be extremely shallow, a preliminary posterior sclerotomy performed ten to fifteen minutes beforehand will often materially deepen it and make the iridectomy easier and safer. This little addition to the procedure has always appeared to be free from risk. Should the surgeon be unfortunate enough to wound the cataract during the iridectomy, he must enlarge his incision and complete the extraction at once. His results in such a case will sometimes prove far better than his expectations. At the same time, the method which has been recommended is much the safest one to adopt. Owing to the rarity with which this condition occurs in Europe the literature is very scanty, but Frenkel and Rosenfeld have both followed a line of practice almost identical with that mapped out above.

Glaucoma following the Spontaneous Absorption of Senile Cataract.—It is obvious that the main indication is to prevent the occurrence of such cases by operating upon senile cataracts as soon as they reach maturity. There is a school of surgeons who believe that when one eye has been successfully operated on for cataract, the second may well be left alone unless and until something goes wrong with the first one. Again, there are those who hold that a cataract in one eye may well remain unoperated indefinitely, so long as the second eye has useful vision. The writer has never agreed with either of the above views, and is more strongly than ever confirmed in his opinion that the most favourable time for extraction of a cataract is as soon as it reaches maturity. This confirmation has been largely derived from the recent writings of American surgeons on the class of cases that fall under the present section.

What is to be done when glaucoma has actually presented itself ? In some of the cases in which signs of iridocyclitis have been present, atropin has proved far more serviceable than meiotics. In several instances the extraction of the cataract has proved successful, not merely in arresting the glaucoma, but also in restoring some measure of vision. In the event of the dislocation of a small lens nucleus into the anterior chamber, the obvious indication is for its early removal.

Secondary Glaucoma following Cataract Extraction.—The treatment indicated will vary with the nature of the pathological condition present.

Anterior synechia of capsule or iris.—Treacher Collins has pointed out that corneal sections are more dangerous than sclero-corneal ones in the above-named operation, for if a capsular synechia forms, the advancement of the capsule and iris is more pronounced in proportion as the incision is placed more anteriorly. Again, when needling for after-cataract, the needle should be introduced at the limbus and not through the cornea, and always if possible at a distance from any existing capsular synechia. The reason for insistence on these precautions is that a capsular synechia may easily be advanced as a result of its continuity with the wound made by the needle, and the onset of glaucoma may thus be determined.

Some surgeons advocate the division of capsular synechiæ by the use of Lang's knives or of some form of needle with cutting edges. The free exhibition of atropin helps to draw the capsule away from the site of its previous attachment. Although good results may sometimes be obtained in this way, it must be confessed that many surgeons have shared the disappointment expressed by A. Knapp in the results of such attempts.

When the glaucoma is due to the impaction of iris in the wound, a good result may be obtained by performing a free iridectomy in the neighbourhood of this impaction, and thereby relieving the iris of the pull upon it. If the glaucoma comes on within the first few days after operation, it is enough to reopen the section and to replace the impacted pillar of the iris, as was done by Posey.

It has been pointed out by various surgeons, that the best method of dealing with the secondary glaucoma which follows cataract extraction, is to prevent its occurrence by a very careful toilet of the wound at the time of operation. Though this is undoubtedly a sound position to take up, the value of such methods is to some extent discounted by the fact, that no matter how carefully we free the lips of the wound of iris or capsule at the close of the operation, one, or other, or both structures may be washed into them under the influence of the subsequent movements of the lids.

Interference with the integrity of the vitreous body is usually the result of the laceration of an after-cataract. Before we discuss the treatment, it is necessary to remind the reader of what has already been said in the previous part of this chapter : Interference with the vitreous body may lead to secondary glaucoma (i.) owing to the presence in the anterior chamber of liquid vitreous, which cannot pass through the filtration angle ; (ii.) owing to the presence of streamers of consistent vitreous, which while remaining attached proximally to the hyaloid body whence they sprang, are sufficiently long to reach into and mechanically block the sinus of the chamber ; (iii.) owing to the pushing forward of the base of the iris, as a result of the rupture of the anterior hyaloid membrane permitting the advance of the front segment of the vitreous, which thus directly closes the sinus of the chamber by pressure from behind ; and (iv.) owing to the bulging vitreous mass contracting adhesions to the margins of the pupil and thus serving to obstruct the flow of fluid forwards from the vitreous to the aqueous chamber.

It will be clear that the treatment called for will vary in each of the above conditions ; thus in the first case, the symptoms may be relieved by tapping the aqueous chamber, whilst in the second the use of eserin, by constricting the pupil, will mechanically draw away the vitreous streamers from the neighbourhood of the angle, owing to their attachments being situate in the vitreous body ; the mechanism of this action is shown in the accompanying diagram (Fig. 140). In the third case nothing short of a filtration operation is likely to be of any use ; whilst in the fourth the indication is for the laceration of the occluding membrane, and the subsequent use of atropin. Unfortunately we cannot always tell in advance the exact cause of the secondary rise in tension, and must therefore lay down certain general lines for our guidance in all cases : If the anterior chamber is deep, and the iris lies flat, we should use meiotics combined with hot fomentations. If these means fail, and especially if vitreous masses can be detected in the anterior chamber, paracentesis should be performed. If the pupil can be seen to be contracted around a bulging mass of vitreous, and if *l'iris bombé* is present, discission of the membrane followed by the use of mydriatics is indicated. Failing success by any of the previous methods, a filtration operation should be performed. For much of the know-

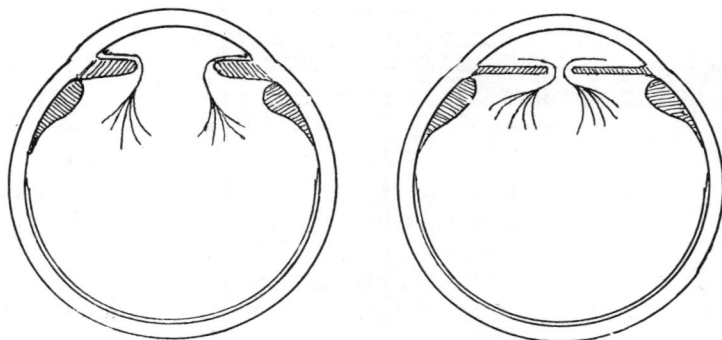

Fig. 140.—To show the mechanism whereby a contraction of the pupil draws on streamers of vitreous which are projecting through a dilated pupil and blocking the angle of the chamber.

The pull of the iris effectively clears the angle of the chamber of the fibrils of vitreous, for the latter are tethered in the posterior chamber and lie loose in the anterior chamber.

ledge summarised above we are indebted to A. C. Hudson, whose original paper will repay careful perusal.

The formation of an impermeable diaphragm, at a late stage, across the front of an eye, as described by Priestley Smith, can sometimes be met by the free laceration of the offending membrane. The communication between the aqueous and vitreous chambers is thus reopened.

The treatment of *annular posterior synechia* following cataract extraction does not differ materially from that of the same condition met with whilst the lens is still present; this has already been discussed. Nor need we delay further over the management of cases in which the glaucoma is secondary to the presence of *irido-cyclitis*, for this subject will receive attention shortly under a section of its own. As to *epithelial cyst of the anterior chamber* producing secondary glaucoma, our only remedy is the removal of the eye.

Our treatment of the subject would be incomplete without a reference to the recent work by [Lloyd (of Brooklyn): In cases of post-operative glaucoma following cataract extraction he has found that, where all other means fail, trephining may prove of great value, but he would add " a caution to avoid trephining over the coloboma of an iridectomy, especially when there is evidence that the vitreous body is pushed forward through this opening, or where there is reason to think that it may be so pushed forward; otherwise the opening made by the trephine may be blocked by vitreous." He adds: " Trephine where the anterior chamber is deepest, and where sound iris can hold back the mass of vitreous, and so allow the aqueous to escape through the opening provided." In support of this suggestion he has published one very interesting, illustrative case of his own and has kindly furnished the author with the notes of two other cases in each of which a suitably placed trephining saved the eye when iridectomy, iridotomy and needling had all failed to do so.

In this connection, he makes the valuable suggestion " that an elevated tension is not infrequently the cause of delayed union after cataract extraction." Again, in another communication he says: " It is probable that in the future, cases which have been classed as delayed union and cystoid wound (after extraction) may find their way into the glaucoma group." These thoughtful views are well worthy of our very serious consideration.

Secondary Glaucoma following Iridectomy.—If the anterior chamber is very shallow, the danger of damaging the lens, when operating for glaucoma, is correspondingly great. Under these circumstances, the obvious indication is to select a method of procedure which carries a minimum of risk of this accident. The author's own preference is for sclero-corneal trephining, but if iridectomy or any similar procedure is decided on, it is well to deepen the chamber by means of a posterior sclerotomy before introducing any sharp-pointed instrument through the limbus.

When glaucoma returns after the failure of an iridectomy, owing to blockage of the angle of the chamber by one factor or another, a sclero-corneal trephining is obviously indicated ; but the surgeon must remember that the condition is then, at the best, a desperate one.

Aniridia.—It has been pointed out that cases of congenital aniridia have analogies with those of buphthalmos. It is obvious that nothing short of an operation designed to produce a filtering scar is of any use under such circumstances.

Intra-ocular Tumours.—The treatment of these is in most cases simple and obvious, viz., the removal of the eye. The surgeon should not forget the possibility of syphilis and tubercle as factors in the production of such growths. He should also learn to regard with suspicion every eye showing a detachment of the retina which does not admit of some simple explanation, and he must not be caught off his guard over cases which at first sight appear to be quite straightforward. The consequences of a failure to detect and remove a malignant tumour are so serious, both for the patient and the surgeon, as to demand the exercise of incessant vigilance.

In excising an eye for new-growth, it is always desirable to meet the contingency that the optic nerve may be involved, and it is therefore well to remove some length of the latter structure. This can, invariably, be very easily done by using the author's optico-ciliary neurectomy hook, described in his book on *Tropical Ophthalmology*. Although such a precaution is often needless, it is so easily taken that it seems a pity ever to omit it.

Detachment of the Retina.—We have referred to the somewhat rare cases in which a simple detachment of the retina is followed by secondary glaucoma. The use of transillumination, and the employment of diagnostic puncture, if necessary, will often settle the diagnosis ; but if any lingering doubt remains, it is better to enucleate without delay. We are fortified in such a course by the knowledge that the eye is useless in any case ; whilst, on the other hand, the coincidence of retinal detachment with increase of the intra-ocular pressure is always suspicious of the presence of growth.

Thrombosis of the Central Retinal Vein.—There is a deep-rooted prejudice against any operative procedure for the relief of glaucoma attended with retinal hæmorrhages. This is undoubtedly due to the fact, that the operation of iridectomy in such cases has sometimes been followed immediately by extensive hæmorrhage and blindness. On the other hand, a search through the literature of the subject will show that the experience of surgeons with this operation has often been astonishingly good ; whilst, since the introduction of sclero-corneal trephining, the confidence in the efficacy of the latter procedure amongst those who have used it, has steadily increased. Wendell Reber and others have laid stress on the fact, that the comparatively slow reduction of pressure is an important point in favour of the use of the trephine in this class of case, and have urged the employment of that instrument.

Much of the uncertainty that clouds the prognosis of operations for hæmorrhagic glaucoma is undoubtedly due to a confusion as to the causes of the condition. For instance, when these hæmorrhages are the result of diseases of the retinal vessels, much must depend on the cause of such diseases and on the manner in which the surgeon diagnoses that cause and applies suitable treatment.

Again, when the bleeding is taking place from a malignant new-growth within the eye, it is obvious that nothing short of prompt enucleation is likely to be of the least value.

Intra-ocular Hæmorrhage, when severe in character, almost certainly demands the removal of the eye. Trephining may first be attempted as a forlorn hope, if the patient is very reluctant to part with the globe, but it is not likely to be of much service.

Irido-cyclitis.—The congestive forms of glaucoma may

sometimes be associated, not merely with congestion of the iris and ciliary body, but also with a definite inflammation of those parts. Indeed, it is often very difficult to say where congestion ends and inflammation begins. The interest of these observations, from the point of view of treatment, is twofold, for (i.) it calls for active antiphlogistic treatment of all congested or inflamed eyes, and (ii.) it shows the need for the most accurate diagnosis possible, since it is obvious that to treat one of these cases successfully, one must have a clear idea as to any causal relationship existing between the glaucoma and the antecedent inflammation, if such has existed. We shall now take these subjects up at greater length :

A glaucomatous eye, showing signs of congestion, should always be actively treated. The patient is put to bed ; morphin is administered for the relief of pain ; active purgation is induced ; the brow and temple are freely leeched ; hot fomentations are applied at frequent intervals ; the room is darkened, and everything possible is done to keep the patient quiet.

So far we are on firm ground, but our difficulties begin when we endeavour to decide whether to use meiotics or mydriatics in a case in which marked signs of iritis are present. We are then between Scylla and Charybdis. Eserin, which is so valuable to us in the treatment of the congestive attacks of primary glaucoma, may prove the worst possible drug in the hypertension which follows an irido-cyclitis, whilst the use of atropin may close the last struggling remnant of the filtration area, and so precipitate a most unfortunate exacerbation of the glaucomatous condition. The result is that many surgeons rely on the antiphlogistic methods we have outlined above, and if they use any drops at all, confine themselves to calling in the aid of dionin.

We have dealt with this subject at some length in the chapter on Ætiology (pp. 144 to 146), and the reader is asked, as a preliminary step, to consider carefully what has there been written. It would, however, be a mistake to suppose that the diseases discussed—influenza, epidemic dropsy, and herpes zoster—are the only, or possibly even the leading, causes of an irido-cyclitis, which may give rise to a secondary rise in tension. Such an assumption would be highly incorrect. We know that a large number of bacterial invasions and of other diseases, caused by less well-known organisms, may be complicated by the presence of irido-cyclitis. To cite only a few of these—syphilis, gonorrhœa, dysentery, tubercle, and leprosy are cases in point. We ask ourselves the question : Why should an irido-cyclitis, the result of the same organism, in one case cause hypertension, in another hypotension, and in a third do neither the one nor the other ? Our inability to furnish a full answer shows us how ignorant we really are, and how tentative must be our deductions as to the correct pathology, and our proposals for the alleviation of the disease. This, however, would be a poor argument against going as far as we can in the light of our present knowledge. Certain practical suggestions may therefore be put forward :

(1) The presence of deposits on the back of the cornea in connection with signs and symptoms of glaucoma, is an almost certain indication that the rise in tension is secondary. This point was insisted on in the American Ophthalmological Society's discussion on ophthalmic zoster (1919). The value of the corneal microscope in such cases cannot be too strongly insisted upon. The author cannot refrain from an expression of surprise at the rarity with which this instrument is used, either in institutions or in private consulting rooms. The introduction of the Gullstrand lamp, as an accessory to the corneal microscope (Fig. 45), has added greatly to the precision of our methods. No hospital and no consulting room is completely furnished without the inclusion of this valuable combination of apparatus. (For details, see references under Gradle.)

(2) The use of mydriatics in place of meiotics, is suggested, if it is not demanded, whenever there is clear evidence of the presence of irido-cyclitis in association with glaucoma. If the surgeon decides to use atropin, he must do it boldly and freely, but he should never take such a course unless he is both ready and able to fall back on

surgical means without any delay, if the exhibition of this drug should result in an increase, instead of in a decrease of the acuteness of the symptoms present. Some would then advocate paracentesis of the anterior chamber; the author finds its results too short-lived, and prefers to perform a sclero-corneal trephining, after which atropin may be freely used, and sometimes with the greatest benefit. A warning is necessary: In consequence of the inflammatory condition present, the trephine hole may close within a few weeks; but, in the meantime, the free mydriasis produced has had the opportunity of arresting the irido-cyclitis, and a second trephining may then be undertaken under much more favourable circumstances. Syphilis and every other possible source of autogenetic poisoning should be sought for and fully dealt with before the second operation is ventured on.

(3) There is another point of interest which deserves mention, and which was brought forward by Lamb during the discussion already referred to. His own words will be given: " I have noted, in connection with increased intra-ocular pressure, not only with herpes, but also with some other conditions of an allied character, that there is a suggestion of what I have called a "funnel-iris." The appearance of depth in the anterior chamber seems to be associated with a narrowing down; and the iris appears to recede toward the pupillary margin. In these cases I have found invariably that I can use a mydriatic without damage. I think they are probably due to an irido-cyclitis." To put Lamb's suggestion in other words, the iris resembles a very widely open funnel, with its apex at the pupil, and its base at the corneal margin. The sign is at least worthy of attention.

Whilst on this subject, it is convenient to discuss Bowman's recommendation that atropin should be used in cases of *l'iris bombé*. It is clear that this is founded on the hope, that in recent cases some part of the ring of attached iris will give way under the strain of a mydriatic, and so re-establish a channel for the passage forward of the aqueous from the posterior to the anterior chamber. The advantage so gained would at the best be only temporary, and it would therefore seem preferable to perform an iridectomy with as little delay as possible. Indeed, as far as the author's experience allows him to decide, there would seem to be one, and only one glaucomatous condition, in which it is justifiable to resort to the use of atropin, apart from the employment of any operative procedure. With this we have dealt above. It is an eventuality which we all fear and which we all hope we may meet as seldom as possible. When it does arise we must take our courage in both hands and act with boldness and decision, feeling that the gravity of the case demands our risking all on a single throw. We shall have done our best, and the result is then in the lap of the gods.

The general prophylactic treatment of those disorders of nutrition, which are believed to be ultimate causes of the onset and progress of the glaucomatous process in many secondary cases, will be dealt with under the chapter on Medical Treatment.

REFERENCES

ELLIOT, R. H.—*Indian Medical Gazette*, 1906, vol. xli. p. 433; *Tropical Ophthalmology*, Oxford Medical Publications, 1920, pp. 373–376.
FRENKEL, H.—*L'Opht. Prov.*, May 1910.
GRADLE, H. S.—" Clinical Observations with the Slit Lamp of Gullstrand," *Amer. Journ. Ophth.*, 1921, vol. iv. p. 427.
KNAPP, A.—*Trans. Amer. Ophth. Soc.*, 1910, vol. xii.
LAMB, R. S.—*Amer. Ophth. Soc. Proc.*, June 1919; and *Amer. Journ. Ophth.*, 1919, vol. ii. pp. 760–763.
LLOYD, R. I.—" Location of Trephine Opening in Glaucoma subsequent to Cataract Operation," *Amer. Journ. Ophth.*, August 1919; and private communications.
REBER, W.—*Ophth. Year Book*, 1914, p. 213.

For references to Black, Bowman, Feingold, Gifford, Hegner, Hudson, Jackson, Mitvalsky, Reuss, Schwenk, and Verrey, see References at end of Part II.

CHAPTER VI

CONGENITAL GLAUCOMA, AND SOME ALLIED CONDITIONS

SUMMARY :—The Nomenclature of the Condition.
  Congenital Glaucoma.
    Signs and Symptoms.
    Clinical Course and Complications.
    Differential Diagnosis.
    Pathological Anatomy.
    Ætiology.
  Experimental Buphthalmos.
  Megalocornea, and Buphthalmos.
  Juvenile Glaucoma.
    Its Relationship to other Forms of the Disease.
    The Types of Glaucoma met with in the Young.
    The Treatment of Buphthalmos and Juvenile Glaucoma.

CONGENITAL glaucoma has figured in ophthalmological literature for nearly one and a half centuries. Excellent reviews of these records of the condition are given by Pyle, Parsons, and others.

Much discussion has taken place as to the best name for the disease. There can, we think, be little dispute that the correct appellation is "congenital glaucoma," for this has not only a definite pathological significance, but it also, with certain limitations, expresses a clinical fact. The matter will be alluded to again later. The principal objection to the term is its clumsiness, and therefore for purposes of convenience, we may speak of the disease as "buphthalmos" or "hydrophthalmos." Of these the former is perhaps the preferable, as it commits us to no theory and has the sanction of very long usage.

To one, who sits down to study the voluminous literature of congenital glaucoma, it comes with something of a shock of surprise to find how widely different are the viewpoints of various writers. It therefore seems necessary, at the very outset, to clarify one's ideas by committing oneself to definitions, which shall be as precise as possible. From birth to advanced senility, no year of life is secure against the attack of one form or another of glaucoma, but surgeons have recognised broad distinctions, which serve to divide the disease into three great groups, viz., (1) congenital glaucoma, (2) juvenile glaucoma, and (3) senile glaucoma. It is easiest, and we think it most expedient, to deal with the poles of life first, and then to group under juvenile glaucoma every case which we cannot include in one or other of the previous classes.

Congenital Glaucoma.—By this we understand glaucoma which is *congenital in origin*. A large percentage of such cases are congenital, not merely in origin, but also in the manifestation of the condition present. The difficulty in their correct classification depends on the following factors : (1) Some parents are unobservant and fail, especially with first babies, to recognise what is obviously an abnormal condition of the eyes, whilst others are reluctant to admit any defect in their offspring. (2) Not a few of the cases require careful inspection and examination for their diagnosis in the earlier stages ; a slight enlargement of the cornea, and a deepening of the chamber may be all that there is to see, and for one reason or another, expert advice may not be called in until months or even years have passed. (3) The congenital defects, which lead to glaucoma, vary enormously in grade ; some are so well marked, that a condition of distension of the eye is pronounced at birth and progresses rapidly in the years that follow it ; in others, the changes may be so ill-defined as to lead only very gradually to the development of the signs and symptoms of glaucoma. Such cases are classified *clinically* as " juvenile glaucoma."

Senile Glaucoma.—When we speak of " senile glaucoma," we understand that form of the disease, which occurs in patients, who are sufficiently advanced in life to have developed those changes, whether anatomical or physiological, which either predispose to, or excite an attack of hypertension in the eye. Senility is, however, a relative term, and there is a deep underlying physiological truth in the saying that "a man is as old as he feels." We know well in our daily experience that one man will present before he is 40 more pronounced stigmata of senility, than another will show at 60. How then can we fix an arbitrary line, where juvenile glaucoma is to cease and senile to begin.? Nor is our problem merely one of the advance of degeneration, for as Priestley Smith has shown, the size and build of the eye and the continuous growth of the lens are determining factors of very great importance.

Juvenile Glaucoma.—Different writers have adopted different standards. Some have considered everything below the age of 35 as juvenile glaucoma, others have taken 40 as their limit. The exact figure we accept matters little, so long as we recognise, that at one pole of life we are dealing with defects of congenital origin, which must at a comparatively early age manifest themselves by glaucomatous symptoms, whilst at the other pole lie a number of cases, the great majority of which are eventually dependent for their genesis on the degenerative and other processes associated with advancing age. Running through the whole, like the web of the texture, is the great factor of the departure of the eye from its anatomical ideal.

If we could judge all cases in the perfect light of full anatomico-pathological knowledge, we could scientifically classify our glaucomas into (1) the congenital, *i.e.*, those due to prenatal defects in the normal development of the excretory passages of the eye ; (2) those in which the degenerative processes, associated with senility, play the leading part ; and (3) those in which the anatomical configuration and development of the eye are such as to pave the way for the onset of glaucoma, with a minimum of assistance from senile degeneration. Unfortunately we have in most cases no means of obtaining such exact knowledge during life ; and on the other hand, it is often a question of the interplay of many factors and not of the evolution of one alone. Thus into the juvenile group, there creep at the one end the slighter congenital cases, and at the other end the more exaggerated instances of structural maldevelopment. The outcome is a confusion, which is rendered worse confounded by the fact, that not one, but many observers have taken a hand in the classification of the cases, and that some, at least, of these have not fully appreciated the difficulties of the task.

It remains then for us, whilst constantly aiming at the attainment of a scientific classification, to bear carefully in mind that the insufficiency of our data too often renders our conclusions open to the suspicion of inaccuracy. To remedy this it is desirable to multiply both clinical and pathological observations, and especially the latter.

Signs and Symptoms of Buphthalmos

Buphthalmos probably always dates from birth, even in so far as its clinical manifestations are concerned, though many of the cases are overlooked in their earlier stages. Gros found in forty-five collected cases, that the condition was noticed at or immediately after birth in 60 per cent. of them, within the first year in 13·3 per cent., from the first to the third year in 17·7 per cent., and later in 8·8 per cent. In dealing with the ætiology and pathology of the question, we shall show reason to believe that buphthalmos is dependent on a defective development of the parts concerned in excretion. It is well known that such defects may be slight or severe. These facts afford a ready explanation of two things, viz., (1) that slight cases of buphthalmos are not always recognised at birth, and (2) that not a few cases of juvenile glaucoma are really buphthalmic (*i.e.*, due to defective development) in origin.

The condition is bilateral in the majority of cases. Gros gave the figure for those affected on both sides at 63·7 per cent. Amongst the unilateral cases neither side is favoured.

The practically unanimous consensus of opinion is that boys are much more frequently affected than girls, thus

404   GLAUCOMA

supporting Gros' figures of 61·2 per cent. in the former and 38·8 per cent. in the latter.

The eye enlarges slowly but steadily, and may attain

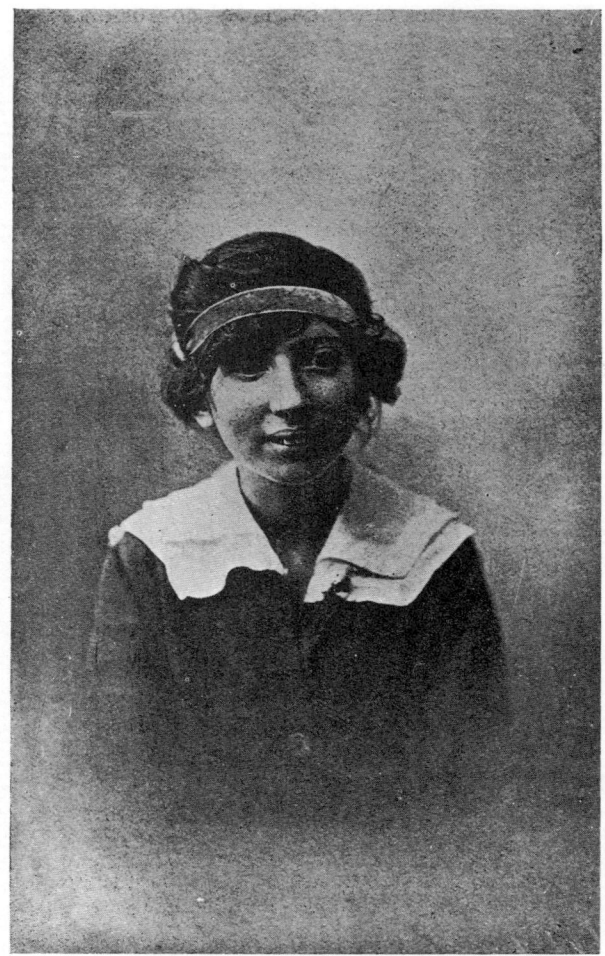

FIG. 141.—Photograph of a young lady (aged 14), suffering from buphthalmos.

Notice that the large corneæ occupy almost the whole of the interpalpebral areas.

CONGENITAL GLAUCOMA

enormous proportions. The most striking feature of the disease is that the whole globe becomes uniformly distended. This is due to the even distensibility of the structures, which is characteristic of childhood. The eye assumes the shape of a much elongated oval, and may fill up all the available space in the orbit, thus leading on the one hand to marked proptosis and on the other to great limitation of ocular movement (Fig. 141).

We may now take the structures seriatim.

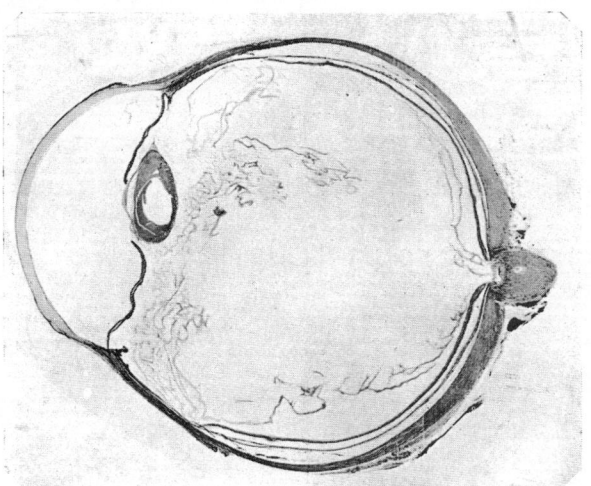

FIG. 142.—Whole section of a buphthalmic eye magnified 2¼ times.

Notice (1) the thinning of the base of the cornea; (2) the large size of the cornea; (3) the stretching of the suspensory ligament; (4) the cupping of the disc; and (5) the enlargement of the eye in all its diameters.

(Photo by E. E. of specimen kindly supplied by Mr. Treacher Collins.)

The Cornea.—No feature of this disease is more striking than that of the enlargement of the corneal base. It is this, combined with the general enlargement of the globe, which has earned for the condition the title of buphthalmos or ox-eye. The cornea appears hemispherical or globular, the anterior chamber being thereby very greatly deepened (Fig. 142). Some idea of the deformity produced may be gathered from the fact that measurements of corneal diameters of over 23 mm. are on record, and that a maximum depth of the chamber of 12·8 mm. as against a normal 2·6 mm. has been observed (Parsons). In association with the increase in the corneal diameter, there is a marked flattening in curvature.

The cornea may be clear and lustrous, or may be the seat of various forms of opacity ; thus (1) it may be steamy

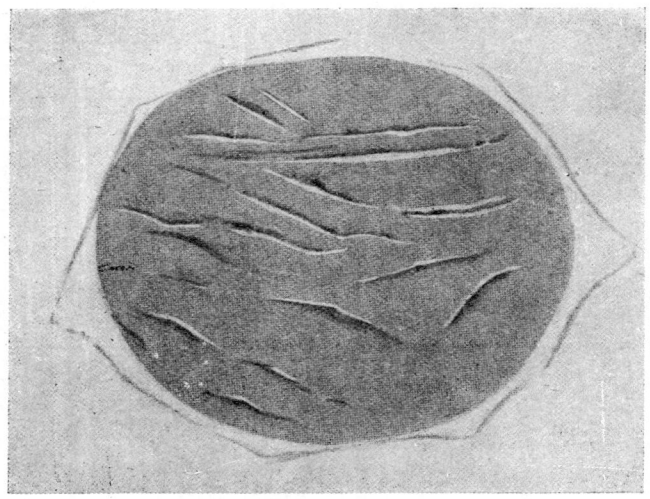

FIG. 143.—Drawing of an excised buphthalmic cornea, showing ruptures of Descemet's membrane, when held before a light and magnified. (Treacher Collins.)

and dull, due to a congestive condition of the globe, strictly comparable with that which is found in senile glaucoma ; (2) opacities may be present due to the overstretching and rupture of Descemet's membrane at various points ; Stähli has calculated that central opacities due to this cause are responsible for an impairment of vision in from 33 per cent. to 50 per cent. of all cases of buphthalmos ; (3) there may be ulceration or degeneration of the surface of the cornea due to defective nutrition and to exposure ; and (4) cicatricial changes may be present as a result of some earlier active inflammatory process.

The ruptures of the membrane of Descemet are of sufficient interest to justify a short description of their clinical appearances. They are, however, not pathognomonic of buphthalmos, for they are seen, though more rarely, in cases of high myopia, of conical cornea, and, it is said, of instrumental birth injuries to the cornea. During life they appear as fine lines, which sometimes branch dichotomously. They are delicate and almost transparent, so that good illumination and examination with the loupe are necessary for their discovery; they are most easily seen against the background of the black pupil (Fig. 143). On ophthalmoscopic examination with a high convex lens, they stand out against the fundus reflex as dark, double-contoured streaks with a red line in the middle. The light and shade on them alter with slight movements of the ophthalmoscope (Coats). Haab compared them to a thread of Canada balsam laid on a glass slide.

In some cases the enlargement and the proptosis of the globe are so extreme that the lids meet with difficulty or not at all. The condition of lagophthalmos so produced is a menace to the safety of the organ, owing to the exposure of the cornea.

The Anterior Chamber.—It has already been said that the anterior chamber is greatly deepened in buphthalmos. At the same time the angle appears (we advisedly say " appears ") to be widely open. This matter will be better discussed under the heading of pathology. It remains to mention, however, that in certain cases of this affection, the anterior chamber instead of being deepened is narrowed or even obliterated. It is probable that these cases do not belong to the same ætiologic class as the commoner ones, which are to be attributed, as has already been said, to defects in the development of the parts concerned in excretion.

The Sclera is nearly uniformly distended in buphthalmic eyes. The result is that the uveal pigment shows through the thin coat, giving the white of the eye a bluish appearance. This is very marked in the neighbourhood of the limbus, where the stretching and consequent thinning of the coat are most pronounced. In some eyes, however, the sclera is found to be thickened, owing to hyperplasia, instead of being thinned. Staphylomata are rarely found to be present, their occurrence being merely accidental.

The Iris is very often tremulous, owing to lack of the usual support from the lens. It is rare to find any evidence of inflammation, but the pattern is often wanting in distinctness, the colour dull, and the lustre impaired. Owing to the displacement backward of the lens system, the plane of the membrane, instead of being convex forward, is usually flat or even somewhat concave forward (funnel-shaped). The typical buphthalmic pupil is round, and is often a little dilated, though rarely it may be normal or even contracted. The pupillary reactions are present, but are decidedly sluggish, sometimes very markedly so; this is to be ascribed to atrophy of the iris tissue, which likewise explains the changes in its appearance enumerated above. Drug mydriasis can readily be obtained, as also can meiosis, up to a comparatively late stage of the disease. Colobomata of the iris and choroid would appear to be not very uncommon.

The Lens is the only ocular structure which is not distended by the increase of intra-ocular pressure; the obvious reason for this is, that the pressure acts upon it from without and not from within. It is usually clear in the early stages, though often cataractous later; it may be of natural size, but is often smaller than normal. On antero-posterior section it presents a spindle shape; this is usually explained by the pull of the overstretched suspensory ligament.

It is obvious that the latter ligament must be put under a condition of strain, from the time that the corneal base first commences to enlarge, and that in advanced cases, the overstretching must be very extreme, and must lead to loss of elasticity in the suspensory fibres, and later still, sometimes even to their rupture. The alteration in the anterior segment of the eye, which we have already discussed, leads to the lens system finding a position farther away from the cornea ; this is equivalent to a posterior displacement of this system. It is stated by Parsons that in addition to the above, there is a slight posterior displacement of the origin of the suspensory ligament in the ciliary body, brought about by the stretching of the globe. At the same time, the lessening in the firmness of the support afforded to the lens renders that structure tremulous and so leads to irido-donesis. In extreme cases, the zonule may rupture, and the lens may consequently become dislocated.

The Vitreous is usually clear in early cases, but later on in the disease, at a time when the retina and the choroid have been affected by the overstretching of the globe, it is common to find floating opacities present. Sometimes they are in such numbers, as to make it very difficult to obtain a clear view of the fundus.

The Choroid, in early cases, appears to be quite normal. Later as the globe stretches, it shares in that stretching, and presents the appearances which we are accustomed to find in the overdistended globes of highly myopic patients. Not only so, but evidence of changes in the uveal coat, is to be discovered in the abundant vitreous opacities, which veil the fundus details from view in late cases.

The Retina is doubly affected, viz., (1) by overstretching, and (2) by the increase in the intra-ocular pressure. We are familiar with the diminished sensibility of the retina which we meet with in high myopia, and which is usually attributed to the abnormal stretching of the membrane ; it must be remembered, at the same time, that there are those who ascribe the unhealthy stretching of myopic globes to an increase in intra-ocular pressure. Nor are we likely to forget that overstretching involves a risk of detachment of the retina. With regard to the second of the two factors above enumerated, the subject has been dealt with at length in Chapter IV. Part V. and need not be again discussed here. Suffice it to say, that what has been written of glaucoma in the adult applies with equal force to buphthalmos, with one important reservation, which will now be set forth. In the adult eye, the investing tunic has attained a texture and a power of resistance, which prevents it from stretching to any great extent under the influence of an increase in intra-ocular pressure. Under the strain of long-continued high tension the adult globe will give at its weakest parts, viz., the intercalary area, the apertures of emergence of the vasa vorticosa, and the optic disc. With the exception of the last-named, which, however, affords very little relief to the pressure present, the yielding of a senile globe is a very slow affair. In the young eye, on the contrary, the whole globe gives before the onset of pathologic pressure, and by so doing, it is held that it keeps the results of the process at bay. To put it colloquially it is Nature's effort to meet the advancing foe, by "yielding to conquer." That some eyes win through to a measure of saved vision is certain, but the greater number yield in the end to the relentless pursuit of the enemy, unless help is available from without. It is the old, oft-told, and melancholy story of "the little nation," battling against odds, whilst waiting for the arrival of relief, an epic as interesting in surgery, as it is inspiring in history.

Incidentally we are here furnished with a very interesting confirmation of the view that has been taken in this book of the true pathology of the field changes in glaucoma : It has been pointed out that those of them which are characteristic of this disease are due to injuries to the nerve fibres at the edge of the disc. The buphthalmic eye is saved for a time from this form of injury by the fact that its coats distend as a whole, and thus the full burden of the pressure is not thrown on the narrow area of the optic nerve-head. If the disease continues, cupping of the disc eventually takes place, but is not, as in senile glaucoma, the primary pathologic feature of the case.

The Optic Disc is sooner or later cupped in buphthalmos, just as it is in senile glaucoma. Essentially the process is the same in both, though in the latter, as has just been pointed out, it may for a while be delayed by the general yielding of the globe. It is not always an easy thing to see the exact condition of the papilla in a late stage, owing to the myopic refraction and to the hazy media. Its brilliant whiteness, due to advanced atrophy, is then much more easily detected than are the details of the cupping of the disc.

The Tension of buphthalmic eyes is raised ; sometimes, and in late cases, it is very markedly so. Owing to the alteration in the curvature of the cornea, the ordinary Schiötz tonometer is unsuitable for recording the intraocular pressure in these cases. We have therefore to fall back on the very unsatisfactory method of digital examination. The stretching of the globe, the cupping of the disc, and other signs seldom, if ever, leave any doubt as to the presence of increased tension.

The Visual Acuity is very rarely normal in buphthalmos and is often much impaired. This is readily understood when we consider the numerous causes that may contribute to such a result, viz., (1) opacities of one kind or another in the cornea ; (2) cataract ; (3) vitreous opacities ; (4) damage to the optic nerve and retina (including retinal detachment) ; and (5) interference with the normal refraction of the eye. The last of these alone remains to be discussed.

From analogy with cases of high myopia, we should certainly have been justified in expecting that the great increase in the size of the globe, and especially in its length, would cause images to be focussed far in front of the retina, in other words, that a condition of high myopia would be imitated. When we consider that the measurement of a number of buphthalmic eyes by Gros yielded a mean of 32 mm. in the antero-posterior diameter, it would seem impossible that any condition, save one of high myopia, could prevail, and yet modern experience would appear to be practically unanimous that in the majority of cases, the myopia present is very moderate in amount. Indeed in rare cases emmetropia and even hyperopia have been recorded by reliable observers. Parsons states that a defect of from -1 D. to -7 D. is relatively common, and he ascribes this diminution of the expected short sight to three factors : (1) Flattening of the cornea ; (2) displacement backward of the lens system ; and (3) flattening and consequent loss of power of the lens itself.

Astigmatism is common and is usually found to be with the rule, thus suggesting that the horizontal meridian of the cornea flattens more than the vertical under the influence of stretching. Irregular astigmatism is not uncommon and may be due either to the condition of the cornea, or to a tilting or partial dislocation of the lens. The satisfactory correction of buphthalmic cases is usually difficult and not infrequently impossible, since the conditions present make a retinoscopy very difficult to perform; nor are these difficulties rendered any the less by the fact that the patient's power of fixation is often indifferent and that nystagmus is not seldom present.

General.—Buphthalmic children are naturally backward and diffident. If the corneæ are exposed, pain frequently makes them fractious and irritable. The limitations in the excursions of the eyeballs necessitate constant turning movements of the head, which impart a characteristic staring look and a somewhat stilted attitude to the patient. The proptosis renders the eyes very liable to damage and the children consequently shun the rough companionship of their fellows. Taken all round, the lot of these little people is a very hard one.

Clinical Course and Complications

In the great majority of instances, an untreated case of buphthalmos goes steadily downhill. The distension of the eyeball increases, bringing in its train the various consequences which we have detailed in describing the signs and symptoms of the disease. On the one hand, we have all the troubles associated with the altered relationships between the globe and the surrounding parts. The proptosis and consequent deformity increase. The cornea may be deprived of the natural protection of the lids, and so become liable to abrasion, ulceration, and even perforation, with consequent panophthalmitis. The increasing limitation of the ocular movements and the pressure on the surrounding parts may be productive of great inconvenience to the patient. On the other hand, the all-important structures of the eyeball itself tend to become steadily disorganised. The media lose their clearness, the retina forfeits its sensibility, and sometimes undergoes detachment, whilst the optic nerve atrophies and loses its function. To this miserable story of progressive ruin there are, however, exceptions. Cases have been published by Axenfeld and others, in which spontaneous recovery from the disease has been claimed to have taken place. More correctly speaking, the progress of the condition has come to a stop. Collins and Mayou have suggested, that the explanation of this arrest is to be sought in the stretching or tearing of the congenital bands in the neighbourhood of the angle of the anterior chamber. They think that possibly in this way, the channels of excretion may be opened up and the cause of the condition thus removed. Fage has pointed out that in those cases, in which a cure of buphthalmos has been claimed as the result of administration of meiotic drugs, a much more reasonable explanation might be, that a favourable ending of the cases would have taken place, whether the drugs had been used or not. It, however, does not seem impossible, that the production of prolonged meiosis may have favoured the happy result by helping to tear the bands to which we have alluded. This is admittedly only a speculation.

There is another side of the question to be remembered, viz., that the buphthalmic eye may be subject to congestive crises, just in the same way as the globe with senile glaucoma. A case in point has recently been quoted by Risley, in which, under treatment, all the signs of congestion cleared up and the tension returned to normal.

The buphthalmic eye is very liable to injury. Subconjunctival ruptures have been reported by Blair, Höeg, and Zentmayer. Such cases appear to do well under a pressure bandage. Ball has recorded the dislocation of one of these large eyes, owing to a blow against the knob of a chair. It was replaced and sutured in position, but later atrophy took place. A stranger accident still is that recorded by Bunge, in which a detachment of the retina and subluxation of the lens followed a jar to the patient's body. Dislocations of the lens are unfortunately far from uncommon, either with or without a history of injury to the eye.

Buphthalmos and Neuro-Fibromatosis.—Fuchs asserts that buphthalmos may be a symptom of neuro-fibromatosis multiplex (von Recklinghausen's disease), which is compounded of a number of changes mostly congenital, viz., multiple neuro-fibromata, mollusca fibrosa, and flat pigment moles in the skin; neuroma plexiforme and lymphangioma of the lids and orbit, and unilateral hypertrophy of the face; lastly tumours of the optic and auditory nerves. Komoto, Weinstein, and Murakami have each published a case of the kind, in all three of which neuro-fibromatosis played a very prominent part. In two at least of the cases, a unilateral affection of the face on the same side, would appear to have been present.

Cabannes met with a case of congenital buphthalmos with striking right-sided hemi-hypertrophy of the face and without obstruction to the excretory passages. He thought the enlargement of the eye dependent on a condition of hyper-nutrition, caused by a large deep-seated angioma of the temporal region. An allied case would appear to be that of Cuperus in which a right-sided buphthalmos co-existed with an extensive telangiectasis, which involved the right eye and right lower lid.

We turn now to the cases published by English writers. These have been comparatively numerous, and some very careful work has been done on the subject. Collins and Batten's case led the former to review a number of previous instances of the affection, viz., those by Alexis Thomson, Sachsalber, himself and Snell, Rockliffe and Parsons, and himself and Marshall. After detailing the changes that have been found in connection with neuro-fibromatosis, he states that all portions of the ciliary nerves supplying the eye may be affected, and that in the uveal tract, as in the skin, there may be a general hyperplasia of the fibrous tissue. The extent of the affection varies in its distribution, sometimes being confined to one set of ciliary nerves, and to the parts supplied by them, and sometimes to another. In some cases, only the terminal filaments and end organs of the nerves are involved ; in others the larger trunks are also affected. Microscopical sections show a marked increase of the perineurium, and endoneurium. The affected nerves may present, even to the naked eye, an appearance of enlargement and of plexiformity.

In Sutherland's and Mayou's case, which was shown as an example of von Recklinghausen's disease, the right side of the face and head was enlarged ; the branches of the third division of the fifth nerve could be felt as so many cords, the lids were hypertrophied, and at one point presented a swelling, which felt like a bag of worms ; white streaks in the cornea were taken to represent enlarged ciliary nerves ; the tension was up, and the disc cupped. The affection dated from six months of age. Verhoeff has stated, that in a case which came under his observation, a number of tortuous, worm-like bodies could be seen clinically on the surface of the eyeball.

The question arises whether the enlargement of the globe is directly connected with the neuro-fibromatosis, or whether it is due, as is the case with other instances of buphthalmos, to some maldevelopment of the channels for the excretion of intra-ocular fluid. Collins appears to incline to the latter view, but does not dogmatise on the subject, and we shall be well advised to imitate his example. Without committing ourselves to any definite expression of opinion, we must at least keep before us the possibility, that the ætiology of these cases may prove to be quite distinct from that of ordinary buphthalmos.

Differential Diagnosis of Buphthalmos

It has been stated by various writers that it is necessary to make a differential diagnosis between buphthalmos and the following conditions : (1) Megalocornea ; (2) juvenile glaucoma ; (3) keratoconus ; (4) keratectasia ; (5) staphyloma ; (6) exophthalmos.

We will take these in turn :

(1) Megalocornea is dealt with in a separate section.

(2) There is no hard and fast clinical line between buphthalmos and certain cases of juvenile glaucoma ; the pathological dividing line need not detain us now.

(3) In keratoconus it is the centre of the cornea which yields, and in advanced cases the appearance, looked at from the side, is characteristic. Further the condition is one which begins to develop in the second decade of life, and not in the first part of the first decade. Most important of all, the base-circle of the cornea is not enlarged, as it is in buphthalmos.

(4 and 5) It is difficult to believe that anyone, grounded in the elements of ophthalmology, could mistake the opaque protrusions of keratectasia or of staphyloma, for buphthalmos, save possibly at a very late stage of the last-named, when the differential diagnosis would be quite unimportant.

(6) The exophthalmos associated with congenital glaucoma is only seen when the disease is far advanced, and is accompanied by such unmistakable enlargement of the cornea, that no difficulty in diagnosis would then be possible.

The Pathological Anatomy of Buphthalmos

In studying the pathological anatomy of buphthalmos, we must take the various structures of the eye in turn.

The Cornea is usually of normal thickness at its centre, whilst its periphery is always found to be thinned, and often to be cellular and vascularised. It is the weak sclero-corneal junction which gives way under pressure from within, and thus bodily displaces the cornea proper forwards ; at the same time the base-circle becomes stretched, and flattening of the cornea results (Parsons).

As has already been mentioned, we find in buphthalmic corneæ, systems of fine lines, which are due to the over-stretching and rupture of Descemet's membrane. The whole subject has been exhaustively dealt with by George Coats. In some cases the membrane is merely thinned

CONGENITAL GLAUCOMA

without actual rupture having taken place. In others, the rupture appears to have been sub-endothelial, though in all probability the endothelium gave way at the time of the break and subsequently closed in and covered the injury. In some instances, the edges of the membrane remain flatly applied to the cornea, though they may become widely separated from each other by subsequent stretching (Fig. 144). More usually one or both edges

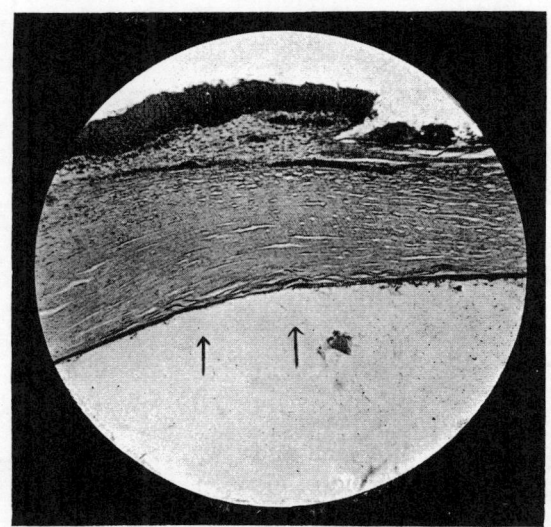

FIG. 144.—Microscopic section of the periphery of a buphthalmic cornea, showing a wide gap in Descemet's membrane.
The two arrows indicate the limits of this gap.
(*Photo by E. E. of specimen kindly lent by Mr. Treacher Collins.*)

show a tendency to roll forward in the manner commonly observed after traumatic ruptures. A definitely spiral arrangement may thus be imitated. Cases are on record, in which the tearing was so excessive, that excrescences appeared on the posterior surface of the cornea, formed by the curled-up margins of the lacerated membrane. Such have been described both by Coats and Rumschewitsch. With regard to the mechanism, whereby ruptures are produced, observers are agreed, that the stretching of the cornea is the essential cause, but as Coats points out, all the phenomena observed indicate that the membrane of Descemet is less elastic and more brittle than the lamellæ of the cornea ; otherwise, it would not tear as it does, and it would not tend to roll up when torn. Experiments on animals have failed to reproduce the characteristic tears, doubtless due to the fact that the overstretching in these cases was far too suddenly applied.

Apparently equally as common as the foregoing changes (though they have attracted less interest, since their genesis has always been obvious) are lesions of the front of the cornea, including Bowman's membrane and the deeper layers. These are a result of trauma of one kind or another. In addition, Takashima has described an interstitial infiltration of the cornea, causing in places breaks in the continuity of Bowman's membrane. These resemble the tears in Descemet's membrane.

The Iris and the Angle of the Anterior Chamber.—In very many cases of buphthalmos, the only points observable in the iris are those atrophic and degenerative changes which are equally found in eyes removed for senile glaucoma. There are, however, not a few cases in which bands, varying in density, in breadth, and in numbers, stretch across the angle of the anterior chamber and tend to occlude it. Round the nature of the origin of these bands a long and vigorous controversy has raged. The earlier view was that they were inflammatory in origin, and indeed for a limited number of cases, this conclusion may be taken to be generally accepted as correct. It applies, however, only to a minority of buphthalmic eyes, for Treacher Collins has urged that these bands, in most cases, are the representatives of a persistent fœtal condition of the pectinate ligament. The case may be summarised thus : (1) In the lower mammals, the pectinate ligament is a much larger and more elaborate structure than it is in man. (2) It is divided up in them into two parts, viz., (a) an outer part, which persists in man as the pectinate ligament, which latter has been described by Arthur Thomson as being fashioned by the breaking up of Descemet's membrane into a number of

CONGENITAL GLAUCOMA

fibrillæ, arranged in brush-like fashion to form a triangular area of trabecular tissue ; and (b) an inner part, presenting large, cavernous, irregular, intercommunicating spaces, the so-called "spaces of Fontana." (3) The very same condition of the parts is found in the human fœtus, but undergoes considerable modification before birth, for the spaces of Fontana disappear, and their place is taken by an extension outwards of the angle, or sinus, of the anterior

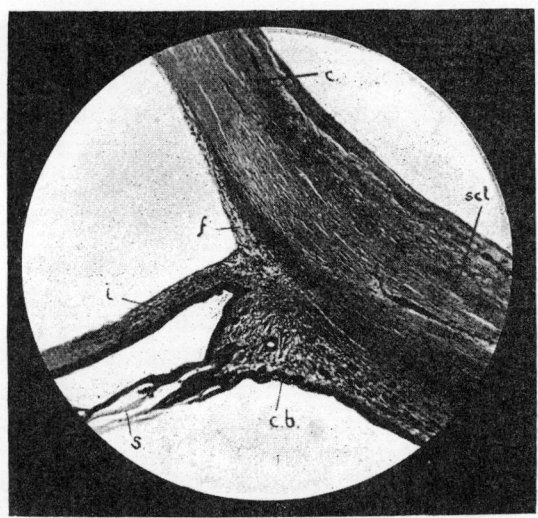

FIG. 145.—The angle of the anterior chamber of the buphthalmic eye shown in Fig. 142 more highly magnified.

The angle, though apparently wide open, is really filled up by fœtal tissue. The canal of Schlemm is absent. c, cornea ; scl, sclera ; i, iris ; f, fœtal tissue in angle ; s, suspensory ligament of lens ; $c.b$, ciliary body

(Photo by E. E. of specimen kindly lent by Mr. Treacher Collins.)

chamber. Should some of the partitions between the spaces of Fontana persist post-natally, they present the appearance of the bands, cords, etc., which have so often been described by pathologists, as filling up the space at the angle of the chamber in buphthalmic eyes (Fig. 145).

It is stated, that in some cases Descemet's membrane does not split up at all to form the pectinate ligament, but that it is continued round on to the anterior surface of the iris. The ciliary muscle then takes origin from the sclera, to which also the root of the iris has been found attached.

It is of interest to remember, that the obstruction to excretion may be present in eyes, which have a deep chamber and an *apparently* widely open angle. It is only when microscopic examination is made, that the true condition of things reveals itself (Fig. 145).

Many congenital defects of the uveal tract have been described as occurring in buphthalmic cases including coloboma of the iris and of the choroid, corectopia, ectropion of the iris, and aniridia. In addition, Mayou has recorded a case of this disease complicated by the presence of pre-natal anterior synechia, and persistent pupillary membrane. All this is only what might have been anticipated, when dealing with a condition, which is so essentially dependent upon a fault in development, as buphthalmos undoubtedly is.

The Canal of Schlemm has been found to be absent or imperfectly developed in a very large number of buphthalmic eyes, which have been submitted to microscopic examination (Fig. 145). These observations have been multiplied by many workers in many lands. The names include those of Rumschewitsch, Gross, Seefelder, R. Cross, Mayou, Stimmell and Rotter, Christel, Spielberg, Nahmacher, Boehm, Zentmayer, Hamburger, and others. The last-named surgeon has estimated that a defect in Schlemm's canal is to be found in 50 per cent. of cases of buphthalmos.

In this connection, it is interesting to record that Rumschewitsch and others have in certain cases observed not merely a defect in or absence of the canal of Schlemm, but a similar want of development of the veins in the anterior segment of the globe. The significance of this observation is obvious, when we remember the intimate developmental and physiological relationships between the canal of Schlemm and its tributary vessels.

The Sclera.—Judging from a general review of the literature of the subject, one would conclude that in the majority of cases, the sclera has been found to be thinned ;

exceptional instances have, however, been recorded, in which a definite hyperplasia of this membrane had taken place, with the result that its thickness was greater than that found in the emmetropic eye.

Takashima devoted a good deal of attention to the measurements of a number of buphthalmic eyeballs, which he examined anatomically. He found that, while the enlargement of the globe was associated with thinning of the anterior part of the sclera, the posterior segment, not only was not thinned, but was usually thickened in comparison with the normal sclera of the same age. He maintained that an analysis of the cases found in literature bore out the correctness of his measurements. In a few cases the posterior segment of the sclera may be thinned, but here, according to Takashima, the true explanation is that the disease is complicated by intercurrent myopia and staphyloma. His view, though he did not press it strongly, was that the enlargement of the globe was to be looked upon, in part at least, as a giant overgrowth of the eyeball, and not simply as a result of stretching.

It is the intercalary [1] region of the sclera which gives way most under pressure, and in association with this, there is said to be a definite set back of the plane of the lens system.

The enlargement of the eye is sometimes very great; thus Coronat and Aurand record a buphthalmic globe, which measured 44 mm. by 30 mm.

The Ciliary Body usually gives evidence of atrophy and degeneration and sometimes of past inflammation.

The Vitreous is often found to be abnormally fluid, as well as being cloudy.

The Ocular Muscles, and even the **Lids,** have been found atrophic and partially paralysed.

The Ætiology of Buphthalmos

It has long been recognised that in the great majority of cases at least, buphthalmos is due to an obstruction to the

[1] Intercalary, pertaining to the region of the canal of Schlemm.

channels of excretion of intra-ocular fluid. Bentzen and Leber proved by experiments on a buphthalmic eye, that the rate of filtration from it was below the normal. The anatomical evidence we have discussed provides ample explanation of the nature of the obstruction. In the earlier years of the study of this subject, pathologists were inclined to explain the anatomical phenomena on the basis of intra-uterine inflammation. Collins' work, abundantly confirmed by that of others, has, however, satisfied most ophthalmologists, that in the majority of cases we have to deal with a condition brought about by an arrest in development rather than with the results of an inflammatory process. It is, however, not only possible, but even probable, that in a minority of instances intra-uterine inflammation is to blame for the condition. Abadie held strongly that buphthalmos was always the result of a specific choroido - retinitis, whilst other writers, including Planchu and Gautier, S. Stephenson, Horton Brown, and Mayou have traced a history of inherited syphilis in their cases. Zentmayer attributes the great frequency of buphthalmos in negro children, to the prevalence of congenital syphilis amongst them.

The suggestion that hyper-secretion may be the cause of buphthalmos would appear to have little to recommend it. Such evidence as is afforded by the condition of the ciliary body is all against such an assumption. Nevertheless so reliable an authority as Fage has quite recently championed the view, that a hyper-secretion, of vaso-motor origin, may be the cause of some of the buphthalmic eyes with which we meet.

It is universally agreed that heredity plays an important rôle in the causation of buphthalmos, but exactly what that rôle is, it is impossible to say. That it acts through inherited disease alone is, we think, a view which may be unequivocally rejected, in spite of the strong support with which it has met from time to time. It is probable that the main factor is the tendency to defective development, and that disease plays a subsidiary and a comparatively infrequent part. Consanguinity has come in for a share of suspicion in this as in so many other congenital conditions.

From time to time, cases are published, in which buphthalmos is stated to have followed an injury to, or an inflammation of the eye. In most of these, the condition is probably quite distinct from that of congenital glaucoma; they really are instances of secondary glaucoma occurring in young and therefore distensible eyes. It is possible that in a few of them, the existence of a congenital want of development of the excretory passages may determine that the effects of injury or of inflammation shall suffice to upset the balance between secretion and excretion, and so precipitate the onset of an attack of glaucoma. Clinically speaking, they are instances of buphthalmos, or ox-eye, but pathologically it is very doubtful if any congenital defect plays a part in the genesis of the great majority of them. It is a question of our use of the terms.

Experimental Buphthalmos

Paul Erdmann in 1908 was able to produce glaucoma in the rabbit's eye by introducing into the anterior chamber a thin steel needle, which formed the positive electrode for a current of 5 ma. The source of the glaucoma was an obliteration of the filtering angle, by the proliferation of the endothelium, caused by minute granules of oxide of steel. In his later experiments, he introduced the prepared electrolytic products into the chamber, and so was able to regulate the reaction.

The resulting condition resembled human buphthalmos; the globe enlarged, the cornea flattened, ruptures of Descemet's membrane took place, and the optic disc was cupped. Meiotics diminished the tension of these eyes, whilst mydriatics increased it. Fluorescein introduced into the blood circulation appeared sooner and more abundantly in the aqueous, than it did in healthy eyes. The albumin content of the fluid in the anterior chamber was raised.

Schreiber and Wengler repeated Erdmann's experiments, and confirmed his findings so far as the rise in intra-ocular pressure was concerned. Their most interesting discovery was, that if this increase in pressure was a gradual one, the optic nerve and retina remained practically unaffected, whilst if the tension was caused to rise suddenly, and was then maintained at a high level, marked degeneration of these structures took place. The condition which they thus produced in rabbits had a distinct resemblance to human buphthalmos; there was a manifest enlargement of all the diameters of the eye with preservation of the anterior chamber.

Terrien and Dantrelle claim to have produced experimental buphthalmos by repeated punctures of the anterior chamber made at short intervals.

It is therefore of interest to recall, that Kümmell has observed, that burns of the limbus are associated with a rise in intra-ocular pressure, accompanied by an increase in the depth of the anterior chamber.

In connection with the above experiments, it is worthy of note that Pichler treated an albino rabbit for enlargement of the globe with hazy cornea and deep anterior chamber. The condition improved somewhat and eventually came to a standstill with excavation of the disc.

Vogt has recently written on hereditary buphthalmos in the rabbit.

Megalocornea and Buphthalmos

Is there a condition, which can be sharply distinguished from the pathological distension of the juvenile globe, which occurs as a result of an increase in the intra-ocular pressure? Kayser is strongly of opinion that there is; that it should be looked upon as a simple gigantism of the cornea; and that for purposes of distinction the name "megalocornea" should be applied to it. Such a view is in opposition to the trend of previous opinion, which regards these cases as instances of infantile glaucoma, which have been fortunate enough to undergo arrest, before permanent damage has been inflicted on the eye. It has been urged in support of this view, that ruptures of the membrane of Descemet have been found in undoubted cases of megalocornea. The assumption that they *are* undoubted cases obviously begs the main question. Kayser's records include seventeen cases occurring in four generations of a family; in all of them, there were perfect transparency of the cornea, increased depth of the anterior chamber, enlargement of the iris, good vision, normal tension, and a natural condition of the optic discs. With rare exceptions, the second generation was missed; males alone were affected, and transmission was through the female line. Kayser gives the following reasons for rejecting the view that these might have been cases of cured buphthalmos : (1) The individual cases differed so little between themselves, as to negative the idea of an arrested disease process. (2) He thought it inconceivable that the process should have developed so far before birth, and then remained stationary in every single case afterwards. (3) No females were affected, whilst in buphthalmos 40 per cent. of the cases are of that sex. (4) Buphthalmos is unilateral in 30 per cent. of the cases, whilst these were invariably bilateral. (5) Ruptures of Descemet's membrane were conspicuous by their complete absence, clearly indicating that no stretching of the eye had taken place after development was complete. Kayser's views had the unqualified support of George Coats, who pointed out that buphthalmos had up till then been regarded as a familial, rather than as a directly heritable disease. Inasmuch, however, as in the vast majority of cases it leads to blindness, the absence of records of direct descent is not astonishing. It is of importance that in not one single one of Kayser's cases was there evidence of any other congenital abnormality in the eyes. The family had lived four centuries in the same neighbourhood, and consanguinity was therefore a possible factor.

On the other hand, it is to be remembered that there are still a number of pathologists, and amongst them men of the reputations of Axenfeld, Elschnig, and Fage, who maintain that a closer examination of cases of so-called megalocornea will reveal changes pathognomonic of infantile glaucoma. Haab has long held a view widely divergent from this, and one more in accordance with Kayser's contention, viz., that these cases of megalocornea are to be looked on as a mixture of hyperplasia and gigantism. Horner shared this opinion and pointed out that when the condition occurs in members of the same family, it never alternates with buphthalmos; this observation was made from his own personal experience. Owuchi found a grandfather, a grandmother, a father, and two sons all suffering from megalocornea. J. Stähli considers that there are numerous transitions from the normal sized cornea to megalocornea, none of which presents any sign or symptom of glaucoma; he cannot see why eyes should be considered glaucomatous, when they have nothing in common with the buphthalmic eye, beyond the large size of the cornea, whilst in all other respects they are normal; the vision, the visual fields, and the condition of the media are all normal; the tension is not raised, and may even be subnormal, and that too after the exhibition of "trial mydriasis." On the other hand, he does not admit, or even suppose, that these cases are not pathologic. Spontaneous dislocation of the lens may, he says, occur in them; an abnormally early arcus senilis may declare itself; and marked alterations in the distribution of the uveal pigment may take place. All these things indicate, according to Stähli, that these cases have a pathologic character.

Before the 1913 meeting of the Ophthalmological Society of the United Kingdom, Treacher Collins showed a lad of 17, whose corrected vision was $\frac{6}{6}$ in each eye; the fields taken with 10 mm. white squares were normal, and the ophthalmoscopic examination showed no cupping of the disc. In discussing the case, Richardson Cross said, that he had recently seen a similar case in a girl of 15, who had full vision after correction of her refractive errors. There was no cupping of the disc, the tension was as nearly as possible normal, and the earlier descriptions of the case indicated that the condition had been stationary for many years. The interest of this communication lies in the fact that it and the discussion which followed it preceded

Kayser's work and Coats' review thereof. The suggestion that arises is, that possibly in the light of later knowledge, these two cases might have been recognised as pure megalocornea. A factor somewhat disturbing to this view, was introduced by C. Killick, who in speaking at the same meeting, quoted a case of his own, in which there was complete excavation of the right optic disc, with bare perception of light in that eye, whilst in the left eye, which was also buphthalmic, there was a normal disc, and normal vision. He concluded that it was a case of double congenital glaucoma, progressive in one eye, and stationary in the other.

It is evident that our views on this subject have not attained to finality, and it is important that in recording future cases, Kayser's observations should be very carefully borne in mind, and especially his contention that ruptures of Descemet's membrane are absent in megalocornea. The importance of this last observation will be obvious in the light of Coats' evidence, that he found these ruptures in all the cases (13 in number) of buphthalmos, which he sectioned, except in one, in which the cornea was too much folded to allow of a satisfactory examination. In none of the 1913 cases, does the report indicate, whether ruptures in Descemet's membrane were present or absent.

The latest convert to the view that megalocornea is a clinical entity distinct from buphthalmos is Seefelder. In a case, which he examined with great care, there were no corneal opacities, no fissures of Descemet's membrane, and no broadening of the limbus ; the sclero-corneal margin was sharp ; the sclera was normal even in the region of the anterior chamber, which was 8 mm. in depth, and bounded posteriorly by sclera. There was no cupping of the disc or evidence of disturbance of the retinal function ; the astigmatism was regular ; the tension was normal ; and the measurements of the two eyes were identical. He suggests a new term for such cases, " gigantophthalmos."

The view would appear to be gaining ground, that a condition exists, which is often confused with buphthalmos, but which differs from it essentially, inasmuch as it is a product of overgrowth and not of overstretching. If this view is established, the name "megalocornea," or some substitute for it, will be justified. But there is still a good deal of spadework to be done before we can rest from our labours, with the confidence that all the difficulties have been cleared up.

Juvenile Glaucoma

Quite recent opinions, expressed by able and competent ophthalmologists, on the subject of juvenile glaucoma, exhibit so wide a divergence, as to suggest that the subject is far from having been mastered even now. On one point, however, there appears to be an agreement, viz., that the group comprehends a great variety of different forms, some few of which should more correctly be classed under buphthalmos, whilst the rest include cases, which imitate and closely resemble every variety of form of senile glaucoma. The views of those, who write on the subject of the juvenile form of the disease, are largely influenced by the nature of the material which they have personally encountered. The condition is not a common one, and the accident of chance may determine that one observer sees a relatively large number of one class of cases, *e.g.*, the late buphthalmic, whilst another's experience lies all in the "precocious senile" forms.

It is generally admitted that juvenile glaucoma is much *commoner in the male* than in the female, thus establishing a bond between it and buphthalmos, and at the same time forming a contrast with what is known to hold in senile glaucoma, in which the sexes are fairly equally attacked. Loehlein found this feature strongly marked in his statistics, which covered a large range of cases collected from literature. Haag, however, whose cases were all drawn from one clinic (Tübingen), challenged this view, and stated that the preference of the disease for one sex was not well marked in his material. Both surgeons appeared to be dealing with large enough numbers to make their conclusions fairly reliable, and one is therefore somewhat at a loss to explain the discrepancy.

The frequent presence of some form of *congenital anomaly* in cases which fall under the juvenile group, is striking and very significant. Loehlein calculates that 50 per cent. of all of them reveal one or another of these signs of hereditary taint. His list includes persistent hyaloid arteries, persistent pupillary membranes, anomalies of the retinal vessels, lamellar cataracts, colobomata, microphthalmos, and other deformities of the globe, and very high myopia. Haag found the same kind of thing in his cases.

Another point of importance as indicating the relationship between buphthalmos and juvenile glaucoma is the frequency with which we find a marked increase in the depth of the anterior chamber in both classes of cases.

In dealing with the subject of senile glaucoma, there is still much difference of opinion as to the part played by *heredity*, but the advocates of the view, that even in adults, inheritance plays a strong part, include such authorities as Priestley Smith, Hirschberg, and Vossius. When we come to consider the juvenile form, we fail to find uniformity of opinion, but at least the great balance of ophthalmological judgment is with the belief, that here heredity shows a more strongly marked influence than it does in the senile disease.

Haag has drawn attention to the common association of juvenile glaucoma with diseased conditions in other parts and especially with *disorders of nutrition*.

All forms of glaucoma, from the simple to the violently acute, are to be found in young people. In this connection Haag makes two surprising statements, viz., (1) that congestive glaucoma is twice as common as the simple form in the young, and (2) that it does not favour either sex in the early decades of life. Loehlein, on the contrary, found that 62 per cent. of all cases in the young were of the simple variety.

The so-called *prodromal stage* is greatly lengthened in juvenile, as compared with senile glaucoma. This is usually explained by the yielding of the tunic of the eye which is possible only in the young.

All writers agree that *myopia* is much more common in juvenile than in senile glaucoma. Thus Haag found myopia in 31 per cent. of his young cases, and in more than half of these (17 per cent. of the total) the short sight was of a high grade. His figure for hyperopia was 28 per cent., the rest being emmetropes. Loehlein found myopia in 50 per cent. of his cases as contrasted with 15 per cent. in the senile form He made the interesting observation, that simple glaucoma was commoner in myopes and emmetropes, whilst the congestive disease bulked larger in the hyperopes, thus establishing a strong bond of resemblance between the juvenile and senile forms of the disease. Numerous observers hold that the tension of many myopic eyes is frequently above the normal. Gilbert has gone so far as to say, that myopia is present in 30 per cent. of his cases of senile glaucoma. His experience would appear to be an uncommon one. It is necessary to remember, that the statistics we have been quoting come largely from Germany, a country in which myopia is believed to be common out of all proportion to what it is in Great Britain.

In connection with this association between glaucoma and myopia in the young, two possibilities present themselves : (1) That the myopia is an expression of the stretching of the globe under the influence of increased intra-ocular pressure, and (2) that both the myopia and the glaucoma may be dependent upon some common cause. In any case we are safe in agreeing with Loehlein, that the relationship between the two conditions is not accidental. Beyond that it would be difficult to go. It is significant, however, that axial myopia of a high degree has been observed in the actual process of development in eyes, the subjects of glaucoma in young people. Such cases have been recorded by Loehlein, Puech, Gilbert, and others.

The closeness of the relationship between the different forms of glaucoma can best be judged by a consideration of the phenomenon of " anticipation " in the hereditary form of this disease. The subject was first discussed by von Graefe, who illustrated his point by reference to families under his observation, in which glaucoma had affected three or four generations, and perhaps more. The symptoms of the disease in the later generations came on between 30 and 40 years of age, whilst in the earlier generations they appeared at 50 or 60. The matter was taken up and carried a good deal farther by Lawford. Some of the pedigrees he quotes are of great interest from our present point of view. In one family the ages of appearance of the disease in three successive generations, were 71 in the first, 40 to 48 in the second, and 25 to 30 in the third. Another record is still more striking; in the first generation the trouble began at 40 years of age, in the second generation at 23 and 25 years of age respectively, and in the third generation five cases commenced between 17 and 28 years of age.

Lawford also gives a summary of the reports of hereditary glaucoma by Mules, Story, and Priestley Smith, in all three of which, " anticipation " was the prominent feature. Of these, Mules' cases stand out, since the age of attack in the first generation was 49, whilst the man's three sons developed signs of glaucoma between 15 and 18 years of age.

Phinizy Calhoun has recently reported eight cases of glaucoma simplex in three generations of one family. In these " anticipation " was a prominent feature of succeeding generations, but the type throughout was steadily that of senile glaucoma. On the other hand. Wallenberg followed a type of juvenile glaucoma through four generations, and in these an increased depth of the anterior chamber was a noteworthy indication of the underlying nature of the affection.

Gilbert met with a couple, both of whom suffered from ordinary congestive senile glaucoma, whilst several of their descendants developed the juvenile form of the disease. Germann's records resemble the preceding : A man suffered from senile glaucoma, whilst his son and two daughters developed the juvenile form.

Loehlein saw three sisters suffering from simple juvenile glaucoma, whilst the fourth was buphthalmic. Hirschberg watched a girl for years with buphthalmos in one eye, and infantile glaucoma in the other.

Not a few efforts have been made to classify **the various types of glaucoma, which we meet with in young people.** Of these the best appears to be that recently enunciated by Fuchs, who recognises the following groups :

(1) True glaucoma with a shallow anterior chamber. The disease tends to occur in several members of a family, and is hereditary ; the patients are comparatively young ; it is clinically, and perhaps pathologically, indistinguishable from ordinary senile glaucoma, with the one exception of the ages of the patients.

(2) Glaucoma caused by congenital malformations, such as defective development of Schlemm's canal, arrest in the development of the pectinate ligament, aniridia, etc. Such are congenital in clinical appearance, or else manifest themselves very early in life. They include buphthalmos.

(3) Glaucoma with a deep chamber and myopia. It may be questioned whether this group is not an artificial one ; but the relationship of myopia to juvenile glaucoma has already been discussed.

(4) Secondary glaucoma, associated with keratitis punctata. The deposit on the posterior surface of the cornea may be so fine as to escape observation, and thus lead to an erroneous classification of the condition as " primary."

Luminous as this schedule is, its defects are obvious, but they have been already dealt with in the preceding pages, and all that can be done now, is to point out once again the need for careful observation of all cases of glaucoma, which occur earlier than ordinary. It seems reasonable to consider any case of glaucoma which occurs before 40 years of age as belonging to the juvenile group.

The Treatment of Buphthalmos

In 1899 Walter Pyle, of Philadelphia, published an exhaustive and luminous article on buphthalmos. His remarks on the subject of treatment are of special interest, as they were made before the day of the modern filtering operations. He considered that the general consensus of opinion was against operative measures, and he pointed out, that though not a few successful cases had been published, there was good reason to believe that they only represented a minority of the operations performed ; and that, if all alike had been placed on record, the results would have been much more discouraging. He laid stress on the difficulty of operating on children, and on the dangers of loss of vitreous, collapse of the globe, intra-ocular hæmorrhage, irido-cyclitis, and panophthalmitis. He discussed paracentesis, the introduction of a seton, the injection of vitreous, iridectomy, and sclerotomy. He commented on the great differences of opinion as to the value of iridectomy, and made the important point, that if an operation is to be done at all, it is imperative that it should be done as early as possible. He looked on the use of meiotics as being of little value, when employed alone, but of the highest service as adjuncts to operative measures. He laid great stress on the careful correction of errors of refraction, and comparatively little on constitutional treatment, though he would by no means neglect the latter.

The next landmark in the history of the subject may, we think, be taken to be Priestley Smith's statement before the International Congress of 1913. He had made inquiries from a large number of British surgeons and summarised their replies in his report. As to the treatment of buphthalmos, the answers he received were very various, and many of them were extremely discouraging. On the other hand, some of his correspondents spoke favourably of the treatment of this condition by iridectomy, by repeated anterior sclerotomy, by Herbert's operation, and by trephining. The interest of these observations is that they were made during a period, when the modern filtration operations were still quite new to the majority of surgeons.

It is of interest therefore to pass on to a review of a number of the more recently expressed opinions on the subject.

The first thing that strikes one in studying this literature, is that the advocacy of medicinal treatment alone, and of the operation of iridectomy has practically dropped out of mention, whilst the references to the newer operations have increased in numbers. Sclerotomy and cyclodialysis appear to have gone out of favour, though Peter and others have had good results from repeated posterior sclerotomies.

The dropping of iridectomy is of the more interest, since it is, after all, merely a harking back to the practice of the old masters of our craft, for de Wecker wrote in 1901: "Von Graefe was in agreement with his colleagues, when he declared that iridectomy was dangerous (in buphthalmos) on account of the defects in the zonule, which laid the eye open to the danger of vitreous escape."

Boehm has pointed out, that the failure of iridectomy to give satisfaction in buphthalmic cases, is to be laid at the door of the absence of the canal of Schlemm; in his own experience the results were good, in two cases in which a cystic scar (presumably with filtration) was accidentally established by the operation.

Jaeger has performed Schloffer's operation (a modified iridencleisis) on five buphthalmic eyes, with an arrest of the condition in two of the cases. Wessely also has published a successful result after an iridencleisis for buphthalmos.

David Priestley Smith advocates his operation of limbal puncture, which he has performed in three cases with one success. Casey Wood speaks well of his thread operation, the histories of which are admittedly very short. Allport, Hay, and Key have obtained good results from Lagrange's method. Weeks has abandoned it in favour of trephining, with a 1·5 mm. instrument, for the reason that he finds it difficult to regulate the size of the opening when using the former method, and he considers the large scleral wound dangerous.

Successful cases of trephining for buphthalmos have been published by Calhoun, Wessely, Zentmayer, Hamilton, Hugh Jones, Buck, Lebensohn, and Dubois. Hallett obtained a good end-result in a child of 7, after trephining

CONGENITAL GLAUCOMA

the eye on three successive occasions. Mayou relieved the tension of buphthalmos by trephining, but the scotoma in one of his two cases continued to advance toward the fixation point. P. H. Adams obtained a good result after double trephining and a Herbert operation in a 5 months old child. Fage, whose valuable work on buphthalmos has already been quoted, lays it down as an axiom, that whatever is done in the operative treatment of buphthalmos, the incision must be kept as small as possible in order to avoid the dangers of vitreous escape, lens luxation, and intra-ocular hæmorrhage. To his mind this rules out the operation of iridectomy. He has sclerectomised 14 cases and considers that the Elliot operation offers the following solid advantages :—(1) Simplicity, (2) the small size of the opening in the tunic, and (3) the possibility of repetition of the procedure if necessary. He lays stress on the rule that whatever operation is done, it must be done early. In giving expression to such a view, he is at one with Pyle and Boehm and, we venture to think, with the great body of sound ophthalmological opinion.

Zentmayer analysed the replies of a number of surgeons, whom he asked to state their opinion as to the best operation for hydrophthalmos. Iridectomy was reported to have given fair results in 42 per cent. and poor in 58 per cent.; sclerotomy fair results in 28 per cent. and poor in 72 per cent.; sclerectomy satisfactory results in 40 per cent., encouraging in 20 per cent. and unsatisfactory in 40 per cent. Meiotics had proved unsatisfactory on the whole and paracentesis was a failure. The Elliot operation was reported as having given the best results of any procedure.

Herbert has opposed sclerectomy on the ground that it is dangerous to empty the large and deep anterior chamber ; in its stead he advocates subconjunctival puncture with a 1 mm. Graefe's knife. In none of his patients was the escape of aqueous sufficient to empty the anterior chamber, yet in all of them there was a temporary fall in vision, which he attributed to circulatory embarrassment from the sudden loss of support to degenerate and weakened blood vessels. He thought that the stasis was incomplete and passed off as the leakage from the chamber lessened. The very same sequence of events, which Herbert here records, may be seen after trephining, not only in buphthalmic eyes, but also, and more frequently, in late senile glaucomatous eyes. A more simple explanation of the phenomena in question, in some cases at least, appears to be, that the refractive power of the lens system is temporarily altered by its advance towards the cornea, and is subsequently restored as the anterior chamber fully re-forms.

The subject of operating for buphthalmos was brought before the Netherlands Ophthalmological Society (March 16, 1918) by Zeeman, who has tried cyclodialysis and trephining in a number of cases. He thinks that operation should only be undertaken in very young children, and that the menace of retinal detachment is of itself sufficient to make the surgeon hesitate how he operates in those who are older. If obliged to operate he would then perform a sclerotomy, but only if driven to it by necessity. Nothing could be more eloquent of the discordance of the views held on this subject at the present time than the discussion which followed. For that reason alone it is worth perusal by anyone who is interested in such cases.

Gifford has not had favourable results in 2 cases in which he trephined for buphthalmos, and suggests that, instead of placing the hole as far forward as the abnormal condition of the parts allows, we should make it as far back as possible, consistent with keeping it well within the anterior chamber. The suggestion is in accordance with the author's experience, and carries out the first principle of a successful sclerostomy, viz., to tap, and to drain sub-conjunctivally the anterior chamber, whilst placing the opening so far forward as to avoid the danger of impaction of the uvea.

The writer has trephined on a number of occasions for buphthalmos, and though he would be very far from claiming that this or any other operation is certain to give invariable success in the treatment of this very difficult disease, he can at least look back on some most encouraging results. Apart from those whose names have been men-

CONGENITAL GLAUCOMA

tioned in connection with published cases, there are quite a number of surgeons, who have trephined successfully for buphthalmos, but who have not considered it worth while to report their results, mainly because their material has not been large. The same is probably true of the other procedures above alluded to. Lastly, Professor Meller has spread the ægis of his advocacy over trephining.

There are some technical points of importance in connection with the operation, when performed on the large buphthalmic eye.—(1) The conjunctiva strips back off the cornea to a very unusual distance and with great ease. There is therefore no difficulty in placing the trephine far forward ; indeed, *the usual step of splitting the cornea is not called for in these cases.* (2) The chamber is so very deep that the trephine can be used with considerable boldness. (3) The tunic of the eye is sometimes very thin, so that it is quickly penetrated. In this connection Hamilton has observed that the tunic of the eye offers little resistance to the cutting blade, and thus makes the operation difficult. Contradictory as this statement may appear to be, there is a distinct element of truth in it, and it is not always easy to cut out a clean disc from one of these eyes. To make a hole, which shall prove to be permanent, is, however, a simpler matter. (4) A real obstacle is sometimes presented by the disproportion in size between the eyeball and the orbital opening. This renders it difficult to get far enough back to make a flap. An anæsthetic must sometimes be used ; assistance may be obtained by having the eye grasped below the cornea and rotated downward by a backward push ; an eyelid retractor for the upper lid may also be of value ; once the conjunctival flap is cut a strabismus hook, or a pair of strabismus forceps, engaging the superior rectus tendon, will prove of great value in the later stages of the operation.

The writer has under his care at the present time a young lady, who had been refused operation by very competent surgeons, and who felt her way into his consulting room with outstretched hands. She had never read a word ; her education was neglected, she was flabby, anæmic, and miserable. Now, over six years after trephining, she has made good some of her lost childhood, she walks with her head erect, rides a bicycle in quiet places, reads, sews, and does her lessons with other girls. Such cases are not uncommon after operation and are amongst the most gratifying that many of us can look back upon.

Be the method what it may, whether iridectomy, subconjunctival paracentesis, Lagrange's operation, trephining, or any other procedure, the writer holds most strongly that the essential factor of success lies in the production of a filtering scar. Our knowledge of the pathology of buphthalmos makes it obvious, that nothing less than the production of a vicarious channel for the escape of intraocular fluid can be of any avail. We know that it is the channels of excretion that are blocked, and if we cannot provide a sufficient safety-sluice, our procedure is doomed to failure. In dealing with senile glaucoma, one may possibly argue as to the rôle of a larger or smaller, a more peripheral or a more central removal of iris tissue ; here we are shut up to a congenital absence of the canal of Schlemm, or a congenital defect in the pectinate ligament. The writer has often contended, on clinical grounds, that the cure of a senile glaucoma by means of iridectomy or sclerotomy is frequently due to the accidental establishment of permanent filtration. If this be so in the case of senile glaucoma, he feels convinced that it will prove at least equally so in the pathologically simplified instances of buphthalmic eyes.

There are many ways of obtaining a filtering cicatrix. Some, such as subconjunctival paracentesis, may require less technical skill than trephining, but the writer believes that there is no surer and at the same time safer method in buphthalmos than the use of the trephine.

Before leaving the subject of treatment, there is a last and a very important word to be said, viz., that we must never forget the possibility that congenital syphilis may be playing a part in any case of buphthalmos, and that we must consequently order our methods of diagnosis and our therapy in the light of this knowledge. The surgeon who relegates this side of the question to the background of his mind is forfeiting some of the power with which modern science has equipped him for the treatment of the disease.

REFERENCES

ADAMS, P. H.—*The Ophthalmoscope*, vol. x. p. 261
ALLPORT, W.—*Brit. Med. Journ.*, March 5, 1911.
AXENFELD, T.—*Klin. Monatsbl. f. Augenh.*, October 1911.
BALL, J. N.—*Interstate Med. Journ.*, vol. xvii. p. 47.
BENTZEN AND LEBER—Von Graefe's *Archiv f. O.*, 1895, vol. xli. p. 3.
BLAIR, C.—*Trans. O.S. of U.K.*, vol. xxx. p. 228.
BOEHM, K.—*Klin. Monatsbl. f. Augenh.*, vol. lii. p. 83.
BROWN, S. HORTON—*Amer. Journ. of Ophth.*, vol. xxx. p. 20.
BUCK, R. H.—*Ibid.*, 1918, vol. i. p. 683.
BUNGE.—*Klin. Monatsbl. f. Augenh.*, June 1909, p. 643.
CABANNES, C.—*La Clinique Ophtal.*, September 10, 1909, and *The Ophthalmoscope*, vol. vii. p. 819.
CALHOUN, F. PHINIZY.—*Journ. A.M.A.*, July 18, 1914.
CHRISTEL, P.—*Archiv f. Augenh.*, vol. lxxi. p. 241.
COATS, GEORGE.—*Trans. O.S. of U.K.*, vol. xxvii. p. 48.
COATS, G.—*Ophthalmic Review*, vol. xxxiii. p. 146.
COLLINS, E. T.—*The Lancet*, 1894, p. 1463.
COLLINS, E. T.—*Trans. O.S. of U.K.*, vol. xxxiii. p. 193.
COLLINS AND BATTEN.—*Ibid.*, vol. xxv. p. 248.
COLLINS AND MARSHALL.—*Ibid.*, vol. xx. p. 156.
COLLINS AND MAYOU.—*System of Ophthalmic Practice*, "Pathology," Rebman Ltd., London.
CORONAT AND AURAND.—*Clin. Opht.*, 1912, vol. xviii. p. 498.
CROSS, RICHARDSON.—*Trans. O.S. of U.K.*, vol. xvi. p. 340.
CUPERUS, N. J.—*Klin. Monatsbl. f. Augenh.*, March 1910.
DE WECKER.—*Proc. Soc. Fran. d'Opht., Congrès de* 1901.
DUBOIS.—*Amer. Journ. Ophth.*, 1919, vol. ii. p. 146.
ERDMANN, PAUL.—*Archiv f. O.*, July 16, 1907, vol. lxvi. pt. 2
FAGE.—*Arch. d'opht.*, vol. xxxiv. p. 574.
FUCHS, E.—*Text-Book of Ophthalmology*, 4th edition (Duane), J. B. Lippincott Co., 1911.
FUCHS, E.—*Report of the Heidelberg Congress of Ophthalmology*, 1913.
GERMANN, D.—*Klin. Monatsbl. f. Augenh.*, July 1909.
GIFFORD, H. A.—*Ophth. Rec.*, August 1916.
GILBERT, W.—*Report of the Heidelberg Congress of Ophthalmology*, 1913.
GROS.—*Thèse de Paris*, 1897.
GROSS, E. G.—*Arch. Ophth.*, November 1909.
HAAG, C.—*Klin. Monatsbl. f. Augenh.*, vol. liv. p. 133.
HALLETT, DE W.—*Ophth. Year Book*, 1919, vol. xv. pp. 109 and 112.
HAMBURGER, C.—*Berlin Ophth. Gesell.*, January 1913.

HAMILTON, R. J.—*Arch. Ophth.*, vol. xlv. p. 372.
HAMILTON, R. J.—*Ophth. Rev.*, 1915, vol. xxxiv. p. 92.
HAY, P. J.—*Ophth. Rev.*, vol. xxxiv. p. 92.
HERBERT, H.—*The Ophthalmoscope*, vol. xii. p. 2.
HIRSCHBERG, J. — *Report of the Heidelberg Congress of Ophthalmology*, 1913.
HÖEG, N.—*Hosp. Tid.*, vol. iii. p. 825.
JAEGER, H.—*Munich Thesis*.
JONES, HUGH.—*Arch. Ophth.*, vol. xlv. p. 372.
KAYSER, B.—*Klin. Monatsbl. f. Augenh.*, vol. lii. p. 226.
KEY, B. W.—*Arch. Ophth.*, vol. xlv. p. 571.
KOMOTO, J. P.—*Klin. Monatsbl. f. Augenh.*, June 1910.
KÜMMELL, R.—*Arch. Ophth.*, vol. xliii. p. 50.
LAWFORD, J. B.—*R.L.O.H. Reports*, vol. xvii. p. 57.
LEBENSOHN, M. H.—*Amer. Journ. Ophth.*, 1918, vol. i. p. 684.
LOEHLEIN, W.—*Report of the Heidelberg Congress of Ophthalmology*, 1913, p. 97.
MAYOU, M. S.—*Trans. O.S. of U.K.*, vol. xxx. p. 120.
MAYOU, M. S.—*Proc. Roy. Soc. Med.*, April 1915.
MAYOU, M. S.—*Trans. O.S. of U.K.*, vol. xxxviii. p. 146.
MELLER, J.—*Klin. Monatsbl. f. Augenh.*, vol. lii. p. 1.
MURAKAMI, S.—*Klin. Monatsbl. f. Augenh.*, October to November 1913.
NAHMACHER, *Ibid.*, February 1912.
OWUCHI.—*Nippon Ganki Gazette*, December 1914.
PARSONS, J. H.—*The Pathology of the Eye*, vol. iii., Hodder and Stoughton, London.
PARSONS, J. H.—*Brit. Journ. Ophth.*, 1920, vol. iv. p. 211.
PETER, L. C.—*Amer. Journ. Ophth.*, 1919, vol. ii. p. 695.
PICHLER, A.—*Arch. f. Vergleich. Ophth.*, vol. i. p. 175.
PLANCHU AND GAUTIER.—*Recueil d'opht.*, vol. xxxii. p. 220.
PYLE, W. L.—*The Philadelphia Monthly Med. Journ.*, April 1899.
RISLEY, S. D.—*Annals of Ophth.*, vol. xxvi. p. 208.
ROCKLIFFE AND PARSONS.—*Trans. Path. Soc.*, vol. lv. p. 27.
RUMSCHEWITSCH, I.—*Klin. Monatsbl. f. Augenh.*, April 1909.
SACHSALBER.—*Beiträge z. Augenh.*, 1897, vol. xxvii. p. 523.
SCHREIBER AND WENGLER.—Von Graefe's *Archiv f. O.*, vol. lxxi. p. 99.
SEEFELDER, R.—*Trans. Thirty-sixth Ophth. Congress*, Heidelberg.
SEEFELDER, R.—*Klin. Monatsbl. f. Augenh.*, vol. lvi. p. 227.
SMITH, D. P.—*Ophth. Rev.*, vol. xxxiv. p. 33.
SMITH, PRIESTLEY.—*Seventeenth Internat. Congress of Med.*, London, 1913, section ix. part i.
SNELL AND COLLINS.—*Trans. O.S. of U.K.*, vol. xxiii. p. 157.
SPIELBERG, C.—*Klin. Monatsbl. f. Augenh.*, September 1911.
STÄHLI, J.—*Arch. f. Augenh.*, vol. lxxix. p. 141.
STÄHLI, J.—*Klin. Monatsbl. f. Augenh.*, vol. liii. p. 83.
STEPHENSON, S.—*The Brit. Journ. of Children's Diseases*, 1905.
STIMMEL AND ROTTER.—*Zeit. f. Augenh.*, vol. xxviii. p. 114.

TAKASHIMA, S.—*Klin. Monatsbl. f. Augenh.*, July and August 1913.
TERRIEN AND DANTRELLE.—*Ophth. Year Book*, 1913, p. 143.
THOMSON, ALEXIS.—*Neuroma and Neuro-fibromatosis*, Edinburgh, 1900.
THOMSON, ARTHUR.—*The Ophthalmoscope*, vol. ix. p. 470.
VERHOEFF, F. H.—*Trans. O.S. of U.K.*, vol. xxiii. p. 176.
VOGT, A.—*Clin. Opht.*, vol. xxiii. p. 667.
WEEKS, J. E.—*Arch. Ophth.*, vol. xlv. p. 372.
WEINSTEIN, A.—*Klin. Monatsbl. f. Augenh.*, November 1910.
WESSELY, K.—*Ophth. Year Book*, 1914, p. 204.
WOOD, CASEY.—*Ophth. Rec.*, vol. xxiv. p. 235.
ZEEMAN, W. P. C.—Neth. Ophth. Soc., Fifty-second Meeting, trans. in *Amer. Journ. Ophth.*, 1919, vol. ii. p. 144.
ZENTMAYER, W.—*Ophth. Rec.*, vol. xxii. p. 25.
ZENTMAYER, W.—Section on Ophth., *Journ. A.M.A.*, 1913, p. 140, and *Ophth. Year Book*, 1914, vol. xi. p. 204.

CHAPTER VII

THE MEDICAL TREATMENT OF GLAUCOMA

IF the surgeon would have clear ideas as to the value of the non-operative treatment of glaucoma, it is essential that he should first understand that several quite distinct conditions confront him in his consideration of this problem. Should he fail to realise this, the result can only be confusion.

Before attempting to discuss the therapeutic means at our command, it is advisable to clear the way by a short statement of what these conditions are :

(A) The prophylaxis of glaucoma.—Under this heading is embraced the consideration of the management of two problems :

(i.) The *prevention of the onset of hypertonus* in the hitherto healthy eye of a patient, in whom we have reason to fear such a complication. That fear may be founded on the family history, on the anatomical configuration of the globes, on the condition of the fellow eye, on a history of vague signs or symptoms possibly indicating the presence of the disease, on the diagnosis, perhaps mistaken, of another medical man, or on any or all of these together.

(ii.) The *prevention of the recurrence of a hypertonus*, which has already declared itself in the past, either by the manifestation of the so-called premonitory signs and symptoms, or by the advent of a distinct and unmistakable attack of congestive glaucoma.

(B) The treatment of an established condition of simple non-congestive glaucoma.

(C) The treatment of an attack of congestive glaucoma.

It will save time and trouble, if before attempting to

discuss the treatment of each of these conditions in detail, we review the various non-operative means which time and experience have placed at our disposal for use in our struggle with glaucoma. There is a strong reason for doing this, since these measures are to a greater or less extent available for the treatment of all the conditions alike.

The Therapeutic Means of Combating Glaucoma

These may be catalogued as follows :—(i.) The production of meiosis ; (ii.) the employment of massage ; (iii.) the use of electricity and of diathermy ; (iv.) the employment of antiphlogistic treatment ; (v.) the production of an increase in the flow of lymph through the eye, or of an alteration in the osmotic properties of the intra-ocular structures ; (vi.) the artificial lowering of the general vascular pressure ; and (vii.) the combating or neutralisation of the various sources of autogenetic intoxication.

(i.) **Meiotics.**—Of these eserin and pilocarpine, with their salts, have proved their efficiency and are widely used. The salicylate of eserin is usually preferred to the sulphate, and the nitrate of pilocarpine to the chloride of that alkaloid. De Schweinitz is of the opinion that the meiosis is due to a direct stimulation of the sphincter muscle fibres, possibly aided by the contraction of the iris vessels. The reduction of intra-ocular pressure which attends it in pathologic cases is usually attributed to two factors : (1) The opening up of the angle of the anterior chamber, which follows the contraction of the pupil ; and (2) the increased surface for absorption presented by the iris under these circumstances. Both explanations appear to be valid. It is, however, worth mentioning that Pissarello has found, that the lowering of tension, produced by the drugs we are considering, is not always in constant relation with the degree of meiosis produced.

A further point of interest is that, when dealing with normal eyes, the production of drug-meiosis produces little if any fall in intra-ocular pressure (Carr, Van Hoorn). The contrast between this fact and the well-known reduction by eserin or pilocarpine of the tension of glaucomatous eyes is highly significant from the point of view of pathology; for the time-honoured explanation that the meiosis produced "clears the angle of the chamber," which is being threatened with blockage in the pathologic eye, fully covers the difference in the behaviour of the normal and glaucomatous globes.

(ii.) **Massage** may be applied to the eye (*a*) with the finger tips (digital massage), or (*b*) by means of instruments, or (*c*) with the aid of suction cups.

(*a*) *Digital massage.*—The great value of massage in glaucoma does not appear to be sufficiently appreciated. The tension of an eye can be quickly and sensibly reduced by digital manipulation, and the patient can be taught to perform the simple movements for himself. These are two in number. The first consists in placing the tips of the two index fingers on the upper lid over the globe (the surgeon standing behind the patient), and pressing with each finger in turn in the direction of the centre of the eye. The movements should be slow at first, and more rapid later, as the operator acquires skill and the patient toleration; the subject must look downward, and gently close the eyes. The period of massage should be short at first (about half a minute), and should be extended until it lasts three to five minutes, thrice daily or more often. The second movement is a gentle, circular, smoothing action performed with three fingers of one hand, through the lightly closed lids. It serves the same purpose as the wide smoothing movements used after massage of other parts, and only needs to be done for about fifteen or twenty seconds. A fomentation given after the massage proves very soothing to the patient, and probably intensifies the effect produced.

(*b*) *Instrumental massage.*—A number of surgeons have advocated the use of this form of treatment. One of the best known instruments for the purpose is that of Maklakow: The point of an Edison electric pen carries a small ivory ball, which is made to vibrate from two or three hundred to as many thousand times a minute in contact with the closed lid. The author used one of these instruments for nearly fifteen years, and found it of considerable value ; it has, however, one great drawback, viz., that it so easily and so often goes out of working order. Some years ago, he got the Dental Manufacturing Company to make an accessory fitting to his pantostat ; this consists of a length of flexible tubing similar to that used by dental surgeons, and capable of transmitting a direct, downward hammer stroke in the direction of the length of the tubing ; into the dental hammer-fitting can be screwed a number of shallow vulcanite cups. These have been made of various sizes so that they can be used on different eyes, and have been moulded on to living globes for the purpose whilst the vulcanite was soft. The length of stroke, that is thus transmitted through the lids to the globe, can be varied within wide limits. The effect of rapidly repeated electric massage is considerable and it is very soothing to the patient. The objections to it are that it can only be administered with the aid of a pantostat, and that the apparatus is expensive. Nor can it be urged that it has any great advantage over carefully applied digital massage.

(c) *Suction massage.*—This is well described by de Schweinitz in the following words : " Another means of reducing intra-ocular pressure is by the suction method, which consists in the use of certain cups, from which air is exhausted by means of a suction apparatus. Domec uses an elliptical eye cup, the concave margins of which fit closely about the globe. The air is exhausted with each respiration of the patient, and from 50 to 200 tractions are made at each sitting. Domec is of the opinion that this method succeeds in two ways, viz., in producing analgesia by traction on the ciliary nerves, and in reducing intra-ocular pressure." De Schweinitz enters a caution against the abuse of these really useful methods at the hands of irregular practitioners.

(iii.) **The Use of Electricity and Diathermy.**—It is stated that the application of high-frequency currents is capable of reducing both the arterial and the ocular pressures. The constant current has also been vaunted for the same purpose, the negative pole being applied to the eye, and the positive one to the neck; a current of 30 to 40 ma. has been used for a quarter of an hour by Le Prince, but Coleman considers that a much lower current should be employed. There are not a few reliable observers, amongst whom is to be numbered de Schweinitz, who have expressed themselves as being doubtful of the therapeutic value of electricity in glaucoma.

The author has no personal experience of diathermy in the treatment of increased intra-ocular pressure, nor has he been favourably impressed by what he has been able to read of the reports of its use by other surgeons.

(iv.) **Antiphlogistic Treatment.**—This includes purgation, the use of leeches, the application of wet and dry fomentations, and the placing of the patient under the most favourable possible conditions for rest both of mind and body. It is obviously applicable only to congestive conditions.

(v.) **The Production of an Increase in the Lymph-Flow or of an Alteration in Osmosis.**—The means which have been recommended to attain these ends have been (*a*) the subconjunctival injection of saline solutions, of which sodium citrate has been the favourite; (*b*) the administration by the mouth, by the rectum, or into the veins, of dialysable substances intended to raise the concentration of salts, etc., in the blood; and (*c*) the local application of dionin.

We shall consider these in turn:

(*a*) The subconjunctival injection of saline solutions has found very few advocates indeed, and not all of these seem very whole-hearted.

(*b*) The administration of dialysable substances by the mouth, rectum, or veins has not received much support. Thomas gives sodium carbonate and sodium chloride in draughts, and at the same time injects 2 tablespoonfuls of sodium bicarbonate, dissolved in 2 quarts of hot water, into the rectum, every morning and evening, with a view to increase the saline concentration of the blood. Alt, following Weekers, has administered 15 grs. of calcium chloride, thrice daily, by the mouth, and has even given bigger doses than this, prescribing the remedy for months at a time, without any inconvenience to the patient, and with marked improvement in the signs of the disease. He quotes Gowland, of Buenos Ayres, as having injected a 2 per cent. solution of the same drug in 2 c.c. doses into the buttock, without pain, and with the reduction of ocular tension. Weekers' latest reports on the method seem less confident than those of Alt. He advocates the use of the drug principally in chronic cases ; he finds that the digestive tract does not tolerate it well in acute glaucoma ; intramuscular injection has not commended itself in his experience. Sansum has employed graded intravenous injections of glucose, and has obtained very striking reductions in intra-ocular pressure thereby.

(c) The local application of dionin is sometimes of real value. The drug can be used either in solution or in ointment ; the latter is preferable, as it largely limits the action of the dionin to the eye, and so spares the nasal passages. It is well, when using it, to begin with weak strengths (2 to 3 per cent.), and to increase the concentration from time to time as required.

(vi.) **The Reduction of the General Blood-pressure.**— From what has been said in previous chapters, the reader will have seen that there is little foundation for the long-cherished belief, that an increase of the general blood-pressure is a serious factor in the causation of glaucoma. It may indeed be questioned whether we are not more likely to do harm than good in glaucomatous cases by drastic measures aimed at the lowering of the general vascular pressure. At the same time, we should of course advise the patient so to regulate his life as to avoid all sources of strain, fatigue, and exhaustion, and we should give him general directions as to his diet, the care of his bowels, and the procuring of regular sleep. Pissarello has found that the ingestion of food lowers the intra-ocular pressure, and on the strength of this observation, he advises the glaucomatous patient to eat little and often, rather than to make few and large meals.

(vii.) **Auto-Intoxication.**—It seems probable that one of the great advances of the future may lie in the direction of the early and scientific combating of the sources of auto-intoxication.

This subject belongs largely to prophylaxis, and will be considered under that head, but it should by no means be forgotten in the routine treatment of cases in which glaucoma has definitely declared itself. Hawley has suggested the irrigation of the lower bowel, in order to remove a possible source of poisoning. Bell, too, has laid some stress on attention to intestinal antisepsis. Brown has seen good result from attention to an unhealthy naso-pharyngeal condition, though he insists much more earnestly on the need for the correction of all errors of refraction in any doubtful case. Homer Smith has indicted the endocrine glands, and entered a plea for the thorough and methodical examination of each glaucoma patient, with a view to the inception of treatment on modern bio-chemical lines. Lamb, who holds similar views, speaks of glaucoma as " the end result of gonadal and renal insufficiency." He suggests the internal administration of adrenalin chloride and pilocarpine.

THE DIFFERENT GLAUCOMATOUS CONDITIONS FOR THE RELIEF OF WHICH MEDICAL TREATMENT MAY BE REQUIRED.

Having dealt with the various therapeutic means at our disposal, we are now in a position to discuss the management of the various conditions, which we tabulated at the beginning of this chapter as possibly calling for the exhibition of non-operative treatment. We shall take them in turn :

The Prophylaxis of Glaucoma.—It has already been pointed out that prophylactic treatment may be thought advisable in patients who have never yet developed an

MEDICAL TREATMENT OF GLAUCOMA

attack of glaucoma, but in whom, for one reason or another, it seems wise to take precautions. It is quite obvious that our position, in dealing with such people, is a considerably weaker one than that which we can take up with patients, who in the past have developed definite signs of hypertension. It matters little whether such signs have been only those which have so misguidedly been branded as "premonitory," or whether they have been sufficiently pronounced to indicate a definite attack of congestive glaucoma. In either case, the surgeon has been placed on his guard, the patient has been alarmed, and the necessity for taking trouble to meet the threatened danger is, or should be, realised by them both. The man, whose future is haunted by the spectre of coming blindness, is much easier to manage, and naturally so, than is he whose fears are founded only on the vague prognostications of a suspicious family history or of deficient corneal measurements. In dealing with both of them the same rules guide us. We must endeavour to regulate our patient's life in such a way as to save him from the results of those perversions of nutrition, which are inseparable from the advance of life. We should eliminate, as far as possible, all causes of autogenetic intoxication; we must cut down the abuse of alcohol, and the grosser indulgences of wrong dietary; and we must insist on regular hours, and sufficient exercise. Again, we should counsel him to avoid want of sleep, constipation, prolonged stooping, overwork, worry, and exhaustion. It may be questioned whether all this good advice will often be of much avail, unless and until the patient has been aroused to a sense of his danger by the onset of definite symptoms. Then, and only then, will he be likely to co-operate with us. Once these have made their appearance, we can count, with reasonable certainty, upon his endeavouring to carry out our instructions, but not before. Then, too, we are in a position to recommend the establishment and maintenance of a constant meiosis, if that course recommends itself to our judgment. The question as to the advisability of substituting operative for non-operative treatment will at once arise. With this subject we shall deal at length in Part II. of Chapter VIII. ; for the present we may concern ourselves simply with indicating the lines along which medical treatment, if decided upon, may best be conducted in the class of case we are discussing.

The maintenance of protracted meiosis.—The advocates of this form of treatment insist that the strength of the instillations should be kept sufficiently low to avoid ciliary cramp, and that the use of the drug should be life-long. Posey, who is one of the ablest, most earnest, and most indefatigable of the champions of prolonged meiotic treatment, has advocated beginning with a tenth of a grain of salicylate of eserin to the ounce, and gradually increasing the strength, so that at the end of some months the patient is using one grain to the ounce of solution. If pilocarpine is used, he doubles the strength. It is simpler to tie oneself to no hard-and-fast rule, but to treat each case individually, using the weakest solution that will maintain meiosis, and only increasing its strength when one finds that it is failing to accomplish its purpose. De Schweinitz, who is distinctly an advocate of early operation, holds that if meiosis can be maintained without causing irritation, the chances of preserving vision are good. He says that " eserin irritation is most successfully avoided, not by preparations of the meiotics in combination with the antiseptics, for example, tricresol, which has been so much advocated, but by ordering very small quantities of the solution, and insisting that it should be very frequently renewed and sterilised at each preparation, and that half an hour after its instillation, during the daytime at least, the eye should be thoroughly flushed with some mild antiseptic solution, for example, boric acid and sodium chloride." He adds, " the great trouble with meiotic treatment is not its lack of efficiency, but the difficulty of carrying it out successfully on ambulant patients, even in the better walks of life. It is hard successfully to maintain in a patient with chronic glaucoma what I may call an eserin life, just as it is hard to maintain in a patient with an enlarged prostate a catheter life and escape infection, resulting, if it occurs, in the one instance in a difficult and stubborn conjunctivitis, and in the other in a cystitis."

The author is not disposed to take such a favourable view of the results to be obtained from meiotic treatment as some surgeons seem to be. There are cases on record in which the glaucomatous process has been long held at bay by non-operative treatment. Individually, the most remarkable of them are those recorded by Lawson and Jackson, whilst Posey has furnished the largest and most detailed statistics on the subject. Lawson's notes, as well as his comments on the case, are worthy of study. He points out, *inter alia*, that instances of this kind are very rare. Of this there can be no question ; on the other hand, every one of us has seen, not one case, but many, in which the desire to hold on to meiotic treatment has resulted in the forfeiture of the patient's sight. Many surgeons' note-books will be found to contain cases of this kind, which come not only from the hands of general practitioners but also from those of able and experienced ophthalmologists. The subject will be dealt with more fully in the next chapter. It will suffice here to make two statements : (i.) The moment that non-operative treatment shows evidence of failing to hold the disease in check, the time has come for surgical interference. (ii.) De Wecker's dictum stands as true to-day as when he first uttered it : " If meiotics have never cured a case of glaucoma, they have prevented many glaucomatous patients from being cured."

In our consideration of this subject, it is important to bear in mind that many of our glaucomatous patients, who will start a prophylactic life with energy and faithfulness, relax in their efforts, as soon as the first fear of consequences passes away, with the result that the regimen we prescribe is not really carried out in its entirety. On the other hand, once a decompression operation has been performed, they are free to live an ordinary life. This is by no means a small matter.

In order the better to estimate what may reasonably be expected from carefully conducted meiotic and general treatment, it is important to realise exactly what meiosis can do for a glaucomatous patient. It can clear the angle of the chamber and thus make physiological filtration as efficient as possible ; and it can augment this effect by increasing the surface of iris available for the absorption of fluid. So much it *can* do, but it *cannot* in any way influence the progress of those anatomical or pathological conditions on which the steady advance of glaucoma depends. Its value is unquestionably greatest in those cases into which an element of congestion enters, for by increasing the outflow of aqueous, it lowers the tension of the eye, removes the obstruction to venous outflow, and thereby helps to cut the vicious circle on which the periodic increases of tension are dependent. In the simple non-congestive cases, all that can be hoped from it, is aid in the prevention of the entry on the scene of the congestive process.

Another point to be kept in view is the period of the twenty-four hours during which the production of meiosis is most likely to be of service to the patient. In considering this important detail, we must remember that two types of condition have to be differentiated : (1) That in which the trouble is primarily due to an interference with the normal vaso-motor mechanism of the eye. The cases coming under this head complain of their symptoms when they are overtired or exhausted, and the indication is to anticipate such a condition by instilling the meiotic beforehand. Inquiry will elicit the best time for the purpose ; usually it will be found that this will be the afternoon, or the late evening. Rest, food, or sleep are of great value in augmenting the effect of meiotic treatment. (2) The type in which the trouble is primarily due to the gradually increasing obstruction to the excretion of intra-ocular fluid next requires consideration. When the patient is moving about and actively using his eyes, he is constantly calling into play that pump action of his iris and ciliary muscles, for the knowledge of which we are indebted to Arthur Thomson. When he falls asleep these movements cease, and then the danger, that deficient excretion will lead to the accumulation of an excess of fluid within the eye, distinctly rises ; the result is a tendency towards the establishment of hypertonus—and this despite the fact that sleep tends to lower intra-ocular pressure, (*a*) by causing a fall in the general blood-pressure, (*b*) by promoting meiosis, and (*c*) by diminishing secretory activity (Gunnufsen). This tendency has long been well known to ophthalmic surgeons, and the consequence has been that it is an established practice to advise the instillation of the meiotic drug the last thing at night. De Schweinitz goes farther than this and recommends a second instillation in the early hours of the morning ; he states that most patients can learn to wake themselves for the purpose. His advice should be taken earnestly to heart.

The author's own practice is to recommend the instillation of as weak a solution of pilocarpine as will keep the pupil contracted, in the morning on awaking, in the afternoon about 4 p.m., and last thing at night. If the onset of the trouble is clearly traceable to fatigue, the patient is directed to anticipate it by an hour with the instillation. If it is a case in which the want of the normal pump action is evidently at fault, the patient is advised to instil an extra drop of the meiotic in the middle of the night, when he or she gets up to pass urine, as the elderly patient usually does.

Some surgeons have suggested that even in those patients who have never yet shown any signs of ocular hypertension, we should institute a course of prophylactic meiotic treatment. To condemn a large body of people to so grave an inconvenience, for long periods of life, in the absence of definite symptoms of glaucoma, does not recommend itself as being in the interests of the greatest good of the greatest number. Meiosis should only be resorted to when there is a distinct indication for it, and not otherwise.

The use of massage.—The value of massage in the treatment of glaucoma, altogether apart from any operative interference, has been greatly under-estimated in the past by the medical profession. The tension of an eye can be quickly, painlessly, harmlessly, and repeatedly reduced by this means without the intervention of a surgeon; for the patient can learn to perform the necessary manipulation without discomfort to himself, and without having to be dependent on the help of another. For these reasons we can employ it even as a prophylactic measure, without the hesitation that we feel in resorting to the use of meiotics.

Medicinal treatment. — From time to time surgeons have recommended the administration of the iodides and of the salicylates in the treatment of the different phases of glaucoma, but it is open to doubt whether these measures are of value. Nor does there appear to be any strong movement of clinical opinion in favour of the injection into the circulation of hypertonic solutions of sodium salts or of glucose. This matter has already been discussed. The idea has proved attractive to some very able ophthalmologists, but has never taken on with the profession at large.

The Treatment of an Established Condition of Simple Non-Congestive Glaucoma.—The progress of a case of simple glaucoma is always slow, and sometimes extremely so. Little change takes place from month to month, and it is consequently very difficult to be sure how far any form of treatment is proving of benefit. The distinction between eyes suffering from this form of the disease and those just dealt with under the heading of prophylaxis, lies in the fact that the former present definite stigmata of disease on examination, whilst the latter, at least at an early stage, may seem quite normal in the intervals between two attacks. This difference depends on the further fact, that in the simple cases the congestive element is so feebly marked as to be recognisable only by the most careful observation; whereas it is by the congestive exacerbations of the condition that we are able so easily to mark the progress of the other cases. The central visual acuity, which is so often impaired, as a result of a congestive attack, is in the simple cases often maintained at a high level to the end. We are thus robbed of all those subjective warnings which drive the congestive patient to the surgeon, and help to determine the undertaking of an operative procedure for the relief of the hypertension. The plain moral of all this is that we must be very much on our guard in these cases, and must take the visual fields at frequent intervals; we should also watch the depth and degree of cupping of the optic disc with especial care; for these observations often furnish our only indications of the progress of the disease. In no case should the periodic use of the tonometer be neglected. If there *is* progress, however slow it may be, we should drop non-operative treatment and resort to the production of a fistulous scar without further delay. For the rest, what has been said under the previous heading of prophylaxis may be repeated here. Most particularly is it to be remembered that meiotic and general treatment is not curative. It may arrest the advance of the degenerative changes caused by the disease, by eliminating the element of congestion, and by lowering the intra-ocular pressure for the time being, but that is absolutely all it can do. When it ceases to do even that, it has been tried all too long, even though the manifestations of congestion are so subdued as to need the most careful examination of the patient for their detection.

The Treatment of a Congestive Attack of Glaucoma.—Such treatment may be designed to prepare the patient for operation, or it may be deliberately substituted for surgical treatment as the result of one or another reason against the inception of the latter. The patient or his friends may refuse consent to any operation, or the state of his health may render it inadvisable to resort to surgery, or there may be some other social or economic factor in the case. If non-operative treatment is to be relied upon, it should be vigorous, and should include purgation, local blood-letting, preferably by leeches, the employment of fomentations, both moist and dry, rest in bed, the relief of pain by morphia or preferably by trivalin-hyoscin, and the isolation of the patient from all worry, anxiety, and work. Hot baths are certainly valuable, and Turkish baths have been lauded by at least one writer. Meiotics should be used in much stronger doses than those recommended for the maintenance of prolonged meiosis. Eserin in strengths of from 0·25 to 1·0 per cent. in combination with a 2 per cent. solution of cocaine should be instilled every three hours or oftener, until the symptoms are relieved, and then less frequently. It is important to employ the solutions fresh.

Von Arlt strongly recommends the combined use of pilocarpine and dionin for the relief of glaucoma. One-thirtieth of a grain of pilocarpine is to be introduced into the conjunctival sac, followed eight minutes later by one-twelfth of a grain of powdered dionin. This process is repeated every third day, and in the interval a 2 to 3 per cent. solution of pilocarpine is instilled every third hour. The use of the dionin is timed so that the maximum effects of both drugs may coincide. The lachrymal canaliculi must be closed by digital pressure during the application of the drugs. Some surgeons, on the contrary, have condemned dionin as dangerous in conditions of ocular hypertension; their view would appear to have been based on the use of dionin alone, and not on its combination with meiotics.

Subconjunctival injections of normal, saline solution and of sodium citrate solution have been suggested, largely on theoretical grounds, for the relief of hypertension, but it cannot be said that they have justified the expectations formed of them, and they have consequently fallen into desuetude.

Massage is of very doubtful value in acute cases; it may do much more harm than good, and it is therefore safer to rely on the other measures we have detailed.

Gilbert has advocated venesection; the idea cannot be said to have ever found favour with the profession.

Sansum has, as already mentioned, reported very remarkable results from the intravenous injection of glucose in acute cases, prior to the undertaking of an operation. The method seems worthy of consideration.

REFERENCES

ALT, A. A.—*Amer. Journ. Ophth.*, 1918, vol. i. p. 184.
BELL, G. H.—*Arch. of Ophth.*, 1920, vol. xlix. p. 341.
BROWN, E. J.—*Amer. Journ. Ophth.*, 1920, vol. iii. p. 669.
CARR, A. M.—*Arch. of Ophth.*, vol. xlvii. p. 177.
DE SCHWEINITZ, G. E.—*Glaucoma, a Symposium*, Nance & Peck, Chicago Medical Book Co., 1914.
DOMEC, T.—*Ibid.*
GILBERT, W.—*Klin. Monatsbl. f. Augenh.*, December 1912, p. 750.
GUNNUFSEN, P.—*Clin. Opht.*, vol. xxii. p. 293; and *Arch. of Ophth.*, vol. xlvii. p. 106.
HAWLEY, C. W.—*Ann. of Ophth.*, vol. xxvi. p. 421.
JACKSON, E.—*Ophth. Rec.*, vol. xxvi. p. 306; and *Ophth. Year Book*, 1917–1918, vol. xiv. p. 84.
LAMB, R. S.—*Amer. Journ. Ophth.*, 1918, vol. i. p. 184.
LAWSON, A.—*Trans. O.S. of U.K.*, vol. xxxiii. p. 194.
PISSARELLO, C.—*Ann. di Ottal.*, vol. xliv. p. 544.
POSEY, W. C.—*Ophth. Rec.*, vol. xxiv. p. 526; *Journ. Amer. Med. Assoc.*, vol. lxiii. p. 219; *ibid.*, 1915, p. 37; *Arch. of Ophth.*, 1920, vol. xlix. p. 293.
SANSUM, W. D.—*Journ. Amer. Med. Assoc.*, vol. lxviii. p. 1885.
SMITH, HOMER E.—*Amer. Journ. Ophth.*, 1920, vol. iii. p. 673.
THOMAS, H. G.—*Ophthalmology*, vol. xiii. p. 582.
VAN HOORN, W.—*Arch. d'opht.*, vol. xxxv. p. 506; and *Ophth. Year Book*, 1917–1918, vol. xiv. p. 80.
VON ARLT.—*Clin. Opht.*, vol. xviii. p. 321.
WEEKERS, L.—*La Clin. Opht.*, June 10, 1912; *Bull. de la Soc. Belge d'opht.*, 1920, p. 39; *Arch. d'opht.*, July 1920.

CHAPTER VIII

IRIDECTOMY IN GLAUCOMA

PART I

The Opinions of the Old Masters

SUMMARY :—Von Graefe.
          De Wecker.
          The 112 Surgeons whom de Wecker addressed.
             (1) The Confusion as to what is to be included in the Term Glaucoma.
             (2) The Variations in the Period at which Operative Interference is undertaken.
             (3) The Variations in the Periods during which the Cases were followed after Operation.
             (4) The Variations in the Technique of the Operation.

FROM the date of the first introduction by von Graefe of the operation of iridectomy for the relief of glaucoma, the merits and demerits of the procedure have been constantly under discussion by ophthalmologists. From time to time the dispute has died down in intensity, only to flare up afresh under the influence of some zealous advocate of the method. At any time we are liable to find ourselves in the midst of one of these periodical outbreaks, and it therefore behoves us to consider the whole question carefully and impartially.

No one who reads the large amount of literature that has appeared on the subject within recent years, can fail to be struck by the fact, that an enormous majority of those who write and speak on it lay very little stress on the magnificent work of the past masters of our craft. To ignore or even to undervalue the work of those, who laid sure and strong the foundations of ophthalmology, would be a mistake in the consideration of any subject, and a very great one indeed in this. For these men worked and wrote under the spell of the enthusiasm cast by von Graefe's great discovery, in the first dawn of the conquest of glaucoma. There were then few ophthalmic surgeons in the field, and operative practice was concentrated in the hands of those few, to the benefit of their surgical skill, and to the multiplication of their professional experience. One point more, and no light one, iridectomy had no serious rival in the field, and reigned a practically undisputed mistress in the domain of glaucoma therapy. It is for these reasons that we shall begin our study of the question before us with the cry " Back to the Old Masters ! " Those who have read, or who will read patiently, what von Graefe, de Wecker, Mackenzie, Bowman, George Critchett, and many another giant of the past had to say on the clinical side of the subject, are bound to rise from their task in a chastened and humble frame of mind. It is true that so far as concerns pathology, these makers of ophthalmic history were dimly groping their way toward the light of a day which has since broken so fully, that the youngest student may learn and clearly understand the facts toward which von Graefe faintly stretched his faltering hands ; but when it comes to clinical observation, the ablest surgeon of the twentieth century may gratefully and profitably learn from the men whose names, now but an honoured memory, were household words in his childhood, or before his birth.

We shall begin with von Graefe. What was his actual attitude towards the advocacy of iridectomy ? It may be summed up in a few short sentences :

(1) The results obtained are in all cases in direct proportion to the promptitude with which the operation is performed.

(2) The more marked the signs of intra-ocular pressure the better the expectation of a happy result, and *vice versa*.

(3) Even when iridectomy offers the least prospect of success, it still remains the surgeon's best hope.

To deal with his views more at length : His all too short experience showed him that the uncertainty of the results obtained by iridectomy in the later stages of glaucoma, was so absolutely opposed to the completeness and durability of the benefits obtained by surgical interference at the earliest possible moment, that he says " the advice to operate immediately and without hesitation cannot be too urgent." Again, " the degree of recovery essentially depends on the length of time the eye has already been affected, and not simply on the condition of the symptoms," and so on all through his writings. Indeed, he went farther than many surgeons are prepared to go to-day, for he advocated most strongly that the operation should be performed in what was then, and we fear is still too often now, regarded as the premonitory stage of the disease. To this recommendation he adds the curious rider that the operation should be undertaken at this stage, " when the other eye has become blind from the same affection."

The qualification is the more extraordinary since it was von Graefe himself who laid down that the existence of " the premonitory stage can never with certainty be denied in the second eye " when the first is severely affected, since the signs and symptoms in the latter overshadow those in the former, and so make them difficult for the patient to recognise.

There can be little doubt, that had von Graefe lived longer, his keen mind would have swept away the artificial and deceptive distinctions, which have been built up between the so-called premonitory and actual stages of glaucoma, and would have launched his operative interference for the first eye as well as for the second at the earliest possible moment. Such would have been the logical evolution, and von Graefe was always logical, of the mind-workings of the man who wrote " iridectomy is obviously most successful during the premonitory period. —The result is still more perfect than when it is performed in the inflammatory stage, soon after the disease has broken out.—The ultimate acuteness of vision very much depends on the period at which the operation is performed."

He was led, in the first instance, to these conclusions by

observing that when he had occasion to operate at one sitting on the two eyes of a patient, in whom the attack of glaucoma had come on in one eye sooner than in the other, it was invariably the eye with the shorter history of the disease, that gave the better result. We shall have many occasions to return to this dictum of von Graefe's. If he had given the world nothing else, he would not have lived in vain. Through all the long years of the half-century that has elapsed since his great work on glaucoma began, the dominant theme in all that has been written on the subject is contained in the two words "operate early." Timid and cautious men have shrunk from the advice, but we believe it remains to-day the clarion call of glaucoma surgery.

The next point, which we must take up and elaborate a little, is that of von Graefe's experience of iridectomy in the more chronic as compared with the congestive forms of glaucoma. Here, again, we shall as far as possible give his own words. He says " symptoms of increased pressure are in favour of the performance of iridectomy since this operation favourably influences cases with high tension," and again, " the more distinct the symptoms of increased pressure are at the time of operation, the more, *ceteris paribus*, may be expected from iridectomy."

Of the results of iridectomy in congestive glaucoma he speaks in glowing terms, but his tone is much less hopeful, when he comes to deal with those obtained by operative measures undertaken for the relief of the chronic form of the disease. This is repeatedly shown throughout his writings, as the following extracts will prove. " Iridectomy exerts a temporary favourable influence even in chronic glaucoma ; since this therapeutic action is at all events superior to the curative effect of any other method of treatment, it is our duty to continue it." And again, he says of iridectomy in chronic glaucoma, " it is indicated, so long as any considerable amount of vision remains, though in many cases negative results, and in others only temporary ones, will be obtained."

There is one very important fact, which must never be

lost sight of, viz., that the great master ruled outside the pale of glaucoma a large number of cases which we to-day would unhesitatingly place in the simple chronic group. On this subject he says, "I never observed any special curative action of iridectomy in amaurosis with excavation of the optic nerve." Those who have studied his writings will probably have little difficulty in agreeing, that under this heading were confused two great groups of cases, (1) that of the simple chronic glaucomas, and (2) that of cases of optic atrophy with shallow cupping of the nerve-head. Von Graefe's classification of glaucoma had not attained the precision of ours of to-day. When he spoke of chronic glaucoma, he would appear to have included a number of cases with subacute exacerbations, and he undoubtedly excluded a large number of those which we should now unhesitatingly include. Only quite recently have ophthalmologists recognised, that there are cases of indisputable, pathological, high tension, which are hidden from digital examination and revealed only to the tonometer. The writer further believes that as time goes on, the view will gain ground that even the most chronic cases have their ups and downs, which are dependent upon vascular storms identical in quality, although widely different in intensity, from those which mark the periodicity of unquestionably congestive cases. At a time when writers are to be found who suggest that iridectomy may be as valuable in chronic as in acute glaucoma, or even more so, it is important not merely to bear in mind what von Graefe said of the success of the operation in the two classes of cases, but also to remember carefully, that his group of chronic glaucoma was a much more limited one than our own.

From the writings of von Graefe, the distinguished introducer of iridectomy for glaucoma, we turn to a consideration of those who were his contemporaries, or who worked shortly after his death. Of these one man stands out pre-eminent, not merely because he was admittedly one of the greatest ophthalmologists of his time, but still more because he was at once the ablest and the most ardent of the partisans whom von Graefe gathered to his standard. His monograph in defence of iridectomy stretched to nearly 200 pages of closely-written matter, and is one of the most valuable contributions that has ever been made to the subject of glaucoma. To the writer it seems that de Wecker first undertook this task with a confidence and an enthusiasm, which could not fail to be modified by the tenor of the remarks, made in reply to his queries, by 112 of the most famous ophthalmic surgeons then living. In those enquiries de Wecker limited himself to the action of iridectomy in simple chronic glaucoma. Before turning to consider what his correspondents had to say, it seems expedient to begin by studying his own conclusions. These may be shortly stated first :

(1) As to the time of operation, he repeatedly endorsed and urged von Graefe's advice " the sooner the better." Like his master he felt the great difficulty of deciding what cases were to be included in the category of simple glaucoma, and he was likewise disposed to exclude a class of case, which we would now unhesitatingly accept as glaucomatous.

(2) Much as he valued treatment by meiotics, he thought it doubtful whether their introduction had not done more harm than good, since it had led surgeons to delay the time of operation. He went on to say "*if meiotics have never cured a case of glaucoma, they have prevented many glaucomatous patients from being cured.*" The italics are our own.

(3) He was a firm believer in the value of general treatment, but only as an accessory to operation, and he went so far as to say that it would become dangerous if it were allowed to delay operative treatment.

(4) With von Graefe he believed that the more acute the form of glaucoma, the better were the results obtained, but he was clearly disposed to attribute the comparatively little success, which attended iridectomy in chronic cases, to the late period at which operation was so often undertaken in them.

(5) It is the crown of de Wecker's glaucoma work, that he appreciated and insisted on the important rôle played

by the filtering cicatrix in iridectomy cases. Von Graefe had observed that a typical filtering cicatrix could be seen after iridectomy in one case in every fifteen, and that "sufficiently marked filtration" could be demonstrated in one case out of every five; but although the possibility that this might be of importance had not escaped him, he had failed to discern its true significance. It was left to de Wecker to bring the filtering cicatrix before the profession as an objective of surgical therapeutics. That he did so must ever redound to his credit.

(6) In his concluding pages, he advocated a combination of sclerotomy and iridectomy as being of more value than either operation alone.

(7) He practically adopted von Graefe's defence of the method, which was, that in the absence of some better method of treating glaucoma, it was the surgeon's duty to perform an iridectomy.

These last two points seem to the writer to be deserving of the most careful consideration, at a time when surgeons are to be found who advocate a surrender of the filtration operations and a return to iridectomy. Let us not forget that the two greatest men of the "iridectomy period" laid stress on the fact that there was then no other alternative available, and that it was therefore the duty of the surgeon to use the operation *faute de mieux*, and let us ponder deeply over the fact that the one to live latest (de Wecker) closed his ardent defence of iridectomy by "hedging" on a combined sclerotomy and iridectomy.

Of the 112 surgeons who replied to de Wecker, 11 did not do iridectomy; 19 had given it up owing to bad results; 10 more had practically done the same; 23 continued to do it *faute de mieux*, in spite of unfavourable results; 17 more continued to do it although they would not commit themselves to any definite opinion as to the value of the method; 3 gave no indication of any kind as to their opinion, beyond stating that they performed the operation; 6 surgeons, who did not give statistics, reported favourably of the operation; 23 (or 20·5 per cent.) furnished more or less definite statistics. Dividing their results into four categories, and counting all doubtful cases as favourable, we find that 6 recorded good results in from 0 to 25 per cent. of their cases ; 5 more in from 26 to 50 per cent. ; whilst 8 claim good results in from 51 to 75 per cent. ; and 4 in from 76 to 100 per cent.

To sum up :—Of 112 surgeons, 74, or 66 per cent., appear to have formed a low opinion as to the value of the method ; 20, or 17·85 per cent., were entirely non-committal, and 18, or 16 per cent., were in favour of the operation. This statement of the case cannot fail to move the careful surgeon to earnest thought when the importance of the subject is taken into consideration.

As one reviews the statements made in the disfavour of iridectomy, and considers that amongst those who obtained poor results are to be numbered men of such outstanding eminence as Axenfeld, Barraquer, Chevallereau, Deutschmann, Dujardin, Galezowski, Krucow, de Lapersonne, Panas, Schmidt-Rimpler, Snellen, Voelkers, and Wicherkiewicz, one cannot be greatly surprised by the pathetic confession of Hansen Grut, himself one of the greatest of the Old Guard of ophthalmology : " La déception que m'a causée le traitement des glaucomateux constitue un des plus grands chagrins de ma longue carrière ophtalmologique."

On the other hand, we find ranked among the champions of the method :—Derby, Haab, Hirschberg, Kuhnt, and Uhthoff. To reconcile the extraordinary discrepancy of the statements seems impossible, but we can with profit consider some of the factors which make the case so difficult of decision. These will be taken in turn.

(1) **The Confusion as to what is to be included in the term Glaucoma.**—As has already been pointed out, von Graefe ruled outside the pale of true glaucoma, all cases in which a distinct rise in tension could not be demonstrated to be presnt. His ideas were confessedly chaotic on this very important point. It was left to de Wecker to discover the path by which surgeons could escape from the enveloping darkness of the confusion which shrouded the subject. That he should have done so at a time when von

Graefe's teaching to the contrary dominated men's minds, must redound to his everlasting credit. None yielded to him in admiration for his *grand maitre*, but whilst his colleagues were urging that the simple forms are not true glaucoma, and should not therefore be treated by operative means, he struck out his own line and blazed the trail for all who came after to follow. His points may shortly be put as follows :

(*a*) Simple glaucoma frequently passes into the congestive form. This statement is not invalidated by the fact that the change often occurs late in the case.

(*b*) In the *same* patient we may meet with simple glaucoma on the one side and congestive glaucoma on the other.

(*c*) In the *same* family, especially among the Jews, one may find some members suffering from simple, and others from congestive glaucoma.

(*d*) The operation of sympathectomy (he might have added " or any other serious operation ") will sometimes cause a simple chronic glaucoma to assume a congestive course.

(*e*) Indisputable cases are on record in which simple chronic glaucoma has been permanently cured by the operation of iridectomy.

The stand which de Wecker took seems the more remarkable, when we consider not merely the attitude of his contemporaries, but that also of a large number of surgeons even at the present time. We will take these points *seriatim*.

During von Graefe's lifetime, a number of his pupils, struck by the difference between the results obtained by iridectomy in simple and in congestive cases, openly abandoned the method in the former, and drew down from their teacher a protest against discarding his operation when they had nothing better to offer in its stead. Eighteen years after his all too early death, his friend and colleague Snellen, in his capacity of opener of the glaucoma discussion at the Heidelberg Congress, rejected iridectomy, and yet no one protested. Later still, in the reports of the distinguished surgeons who placed their experience at de Wecker's disposal, we find abundant evidence of the same spirit at work. Some refused to acknowledge cases of simple glaucoma as such, confusing them with those of optic atrophy; others drew a broad line of distinction between their results in cases in which congestive symptoms had from time to time made their appearance, and those in which the course had been simple throughout. Still others excluded from their statistics all purely simple cases, because they had definitely abandoned the idea of operative interference, unless some congestive manifestations were present. Running through a large number of the reports is the conviction, that the prospect of good results from operation for glaucoma is in direct proportion to the evidence of increased tension present. Czermak crystallised this view in the statement that he never operated for glaucoma, unless (1) the failure of vision had been accompanied by rhythmic evidences of ocular congestion, or (2) the patient assumed the whole responsibility for the results of the procedure.

A confusion in terminology is fatal to clear thinking or to the deduction of reliable inferences, and yet over this most important subject we find such a source of error hanging like a heavy cloud, dimming the light that might have been derived from excellent observations by ophthalmologists of the first class, and extinguishing all radiance from the recorded experience of many others of less distinction. To sum the matter up :—(1) There has been a wide disagreement as to what cases should be included as true glaucoma, and what should be excluded ; (2) of those who have kept the distinction sharp before their minds, some have operated for all conditions, whilst others have limited their active interference to selected cases ; and finally, (3) even the most logical thinkers have not always been careful to reflect clearly in their statistics the distinction which they have drawn in their own minds. It is not then to be wondered at that in this domain of science we still have to confess that " there, among the glooming alleys, progress halts on palsied feet." It is not to be thought that the writer is venturing to criticise these men of the past, who crossed the mountain ranges of difficulty to plant the flag of science in territories of knowledge unexplored before their time. They struggled through the darkness of the encircling night to the dawning brightness of a day of knowledge. Our position is a different one. " Heirs of all the ages," we know what they guessed at ; we can prove where they speculated ; we begin far in advance of where they left off ; and yet, there are many surgeons to-day who appear still to halt between two opinions, as to whether the " glaucomatous process " is one throughout the whole domain of the manifestations of a pathological increase of intra-ocular pressure, or is two or more fold. Be it clearly understood, we make no reference here to the hydra-headed ætiology of the condition, but confine ourselves sharply to a consideration of the process, *qua* process. To the writer's mind it appears to be clearly established that there is no essential difference between the most chronic form of simple glaucoma and the most violent type of the hæmorrhagic affection. The question is one of the " quantity " and not of the " quality " of the elements which enter into the case. The subject has been fully dealt with in a previous chapter, and need not detain us further now.

(2) **The period at which operative interference was undertaken varied enormously in different cases,** and was a primary factor in determining the success or failure of the means employed. We have already shown how strongly von Graefe felt on this subject, and how earnestly de Wecker endorsed his master's teaching, that if operation was to be undertaken, the surgeon's watchword should be " the sooner the better." It matters not what form of the disease we have to do with. In one and in all alike, the results obtained are commensurate with the promptitude with which we act. No one who has carefully read the opinions expressed by de Wecker's brilliant and talented contributors, can have failed to recognise this conviction running through their writings. Like the dominant phrase in a piece of classical music, we find it continually repeated throughout the writings of most of those who have dealt with the subject. Some were con-

tent merely to express their convictions on the importance of early operating; others divided their cases into two groups, according to whether they had operated soon or late; whilst yet others had abandoned surgical interference, unless it could be made before the disease had had time to progress. Thus we see that the same want of uniformity of procedure, which we had cause to regret in our consideration of the previous section, is again to be found here, clouding the issues involved, and sensibly depreciating the value of the statistics furnished.

(3) **The period during which the cases were followed after operation varied immensely.**—There can be no question that this factor is one of very great importance, and much stress was laid upon it, not only by von Graefe and de Wecker, but also by a large number of the latter's correspondents. So strong was the feeling on the subject that some of them, like Landolt, absolutely refused all statistics. Others, amongst whom may be numbered Fuchs, whilst clearly recognising that most iridectomised cases, if given sufficient time, ended in blindness, contended and supported their contention by figures, that the operation, if it did not arrest the disease, at least delayed its progress, and so rendered valuable service to the patient.

The contention that in cases of simple glaucoma, the value of an operative method is only to be decided upon after watching the patient's progress for a period of many years, is up to a certain point a valid one, but it is essential to look at the question from every side before forming a definite judgment. To begin with, it is true that the course of some of these cases is extremely slow, and that most of them would not lead to blindness for a long time, even if unchecked. Moreover, they do not all progress at an even rate, nor is the course of any individual case undeviatingly uniform in the evolution of its signs and symptoms. To attribute a curative action to a method of operative interference may therefore be incorrect.

The next point to bear in mind is that, although the glaucomatous process may be definitely checked by an operative measure, the end the surgeon has in view may yet be defeated by a progressive atrophy of the optic nerve. The writer, in an earlier chapter, has suggested that in such cases the progressive atrophy may sometimes be really quite apart from any influence of the intra-ocular pressure, except possibly in so far as that pressure has injured the nerve and thus rendered it liable to fall a ready prey to any toxic or other influence, which under happier conditions, it would easily have overcome. The moral, that we should, in all such cases, seek for and treat all possible causes of auto-infection, need not be laboured here. The suggestion, if confirmed by the experience of others, will help sometimes to explain the failure of operations, which so far as the reduction of tension is concerned, are technically successful.

Our third point is one that has been powerfully made by Fuchs, and to which not a few others have also called attention, viz., that in view of the advanced age of many of our patients, it will often be sufficient for all practical purposes if we can delay the onrush of the disease, and so slow down its course that useful vision outlasts the patient's term of life. This contention has often been made in favour of iridectomy, and up to a certain point its validity may be freely admitted. If, however, it can be shown that the modern operations give more lasting results, we shall be in a quite different position from that occupied by von Graefe, de Wecker, and their contemporaries, who, having nothing better to fall back upon, were bound to make the best they could of the means at their disposal.

We come now to a point of great importance, and one that, so far as the writer is aware, has never received proper attention, with the result that much unnecessary confusion has arisen. What has been written in the previous paragraphs refers to simple chronic glaucoma. It has little bearing on the prognostic significance of suitable operative interference in that chronic form of glaucoma, which is associated with intermittent, and often more or less rhythmic, exacerbations of intra-ocular pressure. It is necessary to make this point quite clear.

The writer is convinced, and so he believes are most modern ophthalmologists, that there is a form of glaucoma characterised by the manifestation of what may be termed the three cardinal signs of the disease, viz., (1) cupping of the disc, (2) contraction of the field, and (3) (sooner or later) diminution of the visual acuity. These are the cases that von Graefe and many of the surgeons who succeeded him, excluded from the category of glaucoma. In dealing with them, we must bear in mind their slow rate of progress, and suspend our judgment as to the value of our therapeutic measures, but we must not allow their admitted existence to confuse other and more important issues. The whole tenor of the writings of our predecessors has been shown to be that iridectomy was most successful (1) when performed early in the case, and (2) when undertaken in the presence of marked, even if intermittent, exacerbations of tension. The writer is convinced, that in such cases, the value of any method for the arrest of glaucoma can be estimated with considerable accuracy three months after the operation has been performed. If the tension of the eye is then found to be sensibly lowered, the surgeon may in most cases congratulate himself and his patient. It is, however, always necessary for him to bear in mind the danger which has already been alluded to, of what may be termed a collateral atrophy of the optic nerve.

(4) **The Technique of the Operation has an undoubted Influence on the Results Obtained.** — The author has little sympathy with the often used catchword that " the worse the operation of iridectomy is performed, the better are the results." It appears to contain a grain of truth in a mass of error. What does seem of real importance is the exact technique employed. There would appear to be a widespread and very real misconception as to the method adopted by the older surgeons in the performance of an iridectomy. It has been stated by able and distinguished ophthalmologists that the " classical iridectomy for glaucoma " was made in the limbus and was of limited extent. Nothing could be more contrary

to the facts of the case. Von Graefe laid down (1) that the incision should be as eccentric as possible in order to remove the iris as far as its ciliary attachment ; he regarded this as essential to success ; (2) that the excised piece of iris should be as large as possible—the more intense the symptoms the more extensive the incision ; and (3) that the aqueous should be allowed to escape slowly. De Wecker's practice was the same, and a large number of his correspondents laid stress on these features of technique. They did not all do so, and there can be but little doubt that the procedure adopted varied considerably in different cases. Here we meet with another factor, which renders the statistics of various surgeons practically useless for comparative purposes. At the same time, it would be idle to contend that the modern method of performing an iridectomy is much more effective than the old. Such an assumption would be presumptuous to a degree. To understand the real importance of the subject, it is necessary to go back to the already quoted statement of von Graefe as to the frequency (in 20 per cent. of all cases) with which the formation of a filtering cicatrix followed the performance of an iridectomy. We have shown that he commented on, but failed to realise the significance of this form of scar, whilst de Wecker went straight to the heart of the matter. In order to obtain such a cicatrix, it is obviously essential that the wound should be a subconjunctival one. It is possible that many failed to realise this, and that their results were correspondingly disappointing.

It must be admitted that a study of the writings of the past masters of our craft does not make a strong case for the operation of iridectomy in the relief of glaucoma. We shall turn next to a consideration of what has been said or written on the same subject since the introduction of the modern filtering operations.

REFERENCES

DE WECKER, L.—" Valeur de l'iridectomie dans le Glaucome," *Congrès de la Société française d'ophtalmologie*, May 1901.

VON GRAEFE, A.—*Archiv f. O.*, Berlin, 1857 and 1858 ; translated *The New Sydenham Society*, 1859, vol. v.

Part II

The Views of Modern Surgeons

SUMMARY :—Introductory.
        The Relative Value of Iridectomy and Sclerectomy in Glaucoma.
        The *Modus Agendi* of Iridectomy in Glaucoma.
        The Correct Time to select for Operation in Glaucoma.
        The Causes of Hesitation in operating for Glaucoma.
            The Encouragement to delay derived from a limited clinical
                Experience of the favourable results of Meiosis.
            The Fear of an Immediate Bad Result.
            The Fear of Late Infection.
            Professional Conservatism.

Most of the great questions of surgery pass, sooner or later, through a stage of active or even of violent controversy. It is thus that the gold of truth is tried in the furnace of conflicting opinion, and the very fierceness of the discussion may well be a factor in the speed with which a decision is obtained. On the vexed question of the value of iridectomy in glaucoma, there are to-day many widely diverse estimates before us, and the contest of views is decidedly fierce ; but fortunately throughout the discussion the attitude of all alike has been a wholehearted desire to get at the truth, whatever the cost may be. This spirit can only lead to good, and the author's earnest desire is to follow in such worthy footsteps. When he first sat down to the task, the difficulties seemed insuperable ; for it did not look as if it were humanly possible to draw any trustworthy deductions from the tossing torrent of clinical evidence, represented in the writings of recent years. A careful and protracted survey has shown that to some extent these fears were well founded ; it is still too early to hope to attain finality of judgment. In the years to come the river of knowledge will flow broad, strong, and calm, fed by the torrential waters of to-day. We are too near the rapids of strife to hope for a steady even flow of opinion ; but just as some of the great questions, which vexed von Graefe and his colleagues, are to-day matters of established knowledge with us, their successors, so may we hope that a time will come when those who follow us, will find themselves on the calm waters of assured knowledge as a result of our faithful and patient labours. If we may not pass sentence, we may at least calmly and dispassionately weigh the evidence, and we should most assuredly strain every nerve to collect data, which shall accumulate, as the years go by, until a time is reached when we, or perhaps others, can reap where we have sown.

In the following pages then an effort will be made to draw some broad deductions, which shall be of use to us in our search for truth. Details and statistics will for the present be avoided, as it is thought that any close consideration of them can only help to confuse the issue.

THE RELATIVE VALUE OF IRIDECTOMY AND OF SCLERECTOMY IN GLAUCOMA.—Here we are met with a maelstrom of conflicting opinions. Some would perform sclerectomy in all cases of the disease; others would select iridectomy as their universal operation; yet others would continue to do iridectomy in acute and subacute cases, reserving sclerectomy for the chronic disease. Closely connected with the decision as to the operation to be selected, is that as to the time when the procedure is to be undertaken; for whilst there are a large number of surgeons who would follow the rule laid down by von Graefe, that the earlier operation is undertaken in glaucoma the better, there are still many who, for one reason or another, put off the so-called " evil day " as long as possible. Yet another question is entwined with those now before us, viz., that as to the value of medicinal treatment.

How does the performance of an iridectomy reduce the tension of a glaucomatous eye?—It is most important that our answer to this question should be clear and well defined. There are several distinct ways in which iridectomy may act: (1) In early cases, before the angle of the chamber is irreparably sealed, the removal of a sufficient piece of iris mechanically opens up the filtering area in the neighbourhood of the base of the excised portion, and thus permits the escape of a sufficient quantity of fluid to maintain the correct balance between secretion and excretion. This point has been worked out by Treacher Collins. (2) We know that aseptic iris wounds show no tendency to scar formation or healing, but remain indefinitely in the condition produced by the operation. The first hint of this was given by Fuchs at the Heidelberg Congress of 1896, when in speaking of the transfixion of the iris, in operating for *l'iris bombé*, he said : " When I performed this operation for the first time, I asked myself the question : Would these holes (in the iris) remain open ? I expected it, as the holes made in the iris by the passage of foreign bodies not seldom remain open. This expectation has been fulfilled, and the small operation has given me lasting results in this way . . ." Later, Parsons, in his *Pathology of the Eye* (1904), says of wounds of the iris : " There is little or no formation of granulation tissue unless the iris is prolapsed and exposed, consequently also there is no formation of true scar tissue. . . . Uncomplicated wounds of the iris have received scant attention, and it is probable that important facts might be discovered by reinvestigation." Three years later (1907), T. Henderson published a paper on the Histology of Iridectomy, in which he pointed out " that the iris tissue is absolutely indifferent to trauma as such, so long as it is not subjected to toxic or septic agencies." Lastly, Malcolm McBurney, writing on the absence of cicatrisation in the iris after operation or injury, gives an account of a number of cases, in which he, like Henderson, had sectioned the edges of old wounds in the iris, and had found that the " injured iris surface had remained either entirely unchanged, or had merely shown a slight anteroposterior contraction. . . ." He gives to Fuchs the credit of the discovery " that injuries to the iris, in the absence of hæmorrhage and infection, show little or no tendency to scar formation or healing." Thomson Henderson has suggested that the traction on the iris made in performing an iridectomy causes minute rents and lacerations throughout its circumference ; he thinks that these " traumatic crypts " assist the raw edges of the coloboma in bringing the aqueous to the iris veins. (3) As has been pointed out in the preceding part of this chapter, both von Graefe and de Wecker laid stress on the extraordinary frequency with which the performance of an iridectomy was followed by the establishment of a filtering cicatrix. It was the latter writer, however, who first appreciated the deep underlying significance of this phenomenon. Since his time, the observation has become one of the commonplaces of ophthalmic surgery, and to-day the great majority of surgeons accept without reservation the view that one, at least, of the ways in which an iridectomy lowers the tension of an eye is by the establishment of a vicarious channel of filtration between the anterior chamber and the sub-conjunctival space. Any operation, which temporarily relieves a glaucomatous condition, and which at the same time either guides or frightens a patient into taking more care of his eye condition, may easily result in the avoidance of fresh attacks of congestive glaucoma. This is largely a question of prophylaxis. It is, however, quite another matter when we come to discuss operations which are essentially curative in their action, and which rely for their success on the re-establishment of a normal balance between the secretion and excretion of fluids in the eye. The important point to grasp is, that if an iridectomy is to be successful by reopening the normal filtration area in the neighbourhood of the iris base, it is essential that the procedure should be undertaken at an early stage, before the approaches to the angle of the chamber have been obliterated and sealed down by plastic exudate. *It is useless to tear away the iris after the sinus of the chamber is closed.* Moreover, the detachment of the iris no longer takes place along the line of its true and original base, but along that of a new and spurious base, viz., the line of its anterior attachment to the cornea and sclera. When we come to discuss the modern filtering operations, we are dealing with an entirely different set of conditions. We do not aim at opening up old physiological channels, but at forming a new and vicarious conduit for the aqueous. It is admitted that the later the case the worse the prognosis, and that this in part, perhaps in large part, depends on the fact that the advance of the iris, owing to its adhesion to the sclero-cornea, makes the attainment of a uvea-free fistula more difficult and more hazardous ; but there can, we think, be no question that a fistula can be established long after the time is past when an iridectomy would be of any avail. There is thus provided a ready explanation on rational grounds for the strong preference which many able surgeons show towards continuing to perform iridectomy in their acute and subacute cases. We suggest that the real indication lies not in the acuteness of the attack, but in the fact that such acute attacks commonly occur fairly early in the disease. There is another factor which we must leave for the present, viz., the individual preferences of different surgeons for individual methods. This will be discussed later.

If the views above outlined are accepted as correct, it is obvious that they must have a very important bearing on the much discussed and knotty subject of **the correct time to be selected for operation.** If iridectomy is the operation of our choice, it must be obvious that to lose time over general and meiotic treatment is prejudicial to the best interests of the patient, since by allowing the disease to progress, it lets slip the most favourable opportunity for surgical interference. In the previous pages, it was shown that von Graefe, de Wecker, and many others of their leading contemporaries laid the greatest stress on the importance of operating early, if at all. It may be said that the modern operations are on a different footing, and there is a certain amount of justice in this claim. They are not dependent on the reopening of the normal channels, but on the establishment of new and artificial ones. Nevertheless, it is quite certain that the earlier we perform sclerectomy in a case of glaucoma, the better is our prospect of success. **Why then do surgeons hesitate ?** To this question there are several answers. *Firstly*, there are a certain number of cases on record, which have been watched for many years by competent ophthalmologists, and which during that period have remained *in statu quo* under the influence of a suitable regimen and of the instillation of mild meiotics. Many years ago, de Wecker wrote, in bitterness of soul, his opinion that if meiotics had never saved an eye, they at least had lost many. Long before he had read de Wecker's dictum, the writer had put forward his opinion that these occasional cases of success under meiotic treatment had encouraged many ophthalmologists to delay operation, and so had caused a loss of sight totally disproportionate to the meagre gains which can be laid to the credit of what has been termed the "expectant treatment." The writer is convinced that, if taken in the mass, the best results will be found in the clinic of the surgeon who operates the moment that he is satisfied in his own mind that glaucoma is present and progressive in spite of treatment. This is a broad general statement which, however, requires some qualification. Cases must be taken individually and not in a mass, and here, as in every other of the great questions of life, the particular circumstances of the individual must be carefully taken into account. Some few factors may be considered, and of these the one which stands out pre-eminent is that of the age of the patient as affecting his probable expectation of life. An old man, with a very slowly progressive simple glaucoma, would require to be carefully watched. He should only be operated on if he was obviously going down hill at a rate disproportionate to the general failure of his powers. Even then it would be necessary to bear carefully in mind the possible dangers of the course on which we are thinking of embarking. Post-operative pneumonia, insanity, and even comparatively sudden death are possibilities which bulk larger and larger as the sun of life dips towards its horizon. In one case, a man in the eighties may be safely operated on without the least fear of the dangers we are discussing, whilst another, still in his seventh decade, may be in such a condition that it would be very unwise to touch him.

The second reason for hesitation in undertaking an operation for glaucoma, on the part of not a few surgeons, is undoubtedly *the fear of a bad result*. It has been the unfortunate experience of most men in large surgical practice,

and probably still more frequently of a great many who
operate less often, and have therefore less facility of manipulation, that after the operation, be it what it may, the
patient sees less well, and is dissatisfied with the result of
the procedure. Sometimes the failure is due to faulty
technique, and might be avoided; this is probably more
often the case than is admitted. There still remain cases,
in which in spite of an apparently perfectly carried out
procedure, the central vision, or the visual field, or both
are distinctly worse after than before the surgical interference. It is of course necessary to bear in mind that the
full benefit derived from a decompression operation on
the eye cannot be judged till six weeks to three months have
elapsed. The shallowing of the chamber with the consequent advance of the lens system, and the disturbances
of intra-ocular circulation, manifested by choroidal detachments and other phenomena, produce transitory effects
which must be given time to disappear, as they usually will
do. But, apart from these, there remain a certain number
of cases in which the harm done by operation is permanent.
This complication was well known in the days when
iridectomy held undisputed sway. In the majority of
instances, it was met with after operating on late cases,
and especially on those in which the visual field had contracted until its margins closely approached the centre of
vision. It was then found that the relief of tension was
followed by a considerable further loss of field, which frequently invaded and washed out central vision. There
can be little question that this form of post-operative misfortune is very much rarer with trephining than it is with
iridectomy, but it must be admitted that *no* form of operative procedure for glaucoma is quite safe from it in late
cases. There is, however, another side to the question.
If there is one thing more certain than another in the study
of glaucoma, it is that in the vast majority of cases the
condition moves forward, inexorably and steadily, to a
termination fatal for vision. If sight is lost of this most
important fact, the perspective in which the condition is
seen is hopelessly wrong. There are *risks* in advancing to

surgical intervention, and those risks grow greater as the case progresses; but there is the *certainty* of defeat in the vast majority of cases, if the eye is left to fight its own battle aided only by general and medicinal regimen. The number of cases in which glaucoma has been held in check indefinitely by such treatment is very limited. On the other hand, we have all of us seen cases in which a hesitation to operate has resulted in the patient losing all, or nearly all, vision. Such instances are common, but an illustration may not be unnecessary. Within a very short period the writer saw two medical men who were suffering from glaucoma, and who had been advised to "take their chance with meiotics." One of them lost all sight of one eye, which was then removed, as it was painful, and he was told to go on with the same treatment for the second eye. The other lost his field extensively in one eye, and down to within 10° of the centre over part of the second. Both were trephined, the remaining eye in the one, both eyes in the other; both of them have continued in busy practice for well over seven years, *i.e.*, to date, and in both the visual acuity, the fields, and the tensions show that the condition has been definitely arrested. Many of us could multiply such cases, but these are quoted as a protest against the view that "the dangers of operation should make the surgeon very careful how he resorts to the knife or trephine." Rather would one say "the dangers of hesitation are so appalling that the surgeon should weigh well his responsibility before he neglects or hesitates to resort to surgical intervention."

There is one great difference from the surgeon's point of view between the two positions above outlined. If he operates and leaves his patient worse, blame, often very unjustly, falls on his shoulders; whereas, if he refrains from interference and the patient loses all sight, the loss is gradual, and the onus of it is placed by the patient and his friends on the disease or on providence, according to the individual bent of their minds. The lot of the surgeon is a hard one; his critics are often unreasonable and unfair; when he has done his best, and a good best at that, he is open to damage, both material and moral, at the hands of those, who should in reality be his grateful adherents ; and this, because the only standard most of them can judge him by is that of results. Who shall presume to blame the man who, under such circumstances, hesitates to operate on difficult and dangerous cases, or even on those easier earlier cases, before whom he knows stretches out a probably long period of unexpended life, an accident in the course of which may be turned or twisted to the dishonour of his work ? The public in this are reaping what they sow. Despite it all, the greater man is he who can put such considerations from him and act on the probabilities of the case alone. It does not, we fear, follow that he will be the more successful man in a commercial sense.

In the course of the above argument we have touched on *a third cause of hesitation* in operating, viz., *the fear of late infections*. The writer has often maintained, and he still believes that the adoption of a correct technique greatly diminishes the risk in question. He has neither denied nor belittled the danger ; but seen in contrast with the consequences of a policy of " wait and see," it seems to him to be dwarfed by the comparison. This matter will be dealt with at length in a later chapter.

The *last consideration which induces a hesitancy* in operating for glaucoma, is that of undertaking a new form of procedure. Iridectomy is familiar to us all from our professional·infancy onwards ; it is taught, or rather it is supposed to be taught (for it can really only be learnt on the living), in operative surgery classes ; we have had it dinned into us from our receptive student days onwards, that it is a very easy procedure, which it certainly is not. To make an incision in the eye and to get out a portion of iris is easy enough, but to do a neat iridectomy, and to make it exactly as one wishes to in the particular case is *not* easy ; indeed, in a high tension eye, it is a difficult and hazardous procedure for the best operator. On the other hand, the newer operations are surrounded with the dread of the unknown ; the difficulties inherent in them appear to be greater to the unaccustomed operator than have been thought. One thing would seem to be certain, and that is that the results obtained have varied widely in the hands of different ophthalmologists. Allowance must undoubtedly be made for the fact that one style of operation may suit one surgeon, and another another. The man who has carried out a procedure in a large number of cases with excellent results will naturally undertake it with confidence, under conditions which would deter another, whose experience has been less happy, whilst a third who has met, be the reason what it may, with an unusual number of disasters, will refuse to touch the method at all. This rule holds right through all departments of surgery, and explains the extraordinary diversity of means used by those who are working for the same end. Each must find out for himself the method that is best suited to his peculiar surroundings and to his own abilities. What is right for one may well be wrong for another.

A brief summary of the conclusions reached may be given:

(1) If an operation for glaucoma is to be undertaken, the earlier it is performed the better is the result likely to be; therefore it is important to make up one's mind on the subject at the earliest possible moment.

(2) Every case of glaucoma in which operation is postponed should be watched with the utmost care, and the moment that medical treatment fails to hold it in check, surgery should be resorted to *without delay*.

(3) Special watch should be kept on (*a*) the condition of the visual field, (*b*) the tension, and (*c*) the visual acuity. (The order is deliberate.) A departure from the normal in all three, or in any one of them, and especially in the visual field, calls for a decompression operation.

(4) Iridectomy, undertaken with the deliberate intention of freeing the natural channels of excretion, and so of restoring the *status quo antea*, should only be resorted to in those early cases, in which there is reason to believe that such a feat is possible. Once plastic inflammation has blocked the angle of the chamber, the rôle of this procedure ceases.

(5) When it is recognised that the attainment of decompression depends on the opening up of vicarious filtration channels, the obvious call is for one of the newer operations. The fact that an iridectomy or a sclerotomy may be followed by the formation of a filtration scar is beside the point. We should deliberately undertake a well-planned procedure, which aims at the formation of the kind of scar we desire to produce. Any other line of action is bad surgery, since it lacks consistency and clarity of purpose.

(6) Each surgeon must be guided not only by the environment of his patients, but also by his own idiosyncrasies.

(7) Each case must be considered on its own merits. The relative prospects of life and of remaining months or years of sight must be carefully weighed. Against the admitted dangers of operating must be set the inexorable progress and the appalling results of the disease.

(8) Statistics are wanted both of success and failure. If they are forthcoming, as they will be, those who follow us will know what we guess, will walk boldly where we grope, and will owe us a debt like that which we in our turn owe to von Graefe, de Wecker, and the stalwarts of their time.

REFERENCES

COLLINS, E. T.—" Hunterian Lectures," *Lancet*, 1894.
FUCHS, E.—" On the Transfixion of the Iris," *Report 25th Ophth. Congress*, Heidelberg, 1896, p. 179.
HENDERSON, T.—" The Histology of Iridectomy," *Ophth. Rev.*, 1907, vol. xxvi. p. 191.
MCBURNEY, MALCOLM.—"The Absence of Cicatrisation in the Iris after Operation or Injury," *Arch. of Ophth.*, 1914, xliii. p. 12.
PARSONS, J. H.—*The Pathology of the Eye*, Hodder & Stoughton, London, 1904, vol. i. p. 286.

PART III

The Technique of the Operation of Iridectomy for Glaucoma remains to be considered. It is well to premise our remarks by the statement that in congestive cases this may be, and often is, the most difficult and the most hazardous procedure the ophthalmic surgeon ever has to undertake. The man who can perform it easily, smoothly, and safely is a past master of his art.

Many surgeons advocate the use of a general anæsthetic, but this entails serious disadvantages. The assistance that the conscious patient can give the operator is so very great, as to be an important factor in weighing the pros and cons of this question; whilst the elimination of the danger of post-operative vomiting is a valuable asset. There can be no comparison between the difficulties of operating on an eye depressed by its own muscles, and on one artificially pulled down for the purpose. The use of subconjunctival injections of cocaine and adrenalin, or of some similar combination, suffices to make the operation practically painless, and the hypodermic administration of trivalin-hyoscin beforehand quiets the patient and makes him amenable and tractable. There is of course a good deal to be said on either side. The author wishes only to state his own views without offering the least criticism of those of the many who, he has no doubt, will differ from him in this matter.

Another subject on which there is much room for difference of opinion is whether a Graefe's knife or a keratome should be used. Many surgeons and especially those who have not had large operative experience, find the former the safer. The author's strong preference is in all cases for the keratome. In the hand of an expert it is a beautiful instrument, though few can be more deadly if clumsily used. When the chamber is so shallow as not to admit of its safe employment, it is preferable to do a posterior sclerotomy as a preliminary measure, and to await the deepening of the chamber, which usually takes only a few minutes, before proceeding to make the keratome section.

The patient looks down and the conjunctiva is firmly gripped with forceps just below the cornea, and close up to the limbus; a broad, angled or bent keratome is used, and is introduced through the conjunctiva on and at right angles to the median line of the eye a little above the limbus (Fig. 146). The exact distance above it depends on the anatomical configuration of the eye, but care must be taken that the point of the instrument shall emerge anterior to the plane of the iris. The first thrust is made in such a direction that the sclera is penetrated almost at right angles to its own plane ; the moment the point of the blade is through, the direction of the thrust is altered so as to carry the blade on parallel to the plane of the cornea, until a sufficiently large section (about 6 to 8 mm.) has been made. As soon as this is accomplished the keratome is quickly and smoothly withdrawn, along exactly the same plane as that on which it entered. If this manœuvre is rightly carried out, not a drop of aqueous will be lost; its correct performance indicates the high-water mark of finished operative skill.

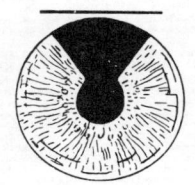

Fig. 146.- Iridectomy for glaucoma, showing the line of the keratome incision, and the resulting coloboma.

With the patient still looking strongly downward, the iris forceps are introduced into the chamber, which up to this moment is still full of aqueous ; the points are allowed to open and a narrow grip is taken of the iris as close up to the pupil as possible. Great care must be taken *not to pinch* the membrane; it should be held quite lightly. The pinching of the iris by the forceps gives rise to pain and provokes the patient to move, whilst if the membrane is lightly, though sufficiently firmly held, no movement of the eye occurs to disturb the operator. The seized portion is drawn out through the wound, and excised by one snip of the scissors. For this purpose the blades of this instrument are pressed firmly against the eyeball, and the cut is made along the length of the incision. A wide iridectomy, which includes the membrane right up to its base, is thus made. Some surgeons recommend dragging the iris out towards each pillar in turn and cutting it off in several snips. Nothing is more provocative than this of the entanglement of the uveal tissue in the section.

A stream of warm, normal, sterile, saline solution

washes the iris back into place, empties the chamber of blood, and completes the toilet of the eye. This question of irrigation will be dealt with more in detail under sclero-corneal trephining.

The coloboma thus produced lies under the cover of the upper lid, and therefore leads to a minimum of dazzling of the eye under conditions of glare. It is, however, a source of very serious trouble to many patients. The glaucomatous subject feels changes of light much more acutely than the ordinary person, even under the best conditions ; and the want of control of the amount of light admitted to the eyes, as a consequence of a large coloboma, is a source of very bitter complaint to the man, who subsequently gets all the advantages of decompression in his second eye from trephining, or other well-planned operation, in which the iridectomy is so small as to make the inconvenience following it negligible. The author sees, from time to time, a patient who, some twelve years ago, was trephined in one eye, and iridectomised in the other ; he never to this day enters the consulting room without a bitter comment on the dazzling due to the coloboma, which resulted from the iridectomy, and he is far from being the only one of the writer's patients who makes this complaint.

Then again, in not a few cases, the edges of the coloboma are tied down to the anterior capsule all round, thus depriving the iris of mobility, and giving the patient a large fixed pupil, with no control whatever over the amount of light entering the eye.

There is a last point, viz., that the astigmatism produced by a wide iridectomy is often severe, and demands correction by cylinders, which, in some cases, are of comparatively high grade, whereas, in trephining at least, the refraction of the eye is little, if at all, interfered with.

Lastly, the fact that the incision is behind the limbus, and therefore under cover of the conjunctiva, as soon as the cut in the latter heals, makes the formation of a subconjunctival filtering scar a possibility. The importance of this feature has already been pointed out.

CHAPTER IX

THE NEWER OPERATIONS FOR GLAUCOMA

SUMMARY

PART I
THE HISTORY OF THE NEWER OPERATIONS FOR GLAUCOMA.

PART II
PREPARATIONS FOR OPERATION.

PART III
SCLEROTOMY FOR GLAUCOMA.
  Anterior Sclerotomy.
  Posterior Sclerotomy.

PART IV
LAGRANGE'S OPERATION. (SCLERECTO-IRIDECTOMY.)

PART V
HOLTH'S OPERATION. (SCLERECTOMY WITH PUNCH-FORCEPS.)

PART VI
HERBERT'S OPERATIONS.
  The Wedge-Isolation Operation.
  The Small Flap Operation.
  The Triple Small Flap Operation.
  The Conjunctiva Infolding Operation.

PART VII
FERGUS'S OPERATION. (SCLERAL TREPHINING WITH AND WITHOUT CYCLO-DIALYSIS.)

PART VIII
THE AUTHOR'S OPERATION. (SCLERO-CORNEAL TREPHINING.)

PART IX
MODIFICATIONS OF SCLERO-CORNEAL TREPHINING SUGGESTED BY VARIOUS SURGEONS.
  Instruments and their Application.
  Modifications of Method.

PART X

COMPLICATIONS WHICH MAY BE MET WITH DURING A GLAUCOMA OPERATION.

PART XI

AFTER-MANAGEMENT OF THE PATIENTS AND TREATMENT OF COMPLICATIONS.

Part I

The History of the Newer Operations for Glaucoma

THERE are few more interesting chapters in the recent literature of ophthalmology than those which record the efforts of surgeons to devise an operation that would be both easy of performance and devoid of serious risk, and that would at the same time offer reasonable prospects of improvement or cure in chronic glaucoma.

Von Graefe's iridectomy held the field practically undisputed for half a century, but whilst it gave general satisfaction in the treatment of the acute and subacute forms of the disease, there had long been a strong feeling of disappointment with its results in chronic cases. This led to the introduction, from time to time, of alternative operations, but although each has had its body of supporters, not one has yet been received as the last word on the surgical treatment of the condition.

Whatever may be the true pathogenesis of the disease, the working hypothesis on which all efforts at treatment are based, is that there exists some abnormal relationship between the intra-ocular pressure, on the one hand, and the resistance of the ocular tunics, on the other. Surgeons have consequently been impelled to seek means whereby the tension of the eye might be permanently reduced by facilitating the outflow of the intra-ocular fluids. This then has been the object kept before the authors of the newer glaucoma operations.

We shall now pass in review these various modern procedures, and in doing so shall adopt as far as possible the wording used by A. J. Ballantyne in his article on the subject published in *The Ophthalmoscope* of July 1910.

The motive for doing so is not merely that the descriptions are excellent, but also that he wrote as a looker-on at the struggle, whilst the author was an active participant in it, and as such might be suspected of finding it difficult to write dispassionately and without prejudice, although this is exactly what he both desires and intends to do.

Sclerotomies

The writings of Lagrange, Herbert, and their followers, first made us familiar with the conception of the " filtering cicatrix," but lest we should imagine that the idea originated with these writers, it is well to recall the fact, insisted on in Chapter VIII., that von Graefe, de Wecker, and others were quite familiar with this form of scar. It was, indeed, de Wecker who coined the phrase. In the discussions which centred round the *modus operandi* of iridectomy in glaucoma, de Wecker held that to explain the apparent success of iridectomy, where the iris was atrophic, one was forced to conclude that the effect depended on the scleral incision, which was followed by a " *cicatrice à filtration*." When it came to be suspected that in chronic simple glaucoma iridectomy was useless or even harmful, de Wecker felt that an alternative operation was desirable, and in 1867 proposed sclerotomy, the cicatrix of which facilitated the filtration of aqueous, and consequently secured a permanent reduction of intra-ocular pressure. Not only did de Wecker aim at the production of a filtering scar, but he also insisted that the sclerotomy wound must be free from incarceration of iris.

Since its introduction, sclerotomy in some form has, next to iridectomy itself, been the operation most largely practised in simple chronic glaucoma. It has been accepted as a safe procedure, although repetition of the operation on the same eye is frequently required owing to the want of permanence of the results. Dianoux reaffirmed its value, but recommended that it should be followed up by massage of the eye, to prevent first intention healing, and to cause the formation of a permeable cicatrix. He was supported by Wicherkiewicz, who recommended the same measure after iridectomy.

The operation of sclerotomy has assumed many forms in the hands of different operators. The two classical methods are those of de Wecker and Quaglino, the former being probably the more popular.

If one may judge from the absence of any expression of disapproval of the newer operations on the part of the supporters of sclerotomy, one is led to the conclusion that in chronic glaucoma, this method, after forty years, has, like iridectomy, failed to give the satisfaction that it seemed to promise. But the belief that it *ought* to be possible to produce deliberately a corneo-scleral wound which will lead to a permanently filtering cicatrix, has never been altogether lost, and was the motive which inspired the newer operations, which will be considered under the heading of Sclerectomies.

In addition to the classical sclerotomies of de Wecker and others, one or two more recent forms may be mentioned.

Querenghi's operation of sclero-choriotomy consisted in paracentesis of the posterior chamber with a perfectly linear Graefe knife, making puncture and counter-puncture immediately behind the insertion of the iris. This author believed that glaucoma was due to an hydropsia of the perichoroidal space, and that his operation overcame this by establishing a communication between the perichoroidal space and the aqueous chamber.

Bjerrum's operation was recommended for simple glaucoma if meiotics failed. With a narrow Graefe knife he made an incision, the puncture and counter-puncture being placed at the limbus and the knife being made to cut out obliquely, so that it emerged through the sclera from 3 mm. to 6 mm. from the upper or lower edge of the cornea. The incision was rendered subconjunctival by making the conjunctival puncture and counter-puncture some distance from the limbus.

Among the sclerotomies should also be included the procedure tried by more than one operator in the past, and revived by Herbert, namely, the infolding of a slip of conjunctiva between the lips of a corneo-scleral wound, with a view to the establishment of a filtering cicatrix.

Still another form of sclerotomy was the *subconjunctival paracentesis* operation introduced by Herbert in 1908. Having subconjunctivally passed a narrow Graefe knife into the anterior chamber, in such a way that it made a short incision parallel to the corneal margin, and 1 mm. from it, he carried the knife from each end of this incision a short distance inwards towards the cornea. In this way he isolated a rectangular tongue of sclero-corneal tissue, the partial shrinkage and displacement of which were said to lead to the formation of a filtering cicatrix. More recently he made a broader tongue, placing it at the upper limbus, and combining it in some cases with an iridectomy.

Abadie's Operation.—In an article which appeared in 1910, Abadie described his operation of ciliarotomy. He had always disputed the claims of Lagrange, chiefly on theoretical grounds. He held that filtration through the cicatrix was not the cause of the reduction of tension after iridectomy or sclerectomy, that a very small iridectomy was as efficacious as a large one, and that the effect was really attributable to division of the nervous circle of the iris.

Believing that in certain cases glaucoma was due to irritation of the nerve plexus in the ciliary zone, he hoped to produce an " anti-glaucomatous " action in such cases by division of the nervous circle. This he did by first dissecting up the conjunctiva and then with a Richter's triangular knife making a 7 mm. to 8 mm. incision through the ocular tunics in a meridional direction immediately behind the root of the iris. The conjunctiva was sutured in place over the wound.

The operation never came into favour with surgeons, and died a natural death.

Cyclodialysis

Heine, of Breslau, introduced this operation to the Ophthalmological Congress at Heidelbeg in 1905. With a straight lance knife he made an incision in the sclera parallel to the corneal margin and 5 mm. or 6 mm. outside of it. A small spatula was then passed through the wound and between the sclera and the uveal tract into the anterior chamber, breaking through the ligamentum pectinatum.

The operation was based largely on the suggestion of Axenfeld, that the choroidal detachment which Fuchs had observed after operation for cataract, occurred also in glaucoma iridectomies, and was responsible for the good results of these operations. Heine believed it possible to set up, by means of his operation, a communication between the anterior chamber and the suprachoroidal space.

The abundance of references to this operation in the literature of the next three years showed that it had excited a good deal of attention, but, of late, it has been comparatively seldom mentioned.

Operations Involving Incarceration of the Iris in the Wound

The operations comprised in this group resemble the most recent procedures of Lagrange and his followers in their aim of ultimately establishing a permanently permeable cicatrix, but the former differ from the latter in that they seek to attain their object by means which are deliberately avoided by the advocates of the iris-free filtering scar.

The authors of the incarceration operations based their proposals on the following three statements : (1) That in such an operation as extraction of cataract, the entanglement of iris in the wound frequently leads to the formation of a cystoid, or, at least, of a fistulous scar, and that the eye in consequence remains permanently soft, with evidence of leakage of aqueous fluid into the subconjunctival tissue ; (2) that in iridectomies done for acute glaucoma the best and most permanent results are found in cases where the iris has become entangled between the lips of the wound ; and (3) that the risk of infection of a prolapsed or incarcerated iris is greatly less in the cases where the latter is covered by conjunctiva. If the beneficial effect of iridectomy in many cases is due, not to the iridectomy but to an accidental inclusion of iris, why not, they ask, set out to produce such an inclusion in a regulated and deliberate manner, adding the conjunctival covering to avoid risk of infection ?

In June 1903, Major H. Herbert communicated the results of no fewer than 130 operations for the production of a *subconjunctival prolapse of the iris* in primary glaucoma. In thirteen the iris was left uncut, in five an iridotomy was added, and in all the others iridectomy was performed. He found that the relief of tension was certain and permanent, although in some cases the reduction was not immediate but was established only after the use of massage and meiotics for periods up to two or three months. The effect on vision was found to be more favourable than could be looked for in the same class of cases from iridectomy, and this was most notable in eyes with advanced failure of vision, for in early simple glaucoma the postoperative astigmatism was apt to disturb the good central vision. He also held that the risk of late infection was very small, and that early serious complications were less frequent than in similar cases operated on by large iridectomies. In 1908, Herbert was still convinced of the value and safety of the operation, but later he abandoned it in favour of a series of other procedures, which he took up in turn.

In 1907, Holth advocated a somewhat similar procedure. He varied his operation somewhat in regard to the form and position of the incision, and the method of producing the incarceration; but in most cases he made either a flap incision at the limbus with a linear knife, covering it with a conjunctival flap, or a 6 mm. incision 1 mm. outside the corneal border with a keratome, which was first made to pierce the conjunctiva 8 mm. to 10 mm. from the limbus, so as to render the corneo-scleral wound subconjunctival. An iridectomy or iridotomy was done before the iris was drawn into the wound. Holth reported that he had done the operation 41 times, in 85 per cent. of which he had obtained persistent conjunctival œdema with normal tension. In a later paper he published the results of a further series of 87 operations with 86 per cent. of filtering cicatrices. He had had no bad results and had not lost an eye. Some of the cases were found still satisfactory on subsequent examinations six months to two years later ; but the author seems to have felt that the results were a little uncertain, and he turned his attention later to the production of a filtering cicatrix by means of sclerectomy. Borthen, in 1909, published the results of 50 operations for establishing a subconjunctival prolapse without previous iridectomy. He claimed that in no case of simple or absolute glaucoma did he fail to obtain the desired results. He still continues to advocate the procedure under the name of iridotasis, and he has some following in so doing. Maher, in the discussion following a contribution by Lawson, stated that he had performed a similar operation combined with iridectomy, and in ten or twelve years had lost only one eye from irido-cyclitis. He thought the benefits outweighed the risks of inflammation or of sympathetic disease.

The fear of disaster from infection of the eye, or from sympathetic ophthalmitis of the fellow-eye in these operations which we have just been considering, rests not only upon clinical experience, but also on the teaching of the pathological findings of Treacher Collins and others. It seems strange that a procedure which is so obviously unsound can find any advocacy at the present time. Much as the author desires to avoid any suspicion of intolerance or bigotry, he feels that there are certain operative methods which are seriously entertained to-day, which stand self-condemned at the bar of modern pathology and surgery. The effort to produce the entanglement of iris in a scar is, in his opinion, one of such.

Sclerectomies

Quite a number of these operations are on trial, but first in point of time come those of Lagrange and Herbert.

Lagrange's Operation.—In May 1906, Lagrange brought forward his epoch-making operation, the details of which have been made familiar through a now fairly large number of papers from the pen of Lagrange and others. He was of the opinion that in iridectomy the removal of iris *per se* was not answerable for the success of the operation. He observed that in operations for glaucoma, hypertension interferes with the co-aptation of the wound, and that the cicatrix consequently allows a certain amount of filtration; and he saw in this phenomenon an explanation of the success of iridectomy. In chronic glaucoma with low tension, operation is valueless because the wound does not give place to a filtering cicatrix. The conditions are strictly comparable to those in the normal eye, in which no form of scleral incision is able to produce a permeable scar (Schoeler). Again, he believed that a filtering cicatrix can be produced either by sclerotomy or by iridectomy, if the iris is involved in the wound; but he deliberately set out to produce an " iris-free filtering cicatrix " and this he succeeded in accomplishing. His operation he called " sclerecto-iridectomy," the sclerectomy being the essential part of the operation, the iridectomy only conditional. He does not recommend his operation for acute glaucoma, but only for cases of simple chronic glaucoma.

Herbert's Operation.—Next in point of time comes Lt.-Col. H. Herbert's operation of " wedge-isolation."

In the argument which preceded his description of the operation he spoke of permeable cicatrices as belonging to three groups, the cystoid, the fistulous, and the filtering. By the filtering, as opposed to the fistulous, cicatrix he appears to mean a cicatrix in which only microscopic channels exist to allow the percolation of fluid. Wilee Lagrange started from the observations that in an eye which is the seat of high tension, sclerotomy is succeeded by a gaping wound which allows of permanent filtration, and that no kind of scleral incision can permit permanent filtration in an eye with normal tension, Herbert took as his starting-point the clinical fact that cataract extractions with a large conjunctival flap return after long periods, with a more or less gaping wound, and with œdema of the overlying, subconjunctival tissue from filtration of aqueous. This he took as his type of *filtering* cicatrix, and he described it as "the condition which has been long desired, but never attained with any approach to regularity in the treatment of glaucoma." From such observations he argued that the iris-free filtering cicatrix is a practical entity, and he aimed at its production in glaucoma.

Herbert's first device to secure delayed union and consequent filtration was his "jagged incision" operation —a form of sclerotomy—dating from April 1906. In this operation he made one or both lips of a small corneoscleral incision as jagged and uneven as possible by means of sawing movements with a narrow Graefe knife. With an experience of sixty cases, he obtained results which were excellent, on the whole, but somewhat uncertain. He also used the operation of Lagrange, both in its original form and combined with the jagged incision, but he soon abandoned these procedures in favour of his "wedge-isolation" operation, first carried out in December 1906. In this operation the intention was to cut out a wedge, or rather a prism-shaped piece of corneo-sclera, the long axis of which was tangential to the corneal margin, its base attached to the under surface of the conjunctiva and its edge towards the posterior surface of the cornea. The isolated wedge was raised a little from its bed by the escaping fluid, and as it had now to depend for its nutrition on the conjunctiva to which it was attached, it shrank sufficiently to provide for filtration from the anterior chamber to the subconjunctival tissue, but not enough to cause an actual fistula. For the operation it was claimed that it permitted of the establishment of different degrees of filtration; that it was safe; and that if it failed to produce the desired result, it did not prejudice the subsequent performance of the usual operations.

The widespread interest which these operations excited led other surgeons to introduce modifications, which, while carrying out the ideas of Lagrange, might be simpler of performance and freer from risk than his opera-

NEWER OPERATIONS FOR GLAUCOMA 497

tion. The first of these modifications was proposed by Holth.

Sclerectomy with Punch-Forceps.—This operation dates from May 1909. The first step, the formation of a corneo-scleral flap, may be carried out either by a Graefe knife or with the keratome. In the former case the conjunctival flap is cut in completing the section, in the latter the keratome is made to enter the conjunctiva some distance above the scleral puncture. Iridectomy follows, and then the anterior lip of the wound is partly cut away by means of punch-forceps, which are a modification of Vacher's or de Lapersonne's irido-capsulectomy punch-forceps.

Brooksbank James's Operation.—In the discussion on Lawson's contribution Brooksbank James referred to a modification of the Lagrange operation practised by him in six cases. A description of his method has more recently appeared in the *Transactions of the Ophthalmological Society*. He dissects down a flap of conjunctiva and then with a Beer's knife makes an incision into the anterior chamber from without inwards, 1 mm. from the limbus. After an iridectomy, a portion of sclera from the lip of the wound is removed by scissors or punch-forceps, preferably the latter.

Sclerectomy with the Trephine.[1]—The latest additions to the list are the two operations in which the trephine is used to remove a segment of the corneo-sclera. These are the operations respectively of Fergus and of Elliot. Both of these operations are based on that of Lagrange, and they have a much closer affinity to that procedure than to the older operations of Argyll Robertson, Fröhlich, and others, in which the trephine was formerly employed.

Fergus's Operation.—Fergus first employed this operation in January 1909, and he demonstrated it before the Ophthalmological Congress at Oxford and the Ophthalmological Section of the British Medical Association at

[1] Ballantyne's original wording has been closely followed in the paragraphs relating to the use of the trephine.

Belfast in July of the same year. The only published account of it was contained in an abstract of the latter contribution in the *British Medical Journal*, until the author took occasion to describe the genesis and the nature of the operation in *The Ophthalmoscope* of February 1910.

The technique of the operation is simple. A conjunctival flap is dissected up towards the cornea and laid over the corneal surface, while with the trephine (Bowman's), a small disc of sclera is removed, a millimetre or two from the apparent corneal margin. At first the operation was completed at this stage by replacing the conjunctival flap, but Fergus soon introduced a modification which now forms an essential part of his operation, namely, the passage of an iris repositor from the trephine hole into the anterior chamber, keeping it in close contact with the sclera and cornea. The conjunctiva is then replaced, and stitched in position.

Elliot's Operation.—About the time that the above operation was on trial, Major Elliot, in Madras, had independently conceived the idea of utilising the trephine in a similar way. He first used the trephine in August 1909, and by the time of his first communication (December 1909) he had operated on 50 eyes.

Elliot also raises by dissection a flap of conjunctiva with its base at the corneal margin. His trephine opening is made as far forward as possible, so as to enter the angle of the anterior chamber. The disc of sclero-cornea is removed, iridectomy is done, if necessary, to prevent incarceration in the wound, and the conjunctiva replaced. Elliot found that in his first 50 cases tension was relieved in every one. While these two operations have features in common, it is obvious, as stated by Sydney Stephenson, that they have marked points of difference. Elliot's operation is as nearly as possible the operation of Lagrange, making allowance for the use of the trephine instead of the scissors, since the opening forms a communication between the angle of the anterior chamber and the subconjunctival tissue, this object being attained by keeping the trephine as far forward as possible. The iridectomy is added, not as an integral part of the operation, but merely to avoid the risk of prolapse.

Fergus's operation, on the other hand, involves an opening up of the suprachoroidal space, to which is added a cyclodialysis. It is true that Lagrange, in stating the aims of his operation, speaks of cutting through the scleral attachment of the ciliary muscle and opening up a communication between the anterior chamber and the suprachoroidal space, but the successful accomplishment of this object must be difficult, and it may be shown in the future that in most cases the incision is purely into the anterior chamber. In any case Lagrange, in his later papers, seems to lay most of the emphasis on the formation of a fistulous track between the anterior chamber and the subconjunctival tissue-spaces. Fergus's operation, therefore, would seem to have a nearer relation to the cyclodialysis of Heine, substituting a trephine opening for a scleral incision with the keratome.

Bettremieux's Operation.—This operation appeared in 1907 under the title of "simple anterior sclerectomy." The author set out from a different standpoint from that of the other operators. He stated that he had been impressed by the following facts: (1) That glaucoma has been caused experimentally by the cautery applied round the cornea, or by tying the anterior vessels, or, accidentally, by burns at the corneo-scleral junction, *i.e.*, by conditions which block the intra-ocular blood circulation; (2) that Exner explains the action of iridectomy in glaucoma on the ground that the arteries and veins in the iris are made to communicate directly with each other; and that this restores the normal circulatory conditions. Taking these as his basis, he operated as follows: The sclerotic having been exposed, with a needle slightly curved at its end, he traversed tangentially to the corneal margin the outer layers of the sclera, which he then excised with a thin and narrow Graefe knife. This was to produce what he called a "filtering zone," but later he laid all the emphasis on the setting up of an anastomosis between the deep scleral and more superficial subconjunctival vessels, which restored the normal blood circulation of the eye. The method was never taken seriously by surgeons.

Lagrange, in speaking of his own operation, warned the reader against confusing it with the simple anterior sclerectomy of Bettremieux, by which, he declared, a filtering scar could not be produced.

REFERENCES [1]

ABADIE, C.—*Arch. d'opht.*, 1909 and 1910.
BETTREMIEUX.—*La Clinique Opht.*, 1907.
BETTREMIEUX.—*Ibid.*, 1908.
BJERRUM, J.—*L'Ophtalmologie Provinciale*, March 1909.
BOLDT, J.—*Beitr. z. Augenh.*, June 1907.
BORTHEN.—*Archiv f. Augenh.*, 1909, vol. lxv.
DEMICHERI.—*Ann. d'ocul.*, 1908, vol. cxl.
DE WECKER, L.—*Manuel d'Ophthalmologie*, 1889.
DIANOUX.—*Ann. d'ocul.*, Feb. 1905, vol. cxxxiii.
DOYNE, R. W.—*The Ophthalmoscope*, 1908, vol. vi.
ELLIOT, R. H.—*Ibid.*, December 1909.
ELLIOT, R. H.—*Ibid.*, July 1910.
FERGUS, F.—*Brit. Med. Journ.*, October 2, 1909.
FERGUS, F.—*The Ophthalmoscope*, February 1910.
HEINE, L.—*Deut. medizin. Woch.*, 1905, No. 21.
HERBERT, H.—*Trans. O.S. of U.K.*, 1903, vol. xxiii.
HERBERT, H.—*The Ophthalmoscope*, 1907, vol. v.
HERBERT, H.—*Ibid.*, Jan. 1908, vol. vi.
HERBERT, H.—*Ibid.*, July 1908, vol. vi.
HERBERT, H.—*Brit. Med. Journ.*, May 14, 1910.
HOLTH, S.—*Ann. d'ocul.*, May 1907, vol. cxxxvii.
HOLTH, S.—*Ibid.*, July 1909, vol. cxlii.
JAMES, G. B.—*Trans. O.S. of U.K.*, 1909, vol. xxix. p. 266.
JOUDIN.—*Westnik. Ophtalmol.*, March 1908.
KRAUSS.—*Zeitschr. f. Augenh.*, July 1908, vol. xvi.
LAGRANGE, F.—*Rev. Général d'Opht.*, 1906.
LAGRANGE, F.—*Arch. d'opht.*, August 1906.
LAGRANGE, F.—*Ibid.*, 1907, vol. xxvii.
LAGRANGE, F.—*Ann. d'ocul.*, Feb. 1907, vol. cxxxvii.
LAGRANGE, F.—*The Ophthalmoscope*, 1907, vol. v.
LAGRANCE, F.—*Arch. d'opht.*, 1908, vol. xxviii.
LAGRANCE, F.—*The Ophthalmoscope*, 1908, vol. vi.
LAGRANGE, F.—*Ann. d'ocul.*, Nov. 1908, vol. cxl.
LAGRANGE, F.—*Recueil d'opht.*, 1908.
LAGRANGE, F.—*Arch. d'opht.*, 1909.

[1] Some of the volumes referred to contain more than one contribution by the same author.

Lawson, A.—*Trans. O.S. of U.K.*, 1909, vol. xxix.
Meller, J.—Graefe's *Archiv f. O.*, 1908, vol. lxvii. part iii.
Meller, J.—*Klin. Monatsbl. f. Augenh.*, December 1909.
Querenghi.—*Zeitschr. f. Augenh.*, Jan. 1908.
Querenghi.—*Annal. d'ottal. e Clin. Ocul.*, 1907, vol. xxxvi.
Rochon-Duvigneaud, A.—*Recueil d'opht.*, 1907.
Rochon-Duvigneaud, A.—*Arch. d'opht.*, 1908, vol. xxviii.
Schoeler.—*Berlin. klin. Woch.*, No. 36, 1881.
Valude.—*Ann. d'ocul.*, 1908, vol. cxl.
Weekers, L.—*Klin. Monatsbl. f. Augenh.*, September 1907, vol. xlv. part ii. p. 230.
Wernicke, G.—*Ibid.*, November–December 1908.
Wicherkiewicz, B.—*Ann. d'ocul.*, Aug. 1905, vol. cxxxiv.

The More Recent History of the Newer Operations for Glaucoma

The later history of the evolution of glaucoma operations must now be told in the author's own words. In 1912, Mayou and Zorab independently and simultaneously advocated the operation of " thread drainage," which consisted in the introduction through the sclera into the anterior chamber of a silk thread, which was then left permanently in place, its end or ends lying buried beneath a conjunctival flap. In the same year Wicherkiewicz introduced his operation of "gridiron sclerotomy," of which little need be said, for it was not founded on any sound principle, nor did it recommend itself to the judgment of the profession. That year was memorable for Elschnig's paper, which dealt its *coup de grâce* to the operation of sympathectomy, a procedure which had outstayed all too long its scanty welcome at the hands of ophthalmologists.

The year 1913 saw the subject of glaucoma operations made the central topic for discussion at the International Congress held in London, when the author had the honour of being associated as an opener of the discussion with those veteran workers, Priestley Smith and Lagrange. One outcome of that Congress was a great stimulation in surgical activity, and during the following years, a large number of papers appeared on the subject, and especially on sclero-corneal trephining. The most important of these latter communications were by Meller, Stock, and Wallis, for these represented the experience of the leading clinics of Vienna, Jena, and London.

Holth's operation also came in for a share of support, whilst Lagrange's sclerectomy declined in favour, on account of the greater risks it involves. About this time too, attention began to be directed to the danger of late infection following the filtration scar operations, with especial reference to trephining.

Zorab and Mayou published (1913) the results they had met with in their thread drainage operation. The former had had one suppuration in 22 eyes operated, and the silk had worked its way out and had to be removed in 9 cases. The latter surgeon's results were less unfavourable, but he had decided to abandon the method in favour of trephining.

The year of the outbreak of the war was prolific of glaucoma literature in its earlier peaceful months. The discussions of the previous year were carried on with unabated vigour, and modifications of the standard operations were still the order of the day, the most notable contributors being Harman and Young. Herbert was still in search of an ideal operation. At the same time, and largely in consequence of the growing dread of late infections, a reaction began to set in in favour of iridectomy. This was almost inevitable, but it may be questioned whether the movement will prove a very serious one; indeed, it appears already to have been checked. It probably attained its maximum in the two following years. The most notable features of 1915, apart from the above, were the advocacy by Casey Wood and others of the "seton operation," and the revival of the flagging interest in "iridotasis." D. Priestley Smith's operation of "limbal puncture" also deserves a mention.

In 1920 Curran brought forward his operation of making a small hole in the root of the iris either by a peripheral iridectomy, or preferably, and in most of his patients, by a peripheral iridotomy. His theory is that in the majority of cases of quiet chronic glaucoma, and perhaps in acute cases also, the immediate cause of the increase of tension is an interference with the flow from the posterior to the anterior chamber, produced by a too close application of the lens to the posterior surface of the iris. The technique consists of introducing a knife needle at the corneo-scleral margin, rucking up the iris with its point, and pushing on the blade to perform the iridotomy. Gifford has warmly championed the method. If this operation succeeds in making an appeal to surgeons, the author cannot but feel that a safer way to perform it would be by making a small peripheral iridectomy through a limited keratome incision.

The most recent tendency, and possibly one of great value, is the effort made by a large number of surgeons to discover whether the various operations may not each have its own proper rôle in glaucoma surgery. Some idea of the enormous interest that these operations have attracted may be gathered from the fact, that during the last three years, there are over 200 references to them in literature, one-half of which are devoted to the trephine operation and its complications. The extraordinary welter of conflicting opinion, that runs all through this mass of valuable writing, leaves one clear-cut impression behind it on the reader's mind, viz., that ophthalmologists the wide world over are very far from having made up their minds on the best surgical means of treating glaucoma. In every country there would seem to be men in totally opposed camps. Cyclodialysis, iridotasis, and iridectomy have their supporters as ardent and untiring as those of Lagrange's operation or of trephining. Under the circumstances all we can do is to wait and work in the sure confidence that, though we may not live to see it, a better day is coming, and one in which general agreement will be reached at least on the great principles involved. Meanwhile, the author has gone steadily on his way, with his confidence renewed and increased in the efficacy of sclero-corneal trephining, a procedure which has its ardent advocates as well as its determined critics. He has no wish to "boost" it, but leaves it in the hands of ophthalmic surgeons, confident that the ultimate verdict will be the right one, however slow it may be reached and whatever it may be.

REFERENCES

CURRAN, E. J.—*Arch. of Ophth.*, March 1920, p. 131; and *Trans. Amer. Med. Assoc.*, 1920, p. 75.
ELSCHNIG, A.—"Sympathectomy," *Klin. Monatsbl. f. Augenheilk.*, May 1912, p. 598.
GIFFORD, H.—*Amer. Journ. Ophth.* 1921, vol. iv. p. 889.
MAYOU, M. S.—*The Ophthalmoscope*, 1912, vol. x. p. 254; and 1913, vol. xi. p. 258.
MELLER, J.—*Zeitschr. f. Augenh.*, vol. xxx. p. 447.
SMITH, D. PRIESTLEY.—*Ophth. Rev.*, vol. xxxiv. p. 33.
STOCK, W.—*Klin. Monatsbl. f. Augenh.*, Oct. 1912, p. 463.
WALLIS, G. F. C.—*The Ophthalmoscope*, 1913, vol. xi. p. 588.
WICHERKIEWICZ, B.—*Arch. de Oft.*, vol. xii. p. 369 (see *Ophth. Year Book*, 1912, vol. ix. p. 208).
ZORAB, A.—*The Ophthalmoscope*, 1912, vol. x. p. 258; and 1913, vol. xi. p. 211.

PART II

Preparations for Operation

(1) **Preparation of the Patient.**—Every glaucoma case should be admitted to hospital or sent to bed, and kept there for at least twelve hours before an operation is undertaken. The routine treatment is to give the patient a free purge of salts and senna, to instil a solution of eserin, to relieve pain and procure sleep by morphia or trivalin-hyoscin, and if the case is acute or subacute, to apply four leeches to the forehead and over the temporal region. To some this may appear to be bad surgery. The author is convinced that it is nothing of the kind. Tension is usually rapidly and distinctly lowered; the congestion of the eye diminishes markedly, and the patient's nervous system quiets down. It may be urged that cases of glaucoma occur in which vision is totally lost within twelve hours. Such must be very rare indeed, and the author can confidently say that he has never yet had cause to regret the delay and that, on the other hand, he has frequently found the operation made much easier by it.

On the evening before operation, the conjunctival sac of the eye to be operated upon, is filled with an ointment of perchloride of mercury of a strength of 1 in 3000, and the same thing is done again very early the next morning, the face being carefully washed with soap and water just beforehand.

Immediately before the operation the lashes of the upper lid are cut close with scissors, the blades of which have been anointed with sterilised vaseline, in order that none of the hairs may drop into the conjunctival sac, and be lost there. It is important to avoid second cuts at the same lashes, for this results in the production of short ends of hair, which are difficult to get rid of, and which may prove very troublesome. The skin for some distance around the orbit is freely painted with tincture of iodine, the lids being included in this application. The upper and lower lids are grasped together between the finger and thumb, so that their free edges are everted, and these edges, together with the lashes, are similarly and carefully sterilised with the iodine. Just before doing this, the Meibomian glands are emptied by firm pressure of the fingers on the two lids pressed together edge to edge, and the expressed secretion is carefully wiped away with sterile swabs. Should a little of the iodine escape into the conjunctival sac, it does no harm, but it is well to prevent any large leakage of the kind, and it is easy to do so.

In the meantime a solution of cocaine (4 per cent.), previously sterilised by boiling, has been instilled four times at 2 minute intervals into the conjunctival sac, and two instillations of adrenalin chloride solution (Parke Davis and Co.'s 1 in 1000) have also been made. A subconjunctival injection of cocaine and adrenalin chloride is next made in the lower *cul de sac*. In order to prepare this, two minims of the cocaine solution (4 per cent.) and two minims of the adrenalin chloride solution ($\frac{1}{1000}$) are mixed with four minims of normal saline solution for the purpose, and one-half or more of this volume of fluid is injected from a freshly boiled, all-glass syringe.

The conjunctival sac is next swabbed out to its farthest recesses by means of sterilised, mounted, wool swabs, under a stream of sterilised, normal, saline solution. All mucus and other exudation is thus completely removed. A speculum is inserted, great care being taken to avoid contamination of it in so doing ; and the conjunctival sac is freely flushed with the same saline solution poured out of a metal irrigator resembling in shape a small teapot with a long spout. If there is much congestion, adrenalin chloride solution (1 in 1000) is once again instilled.

In the case of nervous patients, and in those in whom the eyeball is painful, a hypodermic injection of $\frac{1}{4}$ c.c. of trivalin-hyoscin (The Saccharin Corporation's product) is given about twenty minutes before operation. Chloroform is reserved for children and for hopelessly unmanageable adults. It is very rarely that we meet with a patient of the latter class. If we can dispense with the use of a general anæsthetic, we gain the great advantage of having the patient's co-operation during the steps of the procedure, and we are saved the risks attendant on vomiting and straining after he is put back to bed. Both items are very important. The author has found trivalin-hyoscin greatly superior to morphia ; it is sterile, it very rarely, *if ever*, causes nausea or vomiting, and it keeps the patient drowsy for the next six or eight hours, with a minimum of unpleasant after-effects.

Whereas in dealing with cases of cataract, we must be most careful to bring the adnexa of the eye into a healthy condition before undertaking any operative procedure, the same routine is not considered justifiable in dealing with all glaucoma cases. Obviously an acute catarrh complicating a very chronic glaucoma would require to be dealt with first ; but speaking generally, it is unnecessary to wait, always provided that our antiseptic and aseptic regime is thoroughly carried out.

(2) **Sterilisation of Instruments.**—All blunt instruments should be boiled, and no instrument should be used a second time without fresh sterilisation. Duplicates of all instruments which are likely to be required more than

NEWER OPERATIONS FOR GLAUCOMA 507

once during an operation, should be kept ready. For the cutting instruments, in private work, the author finds absolute alcohol superior to any other form of antiseptic. It leaves cutting edges absolutely undamaged. In dealing with trephines, punch-forceps, keratomes, etc., this is a point of the utmost importance. The author has devised special alcohol sterilisers for the purpose.

(3) **The Surgeon's Hands** should be well washed before operation, but no strong antiseptic need be used. In this way his delicacy of touch is preserved, whilst if care be taken not to handle the operation-ends of the instruments, and to see that these do not come in contact with any foreign matter, no risk is entailed. It is of course essential that the operator's hands should be thoroughly dried on a sterilised towel, and that the trays in which the instruments are kept should be of such a nature as to allow them to dry. These are simple requisites. All dressings are sterilised by heat and are used dry.

(4) **The Apparatus for the Irrigation of the Aqueous Chamber.**—In India, where large numbers of glaucoma patients were operated upon in a single morning, the author always employed McKeown's irrigator, but in English practice he has adopted a simpler but still efficient form of apparatus for the purpose,[1] which can be obtained from any of the leading London firms of instrument makers. It consists of the barrel of an ordinary 2-oz. urethral syringe, to the nozzle of which is securely fastened one end of a piece of fine india-rubber tubing 3 feet in length, whilst the opposite end of the tubing carries a McKeown's irrigator nozzle. The whole apparatus is boiled for 5 minutes before use, and is then emptied and filled with normal, saline solution (0·7 per cent.). A separate assistant takes charge of the apparatus, and gives the nozzle into the surgeon's hand when he is ready to use it.

(5) **Masks.**—For every intra-ocular operation, the surgeon, his assistant, and any bystanders who lean over the table, should wear efficient mouth masks. These should be soaked beforehand in perchloride lotion and then

[1] A modification of Bishop Harman's Undine Irrigator.

put on damp, with a view to prevent dust-droppings from their surface. Sterilised coats should also be worn.

(6) **Arrangement of Patient on Table.**—The patient should be laid on a suitable table or bed with his feet toward the window and his head resting on a small pillow, which is so arranged that its edge is level with his face on the side of the operation. Those surgeons who use an irrigator will find this a not unimportant detail, as it enables the nurse who holds the tray for catching the escaping irrigator fluid, to keep both hand and tray well down out of the way. It is not necessary to cover the patient's face, but his forehead and scalp should be firmly wrapped in a clean, sterile towel, which is pinned in place. Another sterile towel or sheet should cover the patient from his neck downwards.

It is of very great advantage to perform all serious glaucoma operations on the patient's bed if possible, and to leave him lying on his back and wholly undisturbed for the next five or six hours. If trivalin-hyoscin has been used, as above suggested, this will not be found to be a great hardship, and the time will pass quickly and easily.

(7) **Method of Bandaging.**—The bandage employed in Madras was introduced there by the writer in 1897. He has not seen it used anywhere else. It is in his opinion greatly preferable to any other bandage when the two eyes require to be closed (Fig. 147). A piece of bandage cloth is taken, 4 inches broad, and of such a length that it will pass one-and-a-half times round the patient's head. The mid-point of the strip is placed over the patient's external occipital protuberance, and the two free ends are held in front of the face by an assistant ; the position of the two ears and the size of their bases are carefully measured on the bandage. This is now removed, and two holes are cut, one on each side, to fit the bases of the ears. The object of so doing is to fix the bandage so that it cannot slide up or down. Each free end of the bandage is now slit into three tails from before backward to a point opposite the patient's temples ; each centre tail is $2\frac{1}{2}$ inches broad, while the breadth of each of the four remaining tails is $\frac{3}{4}$ of an inch.

NEWER OPERATIONS FOR GLAUCOMA 509

To apply the bandage, the ears are fitted through the holes made for them, and the two upper and two lower tails respectively are tied together, the one pair over the vertex and the other below the chin. The patient is brought on the table with the bandage thus applied. After operation, one of the two broad tails is brought down across the dressings and held in position by an assistant, while the operator brings the remaining tail down on top of the previous one, and fixes the bandage by means of a pin applied at each side.

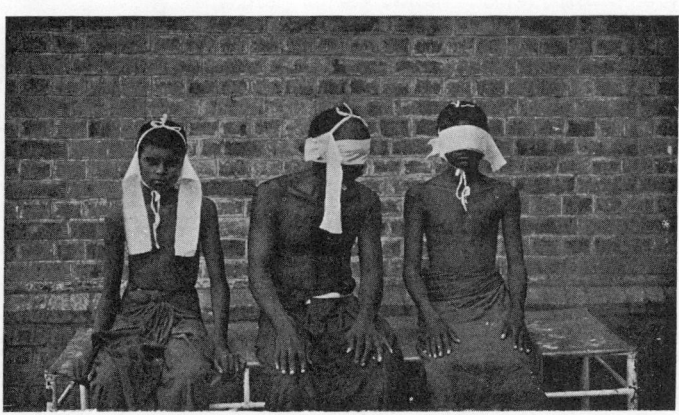

FIG. 147.—The figure to the left shows the patient when he comes on the table ready for operation, except that each tail is rolled up on itself, and fixed with a pin, in order to keep it out of the way until the end of the operation. In the middle figure one tail of the bandage has been pinned in position, the other still hangs down. The figure to the right shows the bandage completed as the patient leaves the operation table.

At each dressing the pins are removed, the two broad tails are thrown backward, and the dressings are changed. The eye is then closed by reapplying the middle tails in the same way as before.

By this contrivance we are able repeatedly to dress our patient without raising his head from the pillow, or in any way disturbing him. Another advantage is that firm and graduated pressure can be very easily applied.[1]

[1] For fuller details as to the preparations for an operation, see the author's *The Care of Eye Cases*, Oxford Medical Publications, 1921.

GLAUCOMA

Part III

Sclerotomy for Glaucoma

Anterior Sclerotomy.—The subject of sclerotomy was discussed when we were considering the history of glaucoma operations. It remains now to give an account of the technique of the procedure as advocated by de Wecker, and as practised by a very large number of surgeons since, especially before the advent of the newer operations.

A narrow Graefe knife is made to puncture the sclera 1 mm. to the temporal side of the limbus, and about 2 mm. below the highest part of the corneal circumference. It is carried on through the anterior chamber to emerge at a corresponding point on the nasal side, just as if the surgeon intended to cut a narrow flap (2 to 2·5 mm. in depth) in the upper quadrant of the eye (Fig. 148). Instead, however, of completing the flap, the puncture and counter-puncture are somewhat enlarged by sawing movements with the knife, and the latter is then carefully withdrawn, without completing the section.

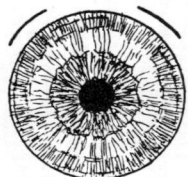

FIG. 148.—De Wecker's sclerotomy, showing the two incisions in the conjunctiva and sclera.

In this way a bridge is left between the two apertures made in the sclera. Should the iris prolapse, it may be replaced with a spud or with a stream of irrigator fluid. If, however, it cannot be satisfactorily got back into position, the prolapsing portion or portions should be excised. If this cannot be done thoroughly, it is better to complete the section with a blunt pointed knife or scissors, and perform an iridectomy, rather than to leave uveal tissue impacted in the wound. Eserin should be instilled before the operation commences, at the close of it, and at intervals during convalescence, in order to keep the iris away from the incisions. The operation can be performed in other quadrants than the superior, but the latter is usually preferred by operators as being the easiest to work in, and the least harmful if an iridectomy has eventually to be done.

Posterior Sclerotomy.—This operation consists in tapping the vitreous chamber through the sclera well behind the ciliary body. The section should be meridional, *i.e.*, it should have an antero-posterior direction, in order to avoid doing more injury than we can help ; the scleral fibres run mostly in an antero-posterior direction, and consequently a section from behind forwards divides as few of these as possible ; the result is that a tendency to gaping of the wound is avoided. A still more important factor is the antero-posterior direction of the vessels and nerves within the eye. The best point to select is one midway between the external and inferior recti muscles about 8 mm. behind the corneal margin. The conjunctiva close to the limbus is seized in the grip of a pair of forceps in the meridian in which we wish to operate. The patient is told to look strongly upward and inward, and the blade of a von Graefe knife is boldly and firmly pushed in vertically at the point already indicated to a depth of about 6 mm., aiming the point as if to strike the very centre of the vitreous body. The knife is then given a quarter turn on its own axis, in order to allow the free escape of fluid from the vitreous body into the subconjunctival space. After a short delay its direction is again rectified, and it is slowly withdrawn. This operation is of value (i.) as a preliminary to iridectomy when the chamber is very shallow, and (ii.) in those rare cases, where something must be done at once but an ordinary set operation is impossible for the time being.

PART IV

Lagrange's Operation (Sclerecto-Iridectomy)

The accompanying illustrations (Figs 149 to 152) will help to explain the steps of the operation. Using a narrow Graefe knife, a small corneo-scleral flap is made above. Puncture and counter-puncture are placed each 1 mm.

outside the corneal margin, and the blade is carried upwards, parallel to the iris and as close to it as possible, the first object being *to sever the scleral insertion of the ciliary muscle.*

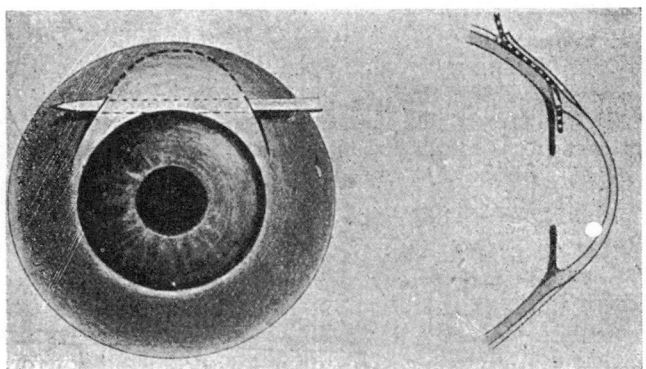

FIG. 149.—Section of the sclera and conjunctiva.

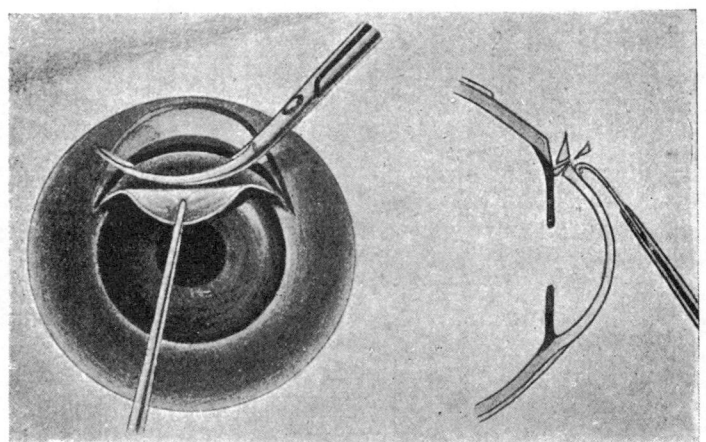

FIG. 150.—Resection of the sclerotic.

The plane of the knife blade is then changed, so that it emerges from the sclera 2 mm. or 3 mm. from the limbus and thus bevels the posterior lip of the incision. The incision is completed by making a large conjunctival flap

(Fig. 149). This flap having been turned down, the corneal lip of the wound is removed with the scissors (Fig. 150).

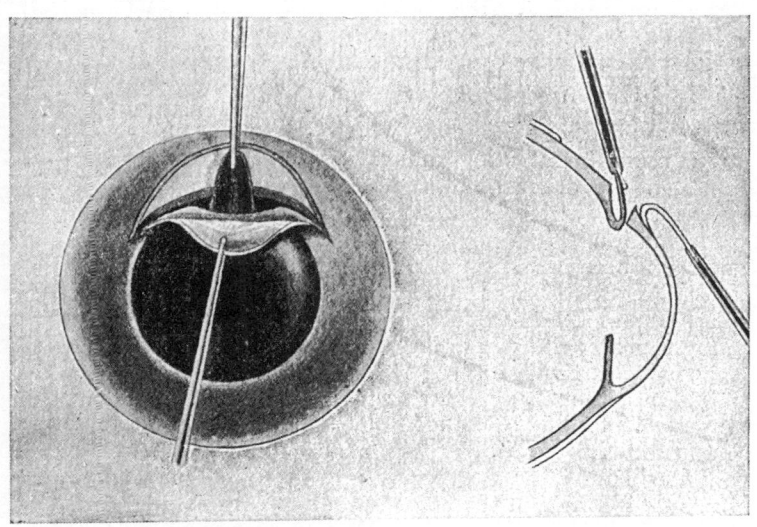

Fig. 151.—The making of the iridectomy.

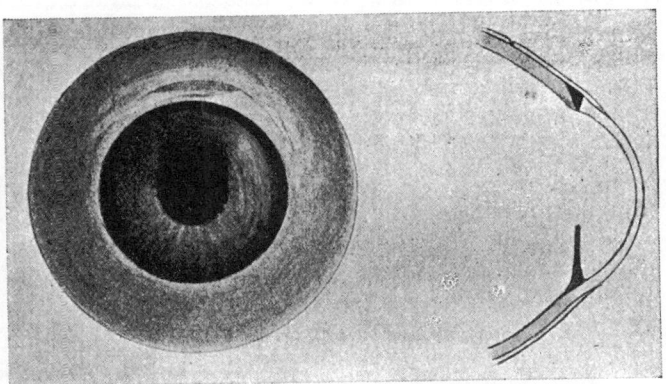

Fig. 152.—The result of the operation.

If iridectomy is considered desirable, it is done at this stage (Fig. 151), and the replacement of the conjunctival flap completes the operation. Iridectomy, although done in all the earlier operations, is not considered essential. It should always be done, where for any reason, such as hypertension, prolapse is feared. No iris must be left between the lips of the wound. The result of the operation is shown in Fig. 152.

From his extensive experience of the operation, Lagrange has reached the following conclusions :—The results of sclerectomy vary according to the degree of hypertension of the eye operated on. Three varieties of cicatrix are distinguishable according to the amount of sclera excised : (1) That in which there is mere thinning of the sclera owing to the excised portion not reaching the posterior surface of the cornea (conjunctiva smoothly covers the cicatrix) ; (2) that represented by a subconjunctival fistulette, due to excision of the whole thickness of the sclera, in an eye with moderate tension (the conjunctiva lies smoothly over the cicatrix) ; (3) the fistulous cicatrix with an ampulliform elevation of the overlying conjunctiva, resulting from excision of the whole thickness of the sclera in an eye the seat of high tension. He believes that in cases of high tension, even a simple sclerotomy will allow ample filtration, owing to the gaping of the wound, while in cases without elevation of the tension, sclerotomy will be quite ineffectual. He therefore proposes the following rules of procedure :—(*a*) If tension is normal to + 1, do sclerectomy without iridectomy, the amount of sclera excised being inversely proportional to the degree of hypertension. (*b*) If tension is + 1 to + 3, do sclerecto-iridectomy, the iridectomy being added to avoid entanglement of the iris. He has never recommended his operation for acute glaucoma, but has strongly advocated it for cases of the simple chronic affection.

Amongst those who still use the method, the unmistakable modern tendency has been to limit the size of this initial incision as severely as possible. This has been due to the dread of the dangers, which are widely felt to be inseparable from any procedure which involves a large and free opening of the globe, especially at an early stage of the operation. To the same fear we owe the efforts by certain surgeons to modify Lagrange's technique.

Modifications of Lagrange's Method.—The principal of these are the operations of Brooksbank James and Foroni. The former has already been described. Foroni's "sclerectomy ab externo" is practically identical with it; it is made at the limbus with a Graefe knife; the aqueous is allowed to escape gradually, a small peripheral iridectomy is performed, and the large conjunctival flap is sutured into place.

Whilst these procedures undoubtedly make the escape of aqueous more gradual and thereby possibly add to the safety of the operation, they would appear to suffer from the disadvantage that the removal of a clean piece of the whole thickness of the sclera is decidedly more difficult in them, than it is by Lagrange's method. They have attracted very little attention from other surgeons, if one may judge from a study of the literature of the subject.

PART V

Holth's Operation (Sclerectomy with Punch-Forceps)

Holth's operation [1] is designed to carry out Lagrange's principle, whilst avoiding that operator's large incision, with its attendant risks of escape of the lens, and of expulsive hæmorrhage. The instruments used are a speculum, a Holth's fixation forceps (Fig. 153), a Holth's bent keratome, with stop, 6 mm. by 6 mm. (Fig. 154), or a Graefe knife, a Holth's double conjunctival hook (Fig. 155), a curved forceps with transversely grooved points, a mouse-tooth forceps, a Dowell's forcep-scissors with both blades blunt-pointed, a Holth's curved iris forceps with stop-screw (Fig. 156), a Holth's punch-forceps (Fig. 157A), a de Wecker's forceps scissors, a repositor, and six mounted cotton-wool swabs.

The operation can be performed by two methods:

(A) *By a linear incision with a Graefe knife.*—The pupil

[1] This description of the operation has been taken practically verbatim from the translation of Holth's original article, which appeared in *The Ophthalmoscope*, vol. vii. p. 774.

GLAUCOMA

being contracted by pilocarpine, a puncture and counter-puncture are made in the sclera 8 mm. from each other, and 1 mm. from the limbus, with the points of entry into and exit from the conjunctiva as far from the limbus as possible. A scleral flap 2 to 2·5 mm. high, and a conjunctival flap extending to 8 mm. from the limbus are now cut (Fig. 158A). The conjunctiva is freed with the scissors from the anterior lip of the scleral flap, and is raised with a forceps, whilst a

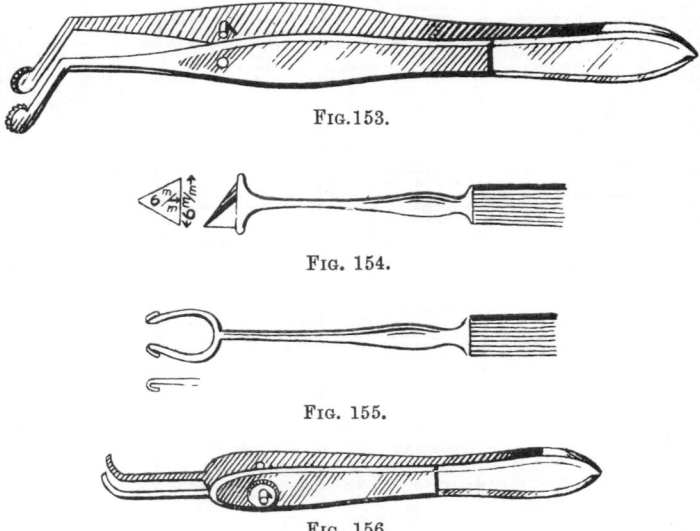

FIGS. 153 to 156.—Holth's instruments (made by Luer).
Fig. 153, forceps.   Fig. 154, keratome.   Fig. 155, double hook.
Fig. 156, iris forceps.

piece of the scleral flap, 3 mm. long by 1·5 mm. broad, is removed with the punch-forceps; a small peripheral iridectomy is performed, unless the iris prolapses, when an ordinary iridectomy is made. The conjunctiva is then carefully replaced, and as a rule does not require a suture. This procedure is suitable for cases with slightly increased tension, and a high degree of direct astigmatism, as it causes considerable inverse astigmatism. It is the easiest operation, and can be performed without an assistant.

NEWER OPERATIONS FOR GLAUCOMA   517

(B) *By a 6 mm. subconjunctival incision, usually upwards, with a keratome.*—The pupil being contracted by pilocarpine, the conjunctiva is punctured 10 mm. from the limbus, and the keratome is passed down beneath it to a point 2·5

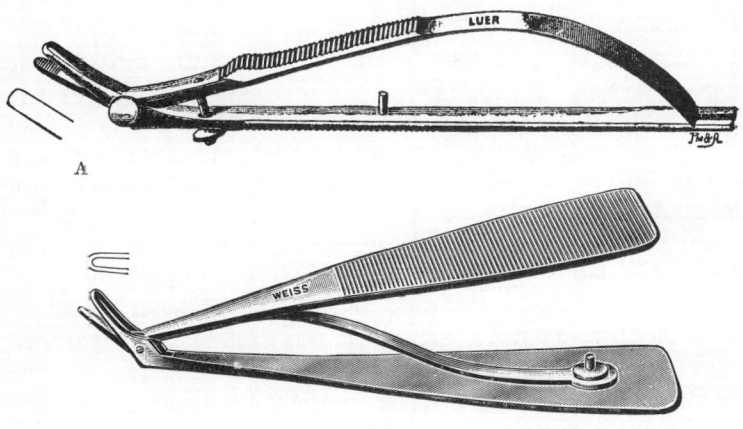

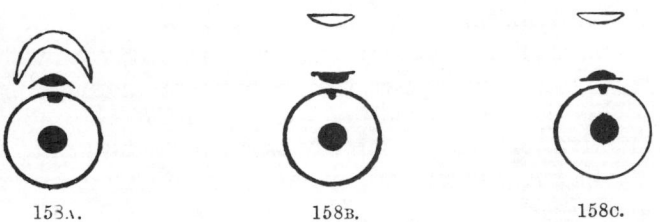

Fig. 157A.—Holth's original punch-forceps.

Fig. 157B.—Holth's new model of punch-forceps, with a blade of 1 mm. for tangential extralimbal sclerectomy.

Fig. 158A.—Diagram of sclerectomy of the anterior lip with a punch-forceps after incision with a narrow Graefe knife.

Fig. 158B.—The same as the above, but through a keratome incision.

Fig. 158C.—Diagram of sclerectomy of the posterior lip with a punch-forceps through a keratome incision.

mm. from the limbus, where it is made to puncture the sclera. The bulbar conjunctiva is then freed with blunt-pointed scissors, between the scleral wound and the limbus. With the help of the curved forceps, the conjunctival flap is caught on the double blunt hook, and pulled down so as to lay bare the scleral wound ; the lower blade of the punch-forceps is introduced into the incision until 1·5 mm. of sclera is seen through the upper blade, when it is cut off rapidly. The blunt hook is then handed over to an assistant, and a peripheral iridectomy is performed, in order to avoid prolapse of the iris. Finally the conjunctival flap is replaced with a spatula (Fig. 158B). A complete iridectomy is done if the iris prolapses, if there is central opacity of the cornea or lens, or if there is a cataract which will require extraction later. The entire subconjunctival pocket can be made with scissors right up to the limbus, and the keratome used for the scleral puncture only. This is more tedious, but probably preferable for lateral operations. In his earlier cases, Holth made his scleral incision 0·5 mm. from the limbus, freed the conjunctiva and pulled it down with the hook, then depressed the corneal edge of the incision with the lower blade of the punch-forceps, which he slipped backwards so that on closing the instrument he excised a piece of the posterior lip (Fig. 158c). The piece of sclera excised by this means was bigger than that removed from the anterior lip, but was not in so favourable a position. In his later cases, the sclerectomy was performed on the anterior lip, and was always successful, provided that a large enough piece of sclerotic had been removed.

It is important to free the conjunctiva thoroughly, as otherwise the flap is cut by the punch-forceps, and the conjunctival epithelium subsequently grows down into the scleral opening, which then cicatrises without producing a filtration scar.

The advantages claimed for the keratome operation are (i.) lessened risk of hæmorrhage or of rupture of the zonule, and (ii.) the production of a lesser amount of astigmatism.

The surgeons who have used Holth's method have been content as a rule to follow his technique, with the exception of the pattern of punch-forceps they preferred to employ. Butler, Johnson, Bardsley, and others have all devised punches of their own. A few, like Butler, perform the

NEWER OPERATIONS FOR GLAUCOMA 519

operation under an Elliot flap. Harman, after an initial keratome section, cuts a flap with his twin scissors, which have been so modified that they free a U-shaped piece, which is left attached to the cornea by a narrow stalk ; this flap is so freely movable that it can be twisted on its pedicle ; the conjunctiva is replaced over it, and an imitation of Herbert's wedge-operation is thus produced ; a basal iridectomy completes the technique.

Whilst these pages were in the press, Holth has published an account of a modified procedure which he has recently adopted. The following description in his own words is taken direct from *The British Journal of Ophthalmology* of December 1921 :

"The idea struck me that perhaps a more peripheral sclerectomy fistula would be better protected against late infection than one close to the limbus. The position of the sclerectomy close to the limbus could not be avoided in my two earlier operations with the punch-forceps removing pieces of sclera from the posterior or anterior lip of the wound. But by putting the 1 mm. wide blade of my new punch-forceps (Fig. 157B) into the anterior chamber in a *tangential* direction from a short incision, 1·5 or 2 mm. from the limbus, an *extralimbal* excision of the sclera can be obtained in the following way :

"Before the anæsthesia the pupil should be well contracted by meiotics. A large curved conjunctival flap 10 mm. from the limbus with the apex somewhat temporally situated is dissected downwards to the limbus, but the ends of the incision should be at least 5 mm. from the corneal margin (Fig. 159).

"An incision 3 or 4 mm. long is made into the anterior chamber ; this is best performed with the keratome ;[1] the

---

[1] " For all keratome incisions upwards I stand in front of the patient, hold the handle with palmarflected, slightly supinated hand and guide the point towards me ; in removing the keratome I have plenty of free movement of the hand for lowering the handle and turning the point sideways in order to avoid any wounding of the lens capsule. By standing behind the head of the patient and holding the handle with dorsalflected and pronated hand, thus guiding the point from him, the operator has very limited hand movement (see W. Czermak, *Augenärztliche Operationen*, Wien, 1893–1904, p. 10,

point of the knife is inserted 1·5 to 2 mm. from the limbus and 3 mm. temporally to the vertical meridian. Before the point of the keratome reaches the chamber, the conjunctival flap is turned upwards from the cornea in order that the point of the knife may be seen in the angle of the chamber ; during this proceeding a good electric sidelight ought always to be used. In removing the keratome from the anterior chamber the handle is lowered and the point turned sideways ; in this way any danger of wounding the lens capsule is avoided. The operator now takes his stand behind the head of the recumbent patient whether

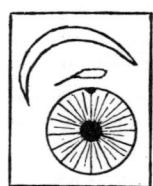 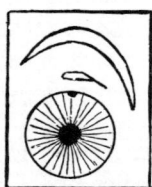

Fig. 159.—Showing the incision in the conjunctiva and sclera in the right and left eyes—somewhat outside the upper vertical meridian. The *tangential* and *extralimbal sclerectomy* is shown at the inner end of the keratome incision in the sclera A small basal iridectomy has been performed. Instead of a conjunctival flap a subconjunctival tunnel may be made to the limbus ; then an assistant, by means of the blunt double hook (Fig. 155), draws down the conjunctival incision exposing the limbus for sclerectomy and basal iridectomy. (Holth.)

the sclerectomy is to be made on the right or the left eye. The 1 mm. wide blade of the punch-forceps is, with the flat part parallel with the sclera in a tangential direction, introduced below the nasal angle of the wound 3 mm. into the anterior chamber. In order to make the scleral opening oblique and so place it farther from the limbus, the handle is lowered till it forms an angle of about 150° with the plane of the iris (see the dotted lines in Fig. 160).

" The piece of sclera is now excised by closing the punch-forceps ; it should be 3 mm. long and the anterior

Fig. 13). For all subconjunctival glaucoma operations the *blades* of the *speculum* ought to be *short* in *transversal direction*. By this means the palpebral fissure can be well opened in vertical direction and plenty of space be obtained for making a conjunctival flap or a subconjunctival tunnel."

edge should be placed rather more than 1 mm. from the limbus. A small basal iridectomy is then performed, but in some cases such as where the iris has completely prolapsed or in some cases of cataract a complete iridectomy is done. The conjunctival wound is then sutured with three fine black silk threads which are tied only with the first half of a surgical knot and removed after forty-eight hours.

" For the left eye the punch-forceps ought to be held

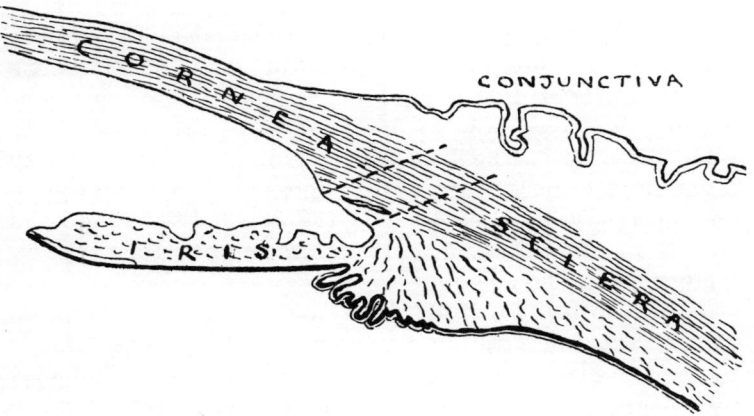

Fig. 160.—The dotted lines show the position, limits, and direction of the tangential, extralimbal 1 mm. wide punch-forceps sclerectomy; in the removed scleral piece is a little of canalis Schlemmii and of the ciliary muscle sinew, while the ciliary body itself is not laid bare. (Holth.)

in the left hand if the operator stands behind the patient; but if he wants to use his right hand he should stand before the patient, preferably on the right side. If the keratome incision in the left eye is made to the nasal side, he may remain standing behind the patient and with his right hand make a tangential sclerectomy to the temporal side; a protruding forehead would, however, during this proceeding present difficulties to the lowering of the handle of the punch-forceps.

" If the patient be a squeezer a transitory paralysis of the m. orbicularis after van Lint (1914) should be made previously by injection of a 2 per cent. novocain solution with adrenalin freshly made with tablets. If the patient constantly turns the eye up, a transitory paralysis of the m. rectus superior may be made previously by injecting 0·5 ccm. of the same solution in the muscle (G. F. Rochat, 1920)."

Part VI

Herbert's Operations

When dealing with the history of the operative surgery of glaucoma, mention was made of some of Herbert's earlier efforts to find a method for the relief of this condition. We have now to detail his later attempts in the same direction. The best course would appear to be to describe each shortly, and as far as possible in his own words, and at the same time to give the original references, so that those who are sufficiently interested can turn to, and study them at first hand.

[1] It is difficult to follow the wedge-isolation operation from a verbal description alone, but the following summary by A. J. Ballantyne, with the assistance of the accompanying diagrams, may make it more or less clear. A very narrow Graefe knife is used. (1) Proceeding as if the intention were to make a shallow corneo-scleral flap, puncture and counter-puncture are made close to the margin of the cornea, the knife point having previously passed through the conjunctiva a little distance above the point of entrance. The upward cut is made with the knife blade bevelled a little backwards, and at this stage the bridge of sclera is left undivided (Fig. 161). (2) The knife is brought down again and its edge turned forward. A forward cut is made perpendicular to the scleral surface, care being taken not to cut through the conjunctiva (Fig. 162). This incision makes the lower boundary of the wedge of tissue. (3) The knife is drawn backwards, and rotated upwards to lie in the original incision, which is continued

---

[1] This description is taken verbatim from *The Ophthalmoscope*, July 1910.

NEWER OPERATIONS FOR GLAUCOMA 523

upwards until the knife edge emerges through the sclera, a millimetre or so from the corneal margin. This completes the isolation of the wedge. The blade of the knife is now turned upwards and backwards to form a long conjunctival flap, which, however, is left attached at its upper extremity. A small basal iridectomy is advisable in order to prevent prolapse.

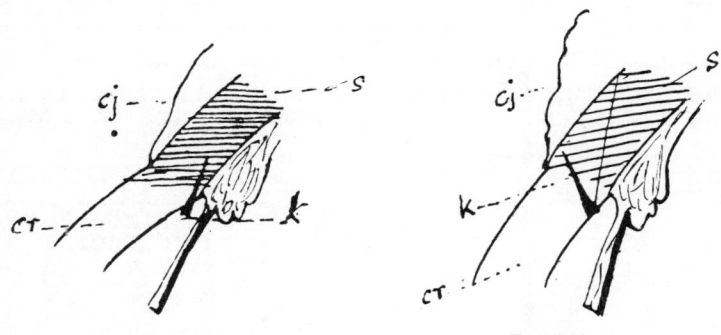

FIG. 161.   FIG. 162.

FIG. 161.—Position of the knife blade in making the first incision.
FIG. 162.—Position of the knife blade in making the second incision.
The thin line in Fig. 162 shows the position of the first incision which has been partly made.
cr, cornea ; *cj*, conjunctiva ; *s*, sclera ; *k*, knife.   (Herbert.)

For full details of this procedure, the reader is referred to Herbert's original description.

The Small Flap Operation.—"The earlier of these operations were performed with a very narrow tapering Graefe knife, either in the lower outer, or upper outer quadrant of the eye. After sliding the conjunctiva on the point of the knife, a 2 mm. scleral incision was made concentric with the corneal circumference, and 1·5 mm. from it (Fig. 163), entering the anterior chamber close to its angle. At the two ends of this small section, the edge of the knife was turned forwards, and incisions were made with slow sawing movements up to the corneal margin (Fig. 164). These two incisions formed the sides of the small flap, the primary incision the end of the flap ; the whole was subconjunctival, the conjunctival puncture remaining small, about 4 mm. from the limbus (Fig. 165). The immediate outflow of aqueous produced considerable temporary conjunctival œdema. Before the operation the pupil was contracted, as far as possible, by physostigmine, and usually one or more instillations of adrenalin were made in addition to cocaine, according to the degree of glaucomatous congestion of the eye." The above description is in Herbert's own words.

Harman modified this operation both in the manner of raising the conjunctival flap, and also in the instrument used for cutting the sclera ; he substituted his twin scissors for the Graefe knife, and he claims that the method he suggests is " elegant and expeditious."

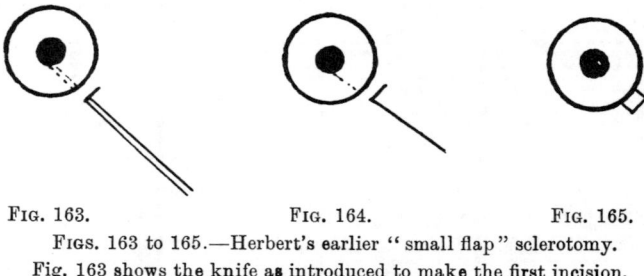

Fig. 163.   Fig. 164.   Fig. 165.

Figs. 163 to 165.—Herbert's earlier " small flap" sclerotomy.
Fig. 163 shows the knife as introduced to make the first incision.
Fig. 164 shows it turned on its edge to cut the first side of the flap.
Fig. 165 shows the flap completed. (Herbert.)

The Triple Small Flap Operation.—Dissatisfied with his previous efforts, Herbert made a further alteration in his procedure which he described as follows :—" The method consists merely in cutting, with modified Bishop Harman's twin scissors, twice instead of once. Instead of two parallel incisions outlining one flap, four incisions are made to include three very narrow flaps (Figs. 166 and 167). A primary incision with a bent broad needle, 3·5 mm. wide, is sufficient to admit of this double cutting by twin scissors with blades 1·5 mm. apart. Personally, I have made this flap section under a conjunctival flap only upon three eyes, but have employed the same incision, cutting with the scissors through the conjunctiva and sclera together in eight eyes ; in these latter cases the primary incision

NEWER OPERATIONS FOR GLAUCOMA

only has been made subconjunctival by sliding the conjunctiva. The operation has been reserved in all but two cases for secondary glaucoma likely to give imperfect or negative results with the small flap sclerotomy. It is obvious that in cases where the conjunctiva is cut through, iridectomy or iridodialysis must usually be combined, lest prolapse of iris should occur, uncovered by conjunctiva."

W. G. Laws has used this operation, but he performed it under an Elliot flap of conjunctiva, in order to place the scleral incision as far as possible from the conjunctival wound (Fig. 168).

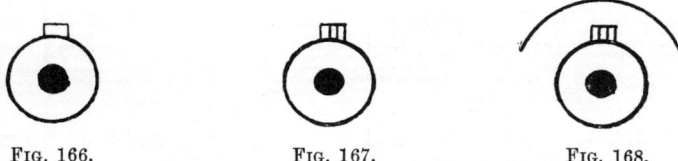

FIG. 166.   FIG. 167.   FIG. 168.

FIGS. 166 to 168.—Herbert's "triple small flap" sclerotomy.
Fig. 166 shows the old operation wound; Fig. 167 the new. Fig. 168 shows Laws' method of performing the above operation under an Elliot flap. (Herbert.)

Herbert's metal rod operation consisted in making a linear sclerotomy subconjunctivally, and then "fixing a small gilded metal rod or knotted thread in the wound for twenty-four hours. The rod or thread lies on the surface of the conjunctiva, depressing the latter into the underlying scleral wound." The method does not appear to have been tried very far, or to have appealed to ophthalmologists. It will be found described in the *Proceedings of the Royal Society of Medicine* for June 1914.

Quite recently, Herbert has taken up an iris-prolapse operation in selected cases. The author has already expressed his opinion on the subject of such procedures, and feels that so far as he is concerned, no good can come of discussing them further. The references to the literature, given below, will enable anyone who is interested in the subject, to read both sides of the question at first hand.

REFERENCES

Elliot, R. H.—*Brit. Journ. Ophth.*, 1921, vol. v. pp. 91 and 237.
Harman, N. B.—*The Ophthalmoscope*, 1911, vol. ix. p. 770.
Herbert, H.—*Ibid.*, 1907, vol. v. p. 292; 1911, vol. ix. p. 76; 1913, vol. xi. p. 398; *Proc. Roy. Soc. Med.*, June 1914; *Brit. Journ. Ophth.*, 1920, vol. iv. p. 550; 1921, vol. v. p. 183.

Part VII

Scleral Trephining (Fergus's Operation)

The author feels that he can best do justice to this procedure by describing it in Dr. Fergus's words, and he does so accordingly. The italics are, however, his own, and are for the purpose of drawing attention to points of importance.

" On the 5th day of January 1909, I did my first operation. I first dissected the conjunctiva from the periphery towards the cornea, and laid the flap of conjunctiva on the surface of the cornea while I used the trephine. I selected for the purpose the medium size of Bowman's instruments. I entirely removed the portion of sclera marked off by the trephine, replaced the conjunctiva, and stitched it into position. . . . As occasion required, I performed the same operation until the spring of 1909, except that *I had introduced another modification which I think of importance* in so far as it is beneficial. I began *to take an iris repositor, and to pass it in at the wound made by the trephine*, keeping it in close contact with the sclera and the cornea till I saw the point of it well in the anterior chamber.

" *Mr. E. Treacher Collins very properly said* in the discussion at Belfast *that my operation, as now performed, was not merely a trephining, but was also a cyclodialysis. I have combined the trephining with cyclodialysis since the month of March* 1909. *I do not remember to have performed a simple trephining since that time.*

" I thought that the largest of these instruments (*i.e.*,

NEWER OPERATIONS FOR GLAUCOMA

Bowman's trephines), the *diameter* of which is *about three millimetres*, was exactly the instrument adapted to my purpose. . . . I feel quite sure that any trephine which is considerably less in its diameter is likely to be too small to give a good result.

"I made my first operation at the upper part of the sclera just above the cornea. A flap of conjunctiva was cut exactly as directed by Lagrange, and was folded over the cornea. I then applied the trephine, but found that it did not grip well, for the simple reason that I had not denuded the sclera entirely of all the conjunctival tissue. That is a step which must invariably be taken in this operation, otherwise the edge of the trephine is apt to slip about and to make the operation unduly difficult. I had therefore to stop the use of the trephine till I had absolutely removed all the conjunctival tissue. There is another danger if this tissue is not thoroughly removed; it is that the conjunctiva as the trephine twists round may be drawn under its edge and torn or cut. . . . Bowman's trephine is certainly the one which I shall continue to use. . . . Another difficulty which occurs is that the eye is movable and therefore is apt to roll about under the pressure of the trephine. That can very largely be prevented by fixing the eyeball above and below the point at which it is proposed to operate. I invariably now use two pairs of fixation forceps, and in that way keep the eye perfectly steady. The trephine as devised by Bowman has another advantage; it has at the other end of it a sort of sharp point which may come in handy in the removal of the little circular piece of sclera as soon as it has been separated.

"In the main I prefer to operate without a general anæsthetic. A few drops of alvatunder put below the conjunctiva render the preliminary stages of the operation perfectly painless. As it proceeds the patient winces, and that at once indicates that you are through the sclera, and that it is time to withdraw the trephine and examine the orifice made. If it has been well made, the piece of sclera should be cut circularly right round. Sometimes it is found that it is not so, but that at one place the trephine has completely divided the scleral tissue while it has not done so at another. In such cases it is generally possible to seize the little piece with a pair of iris forceps and to complete its excision by means of a pair of iris scissors. . . . I dissect up the conjunctiva carefully, but very thoroughly, right to its insertion in the cornea, and the wound made by the trephine is placed as close to the cornea as it can be *without involving the strands of the conjunctiva which are connected with the cornea.* . . . I have thought it right occasionally to modify the operation by combining with it a thorough freeing of the angle of the anterior chamber in the neighbourhood of the operation. For that purpose I take an ordinary repositor and pass it in, keeping the point in close contact with the sclera till I see the point in the anterior chamber. I then move it about from side to side to a slight extent, and in this manner free the tissues considerably. . . . By the procedure thus described *an opening is made right from the anterior chamber into that important space between the choroid and the sclera* on which Mr. Henderson lays so much emphasis, and *that space is in turn drained through an opening which is at least 3 millimetres wide. I regard a small trephine as being entirely out of place,* and further, *the more thoroughly the tissues can be freed in the neighbourhood of the opening the better.*

" But *an objection has sometimes been raised to my operation*, and that is, *that it is done right over the ciliary body*. There still seems to linger in the minds of some operators that the ciliary body is essentially a vital part, the touching of which in an operation may bring on sympathetic ophthalmitis. No doubt the ciliary body is an immensely important structure. On it depends the power of accommodation, and also on it, there is reason to believe depends the whole of the nutrition of the vitreous humour and of the lens. It is further admitted that it is highly vascular, and probably the opinion is quite just that it is very absorbent. . . . I quite admit that inflammation of the ciliary body in any form is a particularly undesirable condition ; I may put it in stronger language and say a somewhat dangerous condition.

"But an inflammation of the ciliary body will not take place unless there be a sufficient determining cause."

It will be observed that a period of nearly five and a half years intervened between the two papers in which Fergus has described his procedure. On the first occasion he stated that it was a combination of trephining and cyclodialysis, and that he had given up simple trephining. His second communication showed that in the course of the intervening years he had modified his practice, for he no longer made a point of the cyclodialysis being a routine step in his procedure, though he still, in certain cases, introduced an iris repositor through the wound in order to effect "a thorough freeing of the angle of the chamber in the neighbourhood of the operation." There are other points of interest to note, viz., (1) that he deliberately trephined wholly in the sclera, though as close to the cornea as possible; (2) that he used a 3 mm. trephine, and condemned the use of any smaller instrument; and (3) that he trephined directly over the ciliary body, and made light of the risks of so doing: it is noteworthy that he referred only to the danger of inflammation due to sepsis, and not at all to that of prolapse of this body into the trephine hole. The author looks upon the latter as far the more serious peril of the two.

These points have been insisted on for the reason that some writers have very incorrectly spoken of "the Fergus-Elliot," or "Elliot-Fergus procedure," whereas the methods adopted by Fergus and by the author have, as shown by our own writings, nothing in common beyond the use of the trephine, a feature in which both were long anticipated by others, since Argyll Robertson used that instrument to operate for glaucoma in 1876, and Blanco and Fröhlich did the same thing in 1903 and 1904 respectively.

Although it is slightly anticipating what is to be said in the next part of this chapter, it seems convenient here to point out the radical differences between the two methods.

Fergus used a large trephine, worked wholly on the

sclera, cut right down on the ciliary body, and, in a number of his cases, deliberately added a further interference with the uveal tissues, in order to open the supra-choroidal space freely. The author's motive, from the first, has been "to reach, tap, and drain subconjunctivally the anterior chamber with a minimum of injury to the structures of the eyeball." To this end the smallest blade (2 mm. in diameter) that can be conveniently used is selected; the junction of the cornea and sclera is trephined as far forwards as possible; the ciliary body is thus avoided; the chamber is entered directly by the trephine; and the iris is only dealt with in order to obviate any tendency it might otherwise have to block the trephine hole, and so to interfere with filtration.

The term "Fergus's Operation" should be held to imply a trephine operation, situate wholly in the sclera, with the use of a 3 mm. trephine, and involving the ciliary body as a routine step. The author's operation, on the other hand, is a procedure that shuns all interference with the uveal tissue, that strives to tap the anterior chamber with a minimum of trauma to the other structures of the eye, and that with these ends in view, limits the diameter of the trephine and pushes the opening right forward so that the disc cut out is half corneal and half scleral. To include two procedures, so different in technique and with such different aims, under a single name, is to create confusion in the minds of surgeons, and serves no good purpose. The difference between them is one, not merely of manipulative detail, but of the principles involved.

REFERENCES

BLANCO.—*Klin. Monatsbl. f. Augenh.*, 1903, vol. xli. pt. 2, p. 150.
FERGUS, F.—*The Ophthalmoscope*, 1910, vol. viii. p. 74; and *Ophth. Rev.*, 1915, vol. xxxiv. p. 202.
FRÖHLICH, K.—*Klin. Monatsbl. f. Augenh.*, May 1904.
ROBERTSON, D. ARGYLL.—*R.L.O.H. Reports*, May 1876, vol. viii. pt. 3.

NEWER OPERATIONS FOR GLAUCOMA

PART VIII

Sclero-Corneal Trephining (Elliot's Operation)

The criticism has been offered that this operation has been said to be easy, but is often difficult. Those with a fair amount of technical experience will probably find it from the start a very easy procedure; but, like all other operations for glaucoma, it may at any time prove a difficult one in advanced and hazardous cases. When the author left India, the Madras figures showed over 900 cases. Since then he has had the opportunity of trephining a large number of eyes in America, in England, and elsewhere, and has had the advantage of receiving valuable suggestions from surgeons, who are trephining all over the world. In the light of this assistance, certain minor details have been modified. Although the technique will now be described in considerable detail, it must not be thought that the operation is a correspondingly complicated one. The author has seen so many instances in which surgeons, who believed that they were adopting his method, were unwittingly omitting or changing important steps in the procedure, that he has decided to describe it as fully and clearly as possible.

(1) **In which quadrant of the eye should the trephining be performed?**—It is obvious that under most circumstances the upper is the quadrant of choice, for (1) the wound is then less exposed to infection; (2) the iridectomy, if one is performed, lies under cover of the lid; (3) the conjunctival flap rarely requires a stitch when made above; and (4) Rochon-Duvigneaud[1] has shown that the measurement from the angle of the anterior chamber to the limbus is greater in the vertical than in the horizontal meridian, and greater above than below the cornea. This is due to the varying distance that the conjunctiva overlaps the cornea, which it does to the greatest extent above. The consequent advancement of

[1] Valuable work on the same subject has also been done by Ducamp, Barraquer, and Sobhy.

the limbus in this direction gives the operator a proportionate increase in the amount of room available for the implantation of the trephine, without risk of doing damage to the ciliary body or to adherent iris. It is not, however, possible to trephine above the cornea in all cases, and it is inconvenient to do so in some others. When a patient is troublesome, and looks obstinately upwards, it may, though rarely, be a convenience to do the trephining below ; the efforts to defend the eye, by looking upward, then aid the operator instead of hindering him. This difficulty usually occurs in those who are already practically blind, and in them the presence of an iridectomy-coloboma within the palpebral aperture is of no consequence.

There are several other sets of conditions in which it would either be difficult or inadvisable to trephine above the cornea, viz., (1) when the operation is undertaken for the relief of staphyloma, and the upper part of the cornea is involved in the swelling ; (2) when, in chronic cases, it is obvious that the chamber is shallower in an upward direction than elsewhere ; (3) when a condition similar to the last named is due to anterior synechia, accompanied by a rise of tension; and (4) when, as pointed out by Lloyd, secondary glaucoma has followed a cataract extraction and there is reason to believe that there is a communication between the aqueous and vitreous chambers through the portal of the coloboma. In most cases of partial staphyloma one can find an area in which the chamber can safely be tapped, and the same applies to the other conditions mentioned above. The difference between the depth of different parts of the chamber in some cases of chronic glaucoma is very striking.

(2) **The nature of the flap, and the method of making it.**—Something has been written about the danger of wounding Tenon's capsule whilst raising the flap ; it hardly seems necessary to take this very seriously ; the suggested danger is not a real one to the man of ordinary knowledge and skill. The underlying suggestion has evidently been that it would be safer to reduce the size of our conjunctival flaps. This is a subject which has engaged

NEWER OPERATIONS FOR GLAUCOMA

much of our attention, and our decision has been to hold on to the large flap for the following reasons : (1) It is a great safeguard against infection of the eye ; (2) a negative point—our observations show us that we do not meet with

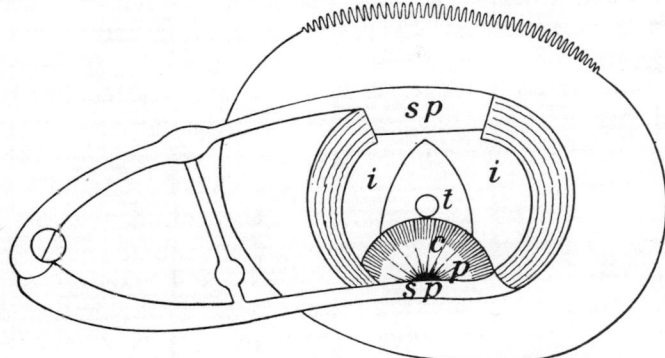

FIG. 169.—The incision, etc., in the early technique.

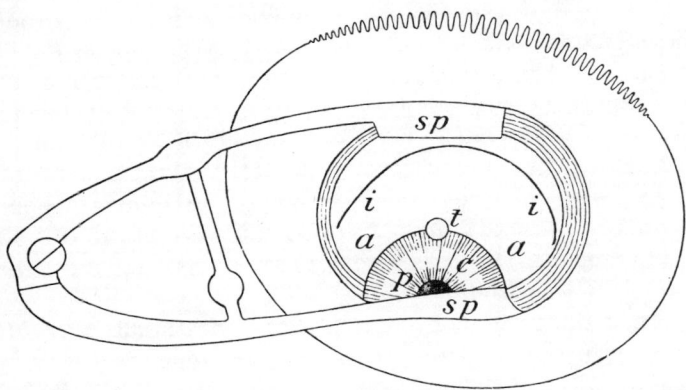

FIG. 170.—The incision, etc , in the present technique.

Sp, speculum ; *ii*, incision ; *c*, cornea ; *t.* trephine hole ; *p*, pupil ; *a a*, channels in conjunctiva along which filtration fluid passes to enter the main area of the subconjunctival space.

any astigmatism in consequence of it ; this has been proved by careful keratometer readings ; and (3) the really important matter—large flaps mean free and easy filtration. A careful study of a number of cases after operation shows that the actual line of the incision is sometimes tied down on to the sclera; if one makes a flap of little length, it tends to curl in on itself; moreover, if the two ends of the incision reach the cornea, and if the line of union then cicatrises, it is obvious that the total area left for filtration is very limited (Fig. 169). A more generous flap is more inclined to lie in place, and is for this reason less apt to cicatrise at its edge, as it unites with the conjunctiva from which it was cut, and not with the subjacent sclera. This helps to provide a larger area of subconjunctival tissue into which filtration can take place. A more important detail still remains to be mentioned. The incision we now employ does not begin and end in the limbus, but runs roughly concentric with it, and ends on either side opposite the highest point of the cornea and about 8 mm. to its inner and outer sides (Fig. 170). The importance of this detail is obvious, for even if the line of incision cicatrises down all round, filtering fluid from the interior of the eye can still find a free exit through the trephine hole into the subconjunctival space outside the incision limits through the areas marked $a\ a$ in Fig. 170. An important confirmation of the value of this form of flap was obtained in an early case, in which we were obliged to open up the wound some time after operation, in order to excise prolapsed iris. The line of incision was bound down to the sclera, but the moment we crossed this line in opening up the flap, free escape of filtering fluid took place into the wound.

In making the conjunctival flap, one should avoid the brow with the scissors; if this be not done, the eyebrows will be cut and dropped on to the wound, thus soiling it. In order to make the description of this important part of the operation clear we may divide the fashioning of the flap into the following stages:

(i.) THE INCISION.—The conjunctiva should be seized as high up as possible on the bulb with forceps, and drawn well down, at the same time asking the patient to look strongly downward; one free horizontal cut, followed by a couple of snips at each side, will often outline the flap throughout its extent; the shape and dimensions, etc., of the flap have already been given.

(ii.) THE DISSECTION OF THE FLAP.—*It is unnecessary, and therefore unsurgical, to dissect up the whole area included in the flap*; moreover, by so doing we rob the flap of the check-ligament-like action of the connective tissue at the angles of the wound (Fig. 171, *eda*). If we leave this tissue intact, the detached conjunctiva tends to spring back into

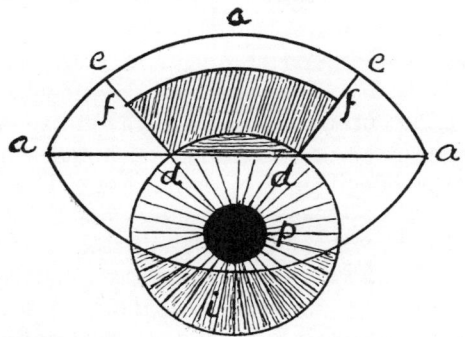

FIG. 171.—Diagrammatic representation of the area laid bare by the conjunctivo-corneal flap.

aaa, line of conjunctival incision; *aia*, flap thrown down on the cornea; above *dd*, dark arc-like area of split cornea; *dd*, straight line of reflection of the flap; *edde*, area dissected up in order to enable the cornea to be exposed; *effe*, area of the upper part of the wound from which the conjunctiva alone is dissected up, when commencing to make the flap; *fddf*, area immediately above the limbus cleared right down to the sclera, in the course of the dissection of the flap; *ade*, the area on each side in which the sub-conjunctival tissue is spared as much as possible in order to preserve the check-ligament-like action, which helps the flap to lie in good position after the operation is finished; *i*, iris; *p*, pupil.

place when released from the downward pull, whilst if we clear the margins of our wound, we find that at the end of the operation, the flap falls limp and inert over the cornea like a loose apron. We should for this reason carry our dissection down to the limbus over the central area only (Fig. 171, *edde*). Such a procedure does not in the least prevent us from exposing the area we require for trephining, whilst it helps very materially to make our flap lie in good position when the operation is finished, and so often enables us to dispense with the use of a suture. In the upper third of the dissection, we do not need to take up anything but the loose conjunctiva. *As we approach the limbus we should work down to the sclera, and should expose the latter bare in the last two-thirds of the wound* (Fig. 171, *fddf*). At the same time the breadth of the dissection should contract as we approach the cornea, so that when we reach the latter, we only expose just such a breadth of it as we mean to split, and very little more (Fig. 171, *dd*). Our *next landmark is the limbus, and we must clearly define this* as a rounded ridge slightly overhanging the adjacent sclera. A failure to do so involves a considerable risk of difficulty when we come to split the cornea in the next stage of the operation. If, however, there has been long-continued chronic congestion, it may be difficult to define this edge, as it then flattens out; in that case the earlier stage of splitting of the cornea must be very carefully conducted, or the flap may be button-holed. *The area over which we are about to apply the trephine must be carefully cleared of all tags of loose tissue*; if this precaution is neglected, the trephine will not bite well, and will tend to shift from its position; moreover, when it does begin to cut, these tags may get caught in the action, and tend to draw the flap into the wound and damage it. The author has seen this happen to beginners. There is a little knack in getting the sclera clear; this consists in closing the blades of a sharp-pointed scissors (those we have used so far in the operation), and making a number of scraping movements *from the centre of the wound out to each side*, close above the cornea; this manœuvre succeeds in clearing the central area of loose tissue, and so provides a clean surface on which to apply the trephine blade at a later stage of the operation.

(iii.) THE SPLITTING OF THE CORNEA—It must first be clearly stated that what we desire to do, is to *split the cornea* and not to cut it. The examination of microscopical preparations has shown that that membrane is really *split*, and that the flap we make includes not merely the anterior epithelium and Bowman's membrane, but also some of the superficial corneal lamellæ, which can be

NEWER OPERATIONS FOR GLAUCOMA 537

traced for a long distance in the sections and can be seen to be separated from the deeper layers. The significance of this observation lies in the fact that we are thus enabled to open up the planes of the lymphatic spaces, and to keep them bathed and unhealed in the fluid which is steadily being poured out from the anterior chamber. The observation has been made by those who cut, instead of splitting the cornea, that if they carry their trephine blade right on to the cornea, the hole tends to fill up. It is suggested that this is due to the cornea having its lamellæ cut clean across, instead of having its inter-lamellar spaces opened up by splitting ; for we have had a more fortunate experience after splitting the membrane in the way we are about to describe.

The conjunctival flap should be drawn gently downwards by traction with closed forceps laid on it, and finding counter-pressure against the cornea ; it must on no account be seized in the grip of forceps and pulled down therewith, or it may easily be torn and rendered useless for its purpose of covering the filtration hole. At the same time, the cornea is split with the scissor points, which are kept closed for the purpose ; or if preferred, a Bowman's needle or a special wedge-shaped splitter, as devised by McReynolds, or any other convenient instrument may be employed. The most important point is to *work at exactly the right place, i.e.,* just behind the line of reflection of the flap ; a number of short well-placed lateral strokes along this line speedily effect our purpose in most cases. If the cuts are made too far forwards, the flap is at once button-holed, whilst if they are made too far back, the surgeon merely wastes his time in an ineffective scratching of the sclera. The instrument is inclined at an acute angle to the cornea, bearing in mind that what we want to do is to dissect off its superficial layers in a thin flap. It is very necessary to have good eyesight and a good light, though granted these two requisites the technique is not difficult. The author's strong preference is to work by daylight, but if an artificial light is used, it is essential to have an additional small hand lamp which can easily throw in a beam sideways when required.

The reflexes obtained by artificial light off the parts are most confusing and annoying, whilst in daylight the work is easy and pleasant. As the dissection proceeds the so-called "dark crescent" of cornea can be seen clearly (Fig. 171) as a dark area convex in outline towards the sclera, and with a straight edge on the corneal side. The figure produced is that of a small segment of a circle, in which the reflection of the flap forms the chord (*dd*), whilst the edge of the stripped cornea corresponds to the arc; a good simile is that of a bow and its string. If in the course of the dissection one sees the line of reflection of the flap no longer curved at the corneal margin but crossing it in a straight line as the string crosses a bow, we may rest assured that the cornea has been split; this suggestion is not without value, for in some eyes the cornea shows up much less dark than it usually does, and an inexperienced operator, unaware of this fact, may fear he has not split the cornea, and may persist till he button-holes his flap. In the very great majority of cases we can split the cornea easily for 1 mm.; in not a few the splitting may be carried 1·5 to 2 mm. on to corneal tissue, but there is nothing to be gained in most cases by going farther in than 1 mm.; in a few cases, and especially in those with long-standing congestion, it is difficult to get a crescent wider than 0·5 to 0·75 mm. Although this latter amount can always be secured, it sometimes is done by tearing rather than by splitting. Such cases are fortunately rare; they occur in eyes which have been the subjects of long-standing congestion, and the prognosis for the maintenance of fistulisation is not so good as it is in the ordinary cases.

There are three other conditions under which one finds a difficulty in splitting the cornea, viz., (1) that in which the conjunctiva is found to be tied down to the sclera, as the result of the use at some previous date of irritating subconjunctival injections in the quadrant we are operating in; (2) that in which a previous operation has been performed in the same neighbourhood; and (3) that in which the subconjunctival tissue of the eye is found to be unusually dense and abundant. In connection with the first of these, our experience has been that any and all of the subconjunctival injections cause the formation of adhesions, but that normal, saline injections do so far less than those of sodium citrate or of the mercurial preparations ; in the case of either of the latter, the adhesions are usually so dense as to make the approach to the limbus difficult, and the splitting of the cornea almost impossible. The obvious lesson is to avoid the injection of any fluids into the area which we may later on need to use for operative purposes. There is an important, clinical point in connection with the second condition above-mentioned, viz., that we must choose the site of our trephining with great care, when a previous operation has been performed on the eye for high tension, or we may find it impossible to reach the limbus at all ; indeed it is sometimes necessary to try in two or three directions before we find a spot at which we can dissect the flap up, as far as is necessary for the successful performance of the operation. As to the third condition above discussed, we have found that there is a very great variation in the amount of subconjunctival tissue in the eyes of patients even of the same age, and that the scantier this tissue layer is, the easier is it to split the cornea and *vice versa*. The author always welcomes the slight increase of difficulty in splitting the cornea in cases where the subconjunctival tissue is tough and abundant ; for this condition carries with it the very material compensation that the resulting flap is thick and therefore little inclined to become vesicular, whereas the thin, brittle conjunctivæ are much more prone to be associated later with this objectionable form of bulging scar.

An important question and one often asked is, How is the operator to tell when he has dissected far enough forward, and when there is a danger of button-holing his flap ? We must bear in mind that the object of splitting the cornea is to enable us to place the trephine as far forwards as we *safely* can. Now an experience of a large number of cases has shown us two things, viz., (1) that on the average, one can safely split the cornea a little over 1 mm., and (2) that such an area of splitting puts us practically in a secure position so far as the danger of trouble from the iris or ciliary body is concerned. To this we may add that it is possibly not desirable to have the whole of our trephine aperture sited on the cornea. Apart from all these considerations, if the surgeon sees that his flap is getting too thin at the edge, he will do well to be content with the amount of splitting he has accomplished, and not to risk button-holing. So much has been written about the latter accident in connection with the splitting of the cornea that it is necessary to point out that the danger of its occurrence is certainly not great at this stage of the operation. It is more likely to occur when the trephine is actually being used, and still more so when the iridectomy is being performed.

In connection with the manœuvre of splitting the cornea, there is a small point of some interest; it will be observed especially in those cases which split easily, that one part of the line we are working on gives more readily than the rest, producing the appearance of a bite out of the straight edge of the flap reflection, or that of a small shallow bay in it. The importance of the observation is that it is much easier to continue the splitting at one of these bays than elsewhere along the line. In conclusion, it is important to lay emphasis on the fact that the split area has a smooth appearance, indicating that we have dissected up along a plane of cleavage. This is what we have always believed we have been doing, and anatomical work has shown this belief to have been justified.

This manœuvre of splitting the cornea has been very minutely described at the special request of a number of surgeons, and it is hoped that it has now been made quite clear. At the same time, one desires to avoid giving any support to the views of those who maintain that splitting of the cornea is a very difficult procedure; it is true that it calls for care and skill, but that is all that need be said of it. To prove this point, we may quote some figures from our statistics in Madras. In 201 consecutive trephinings (between November 1911 and March 1912) the writer damaged his flap on four occasions only (*i.e.*, in 1·99 per cent.), and in not one of these cases was there any evidence that the tiny button-hole made had any influence on the satisfactory course of the case. During the same period ten other surgeons, learning trephining in Madras, button-holed seven times in 124 consecutive operations (*i.e.*, in 5·6 per cent.), and on only one such occasion was it found necessary to shift the area for the application of the trephine.

When we started to practise " splitting of the cornea," the objection that first occurred to us was that the close attachment of the corneal conjunctiva to the deeper layers would cause these parts early to become firmly reunited, and that consequently the corneal area of the wound would be lost for filtration purposes. The experience not only of the author, but also of a number of other surgeons, who have kindly communicated with him on the subject, has clearly shown that such a fear is wholly unfounded. Indeed, the part of the wound overlapping the cornea has proved to provide a free and ready area of filtration with no tendency such as we had feared.

(3) **The Application of the Trephine.**—With increasing experience one thing has become absolutely clear, viz., that if we wish to trephine the chamber, and to establish a permanent filtering channel with a minimum of trouble, we have to be careful to place our trephine hole as far forward as possible.

A failure to observe this rule (1) makes a clean entry into the chamber uncertain ; (2) complicates the free tapping of the aqueous fluid ; (3) leads later on in some cases to an interference with filtration, due to uveal tissue blocking the trephine hole ; and (4) exposes the eye to the danger of vitreous escape. If the trephine hole is far forward, the only part of the uveal coat with which we have to do is the iris, and this can easily be dealt with, as we shall show later on. If the iris base is adherent to the cornea, the advantage gained by placing the trephine hole as far forward as possible becomes still more obvious ; hence the urgency of the need for dissecting the conjunctivo-corneal flap forward in the way already described. In applying the trephine we must not throw away any of the advantage so gained; the flap should be pulled gently towards the centre of the cornea by traction exerted with the points of the closed forceps, and the trephine placed on the prepared corneo-scleral surface so that its edge will *just clear* the flap, thus making use of every fraction of a millimetre of the area which has been gained by the splitting; the dark crescent of corneal tissue bordering the base of the flap can very easily be seen and defined.

The trephine should not be dumped down on the spot on which it is to work, but should be slid into place from the scleral side, the edge of the flap being keenly watched the while; this manœuvre greatly minimises the risk of button-holing the reflected edge.

The beginner may find some difficulty in keeping his cutting edge to one spot at the commencement of the trephining. As a rule, this manœuvre becomes quite easy with a very little practice, especially if a sharp instrument be used. The surgeon may obtain considerable assistance by seizing the trephine blade low down, close to the eye, in the grasp of a pair of conjunctival forceps, and thus fixing the cutting edge of the instrument. With a little practice, however, he will learn to trephine freely and evenly without feeling the need of employing any device to steady his blade.

Some of the surgeons who worked in Madras preferred to discard any trephine-steadier, and instead to fix the eye by gripping it with forceps at one angle of the incision, asking an assistant to draw the flap downwards over the cornea by means of any convenient blunt instrument. There can be no doubt that this modification of technique is greatly appreciated by those who make a practice of using it.

The *exact amount of pressure necessary* can only be learnt by experience; some beginners appear afraid of using enough force and needlessly lacerate their wound by niggling efforts on different spots, the trephine slipping from one place to another each time they reapply it;

others, but they are very few in number, go through with an over-bold confidence and find themselves in the vitreous chamber before they know what they are doing. In order to avoid both these errors, it is necessary (1) to work in a good light *with a very sharp trephine*; (2) to keep the area of operation clear of blood, so that the operator can see exactly what he is doing; (3) to make sure of cutting a definite groove on the first application before raising the trephine to see what has been done; and (4) if necessary, to steady the trephine blade and keep it to one spot by seizing it gently quite close to its cutting edge in the grasp of a pair of conjunctival forceps. Once a definite groove has been started, the blade finds its way into it again with astonishing ease; from this stage onwards the operator, till he has acquired the necessary experience, must raise his blade frequently to see how deep he has cut; with practice this will become unnecessary, and he will then be able to tell when he is through by the sucking feeling which accompanies the completion of the trephining; at the same time aqueous may often be noticed to escape around the instrument or through its lumen, and frequently the patient by a slight movement or by an exclamation shows his consciousness of a little pain; this latter is not severe, and he never starts violently because of it; a movement or an exclamation is all that escapes him. There is a fourth sign to which attention has been drawn by Axenfeld, Hill Griffith, Wallis, and others, viz., the upward movement of the iris at the moment the trephine cuts through, which results in the production of a pear-shaped pupil; this is evidently due to the outrush of aqueous from the chamber, carrying the iris along in the direction of its current. For the detection of this sign it is necessary to hold the flap at right angles to the eye whilst the trephine is cutting its way through. The correct use of the trephine by light, steady cutting strokes requires learning, and can be easily practised on the eyes of animals. The author, when using the earlier form of light handle, worked with the index finger and thumb, and constantly moved his fingers up the instrument as they tended to slide down ; it is this downward slide of the fingers which gives operators most trouble at first, and some require to use a second hand each time they move their fingers back into position again. The adoption of the heavier handle which we now use has greatly simplified this part of the technique. No pressure need be used, as the instrument works by its own weight, and consequently the tendency of the fingers to slip down is practically abolished. All the instrument makers who manufacture the author's trephine have been requested to supply in future the heavier weight of handle, viz., one of 2·5 drachms (9·7 grammes).

The direction in which the blade of the trephine is to be held relative to the corneo-scleral surface is a matter of great importance. It is to be remembered that, in the neighbourhood of the limbus, the cornea is thicker than the sclera. If therefore we hold our blade perpendicular to the surface (*i.e.*, radial to it), we penetrate the coat first on its scleral edge. Now for a double reason this is exactly what we wish to avoid doing, for (1) our one great aim throughout this technique is to place the fistula we are endeavouring to establish as far forwards on the eye as we can ; that is to say, as far as possible from the ciliary body or from adherent iris ; this can obviously be best attained by cutting steep into the anterior chamber on the corneal edge of the wound ; and (2) when we come to speak of the division of the hinge left at the close of the trephining, it will be obvious that so far as the reflected edge of the conjunctivo-corneal flap is concerned, this will be more safely and easily avoided, when we are cutting through the hinge, if the latter lies the breadth of the opening away from the flap, than if the two are contiguous. In the latter case the danger of buttonholing is obviously much increased. Our object should therefore be to make the blade cut through first on its corneal edge, and in order to ensure this, we must slope the upper end of the instrument a little towards the patient's feet. The result will be that as soon as the trephine has cut its way through, the disc, hinged on its scleral side, will be pushed upwards and outwards by a bead of iris tissue, prolapsing through the corneal side of the opening. If the manœuvre is correctly carried out, this prolapse occurs with great regularity. It is, however, dependent on two factors, (1) the presence of a moderately contracted pupil before the operation is commenced, and (2) the use of a sharp trephine. It is important that the pupil be at least *not dilated*, for one finds that when dealing with dilated pupils, it may happen that the iris may bulge through so far that its free edge presents in the hole and allows a free escape of the aqueous fluid, in which latter case the membrane will very likely fall back again into the chamber, making a subsequent iridectomy both more difficult and more hazardous.

The next question of importance is *the size of trephine to use*. We have tried all sizes from 3·5 mm. down to 1 mm., and our personal preference is in favour of a 2 mm. instrument. An opening of this size is practically always large enough, whilst a smaller one has the grave disadvantage—that it does not give room for the use of iris forceps and scissors, should the iris happen to be accidentally dragged into the wound and impacted there.

In our earlier experience with the trephine we found ourselves constantly confronted with the difficulty of deciding whether the whole disc marked out by the instrument should be removed or not; we realised that we were between the dangers of removing too much and too little. If in an early case of glaucoma we take the whole 2 mm. disc away, we may find that the tension remains very low for a long time, possibly indefinitely; on the other hand, if we do not take the whole disc away in chronic congestive cases, the hole is likely to fill up, and filtration may thus cease. With a very little experience of the 2 mm. trephine it will be found possible, provided the instrument is sharp, to detach the disc the whole way round, or to leave it uncut at one small hinge only; in the latter case a single snip of the scissor points does the rest. If we wish, we can cut off any desired portion of the disc, thus removing a third, a half, or more of it at will. The same end may be more neatly and methodically attained by deliberately pressing yet a little more on the corneal edge of our trephine, and so entering the chamber round a half or more of the circumference on that side, thus leaving a comparatively large hinge uncut; in completing the detachment of the disc, we formerly cut across the hinge obliquely with the deliberate intention of leaving the deeper layers of this part *in situ*. Further reflection has shown us that this last procedure is not above criticism, since it must obviously leave the tunic of the eye unnecessarily weakened at that spot. We now determine how much of the disc we intend to remove, and cut it off *at right angles* to the surface, thus leaving the posterior edge of the fistula as steep as its anterior edge, which has been cut with the trephine. There is no difficulty in carrying out this manœuvre; all that it is

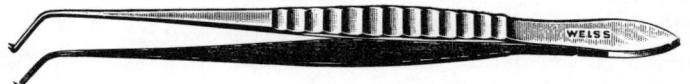

Fig. 172.—Special forceps for helping to remove the deeper layers of the disc, if left behind.

necessary to do is to draw the hinge well away from the eye, and to cut with the plane of the scissor blades at a tangent to the eye, and as close to it as possible. On the contrary, if we do not pull the disc well out, and if we cut with the scissors directed obliquely to the eyeball, we shall evidently cut the hinge obliquely, the very contingency we desire to avoid. It may be urged that we are sacrificing a part of the area of our wound in the sclera, and had much better have diminished the size of our trephine to begin with. The question is, however, not quite so simple as it looks, for we can never in any case say beforehand that the iris will not give trouble by becoming impacted in the wound during or after the performance of the iridectomy; and although this accident is not a frequent one, it must be thoroughly dealt with if met; it is quite an easy matter to resect the deeper layer left, by using a pair of small disc forceps (Fig. 172) and the scissor points, and we are then in the position of being able to deal easily with the offending iris. Similarly, if during the trephining—and with a blunt instrument this may easily happen—we accidentally leave a part of the deeper layers when we meant to remove them, the manœuvre above described enables us to do so quickly and easily. If the trephine blade is sharp, and the operator finds that though he has tapped the aqueous, possibly only at one point, the main circumference of the incision still remains uncut, he may reinsert the trephine, and working with light, quick movements may complete the removal of the disc, even though the chamber may have been practically emptied beforehand. The patient may complain of some pain whilst this is being done, but it will not be severe. In any case the application of cocaine drops (4 per cent.) to the wound right over the trephine hole will soon make the part absolutely anæsthetic.

There is undoubtedly another side to this question, which we may put thus : (1) Since we have made splitting of the cornea a regular feature of our technique, the trouble we formerly had with iris in the wound has practically disappeared ; there can be no doubt that the method of seizing the disc and iris together during the iridectomy has contributed materially towards this happy state of things ; (2) our anatomical measurements of the space available for trephining, without interference with adherent iris or with the ciliary body, have shown that this is limited, and that in case the iris is adherent the limitation becomes still more marked ; (3) a reduction of the diameter of the trephine blade to 1·5, or even to 1 mm., did not prevent our getting excellent and permanent filtration in a number of our early cases ; and (4) we must not lose sight of the fact that for any definite length of wound, a circular incision gives the maximum of surface area, and therefore the minimum possible of weakening of the ocular tunic. It may then be argued that we shall do well to reduce our trephine blades if we possibly can, and in rare cases we have occasionally made a practice of doing so, but rightly or wrongly our leaning is still strongly towards the use of the 2 mm. blade.

(4) **The Iridectomy : its nature and the method of performing it.**—An iridectomy should be made, as a routine step, in every trephining operation, *simply to avoid the risk of iridic tissue becoming impacted in the trephine aperture during convalescence.* The rôle of an iridectomy in this operation is the same as it is in the combined extraction of a cataract ; no more and no less. It provides a sluice-gate through which rushes of escaping fluid can take place, without carrying the iris in front of them on their way out. This view of the case has been combated by certain ophthalmologists, but it is borne out by the fact that our experience and that of many other surgeons has shown that cases in which no iridectomy has been performed, have provided just as efficient filtration as those with iridectomy, provided always that the hole remained iris-free. It also has the sanction of Lagrange's consent. It is obvious that all that it is absolutely necessary to do is to remove a small peripheral portion of the membrane right opposite the trephine hole.

It is a common experience that the trephine disc, when cut by hand, nearly always remains attached at one point to the scleral coat by a narrow hinge. With a little practice it is possible, as indicated in the last section, to enter the trephine in such a manner that the hinge is regularly left on the scleral side of our wound. When this is done with a sharp blade, which cuts its way through, round a large area at once, we find that the iris bulges into the hole as soon as we withdraw the instrument. If this prolapse is watched, it will be observed that the most peripheral part of the iris is the first to pass into the hole ; this is exactly what we should expect from its anatomical position. If the patient squeezes, more and more of the membrane bulges, till at last the free edge of the iris protrudes, the aqueous escapes, and the membrane, now relieved from the *vis a tergo*, drops back into the chamber again. This sequence of events depends to a great extent on two factors, viz., (1) the peripheral position of the wound, and (2) the state of contraction of the pupil. For the prolapsing iris to fill the trephine hole in this way it is a necessary condition that it should be free and untethered ; it must also be in a state of moderate contraction, or the pupillary edge will early present in the wound, the fluid will escape, and the prolapse disappear. The appearance of the little white disc, pushed upwards by the small black bead of iris, is unmistakable, and it is an easy matter to include both disc and iris in one grip of the forceps, and to divide both together with a single snip of the scissor points, thus performing our iridectomy with the same cut that severs the hinge. The great advantage of this is that our grip of the disc steadies the eye, and effectually prevents even a troublesome patient from rotating it until after the portion of iris has been removed. We are thus enabled to avoid all risk of the uveal tissue being dragged into and becoming impacted in the trephine hole.

One finds that one has sometimes made a complete, and at other times a peripheral iridectomy. The former is attended at a later date by certain disadvantages, viz., (1) it tends to cause blurring of images, (2) it may expose the patient to some " dazzling," and (3) it deprives the surgeon of the power of producing strong meiosis, should he subsequently need to do so. When the pupil has been small before operation, and the prolapse of iris is not large, the resulting coloboma will be peripheral, no matter how we make the iridectomy, unless we drag on the iris, which we should of course never do. Unfortunately, the pupil tends to dilate under the influence of the cocaine and adrenalin used for anæsthesia, especially if a subconjunctival injection of the drugs is made. This tendency can and should be combated by the instillation of pilocarpine, started one hour before the operation and repeated if necessary. When the prolapse is free and large, it is necessary to avoid seizing the whole of it in the forceps grip if we would dispense with a complete iridectomy ; it is not difficult to lay hold of just so much of it as lies near the disc, *i.e.*, the peripheral portion only, and we shall thus attain the end we desire. If, however, the whole breadth of the iris has passed through the trephine hole, it is scarcely possible to avoid making a complete iridectomy, especially as we are then pressed for time, and must catch hold of the iris as best we can, before it slips back into the chamber.

We have spoken of the disadvantages of complete iridectomy in trephining, and we must now present its advantages. In cases into which any element of congestion enters, there can be no doubt that to remove a complete strip of iris, favours the free dilatation of the pupil, even if atropin is not instilled at the time of operation; but, what is still more important, it takes away the only obstacle to the free exhibition of this powerful mydriatic within the first few hours after trephining. No one, who has had an experience of the quiet iritis which so often follows operation for glaucoma *by any and every method*, can doubt the great value of the power thus put into our hands by the performance of a complete iridectomy in congestive cases. So far as the simple non-congestive glaucomas are concerned, a peripheral iridectomy is all that is needed, and the advantages of leaving the sphincter intact have already been enumerated.

What are we to do if the iris re-enters the chamber before we can perform an iridectomy, or if it never prolapses from the start? The latter contingency arises (1) if a blunt trephine is used, which either effects an entry into the chamber at one spot only, or at least over too short a circumference to allow of the disc being raised up by the bulging iris; the fluid then drains gently off, the chamber empties, and the pressure behind the iris falls, so that the tendency to prolapse passes away; (2) if the iris is tied down by synechiæ to such an extent as to make prolapse impossible; and (3) if the pupil is widely dilated and rigid before the operation. In order to answer our question, we must consider the pros and cons of the case. In favour of performing an iridectomy, we have to remember that it saves the danger of a prolapse during convalescence, and the necessity, which then arises, of a second operation, always so unwelcome, especially in private work. Against the iridectomy are the following arguments: (1) In endeavouring to seize the iris we may damage the lens, the suspensory ligament, or even the vitreous ; (2) in the event of a sudden movement on the part of the patient, we may get iris tissue impacted in the wound ; (3) experience shows that, provided a prolapse does not occur, we get quite as good a result without iridectomy as with it, indeed we may even get a better ; and (4) the use of a meiotic makes the risk of a secondary prolapse comparatively small ; as has already been pointed out, however, it is greatly preferable to use a mydriatic and not a meiotic, at the close of the operation, whenever possible, or, at the latest, within 24 hours. After very carefully weighing the risks on both sides, it is the author's opinion that if iris fails to present (and in a properly carried out operation, this, in his experience, is seldom the case), it is often better to leave well alone, and to deal with any prolapse at a later stage if necessary. There are, however, cases in which a suitable piece of iris can be easily excised after the removal of the disc by introducing iris or disc forceps into the trephine hole. The author has on a number of occasions elected to take the small risk involved and to do this, and has had no reason to regret it. The question resolves itself into one of deciding which is the lesser of two evils. In this connection it is always to be borne in mind that the narrowness of the trephine aperture markedly increases the danger of impaction and renders replacement of the membrane correspondingly more difficult, thus adding a possible and serious complication to the case and rendering the after treatment more hazardous. The method of performing an iridectomy is consequently of more importance in trephining than in most other operations. It is essential to *put no traction on the iris,* and to carry the scissor points right down into the wound whilst excising the portion of the membrane. When the iris is tied down by synechiæ it is as unnecessary as it is inadvisable to interfere with it ; for the adhesions will prevent it from prolapsing both at the time of the operation and subsequently.

(5) **The Toilette of the Wound.**—It is most important that

the iris should be thoroughly replaced, and that no uveal tags should be left in the wound. If there is any doubt on this head we use the irrigator already described, and placing the nozzle at the entrance of the trephine hole, we direct a bold stream of saline solution into the chamber ; this easily and quickly washes the iris back into place, always provided that it has not been dragged into the wound, and impacted there at an earlier stage of the procedure. At the same time the chamber is washed free of any blood which may have been effused, thus giving us a clear view of details. The presence of a round central pupil affords proof that the iris has been thoroughly replaced. Sometimes when there is a little difficulty, we may attain our object by gentle massage with a spoon over the neighbourhood of the wound succeeded by another irrigation. If we are still unsuccessful, it is probably due to one of two very different conditions, viz., (1) impaction of iris in the wound, as already mentioned, or (2) a return of intra-ocular tension, as the result of the free effusion of fluid into the posterior segment of the eye. The differential diagnosis is easy, for in the former case the eye can still be felt to be soft under the pressure of a spoon applied carefully over the cornea, whilst in the latter the almost stony hardness of the globe is very easily detected. To deal with the former case first : It is quite safe, and, in skilful hands, often not difficult to introduce a spud, with its tip bent forwards, into the trephine hole, and to clear the latter of iris. The use of the irrigator will complete the replacement still more satisfactorily, once the imprisoned iris has been loosened from its attachment to the sides of the tunnel in the sclerocornea. On the other hand, when we are dealing with a hard eye, such manipulation as we have been describing should only be used with the greatest caution. If this rule be disobeyed, there will be considerable danger of damage being done to the deeper parts, for these are packed tight against the hole by the pressure of the fluid behind. The pathology of this condition is discussed at length in another chapter, but the clinical aspect of it may profitably find a place here. It is best understood by reference to a pheno-

NEWER OPERATIONS FOR GLAUCOMA 553

menon which may readily be observed by any surgeon who operates on late cases of glaucoma. Up to a certain stage all goes well. The trephine enters the chamber, the aqueous escapes freely, and the iris and lens move forward in the usual way ; at this stage a spoon placed on the cornea shows that the eye is still soft, and yet in a very short space of time the globe may be found to harden. We have felt this happen whilst the instrument was actually upon the

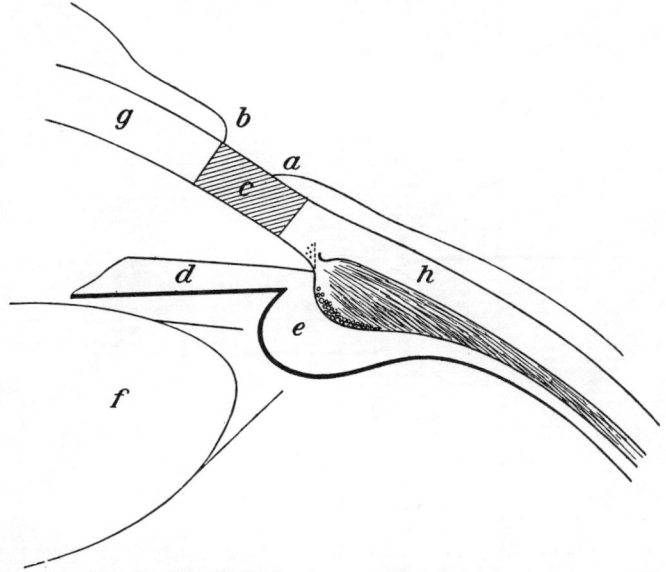

FIG. 173.—Shows diagrammatically the relation of parts in a case of trephining in which the iris base has not adhered to the cornea.

eye, the tension passing from a condition in which the globe could be easily dimpled into hardness within a minute. At the same time, the outflow channel for the escape of aqueous has become blocked ; fluid may actually be imprisoned in the anterior chamber, and yet it cannot find its way out, although a spud bent as above indicated can be seen to pass right into the chamber in front of the iris, and in doing so to give vent to part of the imprisoned aqueous. The lesson is perfectly simple ; a rapid effusion of fluid has taken place into the posterior chamber of the eye, either into the vitreous or between the coats of the globe. This has pushed forward the diaphragm of the eye (iris, lens, and ciliary body) and by pressure of one or more of these deep structures has blocked the trephine hole. If the patient is got back into bed at once, the eye will, after a variable period, and often even after 24 hours, be found to be subnormal in tension and to be filtering freely. The author holds most strongly that it is not in the interest of the

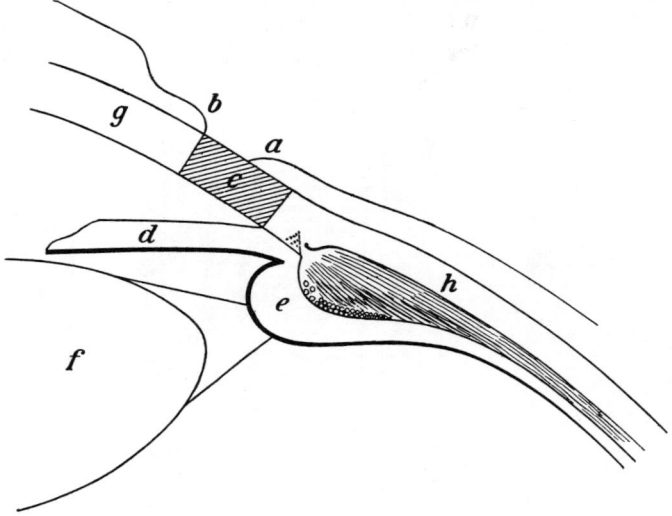

Fig. 174.—Shows diagrammatically the iris base adherent to cornea; the trephine hole lies just in front of the anterior attachment of the iris. The danger of iris prolapse is obvious.

patient to indulge in any manipulation once this hardening condition has manifested itself. He considers that the *patient should be got back to bed with the least possible delay.* It is true that he has at times been able to get a better replacement of the iris by a cautious use of the spud, but he doubts whether even this is justified. To wait and to use meiotics is, he thinks, sounder practice.

There remain to be considered two conditions which were not very uncommon in our earlier experience, but which we have not met with since we took to splitting the

NEWER OPERATIONS FOR GLAUCOMA

cornea, and thus placing our trephine hole farther forwards. In visiting a large number of hospitals in different parts of the world, the author has clearly seen that still, from time to time, surgeons, either through a want of appreciation of the importance of trephining far forwards, or through an inability to carry out the necessary technique on all occasions, make the mistake of placing the trephine hole too far back, either at or even behind the limbus. It seems therefore advisable to deal with the two possible complica-

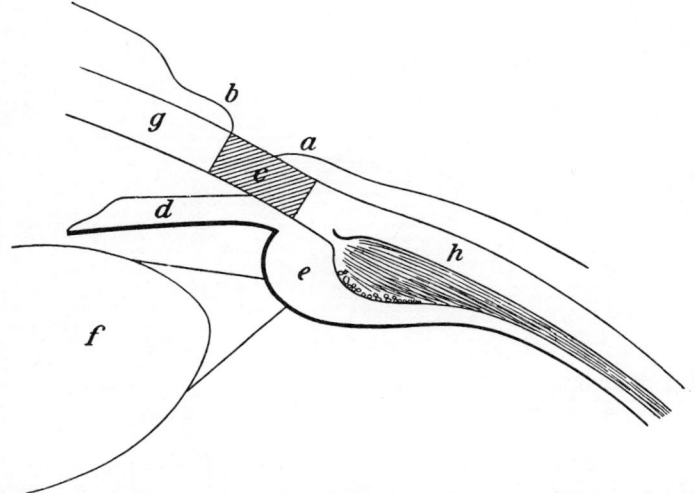

FIG. 175.—Shows diagrammatically the trephine hole entering the chamber at the anterior part of its circumference, the posterior part being blocked by adherent iris.

tions above referred to, which may result from this mistake. They are (1) the effecting of an oblique or valve-like entry into the anterior chamber (Fig. 175), owing to the iris base being adherent to the cornea over a large area of the space covered by the trephine, and (2) the direct entry of the trephine into the posterior division of the aqueous chamber by reason of its cutting through the cornea and the adherent iris as one disc (Fig. 176). We are here dealing with cases, in which the adhesions between the corneal and iridic surfaces have progressed so far forwards, as to place a line of adherent tissue in front of the spot where the trephine has entered the chamber ; we have tapped the posterior and not the anterior division of the aqueous chamber. It is scarcely necessary to insist that the best way of dealing with these difficulties is to avoid them, as may be almost invariably done if the technique advocated in this chapter is carried out. In the last 325 consecutive cases operated on

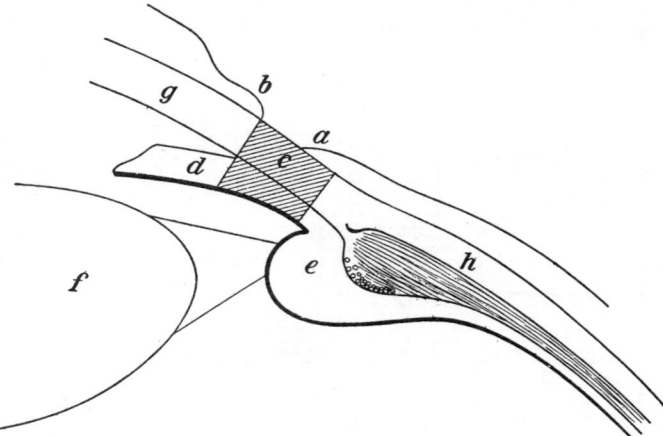

Fig. 176.—Shows diagrammatically the trephine hole passing through the cornea and the subjacent layer of adherent iris, in a case in which the iris is adherent to the cornea far forwards.

The diagrams have been modelled on a drawing of Thomson Henderson's.

Figs. 173 to 176 show diagrammatically the interference of iris with the trephine hole. *a*, Normal position of conjunctiva ; *b*, conjunctiva reflected after dissection off the underlying cornea ; *ab*, represents a section of the crescent seen on stripping the conjunctiva from the cornea; *c*, shaded, represents the piece removed by the trephine ; *d*, iris ; *e*, ciliary body ; *f*, lens ; *g*, cornea ; *h*, sclera.

in the latter part of the author's time in Madras, he found that it was always possible to effect a clean entry into the chamber, and to tap it directly thereby. In the 135 cases operated on in America, and in all those done in England, the same experience has held with very few exceptions. We shall not, therefore, discuss the treatment of a complication which should hardly ever be allowed to occur. Prevention, and not cure, is called for.

NEWER OPERATIONS FOR GLAUCOMA 557

Having satisfied ourselves that the iris is well returned, we next replace the conjunctival flap in good position, by first laying it back over the raw surface from which it was dissected up, and then stroking it well into place with the aid of a spoon or of some similar, rounded and blunt instrument. Two silk sutures [1] will serve to keep the flap in place, and save the surgeon from any anxiety lest it should be rucked up by movements of the lids. In India, we rarely sewed up the wound; in Western practice, we find it expedient to do so, as a routine measure. It is sometimes a little difficult to get hold of the upper lip of the conjunctival incision; the way we have found best is to get the assistant to raise the speculum off the eye, whilst at the same time exposing the upper fornix as far as possible in so doing; a pair of fine conjunctival forceps, passed up under the lid, then secures the edge of the wound without much trouble. An alternative procedure is to pass the two sutures through the upper lip of the incision when it is first made; it is then quite easy to do this. The ends of the sutures are kept out of the way on the sterile head towel during the operation, and to secure their asepticity, they are painted over with tincture of iodine just before they are used for the lower lip of the wound.

Theoretically, there are objections to the use of sutures in a wound, which is kept for a long period in free communication with the interior of the eye by means of the aqueous, since that fluid bathes the whole flap wound right up to its very margin. Practically the risks have proved to be negligible, and the advantage of fixing the flap decidedly outweighs the theoretical disadvantage.

Finally, the upper lid is lifted off the eyeball and brought down to meet the lower one, the patient being at the same time told to look up and to close his eyes. Immediately before doing this, however, we gently stroke the cornea toward the trephine hole with a curette, in order to ascer-

---

[1] When a needle is being used, the assistant has ready a swab soaked in tincture of iodine; this is held about an inch from the eye, and the whole length of the suture is allowed to run over it, before it enters the wound, thus securing its sterility, up to the very latest moment.

tain whether the eyeball is still soft, and whether the escape of aqueous from the chamber is free.

Both eyes are then closed with aseptic pads and a bandage.

(6) **Instillation of Drops.**—The adoption of iridectomy as a routine procedure has considerably modified our practice with regard to the use of mydriatics. If the case is one of simple non-congestive glaucoma, and if only a peripheral iridectomy has been performed, we sometimes delay the instillation of atropin drops (gr. iv ad ʒi) until a few hours have passed, or until the dressing on the morning following operation. If the iridectomy has been complete, and especially if the case is a congestive one, we instil the mydriatic drops before the patient leaves the table. The instillation should be repeated daily until all fear of quiet iritis is past. We have practically abandoned the use of meiotics after trephining. We have formulated these rules because we find in congestive cases a strong tendency to the formation of posterior synechiæ. Moreover, even in non-congestive cases, we have to be constantly on our guard against this quiet iritis which gives so little evidence of its existence and yet is so dangerous to the preservation of sight.

In conclusion it may be permissible to repeat that the operation which the writer has practised, and which he has endeavoured to introduce to the notice of the profession, is that of *simple* sclero-corneal trephining. The motive is to reach, tap, and drain subconjunctivally the anterior chamber, with a minimum of injury to the structures of the eyeball. To this end the junction of the cornea and sclera is trephined as far forwards as possible, the ciliary body is avoided, the chamber is entered directly by the trephine, and the iris is only dealt with in order to obviate any tendency it might otherwise have to block the trephine hole, and so to interfere with filtration. The cardinal rules are few and short, viz.,—(1) dissect the conjunctivo-corneal flap forwards, a full millimetre if possible, splitting the cornea for the purpose; (2) utilise every fraction of a millimetre of the space so gained and apply the trephine as far forwards as possible, consistent with the avoidance of injury to the flap; and (3) use a sharp trephine.

REFERENCES

BARRAQUER.—*La Clin. Opht.*, March 1913.
DUCAMP.—" La Trépanation Cornéo-Sclérale d'Elliot, Etude Technique," *Recherches Anatomiques et Experimentales*, Vigot Frères, Paris.
ROCHON-DUVIGNEAUD.—*The Topography of the Angle of the Anterior Chamber*, Paris, 1890.
SOBHY.—Communication read to the Ophth. Soc. of Egypt, Bulletin of 1921, p. 40.

PART IX

Modifications in the Operative Technique of Sclero-Corneal Trephining, suggested by Various Surgeons

The object of the present chapter is to review the various modifications that have been introduced into the technique of the operation of trephining by various surgeons.

Modified Corneal Trephines, and the methods of using them.—The original Bowman's trephine (Fig. 177) was an extremely crude instrument. It was difficult to obtain a grip of, and it was consequently very unsatisfactory to use. The result has been that a number of new models of trephines have been placed before the profession during the last few years. The illustrations (Figs. 178 to 184) show some of the most popular of these. They demonstrate alike the ingenuity of the surgical mind and the difference in view-point of different operators. Thus, while one man will prefer a bulky handle in order that he may get a good grip and work with firm steady strokes, another sees a great advantage in the thinnest possible grip with a view of obtaining the maximum amount of trephine rotation for a definite movement of the fingers. Again, some surgeons are in favour of the use of a stop on the trephine, whilst others are strongly opposed to it;

and so on with other points. Each surgeon must make his choice. The writer has had a number of successive models made for him. He prefers the conical form of handle with sufficient bulk to provide an easy grip; he

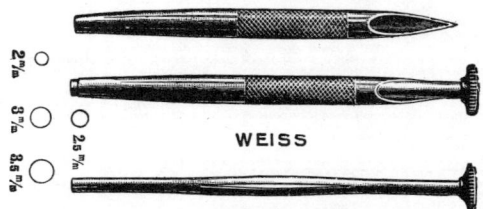

Fig. 177.—Bowman's trephine with roughened handle.

thinks the instrument should be of sufficient weight to cut its own way through with a minimum of manual pressure (9·7 grammes is the weight he has chosen); he prefers a 2 mm. blade in almost every case, but thinks the

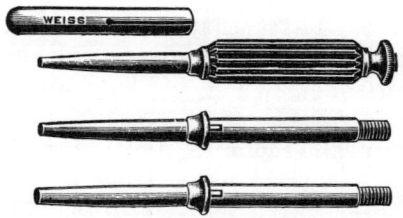

Fig. 178.—Sydney Stephenson's trephine.

handle should be so made as to carry a blade of any desired size at will; lastly, there is possibly some advantage in having the tubular blade long enough to pass right through the length of the instrument, so that the escape of fluid

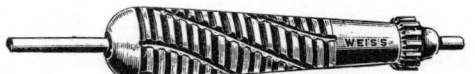

Fig. 179.—Author's trephine.

at its upper end may be clearly seen, and thus may give early notice that the anterior chamber has been entered. Messrs. Weiss have succeeded in making an instrument which complies with all these requirements (Fig. 179).

NEWER OPERATIONS FOR GLAUCOMA

Gray Clegg has suggested the cutting of a slot at the lower end of the blade, a few millimetres above its cutting edge,

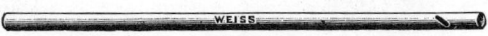

Fig. 180.—Gray Clegg's slotted trephine blade.

in order that the escaping fluid may pass through this, and be easily seen. The author has since used slotted blades on all occasions, but has been struck by the rarity with

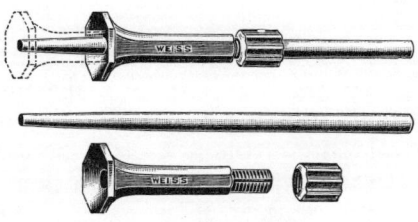

Fig. 181.—Lang's trephine.

The solid part of the upper figure is the instrument ready for use. The blade can be pushed out to suit the operator. The skeleton outline represents the blade drawn into the handle for protection during boiling. The middle figure is the steel tube, and the two lower figures are the handle and its nut, which clamps the blade and holds it firm.

which the exit of the fluid can be observed; this is quite contrary to what might have been expected. Fig. 180 shows such a blade of its actual size.

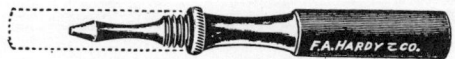

Fig. 182.—Pusey's sclero-corneal trephine.

A number of surgeons have had trephines made for them with a variety of devices to keep the blade to one

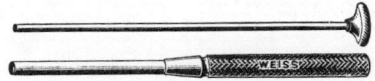

Fig. 183.—Harrison Butler's trephine.

point during the actual cutting of the hole. Some have had a central pin provided, similar to that on the cranial trephines ; others have introduced a hook, or a small corkscrew (Fig. 184), which passes down the blade, and not only seizes the sclera, but also draws it up as the blade sinks into the tissue, thus affording counter-pressure ; others again have used a wavy or toothed blade. The author is not in favour of any of these devices. To begin with, they are in his opinion unnecessary. If one works

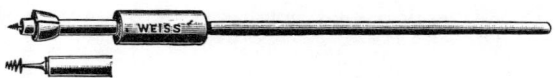

FIG. 184.—George Young's trephine.

with a sharp trephine it is easy to make the blade cut a groove with the very first rotation ; and sharp blades can now be had from any of the first-class instrument makers. Furthermore, these devices make sterilisation more difficult. In the case of the toothed blades, the instrument makers assert that they are difficult to sharpen and unsatisfactory, even when much trouble has been taken over them ; apart

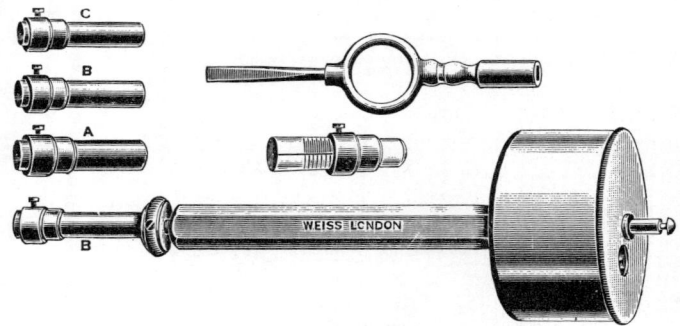

FIG. 185.—Von Hippel's trephine.

from the disadvantages they would thus seem to possess, it may be questioned whether there is any real benefit in using them.

Rollet and Gradle have each brought out a mechanical trephine, which is held in one hand whilst the other rotates the blade by means of a special handle, and a system of cogwheels. These are ingenious, but they keep both the surgeon's hands employed, which is a decided disadvantage.

NEWER OPERATIONS FOR GLAUCOMA 563

Some surgeons have strongly advocated the use of von Hippel's clockwork trephine (Fig. 185). Prominent amongst these have been P. Roemer, Webster Fox, and the late Nimmo Walker. The great objection to the instrument is the difficulty in being sure that it is sterile.

Yet others have preferred a trephine driven by a dental

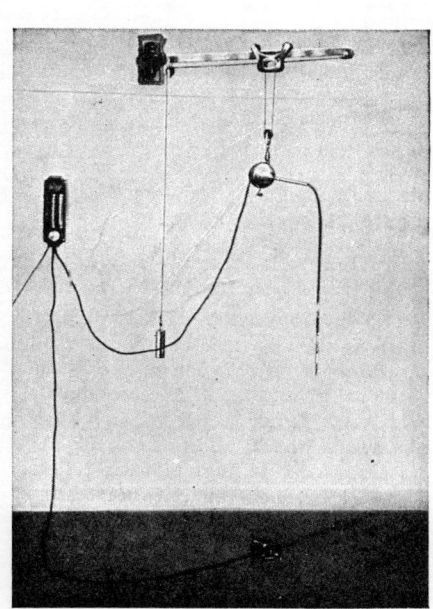

FIG. 186. 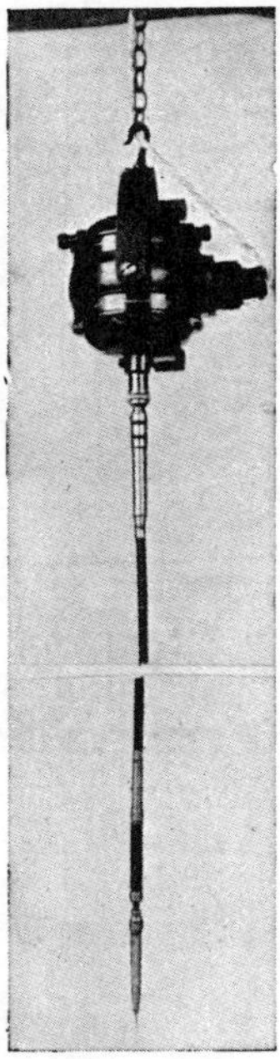 FIG. 187.

FIG. 186.—Vogt's motor trephine, showing wall-resistance foot-control, suspension-bar, etc.

FIG. 187.—Taylor's motor trephine.

engine or by some similar source of power. Figs. 186 and 187 show Vogt's and Taylor's motor trephines. Reber worked with a similar instrument. The advocates of these mechanical devices claim that they can obtain more clean-cut holes than can those who use the hand trephine. The risk of an injury to the deeper structures is undoubtedly greater, and the attainment of perfect asepsis must always be questionable. Moreover, those who have had a little experience with the hand-worked trephine, find no difficulty in cutting out clean discs with it.

Methods of splitting the cornea.—The original instrument employed in Madras for this purpose, was the pair of straight, sharp-pointed iridectomy scissors, already in the

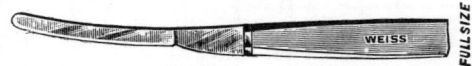

Fig. 188.—Desmarres' secondary knife, used by some surgeons to split the cornea.

hand for the purpose of shaping the flap; in most cases these can hardly be improved upon. Others have thought differently, and quite a number of instruments have been

Fig. 189.—Lang's knife for splitting the cornea.

employed for the purpose. Figs. 188 to 191 will show some of these, which have been specially devised or modified to carry out this step of the procedure. In addition, a number of instruments, originally intended for use in other

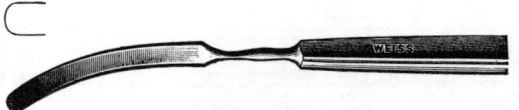

Fig. 190.—Stephenson's knife for splitting the cornea.

operations, have been pressed into service by different surgeons. The list of such includes various knives, needles, and scissors.

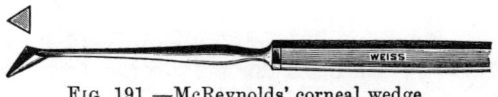

Fig. 191.—McReynolds' corneal wedge.

The modifications of the conjunctival flap which have been suggested by different surgeons.—We shall take these in turn.

Von Mende's flap is shown in the accompanying diagram

NEWER OPERATIONS FOR GLAUCOMA

(Fig. 192). In order to ensure the adhesion of the raw surface of the transplanted conjunctiva to the subjacent cornea, the Russian surgeon removed the corneal epithelium by scraping it with a sharp instrument.

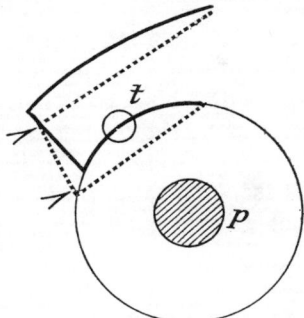

FIG. 192.—Von Mende's flap.

The thick lines show the conjunctival incision and the dotted lines show the flap brought into position and sutured there. t, trephine hole; p, pupil.

Webster Fox uses a very similar technique but does not abrade the cornea, and leaves the flap to take care of itself. Obviously, in such a case, it can heal down to the cornea, only around the edge of the trephine hole.

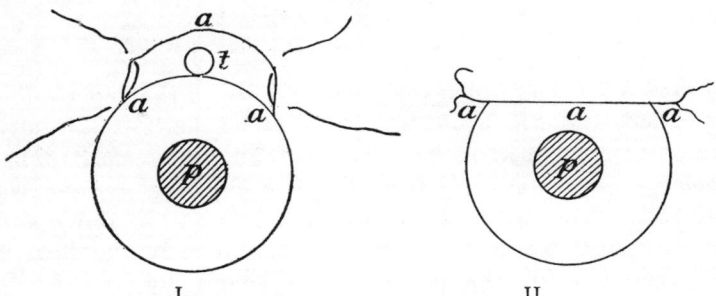

FIG. 193.—Dupuy-Dutemps' flap.

I., flap prepared, and sutures in place for tying. II., flap drawn into place, and sutures tied. aaa, cut edge of conjunctiva; t, trephine hole; p, pupil.

Dupuy-Dutemps employs the sliding flap shown in the accompanying drawings, and places his trephine hole immediately behind the limbus (Fig. 193).

Hill Griffith's original technique was to trephine half on the cornea and half on the sclera without any previous preparation. He then picked up the cut conjunctiva with a fine needle and suture and attached it to the neighbouring cornea, thus drawing down the conjunctiva and thereby covering in the trephine hole (Fig. 194). Later, he modified his technique and used a flap very similar to that of Dupuy-Dutemps with this exception, that his trephine hole was placed astride of the limbus as before.

Without entering into detail as to the exact technique used by each of these surgeons, it will suffice to point out one respect in which every one of the methods so advocated

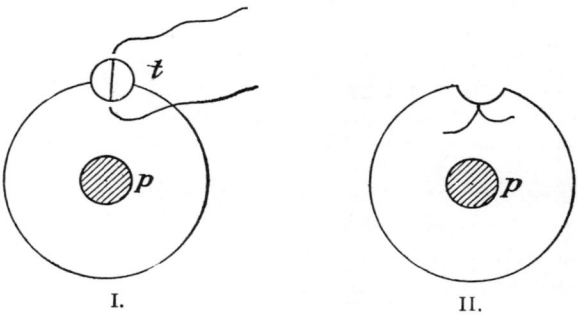

Fig. 194.—Hill-Griffith's earlier flap.
I., showing suture in position. II., showing it tied.

differs from that which the author has from the first recommended, and which he still thinks to be the best. A very important point in our technique is that *we place the trephine hole as far as possible from the breach in the conjunctival surface.* In order to do so, we raise a flap from above and dissect it down to the cornea; consequently the hole is separated from the conjunctival wound by the whole breadth of an extensive flap. On the other hand, the outstanding feature common to all the modifications we are discussing, is that in every case the incision which fashions the flap separates the conjunctiva from its corneal attachment directly over the wound in the sclero-cornea, a wound, be it remembered, which leads into the interior of the eye. It is obvious that in the latter case the risks (1) of septic infection, and (2) of the downgrowth of epithelium through the trephine hole must be greatly enhanced. Nor is this all; the likelihood of early union of the flap to the deeper parts, and therefore of prompt re-establishment of the anterior chamber, is obviously increased when there is a broad space between the point of exit of the fluid from the interior of the eye, and the edge of the flap, as compared to the condition in which that edge lies close to, if not actually over the hole. There is also the danger that the "sliding flap" may slip down and uncover the hole. Should such an accident happen when we are operating by the author's method, it is an easy matter to insert a stitch, and so at once safely and certainly to draw the flap into place, a remedy which cannot so easily, if it can at all, be applied when using one of the modified methods. Furthermore, if the flap is sutured at the time of the operation, it is impossible for it to slip, and this precaution is now always taken by the author.

A last point of great importance remains to be considered. With the author's flap, the corneal filtration area extends anteriorly well beyond the limbus, and there is a distinct area of separated and filtering corneal flap on the pupillary side of that boundary. The photographs (Figs. 195 and 196) illustrate the point. The accuracy of the above assertion has been proved in the experience of a number of those who follow the author's technique. From time to time one sees a contrary statement made, but never, we believe, by any surgeon with a working experience of trephining in his own practice. Suffice it here to say that the flap made by splitting the cornea along its planes of cleavage, and by flushing those planes at once and permanently with isotonic, aseptic, aqueous fluid, does not tend to cicatrise down to the underlying sclera. Very different are the conditions of the modified operation. Even if, as in von Mende's technique, the surface of the cornea is freshened to promote adhesion between it and the under surface of the flap, it is obvious that the latter must heal down to the former, right up to the anterior (or pupillary) edge of the trephine hole. One cannot but look with apprehension on any method which necessarily introduces plastic tissue up to the very margin of the hole which we wish to keep patent for drainage purposes.

In conclusion, it may once again be emphatically stated that the difficulties of splitting the cornea have been very greatly over-estimated, as the author has had the

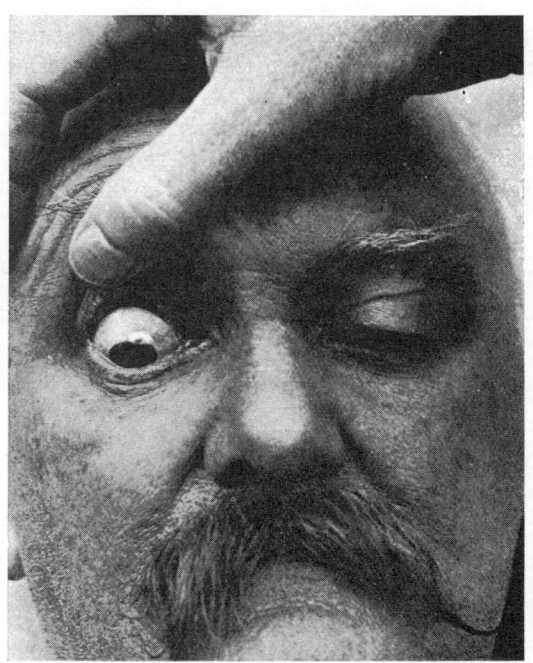

Fig. 195.—T. S.
Over four months after operation. Notice invasion of cornea by the scar and dark trephine hole.

opportunity of showing in many clinics both in Europe and America, as well as in the East. There is no need to resort to modifications of the flap, on the ground that the technique here advocated is too difficult. It is nothing of the kind, and is within the reach of any ophthalmic surgeon of ordinary manipulative dexterity.

The author feels that the best comment he can offer

on the value of these modifications of his original technique is to quote at length the remarks made by Treacher Collins, before the International Congress, in London (1913). He said : " The question to which he wished to direct attention was that of the essential physiological factors which underlie the formation of a filtration. Some years ago he

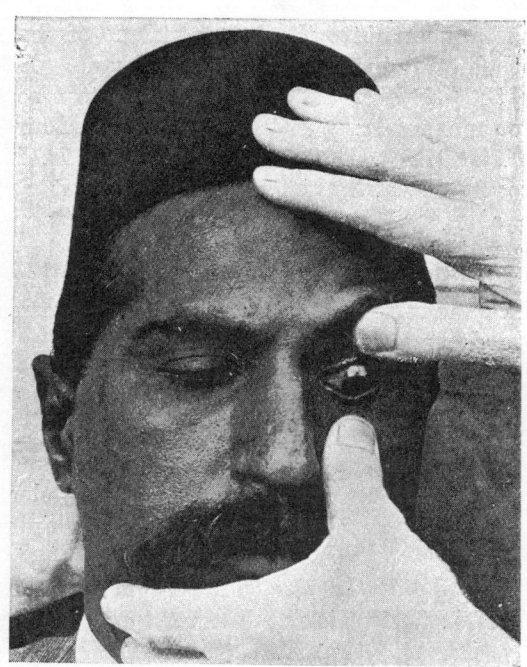

Fig. 196.—P. D.
Three years after operation. Notice prominent bleb, invasion of cornea, and dark trephine hole.

examined several eyes microscopically in which a filtration scar had formed accidentally in connection with an iridectomy for glaucoma, and found that in them a fold of iris tissue had prolapsed into the wound, preventing closure of the sclero-corneal wound and in time stretching and atrophying. For a time he doubted if a filtration scar could be formed without the entanglement of a piece of iris. Some cases shown by Colonel Herbert convinced him, however, that this was possible. Why was it, then, that an opening made at the angle of the chamber did not always become filled with granulation tissue, become covered anteriorly by epithelium, posteriorly by endothelium, and be as impermeable to aqueous humour as the normal corneal tissue ? What prevents the filtration of the aqueous into the normal tissue of the cornea is the endothelium lining Descemet's membrane. He thought therefore that the first essential of a filtration scar was to form a permanent gap in the endothelial lining of the cornea. They knew that wounds of the iris, if aseptic, never became closed by granulation tissue ; it would seem probable also that wounds of the substantia propria of the cornea, if kept bathed by the aqueous humour and aseptic, would also not be closed by granulation tissue. A wound of the surface of the cornea, if kept open, becomes filled by a downgrowth of epithelium, and in an unclosed perforating wound the epithelium would extend down along its margins into the anterior chamber. The third essential in the formation of a filtration scar would seem therefore not to have the opening in the surface epithelium coinciding with the opening in the sclero-corneal tissue. Lt.-Col. Elliot's operation of trephining seems to meet these three essentials in a most satisfactory way ; by removing a circular piece of Descemet's membrane it becomes difficult, if not impossible, for the gap to be bridged across by endothelium. The substantia propria is left exposed to the aqueous humour, and the large conjunctival flap prevents the surface epithelium extending into the substantia propria. He thought it most desirable not to make a button-hole in the conjunctival flap."

REFERENCES

CLEGG, J. G.—*Brit. Journ. Ophth.*, 1917, vol. i. p. 536.
DUPUY-DUTEMPS.—*Proc. de la Soc. d'Opht. de Paris*, March 4, 1913.
FOX, L. WEBSTER.—" A Modified Trephine," *Ophth. Rec.*, 1911, vol. xx. p. 716 ; *Ophthalmology*, Oct. 1912.
GRIFFITH, A. HILL.—*Ophth. Rev.*, January 1914.

TAYLOR, H. H.—" A Trephine, worked by Electric Motor," *The Ophthalmoscope*, 1913, vol. xi. p. 669.
VOGT, A.—*Klin. Monatsbl. f. Augenh.*, April 1913.
VON MENDE.—*Klin. Monatsbl. f. Augenh.*, January 1913.
WALKER, A. NIMMO.—" Sclero-Corneal Trephining," *Medico-Chirurgical Journ.*, Liverpool, July 1911.

PART X

Complications which may be met with During the Performance of the Newer Glaucoma Operations.

Button-holing of or injury to the flap.—This accident may occur during any of the sclerectomy operations, either whilst the flap is being prepared, or later when the piece of sclera is being excised. Those who use large carefully dissected flaps are especially liable to meet with it. During the former step, the conjunctival apron should be dealt with as gently as possible, and should not be roughly seized in the grip of forceps, but drawn gently in the desired direction. Much of the success of this manœuvre depends upon the behaviour of the patient. If he is quiet, it is a very easy procedure ; if he is unruly, it may become very difficult. Again, when we come to the actual sclerectomy, the danger of perforating the flap is considerably accentuated by any sudden movement of the eye. The patient should be warned to lie quiet, and to look down ; and the surgeon should ask his assistant to pull the flap well down out of his way, and should make a point of seeing exactly what he is doing. In dealing with intractable patients, it is advisable to fix the eye by means of forceps, or of a silk thread run round the lower half of the corneal circumference close to the limbus. The two ends of the thread are left long, and the eye can be held down by an assistant whose hand is thus kept well out of the operator's way (Fig. 197). This valuable and little-known method of controlling an eye during operation is applicable to many other conditions, *e.g.*, to the extraction of a cataract ; for it has no tendency to pull open a corneal section in the way that the use of a pair of forceps does. Hence the tendency to vitreous loss is greatly lessened.

The surgeon who takes the precaution of injecting trivalin-hyoscin, in the manner advised in Part II. of this chapter, will very seldom have to complain of difficulty in the management of his patients during operation.

Sometimes, when dealing with the brittle conjunctivæ met with in old people, and in eyes which have long been

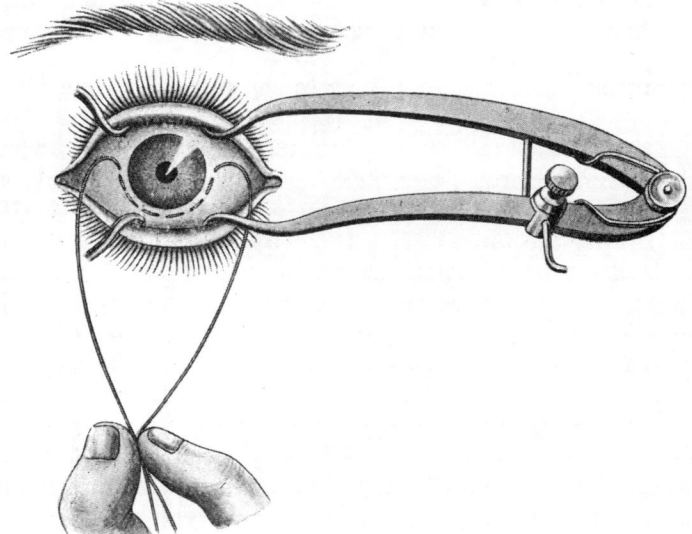

Fig. 197.—Showing the thread, in position for the fixation of an eye, but not yet drawn tight by traction.

subject to glaucoma, the thread method of control is not practicable, and the following device may then be made use of with considerable advantage both to the operator and to the patient. The superior rectus tendon, which has been partly exposed by the throwing down of the flap, is laid bare and is seized in the grip of a pair of Prince's forceps; the eye can thus be easily held in the desired position, without inconvenience to the operator or danger to the patient. If a general anæsthetic is not being administered it is better to substitute a loop of silk for the forceps. The silk is passed under the tendon, and its two ends are knotted together. Simple traction on the loop pulls the globe down into position.

A small button-hole does not appear to constitute a dangerous complication. The author has carefully watched cases in which such an accident has happened, and has fortunately found that the opening becomes closed by cicatrisation and that the eventual result seems to be as good as if no such complication had supervened. It is, however, obviously our duty to avoid button-holing whenever we can; the more so as others have reported bad results, which they have attributed to this complication.

Loss of the Disc in the Anterior Chamber in a Trephine Operation.—This accident happens in about 1·6 per cent. of cases trephined, and can only occur when the whole circumference of the disc is cut through at one time, or when at the most a very slender hinge is left. If, at the conclusion of the trephining, the disc cannot be found, we turn back the flap and can then usually see it lying at the upper part of the chamber and close to the hole. The author has only twice found the disc impacted in the hollow of the blade, and has never heard of such a thing occurring in the practice of any other surgeon; this serves to show the extreme rarity of its occurrence. It is of interest to record that on both these occasions a Gray Clegg's slotted trephine was being used. Care should be taken to avoid all drag on the iris during the iridectomy; this is a very important point, as any impaction of the iris in the trephine hole at this stage makes the subsequent delivery of the disc very difficult. A gentle stream from a McKeown's irrigator will in most cases quickly wash the missing piece of sclera through the hole to the outside, or at least replace it in such a position that its removal proves quite easy. It will often be found that it still remains hinged at one point. A snip with the scissors divides this attachment. The writer has never yet failed to carry out this manœuvre, nor has he experienced any difficulty in effecting his purpose. Should the operator be less fortunate, he need not have the least fear of leaving the disc within the eye, always provided that he has introduced no focus of sepsis along with it. The correctness of this dictum has been established by clinical experience. It is true that on more than one occasion, a surgeon has accused a disc left in the anterior chamber of being the cause of subsequent sepsis, but it would be difficult to eliminate other possibilities of the introduction of septic matter, especially if the operator has " gone fishing " for the disc with various instruments. On the other hand, the author knows of cases n which the disc has been left behind and has done no harm whatever. Indeed, it would be difficult to believe that an aseptic piece of tissue, isotonic with the walls of the eye from which it was cut, could be a source either of irritation or of sepsis.

Holth[1] quotes Elschnig as believing that "the aqueous has tissue-dissolving qualities, which, in his opinion, is proved by the fact that the loose scleral disc, fallen into the anterior chamber during trephining, has completely disappeared in a relatively short time." So far as the author's experience goes, the disc, when it slips into the chamber, slides under the scleral margin of the trephine hole, and is difficult to see even at the time of the operation, until it is washed back into place. As soon as the conjunctival flap is in position, it is quite impossible to see it. He has no experience of the disc being dropped free into the anterior chamber, where it can be observed.

Loss of Vitreous.—This accident is one of the worst nightmares of the operating surgeon. It may occur in any of the procedures undertaken for the relief of glaucoma, but the risk of its occurrence is greater in proportion to the size of the opening made in the eyeball. It is sometimes an indication of intra-ocular hæmorrhage or of the pouring out of a secretion as the result of the sudden reduction of pressure within the eye. It is far more likely to occur in late, and especially in congestive cases, than in early and simple ones. The obvious prophylactic indication would appear to be to keep the wound in the tunic of the

[1] *Brit. Journ. Ophth.*, 1922, vol. vi. p. 22.

NEWER OPERATIONS FOR GLAUCOMA

eye as small as possible. The moment vitreous presents, the surgeon will be well advised, to close the eye as speedily as he can, to get the patient back into bed, and to keep him as quiet as possible there. The prognosis of the case will be materially altered for the worse by the accident.

Intra-ocular hæmorrhage.—The question of a rise in intra-ocular pressure as a result of hæmorrhage has been alluded to in the previous paragraph. It is the most appalling disaster of glaucoma surgery, and may occur either on the table or shortly after the patient has been put back to bed. The operator who has seen the vitreous well up into the wound, burst its limiting membrane and escape freely, to be followed almost immediately by the red stain of hæmorrhage, is little likely to forget the experience. It is equally unfortunate to leave a patient apparently progressing favourably and to be recalled to his side because " the bandages are soaked with blood." Nothing remains but to enucleate the globe, a tragic event indeed alike for the surgeon and the sufferer. The author is persuaded that the danger of this disaster occurring is greatly lessened by reducing to a minimum the aperture in the tunics of the globe, as is unquestionably done in trephining.

Superficial hæmorrhage which obscures the details of the operation.—In operating on congested eyes, the field is often obscured by the blood poured out. In most cases the hæmorrhage can be kept under control by the instillation and injection of adrenalin chloride solution before the operation is commenced, in the manner already indicated in Part II. of this chapter. In any case, the hæmorrhage can be controlled, if need be, by dropping adrenalin solution on the sclera laid bare by reflection of the flap, and by supplementing this action by local pressure with small mounted cotton-wool swabs soaked in the solution. The tendency to troublesome venous hæmorrhage is speedily checked as soon as the scleral coat is pierced, for the resulting relaxation of the tunic of the eye removes the obstruction to the outflow through the large venous trunks. The lesson to learn from this, is not to waste time in endeavours to arrest this hæmorrhage by other means, but to get on with the operation as speedily as possible.

Plugging of the wound by intra-ocular contents.—When the anterior chamber is emptied through the operation wound, the iris, the ciliary body, the suspensory ligament, the lens, and the vitreous body make a movement forward. Under varying conditions any one of these structures may present in and block the opening. Such an accident, as has already been pointed out, is more likely to occur, when, during the operation, the tension of the eye has been raised by sudden exudation from the choroid and ciliary body into the posterior segment of the globe, or by intra-ocular hæmorrhage. Indeed, it may well be doubted whether in the absence of one of these conditions, the incision ever becomes plugged, always *provided that the operator does not drag the uveal tissue into the wound whilst performing an iridectomy.* The plugging of the opening by uveal tissue is, however, much more likely to occur in those long-standing cases in which, beforehand, the iris is adherent far forward to the back of the cornea.

To leave the wound blocked with uveal tissue is a misfortune, and will probably entail the failure of the operation. An effort should first be made by the careful use of iris forceps and scissors to clear the obstruction. In doing so, great care should be taken not to drag on the uveal tissue, and to carry the scissor points right into the wound. When this has been cleared as far as possible, the surgeon takes a curette, or preferably a narrow spud, the last 3 to 5 millimetres of which are bent at an obtuse angle to the rest of the instrument. This is carefully introduced into the chamber, endeavouring in so doing to push the impacted iris back into position. A gush of aqueous and the simultaneous emptying of the chamber may show that our object has been accomplished. If, however, this is not easily effected, and if the tension is still high, it is wiser and safer to abstain from further interference rather than to persist; for we may easily do more harm than good, and may imperil the scanty hope still remaining to our patient.

It can hardly be too strongly insisted upon, that *plug-*

ging of the trephine hole with uveal tissue, at the time of the operation, is an almost wholly avoidable complication. If the technique which has been recommeneed above is carefully followed, this complication will very seldom occur, and only then in the cases in which the diaphragm of the eye is driven forwards *en masse* by exudation or hæmorrhage into the vitreous body, a state of affairs in which masterly inactivity is strongly indicated.

After an iridectomy has been performed, we sometimes find a dark bead projecting through the wound. Transillumination of this through the pupil by oblique illumination reveals that the obstructing substance is translucent and of a greenish colour ; and we then know that we are confronted with a prolapse of the lens or of the vitreous. In either case it is our duty to close the eye at once, for, if the structure has been pushed forward by some effusion, we may find the pressure relieved, and the trouble over within forty-eight hours, owing to the absorption of the effused fluid. If, on the other hand, we are so unfortunate as to be confronted with a dislocation of the lens as a result of overstretching or rupture of the suspensory ligament, the case can just as well be dealt with at a later stage, when all doubts as to diagnosis have been set at rest. This matter will be discussed in the section on Aftertreatment. The surgeon may rest assured that the conditions that we have been dealing with will never arise to trouble him in any early or comparatively early case. They are limited entirely to patients who have long neglected to present themselves for surgical treatment.

Wounding of the Lens.—This accident is much rarer in the modern operations than during the performance of an iridectomy. The risk of it is greatly increased by the introduction into very shallow chambers of pointed instruments, such as knives and keratomes, and especially the latter. The surgeon is often unaware of the accident, and only finds it out as the evidence of it develops later on. Even should he know of it at the time, he will probably hesitate to resort to removal of the lens, which, at the best, is likely to yield very poor results.

Part XI

After-management of Patients Operated on for Glaucoma

The time that it is necessary to keep a patient in bed after operation depends very much on the procedure adopted. It is shortest in the sclerotomies, and longest in those operations which involve a large incision, such as the classical iridectomy, or the Lagrange operation. The author's practice with trephined cases is to operate on them in bed, and to keep them as still as possible for five hours, after which the nurse turns them from side to side at intervals, as they require it ; they remain recumbent for twenty-four hours, and if all goes well, are then allowed to sit up in bed ; they sit up in a chair the following day, move about the room the next day, and leave the Home a week to ten days after operation.

The first dressing of a sclerectomy or sclerotomy case takes place at the end of twenty-four hours, when the following points should be carefully noted : (1) Whether the chamber has re-formed ; (2) whether the pupil is central ; (3) whether the iridectomy is partial or complete, and whether the coloboma is hidden by the lid ; (4) whether the flap is in good position ; (5) whether filtration is free ; and (6) what the tension of the eye is. If the case is in all respects doing well, the opposite eye is now left open. When both eyes have been operated on and the patient is found with the anterior chamber filled, with free filtration, and with the eye normal in appearance, one may sometimes release both eyes of an intelligent patient during the day, from the first dressing on, and only bandage them at night. In any case where the progress is uneventful, both eyes should be released during the day from the fourth day onward.

As indications for prolonged bandaging the following may be recognised : (1) Emptiness of the anterior chamber pointing to a failure in the union of the flap ; (2) the presence of fresh blood in the anterior chamber ; and (3) the existence of iritis or of any other cause of continued congestion of the eye.

Shallowness of the Chamber.—It must be borne in mind that in a certain number of cases the chamber will remain shallow, even though the wound be healed. This may be due to a free filtration into a loose flap. After an interval the chamber will deepen, but in the meantime one need not fear septic invasion of the eye, the interior of which is effectually shut off from the conjunctival sac, if a good flap has been employed.

Whatever operation has been performed, always provided that it has been done under a flap, if the chamber obstinately remains very shallow, the eye should be cocainised, the lids widely separated, the patient told to look down, and the whole length of the incision gently dried by dabbing it with a cotton-wool swab, mounted on a small stick. It will then be found that in some of these cases a small fistulette exists somewhere along the periphery of the flap. Through this tiny opening the fluid can be seen to be escaping in a steady trickle.[1] The spot should be touched with a small mounted swab of wool soaked in a 2 per cent. solution of silver nitrate, and the opening will speedily close.

A quite different condition is that in which the shallowing of the chamber is due to an overstretching of the diaphragm of the eye, as the result of a long-existing hyperdistension of the vitreous chamber. It is here manifestly impossible to do anything but await events.

Displacement of the Flap.—This cannot occur if the flap is sutured in place at the time of operation. If this has not been done, and the conjunctiva be found rucked up or rolled in on itself, it should be stitched in place. The instillation of adrenalin and cocaine usually makes this manœuvre very easy.

Blood in the Chamber.—If a suitable irrigator is used as a routine measure in the toilette of the eye, we comparatively seldom leave much blood in the chamber at the close

[1] Seidel's test consists in placing a drop of fluorescein solution on the wound, and watching any exuding fluid wash the stain away (Holth).

of the operation. Sometimes, however, the iris persists in bleeding, and it is not worth while prolonging the irrigation. At other times the blood poured out early in the operation coagulates freely, and is difficult to wash out. In yet a third class of case, usually due to injury, hæmorrhage takes place into the chamber after the patient has been removed from the table. Whatever may be the source of the blood, the eyes should be bandaged after instilling a solution of atropin sulphate. This régime should be followed until the chamber clears, which, in most cases, it speedily does.

There is a point of practical interest in connection with the presence of blood in the anterior chamber in these cases, viz., that it may cause the patient much anxiety, since he may find that at one time his vision is beautifully clear, and a few seconds later it all clouds over and he sees as through a mist or fog. The explanation of this not uncommon symptom is quite easy : When the patient lies still—as during sleep—the blood corpuscles settle down to the lowest part of the chamber, and are then out of the line of sight. Movements of the head and eyes stir up these corpuscles and cause them to float suspended in the chamber-fluid, thus interfering with the transparent clearness which ordinarily characterises all the media of the eye. It is well for the surgeon to warn patients of this phenomenon in advance. This has the double advantage of preventing them becoming anxious, and of increasing their confidence in a doctor who evidently understands the case with which he is dealing.

Post-operative Iritis.—There is a good deal of misunderstanding in connection with this complication. Several quite diverse conditions seem to have been included under one heading, with the result that differences of opinion, often more apparent than real, have sprung up. Three conditions at least appear to be confused by some recent writers on this subject, viz., (1) the commonly occurring post-operative complication, usually called " quiet iritis," with which every surgeon who has done much operating for glaucoma is familiar ; (2) an exacerbation of, or may be merely a continuance of an acute or subacute condition, which existed prior to the operation ; and (3) a true septic condition of the wound, due to an accidental contamination at or after the operation.

These three conditions must be clearly defined in a surgeon's mind, and definitely separated in his case-sheet analyses. We therefore propose to discuss each head in turn.

(1) *A quiet iritis* is unpleasantly frequent after all kinds of glaucoma operations. The author first called attention to its occurrence in connection with trephine cases, but it is quite as frequently met with after iridectomy or any one of the modern procedures. Its advent is not marked by the incidence of any of the usual signs of an invasion of iritis ; pre-existing pain is relieved by the operation, signs of congestion diminish, vision improves, and the patient appears to be making excellent progress, so much so that unless we are forewarned and thereby forearmed, we discover the complication only when it is too late.

Whilst admitting that this is a form of inflammation, it seems evident that it is a thing apart from an ordinary iritis of septic origin. It is to be remembered that the physical conditions prevailing within the eye are severely changed by an operation for glaucoma. To begin with, such a procedure alters the relations of the parts which border on, or project into, the aqueous chamber. The chamber is, for a time at least, practically empty, with the consequence that the iris lies in direct contact with the lens capsule, the posterior chamber being temporarily reduced to a potential cavity ; at the same time, the long-continued mydriasis has given place to a state of more or less marked meiosis ; so it follows that we have to hand the very conditions which render the formation of posterior synechiæ most easy. Then again, there can be little doubt that the nature of the fluid secreted under the new conditions may be such as to render the deposition from it of fibrin more liable to occur, without in the least premising any access of inflammatory action. Nor is this all that can be said on the subject ; for the recent work on the migration of pigment that has been found to occur at any rate in some cases of glaucoma, even before operation or other forms of treatment have been started, suggests that we have to do, in this disease, with profound metabolic changes, which may easily modify the eye's reaction to interference of any kind, and especially to such as is associated with trauma. The connection is the more significant from the fact that the masses occluding the pupil and the adhesions of the iris to the anterior capsule—met with in glaucomatous cases—are both deeply pigmented.

It has been asked why this quiet iritis is so much more often met with after trephining and other modern operations than it was after the old iridectomy. Is it really the case that it is more frequent ? We may reasonably venture to doubt if it is. It is far from a rare experience to see the iris tied down after an iridectomy for glaucoma, and one of the worst cases of blockage of the pupil and restriction of the iris movement that the author has ever seen, occurred in a case of Herbert's operation performed on both eyes by a surgeon whose claim to be able to carry out the procedure correctly no one would dispute. It must not be forgotten that after a well-performed iridectomy, the chamber will be completely closed in a few hours, and often after only a few minutes. Remember, too, that a wide coloboma makes the effects of posterior synechiæ both less obvious and less injurious to the results, since it leaves a wide area for visual purposes, even should some amount of adhesion take place between the iris and the deeper parts.

The importance of the subject lies in the fact that the fear of iritis may weigh with timid surgeons, and deter them from operating. We have shown most conclusively, over an experience of many hundreds of consecutive cases, that a solution of atropin may be safely used on the second day after a trephine operation, or even immediately after the trephining, and that if this is done, we need no longer dread post-operative occlusion of the pupil. Others have confirmed this statement, and some make a routine practice of instilling the drops at the close of the operation, a procedure which has much in its favour, but which the author thinks is a little too rigid. If an iridectomy—even a peripheral one—has been made, and if the globe at the conclusion of the operation is soft, with no suspicion of iris impaction in the wound, atropin may be safely and profitably used straight away. If, on the other hand, it has proved impossible to remove a portion of the iris, or if uveal tissue has become impacted in the wound, or again if the eye has hardened at the close of the operation —indicating an increase of its fluid contents and pressure on the uveal coat thereby from within—it is safer to withhold the use of the mydriatic and to watch the progress of the case, being careful, however, not to allow the pupil to become dangerously contracted. One thing seems quite certain, viz., that the use of a strong mydriatic is positively harmful, if, on the second or third day, we find iris tissue plugging the wound and causing a rise of tension thereby. Eserin and not atropin is then called for, if reliance is to be placed on drugs at all. One cannot help feeling that if the use of atropin aggravates the blocking of the wound when it is present, it may bring it about when the tendency to the accident is in the ascendant, or even in existence. Whatever the individual surgeon's final decision may be as to the exact date at which atropin should be instilled after operation, there can, we think, be no disputing the fact that the condition which gives rise to synechiæ in this quiet way after one of the modern procedures, and which, for want of a better term, we at present call a " quiet iritis," can, in the immense majority of cases, be controlled and rendered harmless, if the surgeon recognises the risk, and is ready to treat the condition promptly by maintaining full mydriasis, whenever the use of atropin instillations reveals a tendency to the formation of posterior synechiæ in a recently operated patient.

A very different view must be taken of the two other conditions we have still to consider ; we will take them in turn:

(2) *A continuation of, or even an exacerbation of, an acute or subacute condition which existed prior to the operation*, may severely try the nerve and resources of the surgeon. The condition is to be treated on ordinary

lines. A much more important thought is suggested by such cases. Everyone who has dealt with large numbers of glaucoma cases and has pondered over their almost endless variety, has probably come to the certain conclusion, that whilst the term glaucoma is a very convenient label for a huge mass of cases, which all have the common feature of a rise of intra-ocular pressure, the causes which bring about this rise are many and various. In some instances, at least, there is a septic influence at work, and it is of importance that we should ascertain its source. Has it been introduced by the surgeon, or was it there before he stepped in at all ? Is he to blame for it, or is it merely a complication he must expect to meet with, despite the most careful technique ? Speaking from a clinical standpoint, we have no hesitation in affirming that the condition may arise from pre-existent causes, and be quite beyond the control of the operator. The first point is, that the congestion present remains practically unchanged after operation, or at most undergoes the slight aggravation which may be expected to follow mechanical interference. Now this is not consistent with the theory of introduced sepsis, which we know begins to manifest itself about the third day, and rapidly increases in intensity during the few succeeding days. When a more marked aggravation of the signs present manifests itself, the solution of the problem becomes more difficult, but even then we meet with not a few cases in which it is difficult to decide whether such aggravation is due to the amount of interference at the time of trephining, or whether a further explanation is called for. The second point is the frequency with which we find adhesions between the iris and the cornea in late cases of glaucoma, in which there has been no operative interference whatever. Of evidently the same nature is the perilimbal matting, which, when it exists, makes splitting of the cornea so difficult. Again these cases tail off imperceptibly into those of the so-called " quiet iritis " discussed under the preceding heading ; for one meets with an eye in which the marked pre-operative congestion distinctly subsides, and all appears to be going well, and yet close synechiæ may form, and sight be impaired or lost if by any chance the surgeon is caught napping. The third and last point is based on a class of case with which many of us are familiar. A patient, often with a gouty history, develops evidence of raised tension. He is advised to diet himself, to take more exercise, and to be more careful in a variety of ways, with the result that he very speedily improves in general health, and at the same time his signs and symptoms of increased tension disappear, for the time at least, to the great relief both of doctor and patient. Many surgeons will be able to recall such cases. Their meaning would appear to be that the threat of glaucoma was due, in part at least, to a toxic condition which had been removed, or at least ameliorated, by the constitutional treatment employed. We do not pretend to assign the threat of raised tension definitely to bacteria or to circulating toxins, but prefer to leave the matter open. One cannot review the above evidence without a deepening conviction that toxicity, possibly in many forms, is playing a by no means unimportant part in the pathogenesis of some, at least, of the conditions which we now, for convenience' sake, are content to group together under the term " glaucoma." This may appear to be a digression, but it is very important that we should clearly understand the subject, if we are to treat these after-complications of a glaucoma operation intelligently and effectively.

(3) *A septic condition of the eye, due to contamination at the time of operation*, requires little comment here. In nearly 900 consecutive cases trephined in Madras from the first operation of that nature on 2nd August 1909, up to the time when the author left India, we did not meet with a single case of suppuration of the globe, nor with any cases of *severe* irido-cyclitis, which could without hesitation be put down to septic contamination in the theatre. We cannot absolutely exclude an element of sepsis in some of the cases, in which an irido-cyclitis existing before the operation continued thereafter, sometimes in an aggravated form. That would be an irrational claim,

and no one could make good such a position. The author's point is that contamination of an operation wound *depends less on the particular method employed than on the preparatory technique*, especially on conjunctival asepsis or the reverse. These remarks are made because others have attributed their failures after filtration operations to what they consider is the scanty protection afforded by the thin conjunctival flap. Under cover of this explanation, there have been included cases of quiet iritis, of varying degrees of irido-cyclitis, and even losses of the eye due to panophthalmitis. The data on which such conclusions have been founded have sometimes been insufficient for the purpose. We must remember, firstly, that the layer of anterior epithelium suffices, so long as it is intact, to guard the cornea against the inroads of so virulent an organism as the gonococcus; and, in the second place, that the great majority of our conjunctival wounds after trephining are healed, and the chamber thereby sealed, on the first dressing. Finally, our Indian experience of 900 cases, already quoted, shows that the conjunctiva, when properly dealt with, affords sufficient protection to the important structures it covers. It is to be clearly understood that we are not dealing now with cases of " late infection " which are met with months or even years after operation; these will be discussed shortly.

Prolapse of uveal tissue into the operation wound during healing.—This is a comparatively rare complication, and will be still more so in the hands of those surgeons who make an iridectomy a routine step in the performance of their operation. There can be no doubt that the tissue commonly protruded is iridic, though the ciliary body may easily be involved in the misfortune, thus rendering the case more serious. If the ciliary body is pushed far forwards, or if the iris-base is adherent to the corneal periphery, then tethered uveal tissue lies in close propinquity to the aperture in the sclera, and is much more likely to prolapse into the wound than it is when it lies free of abnormal attachments, and with a good space separating its base from the margin of the breach in the sclera. Uveal tissue may be pushed into the wound by a dislocated lens, as we have proved by anatomical examination, but this is a very rare event. It is probable that in the great majority of cases the iris is carried into the wound by the patient squeezing the eye from time to time, and thereby ejecting gushes of fluid from the anterior chamber into the subconjunctival space. The presence of an iridectomy coloboma provides a sluice-gate, through which such gushes of fluid can escape, without carrying the uveal membrane in front of them. In other words, the function of an iridectomy in the modern glaucoma operations is exactly similar to that in cataract extraction. It is not an integral part of the operation, but merely a safeguard.

When a prolapse of iris occurs, the tension of the eye at once rises. The flap, if one has been made, should be raised without delay and the prolapsed membrane freely excised. If care is taken to avoid all drag on the iris during excision, and if no undue delay has occurred in undertaking the procedure, the pupil will return at once to its normal position. A stream from a suitable irrigator may materially assist in its replacement. A very interesting point in this connection is that the protruded iris is very slow to contract adhesions to the sides of the hole. This reminds one of what has already been said (Chapter VIII. Part II.) as to the absence of cicatrisation in the edges of an iris after an iridectomy, and of Sattler's observation of the absence of proliferation in the edges of a trephine wound a fortnight after operation. The clinical importance of these observations lies in the light they throw on the extreme ease with which the impacted iris can sometimes be replaced in the secondary operation.

If the prolapse be a very slight one, as judged not only by the appearance of the operation wound, but also by the amount of displacement of the pupil, and if there be any contra-indication to a second operation, such as the unwillingness of the patient to submit to it, we may first try the free instillation of eserin drops. In a few cases this will prove of decided benefit. We must, however, bear in mind the danger of the prolapse recurring at a later date, after the patient has left our hands. Such an accident would then be very unfortunate, and under the circumstances the surgeon will do well to consider most seriously the advisability of immediate excision in every case of iris prolapse.

Dislocation of the lens or vitreous body into the wound during healing.—It will sometimes happen that, on the day following operation, tension is found to be still high, and a bead is observed bulging into the aperture in the sclera. An immediate diagnosis is called for, since so much depends on the correct treatment of the condition, which may be that of presenting lens or vitreous on the one hand, or of prolapsed iris on the other. As the treatment of these two sets of conditions is very different, it is essential we should make no mistake at this stage. Fortunately, the differentiation is usually quite easy. All that is necessary is either to employ a transilluminator, or to use a lens and throw a strong beam of light into the eye from below (when the sclerectomy has been made above), and at the same time to observe the bulging bead. If this consists of iris, it remains opaque, whilst if the offending tissue is transparent (lens or vitreous body) the bead is illuminated and an opalescent appearance is at once obtained. The diagnosis can be advanced one stage farther, with at least some degree of probability of correctness, if we have observed whether there was evidence of sudden hardening at the time of operation, and if we note the relative depth of different parts of the anterior chamber, when the bulging is under examination. We shall take these two points in turn. (1) When at the close of the operation, the tension of the eye suddenly rises, we may safely conclude that a free exudation from the choroidal vessels or an intra-ocular hæmorrhage has occurred, and though dislocation of the lens is not to be forgotten, the great probability is in favour of vitreous rather than lens having been thrust into the hole. The immediate indication is to close the eye and return the patient as quietly as possible to bed. If, on the other hand, the blockage is first noticed when the eye is inspected on the second or third day, we must think of dislocation of the lens as well as of presenting vitreous. (2) A careful inspection of the aqueous chamber under oblique illumination, will often reveal that its anterior division is shallower in the neighbourhood of the scleral wound than it is in the opposite quadrant. This is a most suggestive sign, and it will usually be safe to conclude that it indicates a displacement and tilting of the lens. What are we to do? We may settle the diagnosis by puncturing the protruding bead with a cataract needle, when the nature of the escaping contents will at once set all doubts at rest. Is this good surgery? It would be a grave mistake to be premature in taking such a step, though one may be driven to it. If the case is one of the impaction of the ocular contents in the wound under the pressure of an intra-ocular effusion, the obvious thing to do is to await the cessation of that effusion and the subsequent absorption of the fluid. This complication is only met with in long-standing and desperate cases, and premature interference will probably aggravate the mischief, whereas if we take the ordinary steps for the arrest of hæmorrhage (both general and local) we not infrequently find that the tension falls, and a less hopeless result is obtained than we would have anticipated. If in the course of three or four days things do not mend, we can puncture the bead of bulging matter, knowing that, desperate as the remedy is, the condition is still more so, and demands drastic action. The escape of fluid vitreous may better the conditions and lead to a fall of tension, though one of course recognises that one is fighting with one's back against the wall. Very strange is the observation recorded by the author in *Sclero-corneal Trephining*, that if the incision of the bead leads to the extrusion of lens matter, the tension is sometimes at once relieved, and yet widespread opacification of the lens does not always occur.

What is the pathological explanation of these cases of presentation of the lens or vitreous body? We had the opportunity of examining two cases in Madras which threw some light on the matter. It will probably be generally admitted that in a large number of instances, the first event of moment in the development of the glaucomatous state is an *increase in the volume of the vitreous body*. How that is brought about does not concern us for the moment. The effect, however, is well known, and consists of a push-forward of the diaphragm of the eye, *i.e.*, of the lens, suspensory ligament, ciliary body, and iris, with a corresponding shallowing of the anterior chamber. Such a condition, if long continued and extreme, must obviously lead to an overstretching of the suspensory ligament, and hence result in the lens possessing an undue freedom of movement so soon as the *vis a tergo* is removed or lessened. Anatomically we have twice observed a dislocation of the lens in sections of frozen eyes removed after trephining, and in both cases it appeared that the ligament was so unduly lax as to have permitted the lens to tilt and move bodily towards the trephine hole. There was nothing to indicate that intra-ocular hæmorrhage had played a part in the phenomenon. In one case the lens was separated from the trephine hole by uveal tissue, whilst in the other it presented directly into the hole.

Three other conditions suggest themselves as likely to cause a blockage of the sclerectomy wound by lens matter or by vitreous, viz., (1) a rupture of the suspensory ligament, (2) an abnormal fluidity of the vitreous, and (3) that fluidity or semi-fluidity of the lens which is associated with the hyper-maturity of a cortico-nuclear cataract. With regard to the first, it is obvious that the relationship of the site of the tear to the position of the wound in the coat of the eye may determine to some extent at least whether the lens drifts towards and blocks the hole, or whether vitreous escapes thereat. If the lens is abnormally fluid, it will easily move out towards, mould itself into, and so block the breach which has been made in the sclera. This is very apt to happen, if a Morgagnian cataract is present at the time of operation. Eyes with such cataracts present especial dangers after a sclerectomy.

The early recurrence of an increase of tension after operation.—The possible causes of this complication are numerous : (1) Failure to enter the anterior chamber freely at the time of operation ; (2) failure to remove a sufficiently large piece of Descemet's membrane in the procedure (Treacher Collins) ; (3) blockage of the aperture by uveal tissue ; (4) the same by lens or vitreous ; (5) the filling up of the wound in the sclera by the proliferation of inflammatory tissue, derived from the sclera, the episclera, or the uveal coat.

Several of these points have already been dealt with from the point of view of treatment. Cases of recurrent tension shortly after operation are amongst the severest trials that a surgeon has to encounter. Whether he decides to await events, or to adopt a new operative procedure, his path is beset with peril. Some surgeons fly to iridectomy, others resort to a cyclodialysis, or to some variety of sclerectomy other than their original procedure. The author, who relies on trephining, repeats the operation at another place, and has even done so on more than one occasion.

Detachment of the Choroid. — Several observers, amongst others Hudson and Knapp, have placed on record cases of this complication following trephining. It is associated with a delay in the re-formation of the anterior chamber, and its prognostic significance does not appear to be serious, the membrane reattaching itself when normal, or nearly normal, tension is restored. A far more serious aspect of the complication is to be sought in the changes secondarily involved : (1) The cornea in these cases may be wrinkled and present striate, ill-defined opacities. Fortunately these usually, if not always, clear up when the chamber re-forms. (2) The shallowness of the chamber favours the formation of adhesions between the iris and the capsule of the lens, since these are not separated from each other by the usual depth of fluid. Moreover, it is sometimes very difficult to obtain mydriasis under these conditions. It is possible that a certain number of cases of this complication occur without being recognised, owing to the fact that the majority of them are very anterior in position. One fact has been overlooked by some recent writers, viz., that detachment of the choroid is far from being peculiar to trephining ; indeed, Meller has found that it occurs in more than 22 per cent. of cases which have undergone Lagrange's operation. Fuchs found it in 4 per cent. of cataract extractions, and in 10 per cent. of glaucoma iridectomies, while Hudson goes so far as to suggest the invariability of its occurrence, in some degree at least, in all cases of perforating lesion of the eyeball involving the escape of aqueous fluid. It may be questioned whether this is correct. The author has not seen reason to believe that it is. He is in accord with Morax's opinion that, as a *clinical* entity, this complication is distinctly rare.

Detachment of the choroid was first described by Knapp nearly fifty years ago. Fuchs considers that it is due to rupture of the ligamentum pectinatum during operation, a channel being thus formed whereby the aqueous humour can escape from the anterior chamber into the suprachoroidal space. Meller holds the condition to be due to a violent exudation from the blood vessels of the ciliary processes. Hudson believes that serous detachment of the choroid and ciliary body is a natural accompaniment of any considerable reduction of intra-ocular pressure, the degree of the detachment varying with the degree of the reduction of this pressure. He considers that the exuded fluid comes from the choroidal blood vessels and not improbably from the veins. There is one point which must be mentioned, viz., that choroidal detachments, which can be recognised ophthalmoscopically, are conspicuous by their absence in a number of very successful cases of trephining, in which the tension has remained markedly subnormal over a period of years. The author has had several such eyes under his observation, in which the most careful ophthalmoscopy has failed to reveal any abnormal condition of the fundus. Schur of Tübingen has reported three cases of detachment of the choroid out of eighty-five trephinings, *i.e.*, 3·5 per cent. ; he quotes these figures and those we have given above in support of Fuchs' view that it is an injury to the ligamentum pectinatum which permits the aqueous to find its way into the supra-choroidal space, and so leads to these detachments of the choroid ; and he points out that such a disturbance of the pectinate ligament is obviously less often brought about by a well-performed trephining than it is by an iridectomy or by a Lagrange operation, since in the first-named procedure this structure is deliberately torn, whilst in trephining it is sedulously avoided.

The obvious treatment for this condition is to keep the patient quiet, and to take steps to heal up any leakage that may be occurring at the periphery of the flap.

Defective Vision after a Decompression Operation.—There are a number of causes of this condition, some of which are so obvious as to call for no comment. It is the purpose of these paragraphs to deal with those cases only in which the blurring of vision is not easily explained : The operation has gone well ; the eye is free of inflammation ; the tension is normal or sub-normal ; such examination as one can safely conduct in the bed does not reveal any gross change ; and yet the patient sees poorly and complains of his defect. We shall consider some possible explanations of the trouble.

(1) *The advance of the lens system* as a result of the free drainage and consequent shallowing of the aqueous chamber makes the patient myopic. This short-sight usually amounts to about $-1\cdot0$ D, but may be a little less, or may run up to $-2\cdot0$ D, or even higher. It is quite unnecessary to do anything more than reassure the patient, as the refilling of the chamber will restore the sight to its former standard ; this usually occurs in a few days or weeks, and almost always within three months.

(2) *Minute quantities of blood in the aqueous chamber* may be just sufficient to " muddy " the fluid and so interfere with clear sight, each time the patient moves about. A corneal microscope will soon show the cause of the trouble.

(3) *Wrinkling and striate opacification of the cornea, as a result of hypotonus*, is a transitory and not uncommon cause of defective vision after operation. As the eye refills, the cornea gets back its pristine lustre and the patient once more sees well.

(4) Retinal changes, which may occur immediately after operation, and which are manifested by a diminution of central vision, by paracentral scotomata, by changes in the peripheral field, or by any or all of these together, constitute the most serious of the defects which we have under consideration, since they are likely to be lifelong. One of the gravest things which a patient can tell us immediately after operation, is that his central vision is gone, or, in his own words, that he cannot see a face or other object when he looks directly at it. It is true that some amount of recovery may subsequently take place, and that, provided decompression has been permanently attained, he may retain enough peripheral sight to enable him to move about, but the prognosis must be extremely guarded. Such a misfortune is only met with in cases in which operation is undertaken very late, and is apparently due to a failure to maintain the circulation over certain areas of the retina, as a result of profound changes in the vasomotor mechanism of the parts.

(5) Detachments of the choroid have been quoted as a cause of interference with vision; but, inasmuch as they are always placed very far forward, it may be questioned whether they have any direct rôle; it is much more likely that they are merely an evidence of hypotonus; we have already discussed some of the ways in which the latter condition may give rise to interference with the acuity of vision.

Late infections following the newer operations for glaucoma.—We must first define the term "late infection," for it has been very loosely used by some writers, with the result that much confusion has been caused. It is very important that such a state of affairs should be put an end to, and this can only be done if those who write, speak, and think on the subject clearly appreciate what they mean when they make use of the expression. All cases in which sepsis is introduced at the time of the operation must obviously be excluded. It is equally apparent that those delayed forms of eye infection, which commence from the first to the third week after an operation, and which may last many months, should be cut out of the category. Nor is this all. Inflammations following an injury to the eye, no matter how long afterwards, whether they be due to a blow, a cut, the sting of an insect, some form of chemical irritation, or any other traumatic cause, must be most jealously scrutinised before acceptance, if we are to appreciate justly the dangers of late infection, properly so called, as a sequela of operation for glaucoma. It will be better first to describe a typical case of the kind : A patient is successfully operated on by one of the newer operations ; for months, or even for years, all goes well ; then he contracts some form of septic infection of the conjunctiva, possibly of a mild type. He thinks very little of this, and neglects it, until he finds that the eye has become red and painful ; then, becoming alarmed, he hastily repairs to his surgeon, who finds the eye congested, especially in the neighbourhood of the filtering scar ; there is evidence of irido-cyclitis, and not infrequently hypopyon is present. Under energetic treatment, full vision may, in rare cases, be restored ; more often sight is permanently damaged to a greater or less extent, whilst a not uncommon event is the loss of all or nearly all vision, and even of the eye as well. If fluorescein is used, it will be found that the conjunctiva is abraded, as it covers the filtering scar, or in the near neighbourhood. If the eye is removed, the path of infection can be traced anatomically from this ulcerated spot to the interior of the globe. The sequence of events is obvious. The factors required are : (1) An infection of the conjunctiva, (2) an abrasion of the surface of that membrane to provide an entry for septic organisms, (3) a suitable path along which such organisms may travel to reach the interior of the globe, and (4) a deficiency in tissue resistance to the onslaught of that particular organism.

Having thus cleared the ground, we may proceed to endeavour to define what we mean by the term late infection : A late infection is the transmission across a filtering scar of septic organisms, which have obtained a foothold on the conjunctiva, and which, on passing into the interior of the globe, give rise to a more or less severe form of uveitis.

It will be observed that this definition in no way excludes the possibility of the sepsis being introduced by the advent from without of foreign matter capable of inflicting trauma on the lining membrane of the eye. It is readily conceivable that when a filtering scar is present, the introduction of a foreign body into the conjunctival sac is a more dangerous event than it is when it occurs in an intact eye. The risk will obviously be enhanced if the invading body is septic, or if septic matter is present in the conjunctiva beforehand. This is a very different matter from including in late infections the results of severe blows on the eye, of burns and chemical injuries, or of the stings of so virulent an insect as a bee. Even a healthy eye may become inflamed, and sometimes severely so, under similar circumstances, whilst one which has undergone any form of operation will probably run greater risks than a globe which has been spared such trauma in the past. It is a question which only time and experience can answer whether an eye, the subject of a filtering scar, runs more risks, under these circumstances, than one which has been operated on without the production of this accessory means of filtration.

It will be obvious from our definition of the term " late infection " that the danger of the occurrence of this complication must be in direct proportion to the efficiency of the scar we establish. A wound, which filters for a short time and then becomes firmly sealed up by the formation and organisation of fibrous connective tissue, cannot be the seat of a true late infection, though this fact has not always been clearly understood by writers on the subject. The form of scar, which filters longest and most freely, will *ipso facto* be that most liable to be the seat of a late infection. This, however, is the very form of scar we are all aiming to produce, since on its permanence and efficiency must always depend the lasting success of the operation we undertake.

It has been contended that it is possible to obtain a

spongy filtering scar as opposed to a fistulous scar, and that the former type of filtration area is safer than the latter (Herbert). On this subject the author has written as follows : " I have . . . pointed out that the conception of a spongy mass of fibrous tissue allowing fluid to filter through it, is absolutely opposed to everything we know of the behaviour of scar tissue. Such a conception could only be justified, if its sponsor could furnish indisputable, anatomical material, demonstrative of the correctness of his theory. Years ago I challenged anyone to bring forward such material, and it has never yet been done." Those who are interested in the subject will find the references to the discussion on it at the end of this chapter. To the author the position has always seemed a perfectly clear one, and the above words express his present view as succinctly as they do those he has always held.

A great deal has been made by some writers of the number of infections which have followed the author's procedure of sclero-corneal trephining, and there have undoubtedly been a number of cases published, and others still unpublished. It is to be remembered that late infections have also followed Lagrange's operation, Herbert's sclerotomies, Holth's punch-forceps operation, cataract extraction, and even iridectomy. If equal volumes of statistics are dealt with, it seems likely that the number of cases of late infection following a procedure is to some extent a measure of the efficiency of that procedure in establishing filtration. Sclero-corneal trephining has appealed so strongly to surgeons that the operation has been performed an enormous number of times in the last few years, as compared with any other method. Its very popularity has thus been somewhat of a handicap to it. There is a still more important point to take into account, viz., the technique adopted by different surgeons. Gifford, who himself met with a case of late infection in his practice, and who is well known as an exceptionally skilful and able surgeon, has, in a very generous article, pointed out that neither Lagrange nor the author has met with one of these late disasters, and has attributed this immunity to our technique of using thick flaps. Lagrange's experience is a very large one, extending over many years, whilst the author is now able to speak from the figures of over a thousand trephinings, amongst which more than two hundred have been followed for periods varying from a few months to seven years. Again Kirkpatrick, whose experience of trephining is probably numerically one of the largest in the world, and who has closely followed the author's technique, cannot recall a single undoubted case of this complication in his own experience. It is not intended to belittle the importance of late infections, or to suggest that such an occurrence constitutes a reflection on a surgeon's method; in the case of operative procedures, of so recent an origin as the newer operations for glaucoma, it is obvious that we all still have much to learn. At the same time, a noteworthy feature in the experience of surgeons who have performed these newer operations, has been the extraordinary discrepancy in their results. One surgeon has had 20 per cent. of late infections, and another has had 10 per cent.; whilst a number of European and American surgeons of large experience, have not had a single case of the kind. It is clear that the factor of the individual operator has something to do with these discrepancies, and it seems possible that there are surgeons who will get better results in their own work by adopting other operations than trephining. The author believes that this number would be greatly reduced, if those who perform his operation would study the technique he has laid down, instead of adopting modifications of their own, as so many seem to have done. This comment is offered in no carping spirit, but as an appeal for a fair trial of a method whose details he has taken great trouble in working out as fully as possible.

It would be both wrong and foolish to make light of the danger of late infection, but it is necessary to look at the whole question in its largest aspects. In treating glaucoma, we are not dallying with a condition of secondary importance. We are fighting desperately for our patient to save him from the horrors of life-long blindness, and in doing so we must take the *pros* and *cons* of the case into account, and must be ready to accept some risks. The author believes that with a suitable technique, these risks can be reduced to very modest dimensions, and that the essential element in such reduction is expressed in the words " use thick flaps." In this connection Wilmer's experience in Washington is highly significant ; for, not only has he had no instance of late infection, but he has had the opportunity of seeing four of the eyes he had trephined suffer from acute and dangerous conjunctivitis during a local epidemic, without any one of them coming to the least harm.

Once a late infection has occurred, we can only treat it on ordinary surgical lines ; but we can do something to make its occurrence less likely and less frequent. Of that there can be no doubt.

The author would suggest that there are two conditions, which may possibly pave the way for the invasion of this form of sepsis. The first of these is the persistence of a leakage somewhere along the line of the original conjunctival incision. In a certain number of cases, one observes that after operation the anterior chamber remains very shallow. It has already been mentioned that if, after an eye is cocainised, the lids are widely separated and a cotton-wool sponge mounted on a stick is applied by gentle dabbing along the periphery of the original conjunctival flap, one will find, in a certain percentage of cases, that a steady escape of fluid is taking place through a tiny fistulette at a point where the conjunctival incision has evidently failed to close. It seems not improbable that this affords an explanation of late infection in those cases in which a shallow chamber has been noted as a prominent feature of the case. Presumably, where fluid can escape from within outwards, accidentally introduced pathogenic organisms may be able to effect an entrance from without. The second condition is that in which the filtration area is found to be covered by a very thin layer of tissue : in such cases the appearance presented is almost vesicular, and in some the vesicle is extremely prominent. An abrasion of the surface epithelium would, under these conditions, not only be likely to occur, but would be of very serious import if it did occur. In any case it is clear, as has already been pointed out, that two distinct and very unfortunate conditions must be present in order to determine the onset of a late infection, viz., (1) an abrasion of the surface epithelium, and (2) a coincident growth of pathogenic organisms in the conjunctival sac. The obvious lessons to be learnt are (1) to aim at forming flaps with thick bases, (2) to protect an operated eye from injury by every means in our power, (3) to impress on patients the importance of remaining for a considerable time at least under medical supervision, and of always looking upon any catarrhal condition of the conjunctiva as serious, and (4) to keep in touch with every trephined eye so long as a catarrh is present, and to give instructions for the treatment of any conjunctivitis which may subsequently arise.

In bringing out the present edition of this work, the author has read very carefully the cases of late infection which have appeared since 1918, and has given attention to the views on the subject that have appeared in the widespread literature of ophthalmology. Having done so, he has left most of what he had to say in the first edition, as it then stood, for the simple reason that he still holds the same views as before, strengthened if possible both by his own recent experience and by that of many others. This seems to him to be one of the questions of surgery on which it is essential to take broad views, and to avoid the evils of panic.

The Vesicular Filtration Scar has been mentioned under the previous heading, and has also received some attention in Chapter IX. Part VIII., but there still remain some matters to discuss in connection with it. It is thought by some to be the *usual* scar that follows a trephine operation. This is totally erroneous. The typical trephine-scar is flat or but slightly raised, resembling closely the Lagrange scar ; when it tends to be raised into a vesicle the probable conclusion is that the technique has been faulty. It is not contended that we never get a vesicular filtration scar after trephining ; we may get such a scar after any procedure that perforates the ocular tunic, *e.g.*, cataract extraction, iridectomy, or any glaucoma operation. Moreover, *with a faulty technique*, it is more likely to follow an operation which drills a clean hole through the eye, as trephining does, than with one which makes an oblique and narrow fistula. In order to avoid this defective form of scar the operator should make his conjunctival flaps as thick as possible, by following out the technique that has been laid down in the chapter already quoted (Chapter IX. Part VIII.).

There is another point to take into consideration, viz., that patients with very thin conjunctivæ are probably more liable to get vesicular scars than those with thick membranes. Experience has, however, conclusively demonstrated that good flat scars may be obtained even in these patients, if proper care is taken in the preparation of the flaps.

Since the author has adopted his present technique of thick-based flaps, he has very rarely indeed met with bulging scars, and he believes that this complication can be practically eliminated by proper care.

There are several disadvantages in the cystoid scar : (1) It can sometimes be seen bulging through the lid, and is then cosmetically objectionable. (2) It may give rise to a sense of discomfort, apparently due to the localised pressure it exercises on the lid from within ; it may be so prominent as to catch on the edge of the upper lid. On one occasion the author saw a very curious accident in one of these cases : The patient was told to look steadily downward for examination of a large bulging cicatrix left by a trephining. Instead of doing so, she looked up suddenly, caught the cyst on the lid edge, and broke it with an audible click, the fluid flowing freely from her eye. She declared that she was then much more comfortable. The cyst leaked for some weeks and she has said ever since that she never was so free of trouble since she first got glaucoma as during this period. (3) It presents but a very thin wall between the intra-ocular fluid within and any dangerous germs without, and so may predispose to the onset of a late infection of the eye; indeed in some of the recorded cases of the latter complication, stress has been laid on the fact that the scar was cystoid. (4) Apart from any actual, physical inconvenience, it may get badly on a patient's nerves, and lead him to fear all sorts of future possibilities.

The treatment of this condition.—Repeated painting of a vesicular filtration scar with a solution of nitrate of silver (gr. x ad ʒi) has in two cases in the author's experience led to a distinct condensation of the overlying tissue together with a shrinking of the bulging cyst, without in any degree interfering with the filtration through the trephine hole. It is important to confine the application carefully to the area of the scar, so as to avoid giving unnecessary pain to the patient.

REFERENCES

COLLINS, E. T.—*Proc. of Seventeenth International Congress of Medicine,* London, 1913.
ELLIOT, R. H.—*Sclero-corneal Trephining,* 2nd edition, 1914, Geo. Pulman & Sons Ltd., London, p. 113.
ELLIOT, R. H.—*Brit. Journ. Ophth.*, 1921, vol. v. pp. 91–95 and 237–238.
FUCHS, E.—*Archiv f. O.*, 1900, vol. li. pt. 2 ; 1903, vol. liii. pt. 3.
GIFFORD, H.—*Ophth. Rec.*, 1914, vol. xxiii. p. 4.
HERBERT, H.—*Brit. Journ. Ophth.*, 1920, vol. iv. pp. 550–555; and 1921, vol. v. pp. 183–7.
HUDSON, A. C.—*R.L.O.H. Reports,* January 1914, vol. xix. pt. 2.
KIRKPATRICK, H.—Personal communication.
KNAPP, ARNOLD.—*Arch. of Ophth.*, 1914, vol. xliii. No. 2.
KNAPP, HERMAN.—*Die intraoculare Geschwulste,* p. 194.
MELLER, J.—*Archiv f. O.*, 1912, vol. lxxx. pt. 1.
MORAX, V.—*Glaucome et Glaucomateux,* 1921, Librairie Octave Doin, Paris.
SCHUR, M.—*Klin. Monatsbl. f. Augenh.*, Sept. 1913.
WILMER, W. H.—*Soc. Med. Journ.*, 1915, p. 419 ; and *Ophth. Year Book,* 1915, vol. xii. p. 168.

CHAPTER X

THE PATHOLOGY OF FILTRATION

Part I

The Filtering Scar in the Treatment of Glaucoma

In the preceding chapters we have spoken often of the filtering scar, and of its rôle in the arrest of glaucoma. To form such a scar, and to ensure that it is permanent in its action, is the aim and object of the modern operations. We have shown that von Graefe appreciated its value in his iridectomies, and that he drew attention to its frequency in his practice; but that it was left to de Wecker to point out clearly that the goal towards which the glaucoma surgeon should press was the attainment of a technique that would ensure *the regular and systematic* formation of the filtering cicatrix, as the result of his operative interference. It is to Lagrange's everlasting credit that, by the introduction of sclerectomy, he was the first to show how this end could be effected. The œdema of the conjunctiva over the filtering scar was well known to von Graefe and to de Wecker in the middle of the last century, and Lagrange was so familiar with it in his everyday work that he hardly troubled to dispute with those who doubted it. Under the circumstances, it cannot but seem strange that in the early years of the present century very few ophthalmologists accepted the possibility of its existence, and that even a decade ago some denied it *in toto*. To-day, the experience of hundreds of surgeons has translated it into the domain of universally accepted facts. At first there was a strong disposition to believe that the entanglement of uveal tissue in the wound was a necessary factor in the establishment of filtration through it. Holth, who was one of the first to make anatomical examinations of eyes which had been subjected to the different forms of modern glaucoma operations, and who found that fistulæ had been established by all of them alike, pointed out that "if the sclerectomy be performed according to Elliot's technique, the iris seldom remains in the wound, but retreats into the anterior chamber. But if the punch-operation be performed . . . it is easy to leave a tag of iris in the aperture, with the result that an iris fistula remains." He believed that the maintenance of continued fistulisation was *dependent upon the lining of the walls of the wound with uveal pigment*. That so able and distinguished an authority on glaucoma as Holth is, should so recently have held such views, shows how wide and deep the cleavage of opinion on this subject has been amongst those who have taken an interest in it. Lagrange and the author have from the first contended that an iris-free cicatrix is the end and aim of the surgeon's effort, that the entanglement of uveal tissue is a misfortune, and that clinical experience has proved these points up to the hilt. It is necessary, however, to pause for one moment to point out the difference between a *clinically* iris-free scar, and the same condition *anatomically*. The latter must be very rarely met with, the former can be attained very frequently by the adoption of a correct technique. Verhoeff was one of the first, if not actually the first, to prove this microscopically. His description is as follows :

"The fistula was filled with an extremely delicate connective tissue, almost free from cells"; this tissue had evidently originated, not from the sclera, but from the tissue of the bleb. Within it were numerous irregular ill-defined empty spaces, which communicated with other spaces, which opened directly into the anterior chamber ; the latter were therefore taken to be analogous to the iris crypts. Neither the free surface of the tissue nor the spaces of the crypts showed any endothelial lining. "The edges of the scleral fistula showed evidences of recent proliferation, with formation of new fibrous tissue, and increase in the number of fixed cells." This was attributed to the trauma of the operation. There had also been some proliferation from the outer surface of the sclera everywhere beneath the conjunctival bleb, which surmounted the fistula. The resulting new tissue had a much denser character than that of the bleb itself, and had, in places, extended as a thin layer over the outer end of the fistula, contracting the diameter of the opening. Descemet's membrane ended abruptly about 0·5 mm. from the edge of the opening, apparently having retracted from it. The conjunctival bleb was not really a bleb, for it consisted of an œdematous delicate connective tissue meshwork, closely similar to iris stroma ; ramifying within this tissue were irregular communicating spaces which were incompletely filled with connective tissue, so extremely delicate as to be scarcely visible. None of them was lined with endothelium or had definite walls ; they evidently resulted from the distension of the tissue spaces by intra-ocular pressure. The œdematous tissue extended down into the fistula for about two-thirds of its depth.

An examination of Verhoeff's micro-photographs distinctly shows the inclusion of uveal pigment in the depth of the wound, although satisfactory filtration had clearly been established. The period after operation was, however, only 52 days. Figs. 198 to 203 are from an eyeball removed over two and a half years after a trephine operation had been performed. Unfortunately, the clinical history of the eye could not be satisfactorily obtained. The filtration scar was perfect, the tension was low, and the eye had to be removed for another reason, independent of the glaucoma. Verhoeff's description of his specimen could be applied almost verbatim to the sections of this eyeball. These two sets of observations (Verhoeff's and the author's) set the seal of anatomical confirmation on the existence of the clinically iris-free filtering-scar.

As a result of his recent valuable work on the histology of filtering scars, Holth has added some details of interest. He writes : " The conjunctiva bulbi has in all the preparations normal and unimpaired epithelium; in the more or less cushion-like part, covering the field of operation, the conjunctival connective tissue is seen to have the fibres somewhat closer together and to be somewhat richer in cells than normally, especially towards the episclera, from which the conjunctiva was loosened . . . in the early stages of the operations. No cells show degenerative changes,

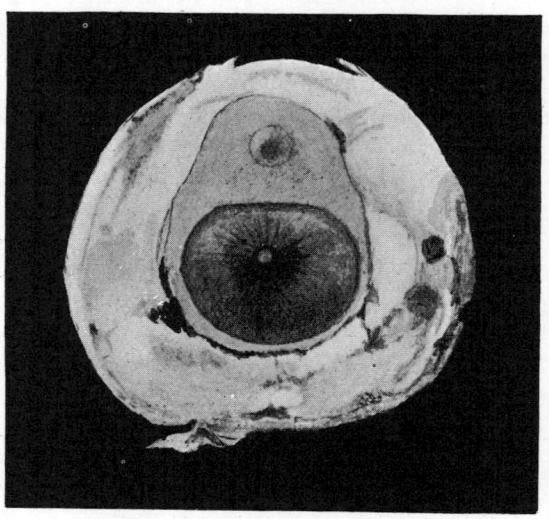

Fig. 198.—An eyeball photographed immediately after removal, and drawn from the photograph by E. E.

The conjunctiva forming the filtering scar was spared at the excision. Notice the flattening of the upper border of the cornea due to that membrane having been split for the trephine operation. The dark area around the trephine hole can still be seen. It was very definite before the removal of the eye. The pupil was occluded.

all are strongly staining . . . in none of the preparations are seen signs of hyaline degeneration."

It may be asked: What is the origin of the view so widely held, that the entanglement of uveal tissue in the track of a wound in the globe favours the formation of a filtering cicatrix? It is admitted that such wounds in which the inclusion of iris tissue has been followed by the

THE PATHOLOGY OF FILTRATION 607

establishment of permanent filtration are not very uncommon; but does this necessarily imply a cause-and-effect relationship between the two things? The following evidence will help to answer this question.

(1) Clinical experience has clearly shown (*a*) that the impaction of uveal tissue in the trephine hole is a great

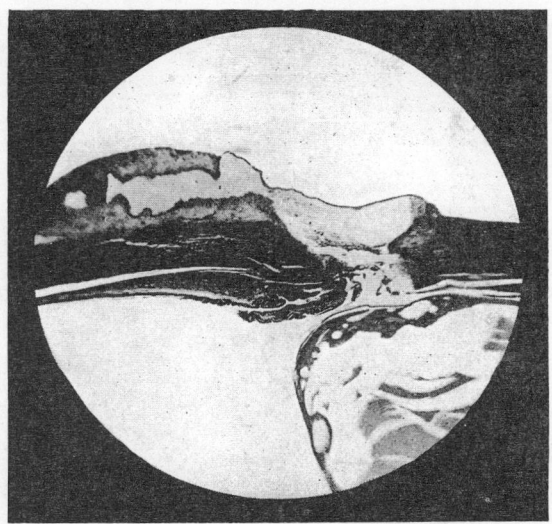

Fig. 199.—A meridional section through the fistula and the filtering scar.

The ciliary body is entangled in its depths; it will be observed in Fig. 198 that the surgeon who performed the operation trephined rather far out, and so lost some of the advantage gained by the splitting of the cornea. The fistulous passage is in free communication with a widely open subconjunctival filtering space. The tissue in both cases is made up of extremely loose connective tissue, very poor in cells, and enclosing a large number of open spaces, which are nowhere lined by endothelium.

(*Photo by E. E.*)

menace to the maintenance, and often even to the establishment of filtration; and (*b*) that the more carefully the trephine hole is guarded against iris invasion the more even and uneventful is the course of convalescence.

(2) Many surgeons have had the opportunity of observing eyes, in which subconjunctival filtration had been

accidentally produced by various operative measures, and had been maintained for years, without there being any *clinical* evidence of the entanglement of iris tissue in the wound.

(3) We have shown that anatomical evidence has been forthcoming of the practical freedom from uveal tissue of fistulæ which had permitted free filtration to occur. On the other hand, the examination of eyes, in which the

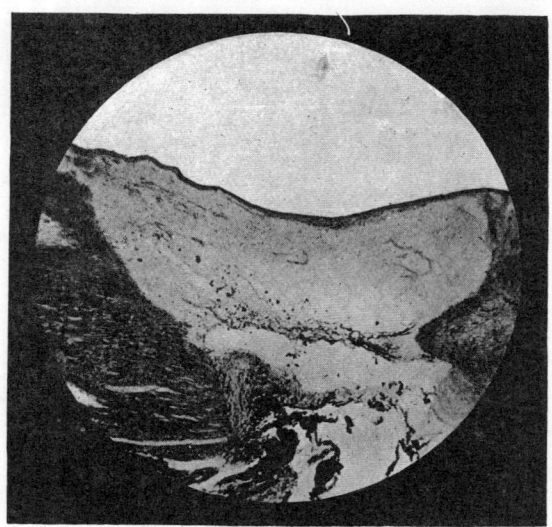

FIG. 200.—The scleral fistula on a larger scale (from Fig. 199). To the left upper corner of the figure is the communication between the fistula and the subconjunctival filtering scar.
(*Photo by E. E.*)

trephine hole had become blocked by the proliferation of connective tissue, has shown the presence of pigmentary tissue in a large number of the wounds, thus suggesting a cause-and-effect relationship between the entanglement of the uveal tissue and the subsequent blockage of the wound.

(4) The question may also be approached from another point of view. It has happened to most surgeons, at one time or another, to have to open a cataract wound in

THE PATHOLOGY OF FILTRATION 609

order to free it of impacted iris tissue. If this be done within twelve hours of the prolapse, or even within twenty-four hours, there is not the slightest difficulty in breaking down the feeble adhesions between the lips of the wound. If, however, we attempt to do the same thing after three or four days, or longer, we find that the most difficult part of the wound to open is that where the iris tissue is

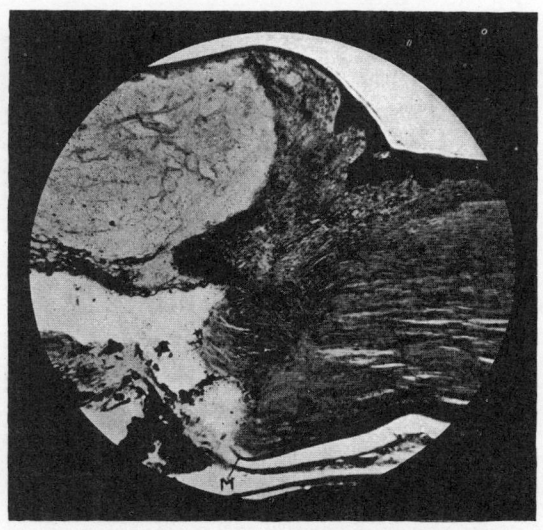

Fig. 201.—The right-hand wall of the fistula.

Notice the thinning of the surface epithelium over the filtering scar, and the membrane of Descemet cut off short in the depth of the wound. *M*, Cut end of Descemet's membrane.

(*Photo by E. E.*)

impacted. This is only what might have been expected, since the vascular iris provides a proliferative exudation more readily than does the much less vascular sclero-corneal tunic. Such an experience suggests that impacted iris does not tend to keep a wound open, but rather helps to seal it firmly up.

One solution that naturally occurs to any thoughtful mind is, that possibly those wounds, which have a predisposition (owing to the fact that they gape, or that they are slow in healing) to become filtering wounds, are the very ones into which intra-ocular tissues, such as the iris, are most apt to prolapse, with the result that they become imprisoned therein. The suggestion is that the impaction of iris in a wound is not necessarily the cause of its developing into a filtering scar, but that it may be an accidental complication, which is more likely to occur

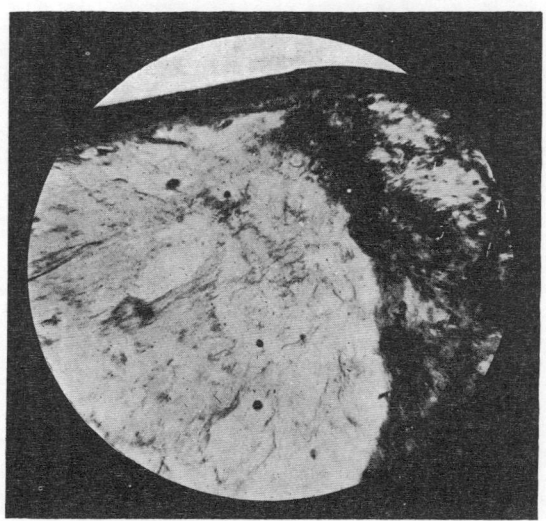

FIG. 202.—The right-hand upper corner of Fig. 201, on a still larger scale, to demonstrate the loose connective tissue which encloses the wide open spaces of the filtering scar.

(*Photo by E. E.*)

in the type of wound which favours the production of such scars. Clinically, the question is one of very great importance, and it therefore merits the most careful consideration.

The author desires to avoid with the utmost care any suspicion of the presentation of an *ex parte* statement on this extremely important subject, which has caused such great differences of opinion among ophthalmologists. He feels that the issues at stake are far too large, and he would therefore invite very special attention to the interesting and valuable writings of Holth to which the reader has already been more than once referred, and to which full references are given at the end of this chapter. In his latest paper (January 1922) Holth has shown photographs from a number of scars, which had continued to filter for comparatively long periods after the performance of iridencleisis, trephining, and the punch-forceps operation. With regard to the first-named operation—there is one feature which at once strikes anyone who studies these photographs, viz., that the track of the fistula is lined on its inner aspect by the opposed surfaces of the posterior layer of the iris, whilst the anterior layer of that membrane is apparently adherent to the scleral and subconjunctival tissue which surrounds it. The transudation of fluid, which occurred during filtration in these eyes, must presumably have taken place across the tissues of the iris. That it could do so will surprise no one who is accustomed to examine the iris in health, under high magnifications of the corneal microscope, and illuminated by a Gullstrand lamp. The sponginess of the iris tissue must be studied in this way to be appreciated. Incidentally, a very interesting point in this connection is the great variation in the relative "sponginess" of different irises. It has often suggested itself to the author's mind that such variations may be a contributory, and perhaps a not unimportant factor in an individual's predisposition to glaucoma. To return to our original subject, it would appear that the difference between the undoubtedly filtering scars we have been discussing and the tightly-closed cicatrices of certain of our cataract extractions—in which iris tissue has accidentally become impacted, with the result that it has helped to seal them up—may lie in the fact that the former include a knuckle of iris whose posterior surface forms the whole inner lining of the wall of the fistula. For the establishment of efficient fistulisation in this way, we may unhesitatingly assume that the one great condition necessary is the absolute asepsis of the technique employed ; indeed, we have had more than one occasion to descant on the absence of any tendency to proliferation, on the part of the iris, sclera, and cornea, when these are cut or injured, always provided that the aqueous fluid which bathes them is aseptic throughout. Holth, as has already been stated, was originally of the opinion that the establishment of a filtering scar depended on the lining of the walls of the sclerotomy wound with uveal pigment. The photographs from trephined eyes in his most recent paper do not appear to bear out such a contention, but rather fall into line with Verhoeff's and the author's anatomical findings. Holth has evidently taken this view in the light of his more extended and very valuable work.

The author in no way challenges Holth's contention that admirable filtering scars can be obtained by suitably performed iris-inclusion operations ; on the contrary, he accepts it unhesitatingly. What he does maintain is that equally good scars, so far as the filtration is concerned, can be got without any inclusion of uveal tissue beyond that which is accidental and unavoidable. He thinks that such anatomical evidence as is available—and it is not by any means negligible—only serves to reinforce the teaching of clinical experience that "the aim of the glaucoma operator should be the establishment of an iris-free filtering scar." This is the doctrine he has preached from the beginning, and he holds it, if possible, more strongly after twelve years' experience of trephining than ever before.

This brings us to a second point on which Holth has expressed himself very clearly. He says "after iridencleisis, as well as after sclerectomies, *a real fistula* through the limbal sclera is seen several years after the operation, *if successful.*" The italics are not in the original. This is a robust statement, founded on anatomical work, and contrasting strongly with Herbert's oft-repeated, but to the author's mind mistaken conception of a *spongy filtering*, as distinct from a fistulous scar. Herbert would postulate as the surgeon's desideratum a sclerectomy or sclerotomy aperture "fully occupied by new fibrocellular tissue." He describes a filtering scar admittedly in the process of contraction, and considers the stage in which he thus encountered it as illustrative of "the final condition of the scars, which are found clinically to filter permanently and satisfactorily." Apart altogether from the fact that such a conception is diametrically opposed to all that pathology has taught us of the behaviour of fibrocellular tissue, the important point remains that *no anatomical evidence* of such a form of scar has ever yet been brought forward, as the end-result of a glaucoma operation which has proved clinically successful. It is both interesting and encouraging to find Holth, the pioneer and the greatest exponent of this line of work, expressing himself in such unhesitating terms as those quoted above ; for, be it noted, this is no academic discussion, but a matter on which the soundness or otherwise of our future lines of operative treatment depend. If the surgeon sees clearly that it is a fistula that he desires, and a fistula that he must have, he will bend all his energies to the attainment of his object under the best possible conditions, and will also be prepared to take certain risks, if necessary, in so doing. If, on the other hand, he allows himself to be misled by the idea that he can relieve his patient by some less drastic procedure, then there is a fear, and more than a fear, that he will be lacking in aim and uncertain in purpose. This is no plea for one form of operation rather than another ; it is an appeal to first principles, which we cannot violate without injury to the heritage we are to hand down to posterity. It is for this reason that so much emphasis has been here laid on the subject.

Holth has pointed out a way in which a successfully established fistula may, at a late date, cease to filter : In his section of a trephine wound he observed scar tissue reaching out " from the posterior (ciliary) wall of the scleral defect after the trephining " into the fine spongy tissue of the fistula itself. He thinks that this process might in time have closed up the whole aperture, and he endeavours to draw a distinction between " the clean-cut keratome incision for sclerectomy with punch forceps from the anterior wound lip " and what he evidently considers is the much less clean-cut trephine wound. In the broad principle involved the author would agree with Holth : Any excess of trauma during the operation would favour the subsequent formation of connective tissue, but there is another side to the question : (1) Might not such an appearance as Holth found in this section have been produced by a transitory reaction immediately following the operation ? Does it necessarily connote a progressive process which would have led to complete obstruction of the filtering channel ? (2) If such a change were progressive, and if it developed at a late stage of the case, it would be difficult to exclude the influence of autogenetic poisoning, and to be sure that the operative conditions were really causal. (3) Holth's assumption that the wound produced by his operation is more clean-cut than that of trephining, will not find acceptance with those who are expert in the latter operation, and who use sharp trephines. If a freshly trephined scleral disc which has been removed in its whole circumference by a trephine is examined under magnification, it will be seen that its edges are as clean and sharp as if cut with a knife. If a hinge is left at the operation and cut across with sharp scissors, that part too of the disc which has been thus cut across is seen to have a smooth sharp edge. One can safely assume that a sharp pair of iris-scissors will cut at least as cleanly as a Holth's punch. The probability is that they cut cleaner. Later on in this chapter we shall have occasion to show photographs of a number of discs removed by trephining. If allowance is made for the effects of shrinkage and of the microtome-cutting of these tiny portions of tissue—a very difficult task—it will be admitted that the surfaces are very clean cut indeed. The author has been able to follow for many years a fairly large number of trephined cases, and he has found them filtering steadily and continuously. What would be the fate of trephine holes cut with blunt instruments—whether trephines or scissors he has no means of knowing, but such a complication can be so easily avoided that it hardly merits serious discussion.

Holth has drawn attention to weeping filtering scars

which can, he says, be detected by Dr. Eric Seidel's fluorescein test [1] "after many cases of sclero-corneal trephining; the aqueous oozes out on the surface of the eye from the thin conjunctival bubble; this bubble at first becomes green by fluorescein, then the oozing aqueous in a slow stream, following the law of gravitation, washes the green colour away." Some eight years ago, when the author was on a visit to America, Dr. Verhoeff drew his attention to oozing from the filtering scar of a trephine wound. This led him to study this matter carefully: A well-made trephine scar does not weep, even when tested a week after the operation—and this is the earliest time that it seems wise and safe to apply such a test. There is in normal cases no staining of the scar under fluorescein, and no evidence of transudation of fluid through the scar as observed under corneal magnification. Rarely one may find cases in which transudation across the scar takes place and in which the patient consequently complains of watering of the eye under conditions of irritation (smoke, dust, wind, etc.), but such transudation may be absent even in thin, vesicular-looking scars. The most important point of all to drive home is that, given a proper technique, the trephine scar should, in nearly all instances, be thick and fleshy; an ectatic, vesicular scar is an evidence, in most cases at least, of faulty technique. It is not contended that such scars can be altogether abolished from our experience, but they should at least be rare, and should be looked upon as defective results. Incidentally we may mention that great improvement may be expected from the painting of such scars with a solution of silver nitrate (grs. x ad ʒi) at weekly intervals.

Holth has drawn attention to two very interesting phenomena: (1) The diminution in apparent size of the sclerectomy defect as seen immediately after the operation and some time later; and (2) the appearance of "a secondary fistula in the subconjunctival tissue communicating with the original one in the sclera." Both these subjects merit discussion.

[1] See footnote on p. 579.

(1) The word "apparent" has been deliberately used above. There can be no question that a number of trephine cases return for later inspection with the trephine hole apparently much smaller and certainly much less distinct than at the time of operation. If, however, these cases are watched from the commencement, it will be observed that the superjacent pad of conjunctiva and subconjunctival tissue which, in some cases, is at first very translucent, and even indeed almost transparent, very soon becomes much denser, and so hides the details of the fistula. The author has observed this to occur over and over again in cases which have continued to filter freely and satisfactorily. At the same time the tendency to marked hypotonus which characterises many trephined eyes immediately after the operation, is steadily replaced by an intra-ocular pressure which much more nearly approximates to the normal. The obvious explanation would appear to be that the flap raised at the time of operation becomes again normally reapplied to its scleral bed, and at the same time undergoes a certain and very desirable amount of condensation.

(2) The appearance of a secondary fistula communicating with the original one in the sclera raises a topic of considerable academic interest. In the second edition of *Sclero-corneal Trephining* the following paragraph appears :

"The author has had his attention called by two surgeons to cases of a very curious nature. The first was reported to him by Captain W. C. Gray, who said 'it looks almost as if spontaneous trephining had occurred.' A definite filtration area was found at the usual seat of trephining. The second case was quite independently reported by an American colleague, whose name the author regrets he has forgotten, but who said he would publish details of the case. The condition closely resembled that in Captain Gray's case. In both, high tension seems to have been relieved by the establishment of filtration ; in both it was apparently quite certain that no operation had been performed ; and in both the filtration area appears to have lain in the neighbourhood of a perforating vessel. The author suggests that a spontaneous relief of pressure had been established by the occurrence of the escape of fluid in some way from the interior of the eye into the subconjunctival area, through one of the apertures of exit of a perforating vessel. It would be of great interest if surgeons would report any cases of the kind in full."

The author has at the present time under his care a lady on whom he performed trephining four years ago. She consulted him recently in a state of anxiety, because she had noticed the appearance of a second dark spot on her filtering scar. This lay to one side of the original trephine hole, and there was a slight increase of filtration immediately over it. The condition of the eye was in all respects satisfactory. It was clear that a small accessory channel, similar to those of which Holth speaks, had been opened up during the previous year, and, though this could not be certainly made out, it seemed probable that the fluid had made its way through the sclera along the channel transmitting a vessel. Holth has suggested that in these cases of accessory fistulisation it may be "that the aqueous has forced its way through the cicatricial roof of the scleral defect and made a secondary fistula in the sub-conjunctival tissue communicating with the original one in the sclera." He admits that this will not explain all cases, as it obviously will not the one quoted above.

REFERENCES

ELLIOT, R. H.—*Brit. Journ. Ophth.*, 1921, vol. v. pp. 91 and 237.
HERBERT, H.—*Ibid.*, 1920, vol. iv. p. 553 ; and 1921, vol. v. p. 183.
HOLTH, S.—" The Anatomy of Successful Glaucoma Operations," *Bericht der Ophthal. Gesell.*, Heidelberg, 1913, p. 355 ; and *The Ophthalmoscope*, 1914, p. 347.
HOLTH, S.—*Brit. Journ. Ophth.*, 1922, pp. 10–22.
SEIDEL, E.—*Arch. f. Ophth.*, 1920, vol. cii. p. 371, and vol. civ. p. 158 (Holth., *Brit. Journ. Ophth.*, 1922, vol. vi. p. 20).
VERHOEFF, F. H.—" Histological Findings after Successful Sclerostomy," *Arch. Ophth.*, March 1915, vol. xliv., No. 2 ; and *The Ophthalmoscope* 1915, vol. xiii. p. 352.

Part II

The Histology of the Trephined Disc in Glaucoma Operations

In the previous Part of this Chapter, we have discussed the gap which is left in the sclera or corneo-sclera after trephining operations for glaucoma, and which has been studied in man by Holth, Verhoeff, Greeves, and the writer. Experimental studies on trephined eyes have been made in animals by Ducamp, Barraquer, Clausen, and Ellett. C. H. Reinhold and W. C. Gray have carried out similar work, which has led to the adoption of conclusions identical with those arrived at by the four writers above named, but they have never published their findings. It will be observed that all this valuable and instructive mass of research work has confined itself strictly to the hole made in the eyeball by the trephine, and to the subsequent behaviour of the edges of that aperture, whilst the condition of the disc removed to form the filtering channel has hitherto apparently received no attention whatever. The writer has had a number of the discs which he has removed by trephining sectioned for examination, and he thinks they present features of sufficient interest to justify a short record of the work.

On purely clinical grounds, he has from the first insisted on the importance of removing the whole thickness of the trephined disc, and has recommended the use of a special pair of forceps to facilitate the seizure of any portion of the deeper layer which might accidentally have been left behind, owing to the trephine having failed to cut through the tunic of the eye with sufficient completeness. Treacher Collins has given a more precise significance to this clinical recommendation as the result of his pathological findings, and has insisted on "the establishment of a permanent gap in the endothelium of Descemet's membrane" as "the most essential feature in the operation" of sclerocorneal trephining. He says : " In a perforating wound of the eye the restoration of the continuity of the endothelium of Descemet's membrane may be impeded in various ways, under which circumstances the filtration of the aqueous humour through it is prolonged or rendered permanent." He goes on to mention the three ways in which this permanence may be brought about, one of which we shall quote : " The gap, formed in the tissue at the seat of the wound, may be so wide that the endothelium is unable to extend across it. The latter is what probably occurs in the operation of sclero-corneal trephining, which renders it so eminently successful. A piece of the whole thickness of the sclero-corneal tissue at the limbus . . . is removed, and the possibility of the endothelium being able to extend round the whole of the inner surface of such a gap is exceedingly unlikely."

It is of interest in this connection to recall Ducamp's observations on the failure of the trephine hole to remain permanent in his experiments on cats. He specially notes that in these operations Descemet's membrane was simply incised and not excised, even when the performance of an iridectomy, made *à ciel ouvert*, proved that the anterior chamber had been perforated by the trephine, and he concluded that the leaving behind of Descemet's membrane was an important factor in the healing of his corneo-scleral wounds in cats, and of those of others in human subjects. It is well known now that trephining experiments conducted on animals are inconclusive and unsatisfactory, and possibly an element in this may be a difficulty in effecting the complete removal of Descemet's membrane in them. As will presently appear, the same difficulty does not hold in operations on man, in whom, granted a proper technique, the whole thickness of the tunic can be easily and certainly removed in the great majority of cases.

This point is well illustrated by Figs. 199, 201, and 203, which present photographs taken from the writer's examination of an eye in which a successful trephine operation had been performed two and a half years earlier. The first of these figures gives a general view of the fistulous track established, whilst the other two, under a higher power, show the membrane of Descemet cut short at the opposite ends of the wound. It will be observed that on the scleral side of the opening that membrane is cut just internal to the point where it breaks up to form the pectinate ligament. Attention is also invited to the irregular hyaline thickenings on its deep surface.

A number of trephined discs have been sectioned and stained in various ways. In all such, the membrane of Descemet, or this membrane and its continuation, the

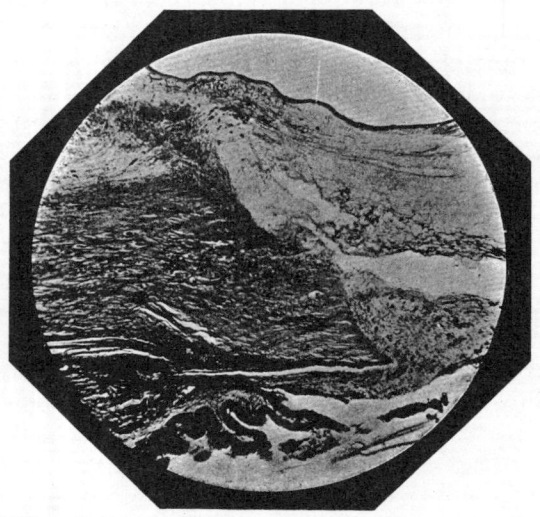

FIG. 203.—The scleral wall of the fistula shown in Fig. 199. The membrane of Descemet can be clearly seen sharply cut across on the edge of the fistula. On tracing it to the left, hyaline excrescences are seen on its surface; farther still to the left, it breaks up to form the pectinate ligament.

pectinate ligament, can uniformly be demonstrated forming a lining of the deep surface of the disc, always provided that a sufficient number of sections are examined, and that the technique has been correctly carried out. A good deal depends on the method of cutting employed, on the sharpness of the microtome blade used, and on the direction in which the cut is made (*i.e.* whether it presses the membrane up against the mass of the section, or tears it away from it).

The examination of a number of sections has shown that a complete 2 mm. disc, cut according to the author's method, often includes an appreciable part of the pectinate ligament. It has also made it clear that the pectinate ligament and that portion of Descemet's membrane close to it, is much more firmly adherent to the subjacent layers of the cornea than is the same membrane farther inward (*i.e.*, farther on to the cornea). This looseness of attachment between the membrane and the cornea is well illustrated in a number of our specimens.

Some stress has been laid by writers on the importance of applying the trephine in such a position that the disc excised shall be lined wholly by Descemet's membrane to the exclusion of the pectinate ligament, and this has been made an argument for the use of smaller trephines than those advocated by the writer. On this subject Treacher Collins writes: " Elliot has frequently laid stress on the importance of making the trephine hole well forwards. . . . It is, I suggest, always desirable that the piece removed should include a complete disc of Descemet's membrane and not encroach on the ligamentum pectinatum, which in many cases of glaucoma has the root of the iris in immediate contact with it. I have found experimentally that the line of junction between clear cornea and opaque sclerotic on the surface of the globe is 1 mm. internal to the position where Descemet's membrane commences to split up into the fibres of the ligamentum pectinatum. If therefore a 1·5 mm. trephine is used, and the centre of it is placed over the margin of the cornea on the surface of the globe, a complete disc of Descemet's membrane will be found on the posterior surface of the piece excised." It is pertinent here to mention Greeves' work on this subject. He has shown that to trephine far out is hazardous, inasmuch as it involves a risk of the implication of the ciliary processes in the trephine hole, and he has suggested that the sudden bulging of the ciliary body into the wound may suffice to rupture the zonule of fibres in the neighbourhood, and so to allow a prolapse of the ciliary processes.

The writer has found that it is easy to split the cornea over a distance of 1 mm. in the great majority of cases. Using a 2 mm. trephine, this technique should just enable the operator to cut through Descemet's membrane all round his disc, assuming Collins' measurements to be correct. The latter does not, however, specify in what meridian of the eye his measurements were made; this point is not unimportant, for Rochon-Duvigneaud has shown that the interval between the transparent edge of the cornea on the one hand and the angle of the chamber on the other varies considerably according to the direction in which the measurement is made; thus, above the cornea in the vertical axis, the average is 2·5 mm., below the cornea 2 mm., and to the nasal or temporal side, in the horizontal axis, 1·25 mm. The writer controlled these measurements on eyes in Madras, and found that the averages were slightly lower than those arrived at by the French worker. This was probably to be expected, as the Southern Indian is on the average a smaller and lighter man than the European.

For the moment we may leave the theoretical method of approaching the question on one side and deal with certain facts which stand out clearly from the examination of a number of trephined discs. These are as follows:

(1) It is not only possible, but it is even easy with a sharp trephine to cut out a portion of disc, which, in the anterior part of its circumference, shall include Descemet's membrane, and in the posterior part the whole thickness of the pectinate ligament.

(2) The deep surface of the disc may be lined (*a*) throughout by Descemet's membrane, (*b*) partly by Descemet's membrane and partly by the pectinate ligament, and (*c*) wholly by the latter structure. We must discuss each of these conditions in turn:

(*a*) In the first case it is obvious that the trephine has been placed well forwards. This is shown by the position of the gap in Figs. 199 to 203, and also by the discs illustrated in Figs. 204 and 205.

(*b*) The relative areas of disc covered by Descemet's

THE PATHOLOGY OF FILTRATION 623

membrane and by the pectinate ligament vary according as the trephine has been placed rather far forward or rather far back. The point is illustrated in Fig. 206 and in a number of the other specimens.

(c) When the whole disc is covered by pectinate ligament the inference is that the trephining has been made too far out, and at the same time either that a small

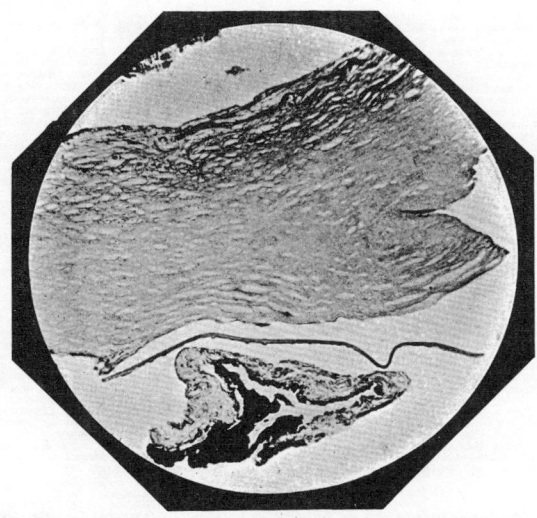

Fig. 204.—A trephined disc covered throughout by Descemet's membrane which has become detached from its base owing to shrinking during the preparation and to the act of cutting. Notice on its deep surface to the left-hand side of the figure (the scleral end) the wart-like excrescences due to deposits of hyaline material. Beneath the membrane of Descemet is seen the knuckle of iris which was cut off by the same snip of scissors that divided the hinge of the disc.

trephine blade has been used or that the outer half of the disc alone has been excised. A third possibility is that the section of the disc has not been meridional.

(3) Always provided that the opening made by the trephine does not become blocked by uveal tissue, or by inflammatory exudate from that tissue, satisfactory filtration may be certainly established when a part, and even a fairly large part, of the lining of the disc consists of the

fibres of the pectinate ligament. This has been shown by the examination of discs of this nature, which have been obtained from eyes in which trephining has proved a perfect success (Figs. 206 and 207).

Moreover, we know that a trephining performed far out may, and often does, yield the most excellent results. This has not only been illustrated in many instances in which the writer's operation has been defectively performed, but it was the procedure advocated as a routine

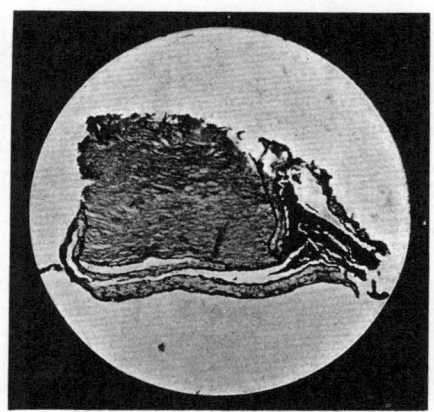

FIG. 205.—A trephined disc which, together with a knuckle of prolapsed iris, was removed with a single snip of the scissors. The membrane of Descemet can be faintly seen lining the deep surface of the disc. The folded knuckle of prolapsed iris can be followed in its whole extent. This specimen clearly shows that when the disc and knuckle are cut away together, the membrane of Descemet cannot escape removal.

measure by Freeland Fergus, who placed his trephine immediately behind the limbus, used a 3 mm. blade, and deliberately laid the ciliary body bare. It is these matters that constitute the radical difference between the Fergus operation and that of the writer. Judging from the results obtained when examining discs from the writer's operation, one may fairly deduce that those yielded by the Fergus procedure would be lined, so far as they lie in front of the angle of the chamber, exclusively, or almost exclusively,

THE PATHOLOGY OF FILTRATION 625

by pectinate ligament. The writer has from the first thought and said that trephining so far back is a mistake, but it would be unscientific and futile to deny that good results and admirable filtration are sometimes obtained by this method.

It has been argued, presumably on theoretical grounds, that it is a difficult thing to remove the whole thickness of the pectinate ligament on the deep surface of the disc by using a trephine. It has been shown by the examina-

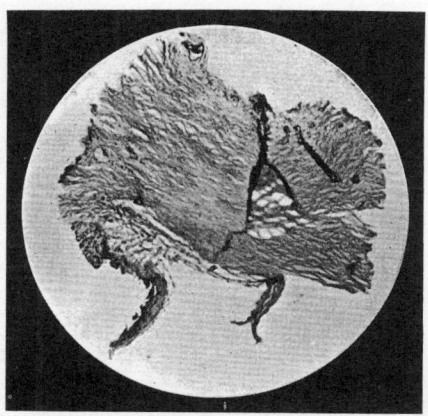

FIG. 206.—A trephined disc on the deep surface of which some layers are seen folded back at right angles. These consist of a few of the deep lamellæ of the cornea, and below this again of Descemet's membrane, with hyaline thickenings on its posterior surface. This membrane can be seen to break up into the pectinate ligament which lies to the left. Deep to this again, on the extreme left of the specimen, is a small portion of the knuckle of iris, which was removed at the same time as the disc.

tion of a considerable number of sectioned discs, that the suggested difficulty is only an imaginary one ; but even should the deepest layers of this structure be left behind, owing to faulty trephining, it may fairly be argued that such a defect in technique would be far less important than that of leaving behind a portion of Descemet's membrane ; for, whilst the latter is impervious to fluid, we know that the meshes of the former transmit it readily.

The real objection to trephining far out is that which has already been indicated, viz., the danger of prolapse of uveal tissue into the wound. The writer has from the first insisted on this from the clinical point of view, and Collins and Greeves have supplied the necessary pathological evidence, as has already been shown. It is not merely that the adhesion of the iris base to the cornea makes it practically impossible to avoid the former structure in many cases; for another element enters into the problem, viz., the consequent dragging forward of the ciliary body with its processes. This brings us to another

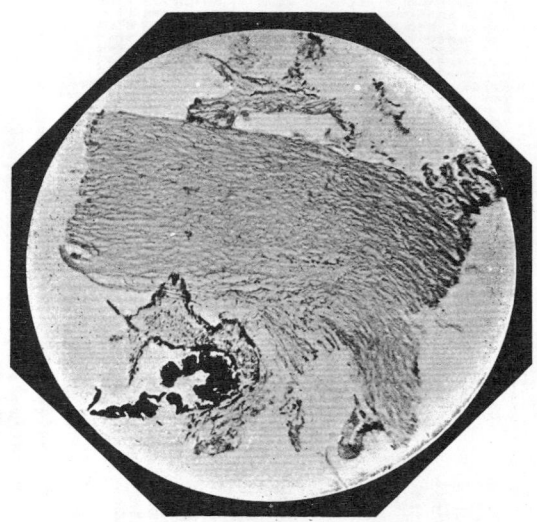

Fig. 207.—A trephined disc, lined on its deep surface to the left (corneal) side by Descemet's membrane, which almost at once splits up to form the pectinate ligament, as can be seen by tracing the membrane to the right. The knuckle of iris, removed with the disc, is also seen in the lower part of the figure.

important anatomical point, for in some of our specimens it has been seen that the iris tissue is tightly adherent to the deep surface of the disc over a greater or less extent of its peripheral circumference. When the trephine blade cuts through such a disc, the anterior part of the opening made is into the anterior chamber, and the peripheral iridectomy, which is performed by seizing the disc and iris in one grasp of the forceps, involves free iris over a corresponding area, whilst the posterior part of the opening goes direct into the posterior division of the aqueous chamber, and removes the whole thickness of the disc (including the pectinate ligament) and the subjacent adherent iris in one block. Clinically, such a procedure may usually be relied upon to produce a good filtering scar.

Allusion has been made to Ducamp's observation that the failure to obtain a good result in cats was due to the membrane of Descemet being left behind, even when an iridectomy had been performed. At one time there was a disposition to argue that because trephining failed in animals, it must necessarily be equally unsuccessful in man. Time and experience have shown the fallacy of such a deduction, but considerable interest centres round the explanation of the discrepancy between the human and animal results. It is, of course, possible that the membrane of Descemet has a greater tendency to repair breaches in its surface in cats and rabbits than it has in man. Again, it is not impossible that faulty technique, and especially the use of blunt trephines, may have been responsible for the failures recorded. The true explanation is, however, probably to be found in Collins' work on the *Anatomy of the Ligamentum Pectinatum*, in which he showed that the angle of the anterior chamber comes far farther forward in animals than it does in man ; this is associated with a corresponding advance in the position of the ciliary body and its processes. At the same time, it must be remembered that it is practically impossible to split the cornea of an animal, although the procedure is quite an easy one in the human eye. Our trephine wound in animals is thus forced far backwards, whilst the angle of the chamber and the site of the ciliary body are both advanced relatively to what is found in man ; this combination makes a successful trephining difficult, if not impossible, in the eyes of sheep, cats, rabbits, etc.

The object aimed at in sclero-corneal trephining, has from the first been to effect an entry directly into the anterior chamber, and so to drain the eye from the reservoir of fluid in that cavity. When the trephine cuts out a neat disc, the moment it is withdrawn the latter is pushed up by a dark bead of prolapsing iris. If the surgeon seizes the disc and the bead of iris in one grip of the forceps, and cuts them off with a single snip of the scissors, he gains two distinct advantages : (1) The patient cannot move the eye away, and thus cause the iris to be drawn into the wound by the hold on the forceps, and (2) it is obvious that *the membrane of Descemet and its expansion into the pectinate ligament must be excised as widely as the limits of the removed*

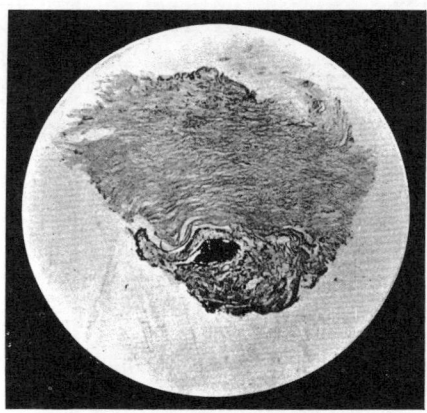

FIG. 208.—A disc lined partly by Descemet's membrane and partly by pectinate ligament, and having on its deep surface the prolapsed knuckle of iris still so tightly adherent to it that both were cut in one solid block.

disc. This is shown in Figs. 205 and 208, in both of which it is seen that the excised knuckle of iris still remained attached to the deep surface of the disc, thus enabling the two to be cut in one block. The commoner occurrence is for the knuckle of iris to float away from the disc as soon as the two are placed in the formalin solution. It must, we think, be obvious that when the iris and disc are removed together there is a moral certainty of the inclusion of the deepest layers of the cornea in the removed disc. Other illustrations of the same thing are to be found in Figs. 204, 206, and 207.

Should the surgeon fail to cut through the disc round a sufficient area of its circumference, he will see a thin, milky-looking membrane blocking the bottom of his trephine-hole after he has excised the disc. A histologic examination of the part removed will show that the membrane of Descemet has been left behind. It is sometimes a very difficult matter to excise the deep layer when so left. The writer has advocated for the purpose a pair of forceps with backwardly projecting teeth, which are often of considerable service. Even with the use of these, great difficulty may be encountered. If this deep layer is left behind, the operation will probably end in failure. It is, therefore, much better to reintroduce the trephine and to complete the removal of the disc therewith, even if some aqueous has escaped. The comparatively thick pad of iris makes the danger of doing so very small, but it is likely that more pain will be inflicted than if the ordinary smooth course of cutting out the disc had been effected in the first instance.

The writer still advocates the technique of directing the trephine at such an angle that its blade first finds its way through on the corneal margin of the disc. In so doing, his object is, not to cut through Descemet's membrane rather than the pectinate ligament—for that point does not seem very important—but rather to ensure that the fistula through the tunic of the eye shall be placed as far as possible from the ciliary body and from the base of the iris ; in other words, his examination of removed discs has only served to strengthen the view that he has held from the first—that the object of getting far forward is to avoid the impaction of uveal tissue in the wound, and so to secure the attainment of what he regards as the glaucoma surgeon's ideal, viz., the iris-free scar.

Hyaline Thickenings on Descemet's Membrane

In the course of examining a number of discs, one interesting feature has presented itself uniformly in the specimens taken from cases of senile glaucoma, viz., the presence of hyaline thickenings on the posterior surface of Descemet's membrane (Figs. 204, 208, 209, 210, and 211). These are especially abundant in that zone of the membrane which lies immediately internal (corneal) to the line at which the breaking up of the membrane to form the pectinate ligament takes place, and have never been found far away from that area. They are very irregular in shape,

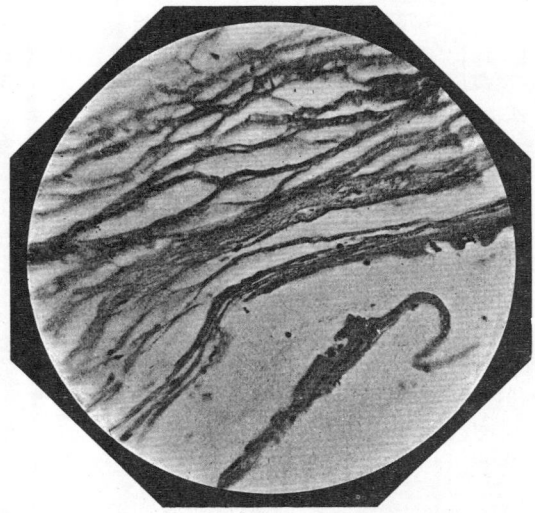

Fig. 209.—This shows the membrane of Descemet splitting up to form a part at least of the pectinate ligament, and closely connected with the deeper layers of the corneal lamellæ. To the extreme right of the figure the hyaline thickenings on the deep surface of the membrane are very obvious, whilst to the left, the splitting up of the membrane to form the fibrils of the ligament is equally clear.

and appear to be scattered erratically in a haphazard manner on the membrane; some of them are covered with adherent uveal pigment, probably due to the accident of adhesion of the iris base to the periphery of the cornea. Struck by the extraordinary constancy with which this phenomenon is met with in his collection of discs, the writer examined a number of sections of glaucomatous eyes, and again found the hyaline excrescences with great frequency. At least two possible explana-

THE PATHOLOGY OF FILTRATION

tions present themselves to start with: (1) That such excrescences may be the rule in elderly people of the glaucoma age; and (2) that there may be some definite connection between them and the presence of glaucoma. Most of the authorities are quite silent on the subject of such excrescences, but Salzmann mentions them and states that the frequency of their occurrence increases with the age

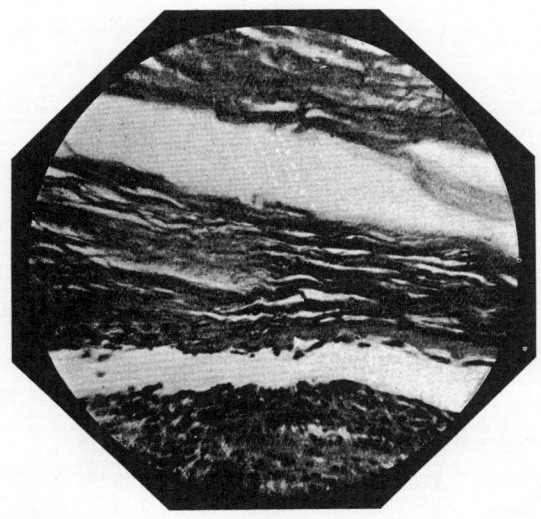

FIG. 210.—This shows the excrescences on Descemet's membrane under a higher power. Toward the left of the specimen the membrane is seen to be breaking up into smaller fibrils.

of the patient. It would be of interest if some pathologist who possesses the necessary material would examine a large number of the eyes of elderly people in whom no suspicion of glaucoma exists, and would thus ascertain the relative frequency of occurrence of the phenomenon in normal subjects. Henderson has maintained that there is a progressive thickening of the fibres of the pectinate ligament, which occurs as life advances and which is due to a definite act of secretion on the part of the cells, which constitute the whole of this structure at birth. He has suggested that the blocking up of the filtering spaces of the ligament, which results from this thickening of its fibres, determines the onset of glaucoma. His main contention as to the thickening of the fibres does not appear to have been either confirmed or refuted by any other observer, but certain points which are not without interest appear to emerge from the present investigation : (1) The hyaline thickening of Descemet's membrane occurs only on the surface which is lined by endothelial cells ; this is in accordance with Henderson's suggestion, and it also supports Collins' view

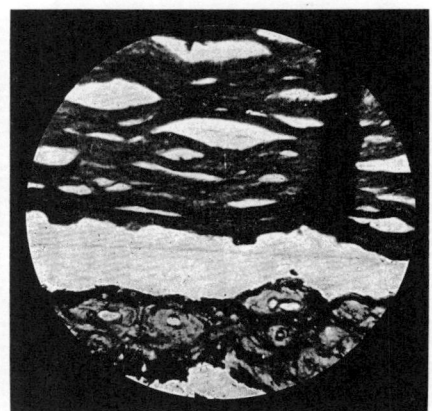

Fig. 211.—This is a higher power magnification of a portion of Descemet's membrane and the adjacent iris, from the same section as Fig. 205. The wart-like hyaline thickenings on the deep surface of the membrane are clearly seen.

that "the elastic lamina itself is originally developed from the endothelial cells which line its posterior surface. (2) The thickenings met with occur over a narrow area, viz., that which is most likely to be influenced by changes in the vascular condition of the parts. (3) No evidence of irregular hyaline thickening of the fibres of the pectinate ligament has been discovered, though a very large number of specimens have been examined. (4) There has also been a total absence of any evidence that the spaces normally occurring in the pectinate ligament are really blocked up by the increased mass of the fibres ; on the contrary, these spaces are always found wide open, unless as a result of pressure from within in late cases. Under these latter circumstances the spaces are indeed closed, but obviously as the result of the pressure referred to, for the area occupied by the ligament is then greatly diminished, and the inward bulge that has accompanied the compression can be clearly seen on the inner surface of the sclera.

It is with some diffidence that attention has been drawn to these hyaline excrescences, as it is obviously difficult to form a definite opinion as to their importance. It hardly seems likely that they have any ætiological significance. If further investigation should prove that they are more commonly met with in the glaucomatous than in normal subjects of the same age, the presumption that will arise will probably be that they are a result and not a cause of those pathological processes which attend a rise of tension in the eye. If one might hazard a guess, it would be that possibly they are due to the long continued congestion, which, in a greater or less degree, is probably inseparable from the glaucomatous condition.

These considerations lead one to make a few observations on another subject, viz., the nature of the pectinate ligament.

The Nature of the Ligamentum Pectinatum

There is a considerable difference of opinion on this subject. The classical teaching is that the ligamentum pectinatum is formed by the breaking up of Descemet's membrane into a leash of fibres, and that the spaces within this meshwork are lined by extensions from the layer of endothelial cells which covers the posterior surface of the membrane. This view has been accepted by most writers on the subject, including Parsons, Schäfer, and Collins, and it has recently been restated as the result of a very careful anatomical research by Prof. Arthur Thomson.

On the other hand, T. Henderson depicts Descemet's membrane as ending abruptly to the inner side of the ligament; he states that "the corneal lamellæ, next to

Descemet's membrane, break up into the innermost fibres of the cribriform ligament at a point just anterior to the termination of the membrane." He believes that the origin of the ligament can be best made out in specimens stained with van Gieson; for, " as Descemet's membrane does not stain the same rich red colour as connective tissue, it stands out under such circumstances quite apart and distinct from the ligament, whose sclerosed fibres are thus easily traced as a direct continuation of the inner corneal lamellæ." More recently, L. Buchanan has supported Henderson, having satisfied himself that Descemet's membrane ends rather abruptly at some little distance from the angle of the chamber. He believes that it plays no part in the formation of the pectinate ligament. Salzmann, too, takes a somewhat similar view, and describes the boundary between the membrane and the ligament as sometimes abrupt and sometimes sloping; he is careful to say that the membrane does not really stop abruptly, but is continued over the trabeculæ of the iris angle as a very thin layer; " the appearance of an ending is," he says, " only brought about by the fact that the membrane thins out so suddenly."

In the course of the present investigation a very large number of sections of trephined discs have been examined, and in most of these the area of junction between Descemet's membrane and the pectinate ligament was demonstrated. Great care was taken to ensure the sections being cut meridionally to the eye, and a variety of stains, including van Gieson's, Weigert's iron-hæmatoxylin, and orcein, were employed. The specimens were cut and prepared by Mr. Chesterman, of Oxford, to whom the writer is much indebted for the great pains and skill he has lavished on them. In no single instance has it been found possible to show an abrupt ending of the membrane of Descemet, whilst in a large number that structure can be clearly seen breaking up into a leash of fibres, just as described by Thomson and others (Figs. 206, 209 and 212). The difficulties of settling histological questions of such a nature are well known, and the pitfalls are many, but one

THE PATHOLOGY OF FILTRATION 635

could hardly rise from the examination of a considerable number of these specimens with any serious doubt in one's mind that the pectinate ligament is formed, to some extent at least, by the breaking up of Descemet's membrane. At the same time many of the sections suggest that the deepest lamellæ of the cornea proper take a part in the enclosing of the spaces of the pectinate ligament. In other words, those spaces seem to lie partly in the meshes of the broken-

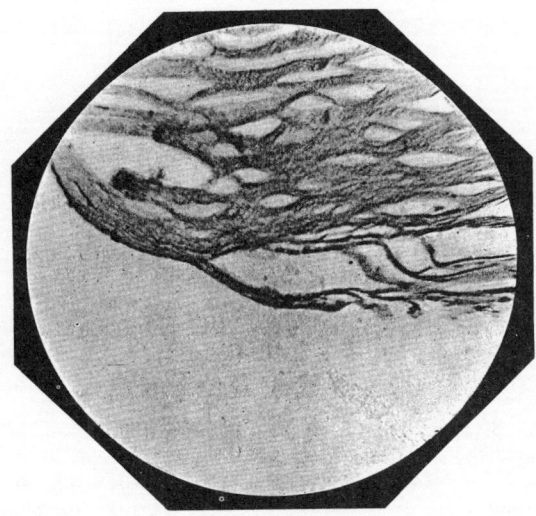

FIG. 212.—From the deep surface of a trephined disc, showing the splitting up of Descemet's membrane to form a part at least of the meshwork of the pectinate ligament.

up membrane of Descemet, and partly in those of the deepest strata of the substantia propria of the cornea. Just where the membrane begins to break up, one can see in a number of the specimens fine fibrils which pass between it and the deepest corneal lamellæ, serving to bind the two together; this explains why, in some of the sections, we find the membrane of Descemet wholly detached and separate from the rest of the disc, but firmly fixed to it at its outer extremity (Fig. 206).

This anatomical discussion is obviously an aside which

is only slightly connected with the original object of the research, but chance has thrown it in our way, and opportunity has brought it into prominence. The writer holds no brief for either theory, but he is the more anxious to get at the truth, because it seems possible that the knowledge so obtained may have a clinical bearing. It has therefore been thought advisable to allude to the appearances observed in the hope that doing so may serve to draw attention once more to what is still undoubtedly a disputed point.

REFERENCES

BARRAQUER, J. A.—" Elliot's Operation," *La Clin. Ophtal.*, March 1913.
BUCHANAN, L.—" The Pectinate Ligament," *Brit. Med. Journ.*, August 16, 1913, p. 399.
CLAUSEN, W.—" Experimental Trephining on Rabbits," *Zeit. f. Augenh.*, vol. xxix. p. 197.
COLLINS, E. T.—" Anatomy of the Ligamentum Pectinatum," *Trans. of Ninth Inter. Ophth. Congress*, Utrecht, 1899.
COLLINS, E. T.—*R.L.O.H. Reports*, vol. xiv. pt. 2.
COLLINS, E. T.—" The Sclero-corneal Trephining Operation for Glaucoma," *The Ophthalmoscope*, 1914, vol. xii. p. 589.
COLLINS, E. T.—*Proc. of Seventeenth Inter. Congress of Med.*, London, 1913.
DUCAMP, A.—" La Trépanation corneo-sclérale d'Elliot," *Etude Technique, Recherches anatomiques et expérimentales*, 1913, Vigot Frères, Paris.
ELLETT, E. C.—" Healing of Trephine Wounds of Sclera and Sclerocorneal Junction," Sect. on Ophth., *A.M.A.*, 1914, p. 390.
ELLIOT, R. H.—" A Preliminary Note on a New Operative Procedure for the Establishment of a Filtering Cicatrix in the Treatment of Glaucoma," *The Ophthalmoscope*, 1909, vol. vii. p. 804.
ELLIOT, R. H.—" Demonstration of a permanently Filtering Trephined Scar," *Oxford Ophthal. Congress*, July 1917.
ELLIOT, R. H.—" The Histology of the Trephined Disc," *Trans. O.S. of U.K.*, 1918, vol. xxxviii.
FERGUS, F.—*The Ophth. Review*, 1915, vol. xxxiv. p. 202.
GRAY, W. C., Major, I.M.S. of Madras.—Personal communication.
GREEVES, R. A.—" Some Observations on Four Trephined Eyes, Examined Microscopically," *Trans. O.S. of U.K.*, 1916, p. 445.
HENDERSON, T.—*Glaucoma*, p. 22, Edward Arnold, London, 1910.
HOLTH, S.—" The Anatomy of Successful Glaucoma Operations," *Bericht der Ophthal. Gesell.*, Heidelberg, 1913, p. 355; and *The Ophthalmoscope*, 1914, p. 347.
PARSONS, J. H.—*Pathology of the Eye*, vol. i. p. 282.

REINHOLD, C. H., Major, I.M.S. of the Punjab.—Personal communication.
ROCHON-DUVIGNEAUD.—Treatise on *The Topography of the Angle of the Anterior Chamber*, Paris, 1892.
SALZMANN, M.—*The Anatomy and Histology of the Human Eyeball*, p. 43, Chicago, 1912.
SCHÄFER, E. A.—*Essentials of Histology*, 1916, p. 501.
THOMSON, ARTHUR.—*The Ophthalmoscope*, 1911, vol. ix. p. 472.
VERHOEFF, F. H.—"Histological Findings after Successful Sclerostomy," *Arch. of Ophth.*, 1915, vol. xliv. p. 129.

APPENDIX

A Microscope for the Measurement of the Cornea has been constructed by Messrs. Zeiss to be used on the small extensible stand of their binocular corneal microscope. It is focussed by means of a rack and pinion movement, and it permits the measurement of diameters up to 20 mm. It gives a magnification of about × 8, and has an exit pupil of about 2 mm.

The eyepiece fitting, containing the micrometer (10 mm.

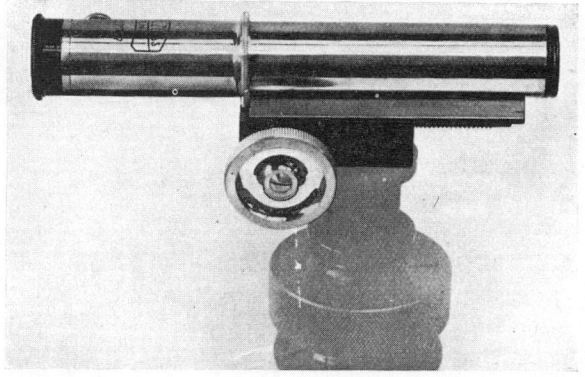

FIG. 213.—The author's microscope for the measurement of the cornea.

divided into 100 parts), can be revolved and clamped so that readings can be taken in any meridian. The actual measurements are ascertained by multiplying the micrometer readings by 2. This has been necessitated by the employment, for economic reasons, of a micrometer scale already in use for others of Messrs. Zeiss' instruments. The spaces are such that there is no difficulty in reading $\frac{1}{20}$th of a mm. or less with great accuracy. The patient's head is steadied on the head-rest of the Zeiss corneal microscope: the eye under examination gazes straight through the tube, and the Gullstrand lamp supplies a full and satisfactory illumination.

INDEX OF NAMES

A

Abadie, C., 422, 491, 500.
Adams, P. H., 435, 439.
Adamük, 36, 39.
Alexandre, 131, 147.
Allport, W., 434, 439.
Alt, A. A., 447, 457.
Axenfeld, T., 91, 413, 425, 439, 465, 492, 543.

B

Baas, K., 235, 240, 243, 294.
Badal, 139.
Bailliart, P., 50, 58, 62, 63, 64, 81, 205, 223, 337, 344.
Ball, J. N., 413, 439.
Ballantyne, A. J., 488, 522.
Bardsley, 518.
Barraquer, J. A., 465, 531, 559, 618, 636.
Beauvieux and Delorme, 338, 345.
Becker, 370.
Bell, G. H., 448, 457.
Bentzen and Leber, 422, 439.
Berry, Sir G., 301, 317.
Bettremieux, 499, 500.
Birnbacher and Czermak, 87, 88, 101.
Bjerrum, J., 21, 123, 147, 253, 256, 267, 268, 270, 286, 287, 290–293, 294, 299, 490, 500.
Black, M., 366, 384, 399.
Blair, C., 413, 439.
Blanco, 529, 530.
Boehm, K., 420, 434, 435, 439.
Boldt, J., 500.
Borthen, 494.
Bowman, Sir W., 19, 21, 368, 384, 398, 399, 459, 560.
Brailey, W. H., 377, 384.
Brown, E. J., 448, 457.
Brown, H., 422, 439.
Buchanan, L., 634, 636.
Buck, R. H., 434, 439.
Bunge, 301, 413, 439.
Butler, T. Harrison, 91, 101, 336, 345, 518, 561.

C

Cabannes, C., 414, 439.
Calhoun, F. P., 431, 434, 439.
Carpenter, J. T., 33, 39.
Carr, A. M., 444, 457.
Carter, R. B., 179, 223.
Casolino, L., 60, 81.
Chance, J. B., 179, 223.
Chesterman, W., 634.
Chevallereau, 465.
Christel, P., 420, 439.
Clark, C. F., 146.
Clausen, 618, 636.
Clegg, J. G., 561, 570.
Coats, G., 380, 384, 407, 416, 417, 418, 425, 427, 439.
Coccius, 19, 21.
Coleman, 446.
Collins, E. T., 44, 47, 52, 53, 58, 114, 177, 368, 370, 372, 375, 384, 390, 415, 418, 422, 426, 439, 475, 483, 494, 526, 569, 591, 602, 618, 621, 622, 626, 627, 632, 633, 636.
Collins and Batten, 414, 439.
Collins and Marshall, 414, 439.
Collins and Mayou, 283, 301, 316, 317, 413, 439.
Coronat and Aurand, 421, 439.
Craggs, H. C., 71.
Craggs, H. C., and Taylor, C. J., 61, 62, 81.
Cridland, B., 334, 335.
Critchett, G., 459.
Cross, R., 420, 426, 439.
Cuperus, N. J., 414, 439.
Curran, E. J., 502, 504.
Czermak, W., 467, 520.

D

De Lapersonne, F., 465.
Demicheri, 500.
Derby, H., 465.
Desai, 139, 147.
De Schweinitz, G. E., 146, 165, 166, 443, 445, 446, 450, 453, 457.

INDEX OF NAMES

Desmarres, 564.
Deutschmann, R., 465.
De Wecker, L., 20, 21, 31, 434, 439, 451, 459, 463–472, 476, 477, 478, 483, 489, 490, 500, 510, 603.
Dianoux, 489, 500.
Domec, T., 445, 457.
Donders, F. C., 19, 21, 123, 136, 147.
Downey, J. W., 344, 345.
Doyne, R. W., 500.
Druault, 179, 223.
Dubois, H., 145, 147, 434, 439.
Ducamp, A., 531, 559, 618, 619, 627, 636.
Dujardin, 465.
Dupuy-Dutemps, 565, 570.
Duverger and Barré, 51, 58, 60, 64, 81.

E

Ellett, 323, 345, 618, 636.
Elliot, R. H., 17, 82, 101, 223, 294, 345, 384, 399, 497, 498, 500, 501, 509, 529, 560, 602, 617, 621, 636.
Elschnig, A., 425, 501, 504, 574.
Emsley, H. H., 173, 181, 182.
Erdmann, P., 423, 439.
Exner, 499.

F

Fage, 413, 422, 425, 435, 439.
Feingold, M., 366, 384, 399.
Fergus, A. F., 497, 498, 499, 500, 526–530, 624, 636.
Fincham, E. F., 181.
Fischer, M. H., 98, 99, 100, 101, 128, 145, 222.
Fleischer, B., 94, 101.
Foerster, 365.
Foroni, 515.
Fourrière, 62.
Fox, L. W., 563, 565, 570.
Francis, L. M., 146.
Fraunhöfer, 183.
Frenkel, H., 389, 399.
Fröhlich, K., 497, 529, 530.
Fuchs, E., 14, 16, 17, 94, 101, 105, 106, 120, 136, 137, 145, 147, 169, 198, 199, 200, 202, 203, 213, 223, 231, 263, 296, 301, 316, 317, 414, 432, 439, 469, 470, 475, 483, 592, 602.
Fumiatzew, 178.

G

Galen, 19.
Galezowski, J., 465.
Gallavardin, 58.

Germann, D., 431, 439.
Gifford, H., 363, 366, 367, 384, 436, 439, 503, 504, 597, 602.
Gilbert, W., 94, 101, 137, 147, 430, 431, 439, 456, 457.
Gowland, 447.
Gradle, H. S., 214, 219, 223, 300, 317, 320, 345, 397, 399, 562.
Grandclément, E., 100, 101.
Gray, W. C., 616, 618, 636.
Green, A. S. and L. D., 145, 147.
Green, E., 297, 298.
Greenwood, A., 146, 313.
Greeves, A., 38, 39, 379, 380, 384, 618, 621, 626, 636.
Griffith, A. H., 543, 566, 570.
Grönholm, V., 118, 120, 142, 147.
Gros, 403, 404, 411, 439.
Gross, E. G., 420, 439.
Grünhagen, 36, 39.
Grut, Hansen, 465.
Gullstrand, A., 188.
Gunnufsen, P., 453, 457.
Gutmann, A., 193.

H

Haab, O., 407, 426, 465.
Haag, C., 121, 138, 147, 428, 429, 430, 439.
Haffmans, 21.
Hallett, de W., 434, 439.
Hambresin, 139, 147.
Hamburger, C., 55, 58, 105, 193, 420, 439.
Hamilton, R. J., 139, 147, 434, 437, 440.
Harman, N. B., 502, 507, 519, 524, 526.
Hawley, C. W., 448, 457.
Hay, P. J., 434, 440.
Heerfordt, C. F., 10, 88, 101.
Hegner, C. A., 363, 384, 387, 399.
Heine, L., 21, 491, 500.
Helmholtz, 19.
Henderson, E. E., and Starling, E. H., 33, 36, 40.
Henderson, T., 64, 82, 95, 96, 101, 120, 338, 475, 483, 528, 631, 632, 633, 634, 636.
Henry, Wallace, 339, 345.
Herbert, H., 21, 26, 435, 436, 440, 489, 490, 491, 493, 494, 495, 496, 500, 502, 522–526, 570, 597, 602, 612, 617.
Hertel, E., 71, 72, 82, 129, 130, 147.
Hess, C., 117, 120, 366.
Hiere, 193.
Hill, L., 66, 82.
Hine, M. L., 333, 345.

INDEX OF NAMES

Hippocrates, 18, 22.
Hirschberg, J., 429, 431, 440, 465.
Höeg, N., 413, 440.
Holth, S., 91, 101, 493, 497, 500, 502, 515–522, 574, 579, 604, 605, 611, 612, 613, 614, 615, 617, 618, 636.
Horner, J. R., 426.
Hudson, A. C., 115, 120, 263, 294, 361, 373, 384, 392, 399, 591, 592, 602.

I

Inouye, 380.
Ischikawa, 94, 101.
Ischreyt, G., 38, 99, 101.

J

Jackson, E., 195, 327, 345, 366, 384, 399, 451, 457.
Jaeger, H., 434, 440.
James, G. B., 497, 500.
Javal, E., 134.
Johnson, 518.
Jones, H., 434, 440.
Joudin, 500.

K

Kagoshima, 122, 133, 143, 147.
Kayser, B., 424, 425, 426, 427, 440.
Keukenschryver, N. C., 380, 384.
Key, B. W., 434, 440.
Killick, C., 427.
Kirkpatrick, H., 44, 372, 384, 598, 602.
Kleczkowski, T., 132, 147.
Knapp, A., 146, 390, 399, 591, 602.
Knapp, H., 592, 602.
Knies, M., 20, 22, 102.
Koeppe, L., 115, 120, 219, 223.
Köllner, 159, 166.
Komoto, J. P., 330, 414, 440.
Koster, W., 37, 38, 40, 88, 101, 117, 120.
Kraemer, R., 131, 147.
Krauss, 500.
Krucow, 465.
Kuemmell, R., 124, 136, 147, 381, 384, 424, 440.
Kuhnt, H., 465.
Kusama and Nakamo, 132, 148.

L

Lagrange, F., 21, 22, 128, 139, 148, 489, 494, 495, 499, 500, 501, 511, 514, 527, 597, 598, 603, 604.

Lamb, R. S., 146, 398, 399, 448, 457.
Landolt, E., 469.
Lang, B., 561, 564.
Lange, 92, 101, 137, 148.
Langenhan and Englemann, 61.
Laqueur, L., 21, 22, 134, 148.
Lawford, J. B., 135, 148, 431, 440.
Laws, W. G., 525.
Lawson, Sir A., 451, 457, 494, 497, 501.
Lebensohn, M. H., 434, 440.
Leber, 20, 22, 102.
Lederer, 36, 40.
Le Prince, 446.
Levinsohn G., 38, 115, 120, 139, 148.
Levitt, 139.
Linstedt, F., 188, 223.
Lloyd, R. I., 383, 393, 399, 532.
Lobo, 62.
Loehlein, W., 132, 137, 148, 428, 429, 430, 431, 440.

M

McBurney, M., 475, 483.
McCaw, J. A., 100, 101.
Mackenzie, W., 19, 22, 459.
McLean, W., 51, 61, 82, 320, 322, 324, 331, 335, 345.
Macrae, A., 63, 82.
McReynolds, J. O., 564.
Maggiore, L., 3, 4, 17.
Magitot, A., 11, 17, 34, 40, 51, 55–58, 63, 64, 82.
Maher, O., 494.
Maklakow, 444.
Manson-Bahr, P., 146, 148.
Marbaix, 328.
Marks, E. O., 253, 255, 294.
Marx, E., 253, 294.
Maynard, F. P., 99, 101, 143, 145.
Mayou, M. S., 381, 384, 420, 422, 435, 440, 501, 502, 504.
Meller, J., 437, 440, 501, 502, 504, 592, 602.
Meller and Fuchs, 368, 384.
Menacho, M., 145, 148.
Minor, J. J., 384.
Mitvalsky, 366, 384, 399.
Moore, F., 62, 82, 206, 223, 331.
Morax, V., 10, 18, 118, 120, 145, 148, 171, 176, 177, 179, 201, 211, 212, 223, 224, 225, 226, 228, 329, 345, 592, 602.
Mules, P. H., 431.
Müller, H., 19, 22.
Munns, S. B., 145.
Murakami, S., 414, 440.

N

Nahmacher, 420, 440.
Natanson, A. N., 368, 384.
Nordensen, E., 379, 384.
Norman, 187.

O

Oeller, 211.
Orcutt, D. C., 145, 148.
Owuchi, 426, 440.

P

Panas, 465.
Parker, W. R., 49, 58, 146.
Parsons, J. H., 36, 40, 111, 123, 148, 376, 379, 381, 384, 400, 406, 409, 411, 416, 440, 475, 483, 633, 636.
Paulus Ægineta, 19.
Percival, A. S., 339, 343, 345.
Peter, L. C., 236, 254, 294, 434, 440.
Pichler, A., 424, 440.
Pickard, R., 216, 223.
Pissarello, C., 443, 447, 457.
Planchu and Gautier, 422, 440.
Posey, W. C., 390, 450, 451, 457.
Puech, 430.
Pusey, B., 561.
Pyle, W. L., 400, 432, 435, 440.

Q

Quaglino, 490.
Querenghi, 490, 501.

R

Raeder, G., 188, 223.
Reber, W., 395, 399, 563.
Reinhold, C., 618, 637.
Reuss, 366, 384, 399.
Risley, S. D., 128, 148, 413, 440.
Robertson, D. Argyll, 497, 529, 530.
Rochat, G. F., 522.
Rochon-Duvigneaud, A., 8, 51, 58, 501, 531, 559, 622, 637.
Rockcliffe and Parsons, 414, 440.
Roemer, P., 40, 58, 71, 82, 563.
Roemer and Kochmann, 60, 71, 82.
Roenne, H., 21, 22, 245, 267, 268, 292, 294, 296, 299, 303, 317.
Rollet, 562.
Rollet and Curtil, 60.
Rosenfeld, M., 389.
Ruben, L., 99, 101.
Rufus, 19.
Rumschewitsch, I., 417, 420, 440

S

Sachsalber, 414, 440.
Salus, R., 366, 384.
Salzmann, M., 13, 14, 70, 82, 201, 223, 631, 634, 637.
Sansum, W. D., 447, 456, 457.
Sattler, C. H., 38, 62, 72, 82, 587.
Scalinci, N., 100, 101, 126.
Schäfer, E. A., 633, 637.
Schieck, 115, 120, 219, 223.
Schiötz, H., 51, 179, 223, 318, 321, 323, 326, 334, 335, 345.
Schipfer, 145, 148.
Schmidt-Rimpler, H., 240, 465.
Schnabel, W. J., 90, 93, 94, 101.
Schoeler, 495, 501.
Schönberg, M. J., 33, 40.
Schreiber, L., 381, 384.
Schreiber and Wengler, 423, 440.
Schur, M., 592, 602.
Schwenk, P. N. K., 367, 384, 399.
Sedwick, W. A., 100, 101.
Seefelder, R., 420, 427, 440.
Seidel, E., 53, 59, 255, 268, 270, 272, 294, 579, 615, 617.
Sheard, C., 175, 179, 183, 224.
Sinclair, A. H. H., 229, 230, 250-252, 253.
Sinclair, W. W., 339, 345.
Smith, D. P., 434, 440, 502, 504.
Smith, H. E., 448, 457.
Smith, Priestley, 20, 22, 45, 48, 50, 59, 62, 64, 67, 96, 102, 103, 105, 106, 109, 112, 113, 116-120, 121, 122, 123, 125, 127, 133, 134, 136, 137, 148, 221, 254, 256, 276, 294, 324, 348, 355, 356, 358, 359, 364, 368, 374, 377, 379, 383, 384, 392, 402, 429, 431, 433, 440, 501.
Snell and Collins, 414, 440.
Snellen, H., 21, 465, 466.
Sobhy, 531, 559.
Spicer, W. T. H., 381, 384.
Spielberg, C., 420, 440.
Stähli, J., 406, 426, 440.
Starling, E. H., 32, 40, 70, 82.
Stellwag, 20.
Stephenson, S., 422, 440, 498, 560, 564.
Stilling, 201.
Stimmel and Rotter, 420, 440.
Stirling, A. W., 88, 101.
Stock, W., 502, 504.
Story, J. B., 431.
Straub, M., 366, 384.
Sutherland and Mayou, 415.
Sym, W. G., 230, 251, 294.

INDEX OF NAMES

T

Tacke, D., 366, 384.
Takashima, S., 418, 421, 440.
Taylor, H. H., 563, 571.
Ten Doesschate, G., 145, 148.
Terrien and Dantrelle, 424, 441.
Thienpont, 141, 148.
Thomas, H. G., 100, 101, 446, 457.
Thompson, A. Hugh, 214, 224.
Thomson, Alexis, 414, 441.
Thomson, Arthur, 5, 18, 70, 73–81, 82, 97, 98, 101, 120, 128, 142, 148, 171, 307, 418, 441, 452, 633, 634, 637.
Toczyski, F., 61, 82.
Traquair, H. M., 230, 294.
Treitel, T. T., 241.
Tristaino, B., 72, 82.

U

Uhthoff, W., 465.
Ulbrich, C., 43, 44, 59, 188.
Uribe-Troncosco, M., 126, 327, 329, 345.

V

Valude, 501.
Van der Hoeve, J., 245, 285, 289, 290, 291, 292, 294.
Van Hoorn, W., 444, 457.
Van Lint, 521.
Vaughan, H., 61, 82.
Veasey, C. A., 145, 146, 148.
Velter, E., 60, 64, 82.
Verderame, F., 71, 72, 145, 146, 148.
Verhoeff, F. H., 124, 148, 415, 441, 604, 605, 612, 615, 617, 618, 637.
Verrey, L., 366, 384, 399.
Voelkers, 465.
Vogt, A., 239, 424, 441, 563, 571.
Vogt, A., and Jaffé, B., 132, 148.

Von Arlt, 456, 457.
Von der Heydt, R., 239, 294.
Von Graefe, A., 19, 20, 21, 22, 89, 91, 101, 123, 184, 185, 209, 224, 431, 434, 458–472, 473, 474, 476, 477, 483, 489, 603.
Von Hippel, E., 36, 40, 130, 148, 562, 563.
Von Mende, 564, 571.
Von Schultén, 67, 82.
Vossius, 429.

W

Walker, A. N., 563, 571.
Walker, C. B., 230, 294.
Wallenberg, 431.
Wallis, G. F. C., 502, 504, 543.
Weber, Adolph, 19, 20, 22, 102.
Weekers, L., 72, 82, 447, 457, 501.
Weeks, J. E., 145, 146, 148, 434, 441.
Weidler, W. B., 379, 380.
Weinstein, A., 414, 441.
Wernicke, G., 501.
Wessely, K., 60, 82, 127, 434, 441.
Wicherkiewicz, B., 465, 490, 501, 504.
Willbrand, H., 230, 231, 294.
Wilmer, W. H., 599, 602.
Wood, Casey, 434, 441, 502.
Woods, Hiram, 146.

Y

Young, G., 339, 345, 502, 562.

Z

Zeeman, W. P. C., 436, 441.
Zentmayer, W., 413, 420, 422, 434, 435.
Zorab, A., 501, 502, 504.

INDEX OF SUBJECTS

A

Abadie's operation, 491.
Abderhalden reaction, 130.
Absence of proliferation in edges of trephine wound, 587.
Abuse of mydriatics, 110, 138.
Accommodation, influence of, on glaucoma, 76, 142, 452.
   weakness of, 192.
Acute glaucoma, 2, 160, 317, 477.
Adrenalin, 484, 505, 575.
   in blood, 132.
Ætiology of glaucoma, difficulty in tracing, 84, 111.
African arrow-head poison, 177.
After-cataract, 368, 373.
After-management of patients, 578.
Age, a cause of glaucoma, 121, 122, 130.
Anæsthetics, general, 484, 506.
   local, 484, 505.
Anatomy, 3.
Angle of chamber, 8.
   closure of, 9, 20, 108, 111, 370, 418, 476, 482.
   measurements of, 531.
   methods of examination of, 187.
   obliteration of, 4.
   open in glaucoma, 113, 370.
Animal experiments, 619.
Aniridia, 375, 394, 420.
Annular scotoma, 285, 294, 304.
Anterior chamber, anatomy of, 8.
   contents of turbid, 189, 593.
   depth of, 115, 187.
   in buphthalmos, 407.
   shallowing of, 108, 111, 115, 117, 160, 164, 186, 349, 370, 579, 591, 599.
   shallowing of, senile, 116.
Anticipation, in glaucoma, 430.
Antiphlogistic treatment, 396, 446, 455.
Apparent discontinuity in course of retinal trunks, 202.
Aqueous humour, Magitot's views on the, 56.

Aqueous humour, qualities of, 574.
Arterial pulse in retina, 204.
Arterio-sclerosis, 62, 64, 81, 131, 206.
Asepsis, 584, 585.
Astigmatism, absence of, after trephining, 533.
   after iridectomy, 486.
   in buphthalmos, 412.
   post-operative, 493.
Atrophic cup, 210.
Atrophy of iris tissue, 106.
   of optic nerve, 216, 304, 338.
      cavernous, 90.
      progressive, in spite of relief of tension, 91, 92, 244, 470, 471.
Atropin, abuse of, 139, 141, 381, 396, 583.
   use of, 397, 398, 558, 580.
Atypical cases of cupping, 212.
Author's extension of Seidel's sign, 270.
   forceps, 629.
   large perimeter, 263.
   light sense apparatus, 341, 342.
   massage apparatus, 445.
   optico-ciliary neurectomy hook, 394.
   photometer, 340.
   pointer, 259.
   scotometer, 257, 260, 286.
Auto-intoxication, 93, 128, 383, 448, 470.

B

Baas on the visual field in glaucoma, 240, 243.
Bailliart's ophthalmo-dynamometer, 337.
Bandage, Madras eye, 508.
   pressure, 36.
Bandaging, prolonged, indications for, 578.
Basedow's disease, 205.
Bee-sting, 596.
Bettremieux's operation, 499.
Bilaterality of glaucoma, 157, 166.

INDEX OF SUBJECTS

Bjerrum's method, 253, 303.
  operation, 490.
  scotoma, 245, 254, 270, 287, 315.
    development of, 270.
  screen, 253, 286.
  sign, 164, 267, 306, 314.
    in non-glaucomatous conditions, 268.
Blind painful eyeball, 166.
  spot, enlargement of, 254, 268.
    the normal, 274.
Blood-pressure, general, reduction of, 447.
  intra-ocular, 30, 64, 131.
    and venous congestion, 64.
    laboratory experiment on, 66.
  retinal, 65, 89, 311.
  systemic, and intra-ocular pressure, 59, 62, 64, 89, 131.
    and retinal blood-pressure, 66.
    measurement of, 65, 67.
Blows on eye, 596.
Borthen's operation, 494.
Bouncing of hard eyeball, 35.
Bowman's membrane, ruptures of, 418.
  trephine, 526, 527, 559, 560.
Brittle conjunctivæ, 572.
Buphthalmos, 400, 403.
  ætiology of, 421.
  astigmatism in, 412.
  changes in anterior chamber, 407, 418.
    in choroid, 409.
    in ciliary body, 421.
    in cornea, 405, 416.
    in iris, 408, 418.
    in lens, 408.
    in lids, 421.
    in ocular muscles, 421.
    in optic disc, 410.
    in retina, 409.
    in sclera, 407, 420.
    in vitreous, 409, 411.
  clinical course of, 412.
  complications of, 412.
  differential diagnosis of, 415.
  dislocation of lens in, 414.
  enlargement of eye in, 404, 421.
  experimental, 423.
  fœtal condition of anterior chamber in, 418, 419.
  general health in, 412.
  inherited syphilis in, 422, 438.
  interference with media in, 411.
  operations for, 433.
  pathological anatomy of, 416.
  proptosis in, 405, 412.
  rate of filtration in, 422.
  spontaneous recovery from, 413.

Buphthalmos, technique of trephining in, 437.
  tension of eye in, 411.
  tonometer readings in, 411.
  traumatic, 423.
  treatment of, 432.
  visual acuity in, 411.
Burns of limbal region, 136, 424.
Butler's tonometer chart, 336.
  trephine, 561.
Button-holing of flap, 538, 540, 541, 570, 571, 573.

C

Capillary pressure, intra-ocular, 59, 59.
Cataract, 194.
  an accidental complication of glaucoma, 195.
  diagnosis of, 194.
  extraction of, 363, 390, 391, 597.
  extraction, intracapsular, 373.
  intumescent, 365, 388.
  secondary to glaucoma, 194.
  spontaneous cure of, 366, 389.
Causes of glaucoma, 84, 110, 121, 131, 133, 134, 136, 138, 143, 144, 146, 366, 389.
  exciting, 130, 138, 143, 144, 146.
Cavernous atrophy of the optic nerve, 91.
Central scotomata, 274, 279, 283, 284, 291, 314, 315, 317.
  vision, impairment of, 156, 164, 279, 284.
Channels, additional, for excretion of aqueous, 31.
Charts for scotometry, 260, 287, 308.
Chemosis, 163.
Chibret's photometer, 343.
Chloroform, 506.
Choroid, atrophy of, 218.
  damage to, in glaucoma, 218.
  detachment of, 591, 594.
  tumours of, 377.
Choroidal circulation, 10, 303, 309.
  Magitot's views on, 56.
Choroiditis, 383.
Chronic glaucoma, 2.
Ciliarotomy, 491.
Ciliary body, 192.
  congestion of, 192.
  glands of, 9, 52.
  interference with, 528, 529, 530.
  secretion from, 9, 20, 52, 53, 123, 126, 144.
  swelling of, 8.
  tumours of, 376.

INDEX OF SUBJECTS

Ciliary irritation, 372.
processes, drag on, 372.
retraction of, 106.
swelling of, 117.
wedge-like shape of, 108.
Circular method of examining visual field, 256.
wound in sclerectomy, advantages of, 547.
Circumlental space, 47, 117.
Climacteric, influence of, on glaucoma, 133.
Clinical course of congestive glaucoma, 159.
of simple glaucoma, 155.
Closed, 25.
sphere, 27, 39.
Cocaine, 139, 484, 505.
Coloboma of choroid, 420.
of iris, 420, 475, 486.
of optic nerve, 211.
of sheath of optic nerve, 212.
Colour fields in glaucoma, 248.
Complications of glaucoma operations, 571.
Cones, retinal, 305.
Congenital glaucoma, 400, 401.
Congestive glaucoma, 2, 11, 108, 110, 111, 115, 117, 126, 135, 139, 151, 152, 157, 160, 167, 224, 307, 343, 396, 413, 442, 455, 461, 466.
Conjunctiva, 3, 167, 506.
Conjunctiva-infolding operation, 490, 527.
Conjunctival pitting, 34.
Consanguinity, 422.
Contra-indications against operating, 455.
Convergence, effect of, on intra-ocular pressure, 333.
Corectopia, 420.
Cornea, 168.
anaesthesia of, 164, 165, 170, 185.
changes in, in buphthalmos, 405, 406.
measurement of, 135, 221.
author's instrument for, 222, 639.
perforation of, 348, 349, 385.
splitting of, 3, 437, 536, 538, 564, 567, 622.
steamy, 160, 163.
ulceration of, 186, 349.
wound of, 348.
Corneal microscope, 187, 194, 397, 611.
oedema, 169.
opacification after operation, 593.
opacity, the detection of, 170.
Couching of cataract, 354, 360, 363.

Crescent, corneal, 538.
Cupping of optic disc, 12, 157, 197, 201, 208, 213, 214, 296, 313.
disappearance of, 91, 92.
Curran's operation, 502.
Cyclodialysis, 9, 434, 436, 491, 499, 503, 526, 591.
Cyst, epithelial, of anterior chamber, 368, 370, 393.

D

Debilitating conditions, a cause of glaucoma, 62.
Degenerative changes in eye, 123, 125, 126, 161, 165, 166, 168.
Descemet's membrane, breach of, in trephining, 570, 605, 618, 627, 628.
hyaline thickenings on, 629.
ruptures of, 407, 416, 423, 427.
Desmarres' knife, 564.
Device for demonstrating cupping, 201.
De Wecker's correspondents, 463, 465, 466.
sclerotomy, 31, 490, 510.
views on iridectomy, 463.
De Zeng perimeter, 231, 263.
Diagnosis of glaucoma, difficulties in 149.
Diaphragm, impermeable, across eye, 374, 392.
Diathermy, 445.
Digital massage, 444.
pressure on eye, results of, 30, 65, 299.
Dilatation of pupil, 8, 160, 163, 164, 189, 191.
cause of the, in glaucoma, 191.
Dimpling of normal eye, 30.
Dionin, 141, 396, 447, 456.
Disc forceps, 546.
loss of, 573.
Discission of cataract, 365.
Distribution of nerve fibre bundles in retina, 233.
Downey's photometer, 344.
Druault's test for physiological halos, 181.
Dupuy-Dutemps' flap, 565.

E

Early operation in glaucoma, 460, 463, 468, 471, 477, 482.
Ectropion of iris, 420.
uveae, 165, 190.

INDEX OF SUBJECTS 649

Edridge Green on retinal lymph circulation, 297.
Egyptians, glaucoma among, 134, 136, 222.
Elasticity of eye, 28.
Electricity in treatment of glaucoma, 445.
Elementary features of glaucoma attack, 155.
Elliot's light sense apparatus, 341, 342.
  operation, 435, 436, 437, 498, 499, 503, 531, 570, 597, 601.
  motive of, 530.
  perimeter, 263.
  scotometer, 257.
  sign, 272, 275, 279, 281, 283.
  trephine, 530, 560.
Embolism of central artery of retina, 268.
Emsley-Fincham test for physiological halos, 182.
Endocrine glands in relation to glaucoma, 130, 448.
Environment, 135.
Epidemic dropsy, 99, 146.
Erdmann's experimental buphthalmos, 423.
Eserin, 396, 443, 450, 456, 583, 587.
  irritation, 450.
Established glaucoma, 161.
Euphthalmin, 139, 194.
Excretory channels, mechanical blocking of, 348.
Exercise, effect of, on intra-ocular pressure, 62, 142.
Exophthalmos, 416.
Eye, anatomical changes in, predisposing to glaucoma, 122.
  defective development of, 118.
  development of, 118.
  feel of the, 28.
  fluids of the, 11.
  size of, in glaucoma, 108, 111, 118, 134, 137, 221, 404.
  influenced by sex, 118.
  volume of contents of the, 39.

F

Failure to diagnose glaucoma, 148.
Family, influence of, on glaucoma, 135.
Fatigue, as a cause of " coloured rings," 177.
  easily induced in glaucoma, 230.
Febrile diseases, causative of glaucoma, 144.
Fergus's operation, 497, 499, 526, 530.

Fergus's operation contrasted with Elliot's operation, 529, 624.
Filtering scar, 20, 26, 438, 472, 474, 475, 476, 483, 486, 489, 491, 495, 596, 600, 603, 612.
  anatomical examination of, 599, 604.
  essentials of, 570.
Filtration angle, closure of, 20, 102, 108, 110, 117, 348, 360, 382.
Fistula of cornea, 113, 351.
  secondary, 616.
Fistulettes along margin of sclerectomy flap, 579, 599.
Fistulous scar, 26, 492, 604.
Fixation of eyeball, thread method of, 571.
Fixed contents of globe, 27, 39.
Flap in sclerectomy wound, displacement of, 579.
  dissection of, 535.
  incision for, 531, 533.
  nature of, 532.
  replacement of, 557.
  size of, 533.
  to be made thick, 585, 599, 601, 615.
Flashes of light, 160, 226.
Fluid, effusion of, into posterior segment of eye, 552, 553.
  intra-ocular, alterations in, 123, 123, 347.
  escape of, osmosis in relation to, 71.
  flow of, through eye, 40.
  obstruction to, 48.
  function of, 49.
  increased secretion of, 123.
  rate of escape of, 38, 41, 488.
  source of, 49, 52, 53.
Fluorescein, an aid to diagnosis, 193, 423, 595, 615.
Foerster's operation, 365.
Fontana, spaces of, 419.
Food, influence of, on glaucoma, 135.
Foramen scleræ, 296, 303, 316.
Foroni's operation, 515.
Förster's photometer, 343.
Fuchs on the cupping of the disc, 198, 199, 200.
  on fibres of the optic nerve, 300, 316.
  on the lamina cribrosa, 14–17.
  on perimetry, 231.
Fulminating glaucoma, 155, 298.
Funnel iris, 398.

G

Gait of glaucoma patient, 156.
Gigantophthalmos, 427.

Glands, ductless, in relation to glaucoma, 130.
Glaucoma, analogy with hernia, 153.
  a bilateral disease, 157, 166.
  causes of, 121, 132, 327.
  confusion as to term, 465, 467.
  definitions of, 128, 129.
  diagnosis of, 149, 275.
  early, 152, 160, 161, 168, 170, 224.
  from the use of drugs, 139, 140.
  irritative, 100.
  late, 164, 168.
  medical treatment of, 442.
  post-operative, 368, 374.
  secondary to cataract, 195, 366, 389.
  signs of, 157, 164, 165, 327.
  stages of, 152, 160, 162, 164.
  symptoms of, 152, 164, 165 et seq.
  types of, in young people, 432.
  various forms of, 430, 432, 465.
  visual fields, factors in production of, 286, 298.
    shapes of, 284.
Glaucomata, or suffusions, 18.
Glaucomatous cup, 91, 208.
  halo, 218.
Glaucoses, 18.
Glial tissue, changes in, in cupping of disc, 198, 199.
Glioma of retina, 379.
Glucose, intravenous injection of, 456.
Gradle's tonometer, 320.
  trephine, 562.
Graduation of sclerectomy wound, 32.
Gray Clegg's trephine, 561, 573.
Green reflex of glaucoma, 163, 194, 195.
Gridiron sclerotomy, 501.
Griffith's flap, 566.
Gullstrand slit-lamp, 219, 397, 611.

H

Hæmorrhage into anterior chamber, 124, 579, 580.
  intra-ocular, 166, 382, 395, 575.
  superficial, during operations, 575.
Halos, 173.
  clinical test for, 174, 181.
  measurement of, 173, 181, 184.
  physiological, 176, 178, 181. And see under Rainbows.
Handle of trephine, conical, 560.
Hardening of globe during operation, 552, 553.
Hardness of glaucomatous globe, 35, 163.
Harman's operation, 519, 524.

Headache, 160, 225.
Heine's operation, 491.
Hemianopia, 284, 292, 294.
Herbert's operations, 31, 433, 435, 436, 491, 493, 495, 522, 525, 597.
  modifications of, 522, 523.
Heredity, influence of, on glaucoma, 134, 422, 425.
Hernia, analogy with glaucoma, 153.
Herpes zoster, 146.
Hiere's method of diagnosis between glaucoma and iritis, 193.
High-frequency currents, 446.
Holocaine, 139, 332.
Holth's instruments, 515.
  operation, 31, 365, 493, 497, 502, 515, 597, 614.
  modifications of, 519.
Homatropin, 139, 194.
Hudson's perimeter, 263.
Hydrodynamics of eye, 48, 54.
Hydrophilism, 98, 127, 145.
Hydrophthalmos, 400, 435.
Hydrostatics of eye, 48, 54.
Hyperopia in relation to glaucoma, 136.
  senile, 136.
Hypersecretion, a cause of buphthalmos, 422.
Hypertension, distinction between, and glaucoma, 327.
Hypertonus of eye, 29, 30, 71, 380, 442.
Hypotonus, 29, 31, 71, 442, 593, 616.

I

Incarceration of iris (or capsule) in wound, 370, 372, 551, 582.
  operation for, 492, 493, 494.
  of vitreous in wound, 373, 588.
Index of filtration, 34.
Indians, incidence of glaucoma in, 134, 136.
Inelastic eye, 37.
Infero-temporal bundle of optic nerve fibres, 235.
Influenza, 145.
Injuries, causative of glaucoma, 146.
Intermissions in the advance of glaucoma, 158.
International Congress, 1913, 501, 569.
Intoxication, autogenetic, 128.
Iridectomy, 20, 375, 386, 388, 393, 434, 435, 438, 458, 463, 464, 471, 481, 488, 503, 548, 593, 597.

INDEX OF SUBJECTS 651

Iridectomy, advantages of, in trephining, 550.
  and sclerectomy compared, 474.
  complete, 549, 558.
  difficulties of, 186, 470, 481, 483.
  disadvantages of, in trephining, 549, 550.
  in sclerectomy operations, 497, 499, 513, 548, 549, 550, 587.
  modern surgeons on, 471.
  modus agendi of, 474, 475.
  peripheral, 548, 549, 558.
  technique of, 471, 483, 548.
  the Old Masters on, 458.
Iridencleisis, 434, 611, 612.
Irido-cyclitis, 367, 372, 382, 393, 585, 586.
  a cause of glaucoma, 113, 127, 146, 374, 382, 383, 395.
  septic, 585.
Irido-donesis, 409.
Iridotasis, 494, 502, 503.
Iridotomy, 386, 493, 502.
Iris, atrophy of, 106, 164, 165, 190, 368.
  base of, adherent to cornea, 103, 108, 353, 476, 555.
    pressed against cornea, 102, 105, 111, 370.
  bombé, 42, 353, 354, 374, 379, 392, 398, 475.
  changes in, 189.
  crypts of, 9, 102, 106.
  discoloration of, in glaucoma, 163, 164.
  entanglement of, in scar, 385.
  -free scars, 604.
  prolapse of, 348, 493, 587.
  retraction of, 106.
  spaces of, occluded, 105, 108.
  tumours of, 376.
  veins, 69.
  wounds, aseptic, 475, 584, 585, 611.
Iritis, post-operative, 580.
  quiet, 550, 558, 580, 581.
Irrigation of aqueous chamber, 486, 507, 552, 553, 573, 579.
Irrigator, McKeown's, 507, 573.

J

Jackson's use of mydriatic in diagnosis of glaucoma, 195.
Jagged incision operation, 496.
James's operation, 497, 515.
Japan, glaucoma statistics in, 133.
Jews and glaucoma, 134, 466.
Juvenile glaucoma, 402, 416, 428.
  associated with disorders of nutrition, 429.

Juvenile glaucoma, congenital anomalies in, 438.
  forms of, encountered, 429, 431, 432.
  heredity in, 429, 431.
  myopia in, 430.
  pedigrees in, 431.
  prodromal stage in, 429.
  sex predisposition in, 428.

K

Keratectasia, 416.
Keratitis punctata, 186.
Keratoconus, 416.
Keratome, advantages of, 484.
  dangers in use of, 365.
  method of using correctly, 485.
Keratometer, 135.
Kink of retinal vessels in glaucoma cup, 202, 209, 296.
Koeppe's sign, 219.

L

Lachrymation, 225.
Lagophthalmos, 407.
Lagrange's operation, 31, 434, 438, 495, 500, 502, 503, 511, 578, 592, 593, 597.
  dangers of, 502, 514.
  indications for, 514.
  modifications of, 515.
  size of incision in, 512.
Lamb's sign, 398.
Lamina cribrosa, 14, 196, 198, 208.
  resistance to pressure of, 16, 198.
  variations in anatomical structure of, 17.
  yielding of, 198, 208, 315.
Lang's discission knives, 390.
  knife for splitting cornea, 564.
  trephine, 561.
Late infection, 481, 585, 594, 596.
  conditions favouring, 599.
Laws' modification of Herbert's operation, 525.
Leakage, conjunctival, 599.
Lens, 193.
  accidental wounds of, 363.
  appearance of, in glaucoma, 163.
  dislocations, 355, 588, 589.
    anterior, 355, 357, 386.
    into vitreous, 115, 577.
    lateral, 358, 387.
    operative, 577.
    posterior, 359, 387.
    spontaneous, 355.
    traumatic, 357, 363.

INDEX OF SUBJECTS

Lens, fluidity of, 590.
　growth of, 8, 108, 116, 117, 119, 122.
　in buphthalmos, 407.
　operative injuries of, 364.
　wounds of, 363, 388, 577.
Life, prospects of, in relation to operation, 470, 478, 483.
Light, influence of, on glaucoma, 142.
　sense, 338.
Light sense apparatus, author's, 341, 342.
Limbal puncture, 434, 502.
Lindstedt's method of measuring depth of anterior chamber, 188.
Lymphatic circulation in the eye, 56.

M

McLean tonometer, 321, 335.
McReynolds' corneal splitter, 537, 564.
Magitot's views on intra-ocular tension, 55.
Maklakoff's massage instrument, 444.
　tonometer, 318.
Manometer for estimation of intra-ocular pressure, 25.
Manometry, 29, 36, 42, 43, 45, 324.
Marks on perimetry of glaucoma, 253.
Marx' method of perimetry, 253.
Masks, operation, 507.
Massage apparatus, author's, 445.
　digital, 444.
　instrumental, 444.
　of eye, 33, 444, 453, 456, 489, 493, 552.
　suction, 445.
Mechanical trephines, 562.
Medial causes of diminished visual acuity, 227.
Medical treatment of glaucoma, 434, 442, 454, 463.
Megalocornea, 38, 416, 424.
Meiotics, 21, 140, 225, 391, 397, 433, 435, 443, 449, 450, 451, 452, 456, 478, 549, 558.
　caution as to use of, 451, 463.
　effect of, on depth of glaucoma cup, 92.
Memory sight, 165.
Metal rod operation, Herbert's, 525.
Microphthalmos, 118, 429.
Mists of vision, 160, 168, 171, 172.
Morgagnian cataract, 590.
Morning mists, 171, 172.
Motor trephines, 563.
Mydriasis, due to exclusion of light, 142.

Mydriasis, trial, 195, 426.
Mydriatics, 110, 139, 397, 558, 583.
　abuse of, 110, 138, 583.
　care in use of, 138, 140, 194.
　in relation to venous pulsation, 206.
Myopia and glaucoma in the young, 137.
　and intra-ocular pressure, 38.
　high, 380, 411, 429.
　in glaucoma, 137, 193.
　in juvenile glaucoma, 430.
　post-operative, 593.

N

Nasal field, restriction of, 240, 307.
Nausea in glaucoma, 226.
Negro children, syphilis in, 422.
Negroes, incidence of glaucoma in, 134.
Nerve fibre bundles, anatomical variation in, 298, 314, 316.
　in retina, 233, 315, 316.
　in retina, arcuate curves of, 325.
Nerve fibres, conductivity of, 306.
　injury to, 208, 209, 296, 303, 305, 306, 313.
　of disc, atrophy of, 196, 212, 215.
　optic, support from vessels' sheaths, 313, 315.
　overstretching of, 218, 296, 313, 315.
Nerves of ciliary body, 10, 192.
　of iris, 10.
Nervous disturbances, influence of, 110, 132, 143.
Neuralgia, trigeminal, 162, 224.
Neuro-fibromatosis, 414.
Neuro-retinal causes of diminished visual acuity, 227.
Norman's method, 187.
Nutrition, disorders of, 399.
Nystagmus in buphthalmos, 412.

O

Opacity, corneal, 170, 406, 591.
Operations for glaucoma, dangers of, with restricted field, 245, 285, 292.
　newer, 488, 501.
Operation-table, arrangement of patient on, 508.
Operative interference, rules for determining, 468, 482.
Ophthalmia, 136.

INDEX OF SUBJECTS

Ophthalmic zoster, 397.
Ophthalmo-dynamometer, Bailliart's, 50.
Ophthalmoscopic appearances in glaucoma, 164, 196, 201, 204.
Optic disc, cupping of, 12, 19, 197, 201, 410.
　differential diagnosis of cupping of, 201.
　pallor of, 196.
　nerve, anatomical distribution of, 300.
　atrophy of, 185, 234, 248, 470, 471.
　changes in, in glaucoma, 195, 309, 312.
　entrance canal of, 11.
　progressive atrophy of, 91, 92, 244, 470.
Optico-ciliary neurectomy, 394.
Optic vesicle, primary, 297.
Oriental practice, ulceration of cornea in, 350.
Osmotic action, 44, 47, 48, 70, 73, 81, 129, 446.
　in eye, researches on, 71.

P

Pain in glaucoma, 152, 162, 166, 224.
　explanation of, 225.
Panophthalmitis, 166, 186, 412, 586.
Papillo-macular bundle, 234, 236, 309.
Papillo-retinitis, hæmorrhagic, 268.
Paracentesis, 19, 36, 433, 490.
Paracentral defect, explanation of detached areas of, 283.
　scotoma, 272, 279, 287.
Parallactic displacement of vessels, 202.
Pathological anatomy, 87.
Pectinate ligament, 3, 76, 97, 362, 418, 627, 633.
　fibrosis of, 95, 123.
　injury to, 592.
Perilental space, 48, 117.
Perimeter, author's large, 263.
Perimeters of various kinds, 230, 231, 263.
Perimetric results, methods of recording, 259.
Perimetry, large object, 229, 240, 247.
　small and large object, 229, 240.
　small object, 249, 262.
　features of, in glaucoma, 249.
Period of disease, 298, 299.
Peter on scotometry, 254.
Photometers, 340, 343, 344.

Photopsiæ, 160, 226.
Phthisis bulbi, 166, 186.
Physiological cupping, 200, 208, 209, 216.
Pigment granules, Koeppe's, 219.
Pilocarpine, 443, 450, 453, 456, 549.
Porcelain-like appearance of sclera, 165, 168.
Posterior chamber, entered by trephine, 556.
　staphyloma, 203.
　synechia. See Synechia.
Post-operative complications, 368, 375, 478, 481, 580.
Precautions after sclerectomies, 578, 599.
Pre-glaucomatous stage, 219.
Preparation of patient for operation, 504.
Presbyopia, increase of, 161, 193.
Pressure, 24.
　amount necessary during trephining, 542.
　capillary, intra-ocular, 50.
　in aqueous and vitreous chambers compared, 40, 42, 43, 45, 48, 111, 117, 127.
　in relation to intra-ocular contents, 37, 56.
　intra-ocular, 24, 32, 36, 132, 296, 334.
　　estimation of, 24.
　　influence of age on, 61, 127.
　　of drugs on, 60.
　　of hæmorrhage on, 382.
　　normal limits of, 335.
　　physical conditions regulating, 27, 56.
　　relation to systemic blood-pressure, 59, 60, 61, 63, 64, 204.
　　to tension, 327.
　rise in, 1, 88, 151, 327.
Priestley Smith on scotometry, 254.
Primary glaucoma, 2, 108, 116, 121, 347.
Principle of modern operations for glaucoma, 31, 33.
Prodromata, 152, 160.
Prognosis of glaucoma, 478, 479.
Progress of glaucoma case, necessity of watching, 208.
Prophylaxis of glaucoma, 162, 442, 448, 453, 476.
Proptosis, 405.
Pseudo-cornea, 113.
Pulsation of retinal vessels, 65, 204, 206.
Pulse, retinal, 19, 65, 164, 204.
Pump action in eye, 5, 70, 73, 81, 97, 98, 142, 171, 307, 452.

INDEX OF SUBJECTS

Pump action in eye, muscles producing, 73.
Punches for sclerectomy, 497, 518.
Pupil, artificial, 386.
  dilatation of, 8, 160, 163, 164, 189, 191.
  oval, in glaucoma, 164, 191.
  post-operative occulsion of, 583.
Pusey's trephine, 561.

Q

Quadrant of eye selected for trephining, 531.
Quaglino's sclerotomy, 490.
Querenghi's operation, 490.
Quiet iritis, 550, 558, 581.

R

Race, influence of, in glaucoma, 135.
Raeder's corneal microscope, 188.
Rainbow rings, 160, 168, 173, 174, 175, 227.
  causes of, other than glaucoma, 176, 178, 182, 183.
  differential diagnosis of, 178.
  in cataract, 178.
Raphé, horizontal, in retina, 235.
Recklinghausen's disease, 414.
Refraction, alterations in, 193.
  errors in, 136.
Results after sclerectomy, discrepancies in, 598.
Retina, damage to, in glaucoma, 207, 217, 296, 304, 305, 409.
  detachment of, 377, 379, 394, 413.
  glioma of the, 379.
Retinal artery, pressure in, 50.
  changes after operation, 10, 594.
  circulation, 303.
  lymph circulation, 297.
  nerve fibres, 233.
  vein, thrombosis of central, 380.
  vessels, changes in calibre of, 207.
  interference with, 296.
  level of, 201.
  pulsation in, 196, 204.
  causes of, 204.
Retinitis pigmentosa, 304.
Retino-choroidal circulation, 303.
Retino-choroiditis juxta-papillaris, 268.
Revolving spectra, 184.
Rigid, 25.
  walls, 27, 28, 36, 37, 38, 39.
Rigidity of eye, 36, 324.
Ring scotoma, 285, 294, 304.

Rods, retinal, 305.
Roenne's step, 240, 245, 267, 268, 275, 288, 293, 299, 303, 312, 314.
Rollet's trephine, 562.
Ruptures of globe, subconjunctival, 413.

S

Salzmann's method, 187.
Sarcoma of choroid, 379.
Schemata, 23, 26.
Schiötz' tonometer, 320, 322, 323, 334.
Schlemm's canal, 3, 70.
  anatomy of, 5, 75.
  circulation through, 5, 70, 71, 76.
  imperfect development of, 420, 434, 438.
Schloffer's operation, 434.
Scintillating scotoma of migraine, 177.
Sclera, 165, 167.
  change of colour of, 165, 168, 407.
  growth of, 119.
  in buphthalmos, 407, 420.
  thickness of, in glaucoma, 99, 201.
Scleral foramen, shape of, 198.
  spur, 5, 73, 75.
  trephining, 526.
Sclerecto-iridectomy, 495, 511.
Sclerectomy, 435, 612.
  ab externo, 515.
  simple anterior, 499, 510.
  with punch-forceps, 515.
  with the trephine, 497.
Sclero-choriotomy, 490.
Sclero-corneal trephining, 32, 365, 393, 398, 434, 435, 437, 498, 531, 558, 591, 593, 597.
Sclerotomy, 20, 31, 433, 434, 436, 464, 489.
  anterior, 510.
  gridiron, 501.
  posterior, 394, 484, 511.
Scotoma, Bjerrum's. See Bjerrum's scotoma.
  Elliot's, 272, 275, 279, 281, 283.
  Seidel's, 270, 284.
Scotometer, author's, 257.
  Priestley Smith's, 254.
Seasons, influence of, on glaucoma, 143.
Secondary cataract, 194.
  glaucoma, 2, 108, 195, 347, 390, 393.
  ætiology of, 347, 354.
  treatment of, 385, 393.

INDEX OF SUBJECTS

Seidel's sign, 254, 268, 270, 275, 281, 284, 314.
    author's extension of, 255, 314, 615.
Self-lit perimeters, 230.
Senile glaucoma, 401.
Septic conditions in relation to operation, 584, 585.
Seton operation, 502.
Setons, 433.
Sex, influence of, in glaucoma, 133, 403.
Silver nitrate, effect of, on cornea, 177.
Simple glaucoma, 2, 10, 103, 108, 109, 115, 121, 132, 137, 152, 153, 155, 157, 158, 307, 442, 454, 466, 470, 489, 490, 495, 550, 558.
Sinclair on small-object perimetry, 250.
Sleep in relation to glaucoma, 80, 172, 225, 307, 452.
Sliding flap, 565.
Slit-lamp, Gullstrand, 219, 221.
Small flap operation, 523.
Splitting of cornea, 3, 437, 536, 538, 564, 568.
Spud, use of, in sclerectomy, 552, 554, 576.
Stages of glaucoma, 152.
Staphyloma of cornea, 166, 168, 350, 416, 532.
Stephenson's knife, 564.
    trephine, 560.
Sterilisation of instruments, 506.
    of surgeon's hands, 507.
Subacute glaucoma, 2.
Subconjunctival injections, 446, 456, 539.
    puncture, 435, 438, 491.
Suffusions, 18.
Sunlight, brilliant, 136.
Supero-temporal bundle of optic nerve fibres, 235.
Suprachoroidal space, opening up of, 490, 492, 499, 528, 530, 593.
Suspensory ligament, rupture of, 577, 590.
Suturing of flap, 557.
Sym on the visual field in glaucoma, 251.
Sympathectomy, 420, 466, 501.
Sympathetic, cervical, stimulation of, 36.
Synechia, annular posterior, 352, 370, 374, 386, 392.
    anterior, 348, 364, 390, 532.
    posterior, 364, 581.
    ring, 42.

T

Tangent rule, 253.
Taylor's motor trephine, 563.
Telescopic vision, 242.
Tenon's capsule, 532.
Tension, 1, 24, 327, 333.
    as affected by fistulisation, 31.
    increase of, 158, 164, 307, 585.
    recurrence of, after operation, 590.
Terms, 1, 24, 25, 84, 464.
Therapeutics of glaucoma, 443.
Thread drainage, 434, 501, 502.
    fixation of flap, 571.
Thrombosis of central retinal vein, 380, 394.
Toilette of wound, after trephining, 551, 573.
Tonometer, 24, 462.
    method of using a, 329.
    Schiötz', 318, 320.
        application of, 320.
        precautions in use of, 322.
        rôle of, 323, 325.
Tonometry, 317.
    digital, 19, 28, 318.
    limitations of mechanical, 326.
Toothed trephine, 562.
Trachoma, 136.
Transillumination, 187, 394, 577, 588.
Transilluminator, Würdemann's, 187.
Transition from simple to congestive glaucoma, 157, 160.
Trephine, application of, 535, 541, 550.
    blade, direction of, during operation, 544.
    hole, placed too far back, 555, 621, 625.
    methods of steadying, 542, 543.
    size of, 527, 529, 530, 544, 545, 547.
Trephined disc, hinge of, 544, 545, 548, 573.
    histology of, 618, 622.
    method of dealing with, 545, 546, 548, 549.
Trephines, sharp, 559.
Trephining, completion of, 546.
    incomplete, 548.
    scleral, 526.
    sclero-corneal, 31, 365, 393, 398, 434, 435, 437, 498, 531, 591, 593, 597, 600.
Triad of glaucoma signs, 157, 471.
Triple small flap operation, 524.
Trivalin-hyoscin, 455, 484, 504, 503, 508, 572.
Tube-vision, 242.
Tumours, intra-ocular, 376, 394.
Turkish baths, 456.

INDEX OF SUBJECTS

U

Ulbrich's method of measuring depth of anterior chamber, 188.
Ulcus serpens, 166.
Use of keratome, 484.
U-shaped scleral flap, Harman's, 519.
Uvea, ectropion of, 165, 190.
Uveal pigment in filtration scars, 604.
    tags in trephine wound, 551, 552.
    tissue blocking sclerectomy wound, 541, 576, 577, 586.
        impaction of, in trephine hole, 607.
        interference with, 529, 547.

V

Van der Hoeve on early recognition of scotomata, 292.
Vasa vorticosa, 66, 87, 379.
    ligature of, 117.
Vascular system, changes in, 130, 152.
    systems of eye, 11.
Vaso-motor changes, intra-ocular, 153, 154, 191.
    control, general, 132, 152.
    intra-ocular, 125, 151.
Venesection, 456.
Venous pulse, retinal, 205.
Vesicular filtration scar, 600.
Vessels, alteration in apparent direction of, on disc, 202.
    disease of, in glaucoma, 89.
    of ciliary body, 10.
    of iris, 10.
    perforating, 10.
    retinal. See Retinal Vessels.
Vision, central, impairment of, 156, 164, 245, 306, 479.
    defective, after operation, 593.
    improvement of, after operation, 245, 480.
Visual acuity, diminution of, 227, 339.
    field, changes in, in chronic glaucoma, 163, 229, 287, 295, 299, 300.
        loss of, after operation, 480, 593.
        shrinkage of, 156, 164, 240, 242, 300, 307.
        atypical, 242.

Visual fields, normal, 229.
    variety in shapes of glaucomatous, 293, 298.
    purple, 297.
Vitreous masses blocking angle, 115.
    blood in, 382.
    dislocations of, into wound, 588.
    escape, 541, 574.
    fluid, source of, 44, 46.
    fluidity of, 590.
    injection of, 433.
    interference with, 361, 362, 391, 541.
Vogt's motor trephine, 563.
Volume of contents of eye, alterations in, 28, 30, 35, 37, 38, 39.
Vomiting in glaucoma, 225, 226.
Von Graefe on iridectomy, 459.
Von Hippel's trephine, 562, 563.
Von Mende's flap, 564, 565.
Von Recklinghausen's disease, 414.

W

Webster Fox technique of trephining, 565.
Wedge, McReynolds' corneal, 564.
Wedge-isolation operation, 495, 520.
Weight of trephine, 560.
Wicherkiewicz' operation, 501.
Wilmer's experience of trephined eyes in epidemic, 599.
Wounds of iris, delay in healing of aseptic, 475.
    sclerectomy, plugging of, from within, 576.

Y

Young's threshold test cards and rings, 339.
    trephine, 562.

Z

Zeiss' visual photometer, 343.
Zonular opacity of cornea, 166, 186.
Zonule, slackening of, 122, 187.
Zoster, ophthalmic, 397.

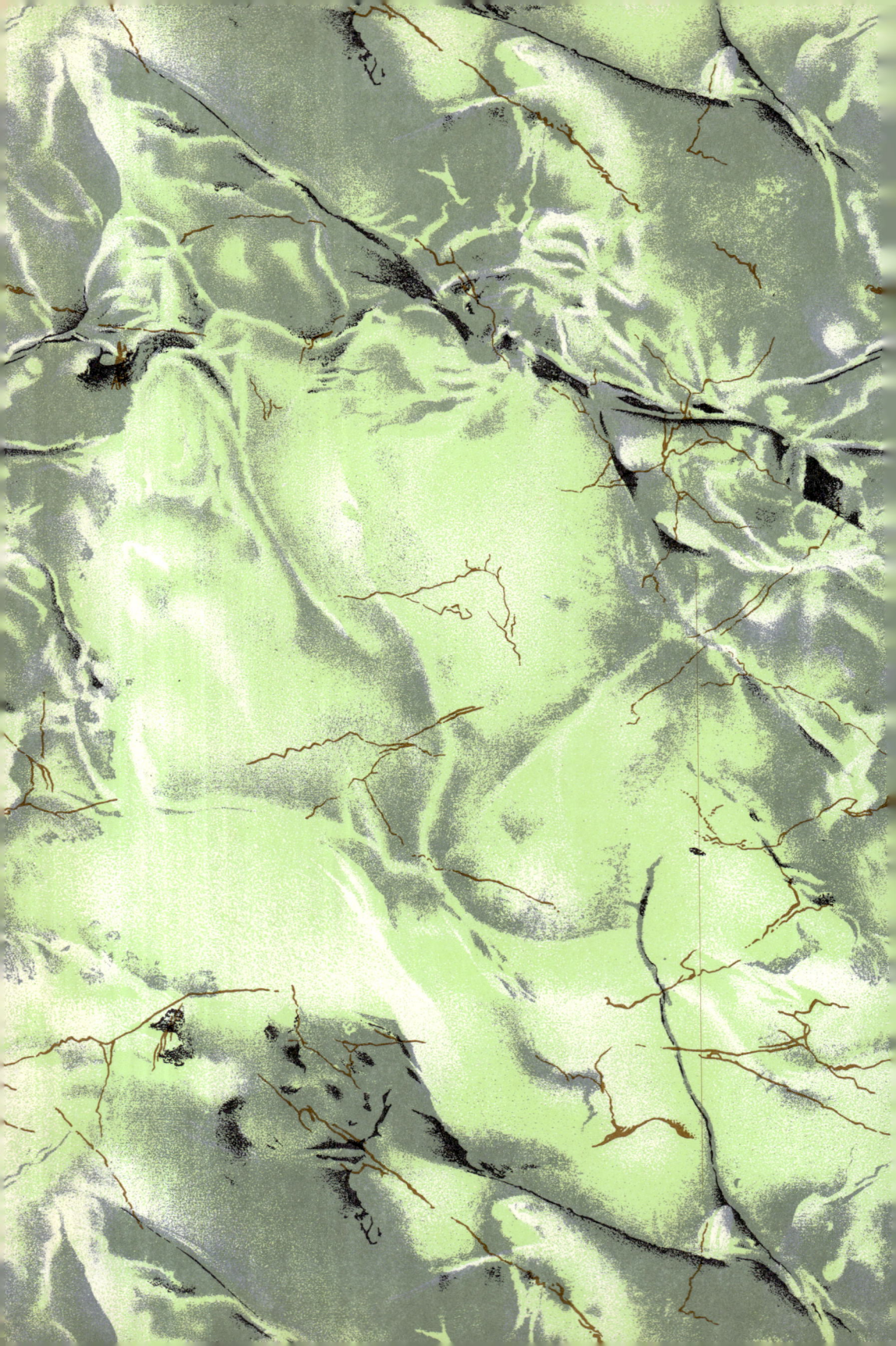